D1030941

DAIRY PRODUCTS IN HUMAN HEALTH AND NUTRITION

PROCEEDINGS OF THE 1ST WORLD CONGRESS OF DAIRY PRODUCTS IN HUMAN
HEALTH AND NUTRITION / MADRID / SPAIN / 7-10 JUNE 1993

DAIRY PRODUCTS IN HUMAN HEALTH AND NUTRITION

Edited by
M. SERRANO RÍOS, A. SASTRE, M.A. PEREZ JUEZ, A. ESTRALA
& C. DE SEBASTIÀN

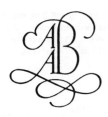

A.A. BALKEMA / ROTTERDAM / BROOKFIELD / 1994

Our very special thanks to the European Community Commission which, across D.G. VI, (Agriculture), offered the best support towards the organisation of this congress.
Their suggestions, encouragement, financial aid and participation, have been fundamental factors in the congress achievement.
We hope this pioneer enterprise will continue to find in them support for future events which will convey us towards a better knowledge of milk and dairy products in health and nutrition.

The Organising Committee

Sponsored by the European Community E.C.

Under the special patronage of

Sociedad Española de Nutrición
Básica y Aplicada (S.E.N.B.A)

and the patronage of

Asociación Española de Pediatría
Asociación Hispana de Osteoporosis y Enfermedades Metabólicas Oseas
Asociación Latinoamericana de Pediatría
Grupo Mediterraneo para el Estudio de la Diabetes
Sociedad Española de Arteriosclerosis
Sociedad Española de Cardiología
Sociedad Española de Dietética
Sociedad Española de Endocrinología
Sociedad Española de Higiene y Medicina Social
Sociedad Española de Nutrición
Sociedad Española de Nutrición Parenteral y Enteral
Sociedad Española de Obesidad
Sociedad Española de Patología Digestiva

Published by
A.A.Balkema, P.O.Box 1675, 3000 BR Rotterdam, Netherlands
A.A.Balkema Publishers, Old Post Road, Brookfield, VT 05036, USA

ISBN 90 5410 359 0
© 1994 A.A.Balkema, Rotterdam
Printed in the Netherlands

Dairy Products in Human Health and Nutrition, Serrano Rios et al. (eds) © 1994 Balkema, Rotterdam, ISBN 90 5410 359 0

Table of contents

Dairy Products in Human Health and Nutrition, Serrano Rios et al. (eds) © 1994 Balkema, Rotterdam, ISBN 90 5410 359 0

Preface

The First World Congress of Dairy Products in Human Health and Nutrition was held in Madrid, Spain, on June 7-10, 1993. The event was an initiative of the European Community which sponsored the multidisciplinary efforts of the Dairy Industry and of scientists in the different disciplines in the field of nutrition.

More than 700 people attended this major meeting devoted entirely to the scientific discussion and updating of virtually every issue related to the impact of milk and dairy products consumption on human health, at any age and/or sex, worldwide.

The preparation of the Congress was a painstaking endeavour carried out with perserverance and enthusiasm by, both the Scientific and the Organising Committees, which led to a most stimulant scientific programme, conceived in such a way that every delegate to the Congress could have the opportunity of learning the most updated research; to get accounted with current opinion of leading authorities on such debatable issues as the influence of dairy products intake and the prevention of osteoporosis, or about the realities and fancies on the controverted relationships between cancer and dairy products consumption. These and many other problems of current interest were critically presented, vividly discussed, usually followed by clear unbiased conclusions offered by the chairmen of each session. The editors are pleased to present here the unabridged version of the main Lectures and Round Tables. The Congress Programme was preceded by one morning session on Diet and Atherosclerosis, under the chairmanship of Prof. M. Pocoví from the Department of Biochemistry and Molecular Biology at the University of Zaragoza, Spain.

The revolution introduced by Modern Molecular Biology concepts and technologies is also influencing the research and industrial strategies in the field of dairy products. We felt that this Congress could not be representative of current trends in the Science of Nutrition without an authoritative discussion of some of its most relevant contributions to our field. Three major papers made up this basic background: 'Lactation, comparative molecular physiology and molecular biology' by Prof. L.M. Houdebine; 'Milk composition in animals and in humans – Nutritional aspects' by Prof. L. Hambræus; 'The milk gland as a bioreactor for therapeutic and nutritional proteins' by Dr Hennighausen.

Dr Houdebine's paper contains a clearly written updated review of the developmental aspects of milk production by the mammary gland. The authors describe the control of the mammary gland functioning both by 'classic' hormones (prolactin, glucocorticoids, estrogens, progesterone) and by numerous other growth factors, acting partially through autocrine mechanisms in concert with estrogens or other hormones. Special attention is given to the increasingly recognized importance of the extra cellular material (ECM) and of some of its components (Collagen IV, laminia, proteoglycans) on the organisation of the mammary tissues that grant an appropriate functioning of the gland. It appears as the discussion pursues that the 'organisation' of the mammary tissue is the result of a subtle balance between proteolytic and antiproteolytic activities.

Also the major effects of prolactin on milk synthesis/secretion start to be better understood after the recent identification of the prolactin receptor gene as a member of the cytokine family likely transmitting their cellular messages through activation of the kinase system. The author also touches upon other fascinating new developments concerning the identification of the major milk protein genes in several species; as well as the type of cellular signals that may stimulate their expression at the level of the mammary tissue. In its conclusions the authors emphasized that: 'there is little doubt that transgenic mammals will be used in a near future to produce various recombinant proteins'. Interesting new data on transgenic animals are to be found in the paper by Prof. L. Hennighausen 'The gland as a bioreactor for therapeutic and nutritional proteins'. The basic idea is that modern technologies in molecular biology allow researchers to 'convert' milk glands of transgenic animals into Bioreactors capable of producing pharmaceutical and, of course, many proteins of nutritional value. The term 'molecular pharming' is coined to describe the generation of these 'bioreactors'. Reading this paper is intellectually most motivating. In an attractive style Dr Hennighausen tells us numerous success stories, describing the impressive impact of cloning technologies (since the mid eighties to present) on our knowledge of the mammary gland and of its main secretory product: Milk. Among many of these achievements some of them are to be stressed; the isolation of the milk gene protein of several species, such as protein WAP, X-Lactoalbumian and several caseins. All this represent the 'step from mice to farm animals' that has allowed scientists to produce human pharmaceuticals by the mammary glands and its secretion into milk. In this context the use of designed genes using defined sequences (promoter/upstream) from WAP and other milk proteins has been used to direct the synthesis of forming proteins by the mammary tissue in the transgenic mice and from other species. The evaluation of the potential hybrid genes and other future developments close this exciting chapter. As a conclusion we may very well quote here the authors words at the summary of his paper: 'Given the speed with which molecular pharming technology is being developed barnyard biotechnology should soon find its place alongside of conventional technologies for pharmaceutical production'. An important contribution to the Background Basic Science, included in this book, is the paper on 'Milk composition in animals and in humans – Nutritional aspects' by Prof. L. Hambræus, who closely examines the interspecies variations, from the seal to the human with a minute analysis of the relative nutritional value of macro/micronutrients contained in milk from the different species. Milk is studied as an energy source; and as an important protein source. Special attention is given to 'Calcium, the third macronutrient of concern'. A scholarly written consideration of milk in its physiological/nutritional values clearly establishing that milk proteins act simultaneously as a source of essential aminoacids for protein syntheses, for specific physiological functions (e.g. defense against microbial infections) and as growth factors and modulators. A relatively wide attention is given to lactoferrin (milk iron-binding protein) stressing its major antimicrobial/nutritional, mitogenic and trophic properties, and even its potential as a defense against the generation of free radicals in any organisms. Furthermore, fats in milk, vitamins and minerals, deserve due attention in this paper whose succint conclusion remarks that: 'There are many interesting differences in the composition of milk at the macro/micro levels, though we are still far from understanding their physiological background'.

The industrial production of milk and dairy products as well as their situation in the world, occupy a significant part of the contents of this book. Dr F. M. Luquet, in his work entitled 'Technological evolution in dairy products, from craftmanship to biotechnology'; Dr Gemperle in 'Dairy products and milk production tendencies and strategies in the world'; and Dr Schelhaas in 'The economy of milk production – A worldwide overview'.

The article by Dr Luquet is an exciting travel through the history of milk and milk derivatives that human beings have been using as essential ingredients of their nutrition since the eve of mankind.

The history goes back to 10 million years, when glaciers melted down and farming was started, with milk producing animals; sheep, goats, bovine. Since the discovery of 'fermented cheese' and the first cheese making industries which we are told by Dr Luquet were set in ancient Rome. People with different cultures (Hebrews, Mongols, Turks, ...) have had milk and cheese not only as a favourite nutrient but also as a cultural identification marker. Many other fascinating stories on milk and milk products are to be found in this paper. Particularly interesting are the three last: 1) Major events of the last decades; 2) The biotechnology of a modern product: 'Yoghurt'; 3) Points concerning the future.

An item of major focus is: The economic problems of the western countries where Dr Schelhaas identifies three determining factors. The strong protection enjoyed by the industry in the recent past, the strong growth of production technology, and the generally stagnating demand. His detailed analysis of the changing policies in the dairy industries is very illuminating of the present and prospective problems faced by the dairy sector. The extreme importance of GATT negotiations for the western dairy sector is lucidly reasoned. Many other important items such as the future developmens for 1994, the economic situation in Eastern Europe and the crisis in the dairy industry are some of the most appealing parts of this highly elaborated chapter. In Dr Schelhaas' article one will find matter enough for reflexion particularly by those concerned about dairy industry and its present/future problems.

Moreover, Dr Gemperle's most informative paper on 'Dairy products and milk production tendencies and strategies in the world', discussed the world geography of the dairy industry in terms of comparative production/consumption by regions and populations, the differences in cow milk yield's throughout the world and the wide variety of factors that influence those processes worldwide. This paper gives a global scope of the world dairy products with abundance of data collected in virtually every country of the world. The author also cogently stimulates the convenience of milk consumption during adolescence as a necessary ingredient of a well balanced diet, thus creating a 'new balance for health'. One may add the exhaustive information on 'Meeting dietary nutrient requirements with cow's milk and milk products' co-authored by Drs D.J. Brisonnette and K.N. Jeejeebhoy. A detailed account of energy and nutrient requirements at different ages (children, adolescents, elderly, both men and women) as well as the individual components of milk (carbohydrates, proteins, aminoacids, vitamins, minerals, micronutrients) and its relative contribution to the global nutritional values of milk and its derivatives, is very thoroughly discussed. The first conclusion of the authors is unequivocal: 'The value of milk in human nutrition is vital and necessary as it completes the diet of the young and the elderly; in particular from the perspective of protein qualities. A diet combining cereals of grain and milk would be a great benefit. In fact cereals/ vegetables may contribute to that mixed diet, some of the micronutrients (iron, copper, manganese, folic acid, vitamin E) defective in milk, whereas the latter will increase the whole biological value of protein in that dietary composition'.

The paper by Drs P.F. Fox and A. Flynn, on the biological properties of milk, focus preferentially on the physiological significance of: 1) Enzyme and enzymes inhibitors; 2) Binding proteins (casein, lactoalbumin, serum albumin, lactotransferrin, vitamins); 3) Immunoglobulins; 4) Bifidus factors; 5) Growth factors; 6) Casein hydrolyzates; 7) Platelet modifying factors: Angiotenting converting enzyme (ACE) inhibitor. The paper is a clearly written account of the most relevant literature on each of the aforementioned items.

A global, critically written review of the 'Positive health benefits of consuming dairy products' is that of Prof. M.I. Gurr. In this paper the author examined the qualities of milk and its many nutrients in a very dynamic way ('the rise and fall of milk'). The traditional roles of milk as 'nutrient provider', and its impact on several areas of normal health and pathology (dental, lactose, digestion, ulceration, diarrhoea, immunity, hypertension, hyperlipidemias and coronary heart disease, cancer) are reviewed. In the field of cancer Dr Gurr remarks that 'the most promising area of current research is in regard to a protective effect of calcium in relation to colon cancer'. Most provocative is Dr Gurr's statement: 'There is now sufficient evidence from epidemiology from human intervention studies and animal experiments taken together, that consumption of milk products, even those containing milk fat *does not* result in hyperlipidemia', and continues with 'This is consistent with a strategy to promote milk as part of an integrated health lifestyle in which diet and other factors play a part'.

Moreover interesting data about 'The evolution of the nutritional impact of milk and dairy products in Spain' are given by Dr G. Martí Henneberg et al. through a well designed population-based, randomized (the family as the randomization unit) prospective study conducted at the city of Reus, Catalonia. The main results of this study indicate that: 'Spain is still a moderate consumer of milk and dairy products... despite the fact that during the last decades the intake has been on the increase ...; only during the first years of life do the dairy products have a significant place in the lipid contribution to diet'.

Furthermore, the article by Dr F.J. Kok, widens the epidemiologist's perspective in his short review of the 'Epidemiological topics in nutrition and health relevant to dairy industry'.

A most important complementary information is to be found in the paper by Dr F. Monckeberg on 'Dairy products in the third world – An overview' with more focus on Chile and other Latin-American countries. The authors properly presented the prevalence of under/malnutrition in underdeveloped countries, reviewing their characteristics, and the importance of milk as a nutrient, under the precarious living conditions in those countries. Some data are amazing, such as those from the last report of FAO: an estimated 1.156 million human beings are living in poverty! Undernutrition however, as Dr Monckeberg points out, is often present 'not because they (the people) do not have access to adequate amounts of their usual diet but mainly because they do not have enough income to obtain a qualitative and quantitatively adequate diet. By contrast Dr Monckeberg describes in detail the positive experience in Chile by programs from the National Health Service, aimed to improve health and nutrition in infants and pre-school children. In this study free distribution of powder milk, cereals, vitamins and minerals was an essential component of foods provided to the infant population and also to lactating and pregnant women. It seemed that the consequences of such an enterprise have been dramatically favourable since no more than 4% of infants in Chile (1992) in their first year of life showed signs of malnutrition. This positive Chilean experience should be expanded to other countries where infant malnutrition is still a major health problem.

The consumption and expected effects of milk and milk derivates on health widely varies along the human vital cycles as it is extensively considered in the following papers: 1) 'Metabolic interactions during pregnancy in preparation for lactation' by Prof. E. Herrera Castillón and co-workers; 2) 'Dairy products during the perinatal stage – Relevance of their calcium and long chain polyunsaturated fatty acids contents' by Prof. M. Moya; 3) 'Dairy products in infant nutrition', co-authored by Prof. E. Casado de Frías, Drs Maluenda and Marco; 4) 'Dairy products and adolescent nutrition' jointly written by Prof. M. Giovanni, Drs Rottoli and Agostini; 5) 'Dairy products and the elderly' by Dr G. Schaafsma; 6) 'Nutrition with milk and dairy products'. Recent aspects of nutrition with milk and dairy products' by Prof. C.A. Barth; 7) 'Milk consumption and level of risk on health and nutrition in grouped countries in the world' by F. Mardones Restat; 8) 'Dairy products and physical activity' authored by Dr P.W. Lemon.

Dr P.W.R. Lemon writes a most interesting overview of the physiological/biochemical bases supporting the chronic effects of exercise nitrogen/protein metabolism in humans with different states of physical training, as well as the possible adverse effects of sustained high protein intake.

The author summarizes his views by advising: 'Care must be taken to consume adequate total energy (carbohydrate is very important because it is the major source of exercise fuel) to cover the high expenditures of training as insufficient energy intake will further elevate dietary protein requirements'.

The biochemical and physiological overview on the nutrient traffic across the placenta and the motherfoetus metabolic interactions is masterly described by Prof. E. Herrera Castillón and colleagues, mostly based on their extensive research in rats. The critical analysis of their own results and those of the literature entitle the authors to give clearcut meaningful conclusions, the first one reading '... although the placentary transfer of lipids is small, sustained maternal hypolipidemia during late gestation is of prior importance for the metabolism of the mother and of her offspring'. Lastly the authors warn that deviation from the finely tuned hyperlipidemia may alter her lipoprotein profile and even be responsible for an alteration in the composition of the milk.

'Milk consumption and level of risk on health and nutrition in grouped countries in the world' by Dr Mardones Restat, adds further information on the impact of milk consumption on health and nutrition levels in the most vulnerable human groups in the third world (Africa, Asia, Latin America). The positive Chilean experience is briefly recalled as an encouraging example.

Prof. Moya and Prof. Casado de Frías et al., independently discussed the use of dairy products in Spain at the perinatal and childhood cycles respectively. The relevant positive role of calcium and poliunsaturated trans fatty acids is stressed by Prof. Moya. Prof. Casado de Frías et al., make a thorough account of the impact of natural and artificial lactation upon growth in children. A detailed critical analysis of the most varied (milk) feeding formulae is the core of these papers.

Nutrition imposes difficult challenges during adolescence, 'a very intense anabolic period' as stated by Dr Giovannini et al. The authors present a comprehensive view of the nutritional problems peculiar to the adolescent from their eating habits, tendency to obesity and growth. The authors emphasize the importance of calcium intake whose impact in the different phases of skeletal growth (height, volume, weight, maturation, modelling, redistribution, repair) is of primary importance.

Even a more difficult problem in practice is nutrition at the old age. On this subject Dr Schaafsma's paper is an updated critical overview of the topic. His conclusions are: 'That the considerable nutrient density of dairy products fit excellently in the diet of the elderly', and that milk consumption is essential for the prevention of osteoporosis and probably also, for that of hypertension and colon cancer. Finally, he states that 'fermented milk can exert beneficial effects on the immune system and the intestine' but the nutritional significance has not yet been completely established.

Furthermore, in this book the properties of the potential therapeutic significance of peptide hormones (e.g. BGH) and growth factors found in milk and milk derivatives (e.g. IGF 1) of bovine origin are concisely introduced by Dr O. Koldovsky in the paper 'Peptide hormones and growth factors in bovine milk'.

See also the interesting paper 'Nutrition with milk and dairy products' by Dr C.A. Barth, for modern aspects of its use in nutrition.

Numerous other topics dealing with human disease and dairy products, covered the problem of liver disease (Dr S. Hirsch); 'Nutrition and immunity' by Dr F. Ortiz Masllorens; 'Nutrition and immunity, the therapeutic impact' by Dr J.W. Alexander; 'Malnutrition and the immune response' by Dres. Suskind et al.; 'Dairy products, calcium and colon cancer' by Dr M.J. Wargovich. Dr Hirsch gives a clear overview of the multifactorial ethiopathogenesis of malnutrition in chronic liver disease and of its frequent complication of hepatic encephalopathy. The classic 'blood ammonia' and the false 'neurotransmitters' hypothesis held for the pathogenesis of the latter conditions are critically discussed at the light of recent research data. A major point is the focus on the real impact of the nutritional support to reduce, and or prevent, the incidence of nutrition associated complications to chronic liver disease. The author concludes that artificial aminoacid mixtures, 'are not better than natural proteins' while emphasizing that some milk delivered nutrients (e.g, casein, lactose) appear to have a definitive beneficial effect.

The use of dairy products in artificial nutrition, is introduced in 'The historical account of the evolution of artificial nutrition' by Prof. H. Joyeux. The milestones in the steady progress of artificial nutrition since the most remote times to present, is pointedly recorded. Artificial nutrition stands today as a full clinical/experimental science that confirms Hippocrates theme 'be your food your medicine'. Furthermore a detailed account on 'Milk and dairy products as dietary supplements' is given by Dr A. Gil. The paper provides an unbiased description of the physiological and nutritional value of cow/human milk and milk by-products; their use as dietary supplements as well as a destiller of important formulas and enteral supplemented diets in adult life. Moreover, the paper by Drs J. Reilly and Tombea, expand the current information on the strategy used for providing optimal enteral provision of proteins in intestinal mucosa.

Dr Brisson's paper is an exhaustive review of the available data, (including his own) on potential health risks involved in the excessive consumption of trans-fatty acids. The message seems to be that the field is still to be clarified by further research. However it appears that the trans-fatty acids from partially hydrogenated vegetable oils do not have greater cancerogenic potential than the 'cis' isomers.

Dr Ortiz Maslloréns, a basic research immunologist himself, discusses the specific as well as the non-specific barriers against external offensors (bacterioviruses, fungi and parasites) and its relationship to the pathogenic pathways by which malnutrition may have defective immune response.

In a similar vein Dr R.M. Suskind et al. contributes with a thorough review of clinical/epidemiological and immunopathogenic aspects of malnutrition in children.

Dr Alexander, a highly regarded expert in the field, updated the state of the art on nutrition and immunity. The author overviews the basic immunological mechanisms (cell-mediated humoral responses) underlying malnutrition.

Dr Wargovich's paper offers a well balanced view of the controversial issue of 'Dairy products, calcium and colon cancer' summarizing the available epidemiological, experimental and clinical data on the effects of calcium intake to the risk of colon cancer.

Dr J.M. Ordovas, a well known Spanish research worker, based at the Lipid Laboratory at Tuft's University, Boston, USA, lucidly discussed the importance of early dietary treatment in children by reduced intake of saturated fats to diminish the risk of developing coronary heart disease in adulthood. Dr Ordovas cautioned against using indiscriminatively the low fat, low cholesterol diet in children under the age of two. In his lecture on 'The interplay of genetic and environmental factors: Effects on plasmalipoproteins', Dr Ordovas showed that general candidate genes (Apo A.I., A.IV, B and E) have a significant importance in regulating the levels of plasma lipids in response to diets with variable content of those and other nutrients. A most comprehensive paper on 'Current issues on the management of cholesterol in high risk adults' is that of Drs G.L. Vega and M. Grundy, who reviewed current epidemiological evidence that justifies aggressive lowering of cholesterol both in primary and secondary prevention of CHD in several special groups at risk.

Also an authoritative view of the rationale underlying the prevention and treatment of CAD by nutrition modification is given in the article by Dres. S.L., and W.E. Connor. Other specific topics of high interest such as 'The effects of fatty acids and cholesterol on serum lipids' by Dr D.M. Hegsted; 'The effects of monounsaturated fatty acids on serum lipoproteins' by Dr R.P. Mensink; and the 'Analysis of cardiovascular risk factors in the Spanish Community of Navarra' by Dr I. Villa Elizaga et al., add further important information. Decreased physical activity may add to the cluster of cardiovascular risk factors such as lipids, as reviewed by Dr U. Ravnskov.

An excellent plenary lecture on 'Micronutrients, antioxidants and general mechanisms of disease' was given by Dr N.W. Solomons. This paper is an attractive essay of 'the consequences of living in serobic environment'. Dr Solomons addresses the interactions between host and environmental factors as determinants of the effects of oxidants on human health from an epidemiological and ecological perspective. The role of antioxidant micronutrients in milk (riboflavin 'fortified' with vitamin A) and its potential benefits on human health is clearly discussed.

The Disaccaorde Lactose is the typical representative of mammalian origin. The relationships between lactose intestinal flora, and the syndrome of lactose intolerance are the subject of the paper by Dr J.C. Rambaud et al. in 'Dairy products and intestinal flora' and by Dr D.A. Savaiano in 'Lactose intolerance: Dietary management'. Among other conclusions Dr Rambaud et al. remark the importance of using fermented dairy products as probiotics to promote lactose adsorption in the small gut in changes in the colonia flora eco system. The authors indicate 'that the application of genetic engineering to select new micro-organisms which would transmit at a high rate in the gut would be scientifically most rewarding'.

According to Dr Savaiano's review of the most recent research findings relating lactose intolerance to development of symptoms 'the uniform conclusion is that only one fifth to one third of maldigesters will develop symptoms following consumption of one glass of milk'. The paper ends with a concise discussion on colonic adaptation to lactose, whose physiological significance and diverging results in aging (worsening when milk consumption diminishes) and pregnancy (improving when milk intake increases) deserves further research.

Finally the use of milk based hypoallergenic infant formula, was the main topic at the Round Table on Intestinal Flora, Lactose and Hypoallergenic formulas, and is herewith presented in the paper by Dr J.C. Monti.

'The calcium requirements for optimal skeletal health in women' by Dr J.A. Kanis; 'The importance of vitamin D for the prevention of osteoporosis', by Dr L.H. Allen; and 'Nutrition and bone', by Dr Burckhardt, were presented at a most exciting session under the heading 'Calcium, osteoporosis and dairy products'. Dr Kanis defined the calcium requirements for appropriate skeletal health, thoroughly reviewing the existing data and the delaying effects of pharmacological doses of calcium on bone calcium losses in post menopausal or castrated women. The paper of Dr L.H. Allen also reinforces the important therapeutic role of vitamin D administration to maintain mineral bone mass after menopause.

'Dietary calcium as a possible antipromoter of colorectal carcinogenesis' by Dr R. van der Meer et al., provides biochemical and nutritional data suggesting that supplemented calcium in the diet may be protective against colorectal carcinogenesis by increasing colonic precipitation of bilec fatty acids, and inhibition of luminal citolytic activity.

Two outstanding contributions were those of two top Spanish scientists Prof. F. Mayor Zaragoza and Prof. F. Grande Covian. The Organising and Scientific Committees felt most privileged to have Prof. Mayor Zaragoza delivering the Introductory Plenary Lecture on 'Dairy products in human nutrition – Present and future'. From his unique position as a basic researcher of well recognized reputation and as General Secretary of the UNESCO, he offered a most exciting view of the problems of health and education throughout the world and stressed the need of a greater solidarity across the world to solve the appalling problems of health and education of a significant fraction of our less favoured human fellows.

Prof. F. Grande Covian, one of the founders of Modern Nutrition, brilliantly closed the Congress offering a magnificent lecture on 'Dairy products in human growth and development – A worldwide overview', where he offered his personal views on the comparative aspects of nutrients and nutrition throughout the animal kingdom as they may help to set up the scientific bases for a better planning of human nutrition.

More than first hand science was offered during the Congress days. Enjoyable dinners and cocktail receptions, favoured with the warm hospitality of our City of Madrid, completed a most rewarding human and scientific experience. However the organisers were ready to offer their apologies for any failure that might have been detected.

The Editors would also like to end this introduction by thanking all those that have contributed to the scientific and social success of this unique occasion. The excellent organisation by Tilesa is to be commended, as well as that of our publishers, A.A. Balkema.

Let us make a final reflection on dairy products in health and human nutrition, the Madrid meeting clearly showed that the interest in the field of dairy products is, indeed, universal; and that no one can claim exclusivity in dealing with it. The multidisciplinary and unbiased approach of our meeting should not be dismissed. The First World Congress is indeed over, but the challenge for its continuity should be responded by those, scientists, health professionals and representatives of the dairy industries who have a serious commitment to develop this field for the best of human nutrition and health.

The Editors

1 Lactation, milk composition, biotechnology and industrial production

1. Lactation, milk constituents, colostrum and nutritional products.

Dairy Products in Human Health and Nutrition, Serrano Ríos et al. (eds) © 1994 Balkema, Rotterdam, ISBN 90 5410 359 0

Lactation: Comparative molecular physiology and molecular biology

L. M. Houdebine

Institut National de la Recherche Agronomique, Jouy-en-Josas, France

ABSTRACT : Milk secretion starts at parturition after mammary gland growth which takes place essentially during pregnancy. Estrogen is one of the major signal which triggers mammary development. It acts by degrading locally extracellular matrix and by sentisizing the cells to growth factors. A large part of mammary growth factors (TGFα, MDGF1, IGF1, ...) are produced within the mammary gland. During pregnancy, progesterone and TGF-β prevent the induction of milk secretion while favoring mammary gland growth. In the developped gland, the epithelial secretory cells are polarized and organized in alveoli.

The extracellular matrix composed mainly of collagen I and IV, laminin, fibronectin and proteoglycans plays an essential role in the cell organization and differenciation. Prolactin alone can induce milk secretion to variable degrees according to species. This action is amplified by glucocorticoïds and IGF1 or insulin. During lactation, several metabolic hormones favour milk secretion. In this respect, GH plays an essential role in ruminants and GH injections greatly enhance milk production in these species.

Prolactin receptor gene has been identified. It contains no protein kinase activity but the transduction of the prolactin message to milk protein genes seems to involve a cascade of Ser/Thr but not Tyr kinases. Several milk proteins genes have been cloned and sequenced. Their regulatory elements located in the upstream of their coding region are being studied. Several of the regulatory regions are being used to tentatively produce recombinant in milk of transgenic animals and to modify milk composition to improve its quality.

I - INTRODUCTION

The onset of milk secretion after parturition is the final step of a complex process which includes epithelial cell multiplication, organization of the cells in aveoli, specific induction of milk protein gene expression, hypertrophy and polarization of the epithelial cells. These events which take place in the mammary gland are accompanied by profound changes in the metabolism of the female. In non-pregnant and non-lactating female, the mammary gland is almost inexistent and it is very silent in the animal. In contrast, this organ utilizes a very significant part of the body energy throughout lactation. These multiple and complex process are controlled by many factors. The importance of hormones and particularly of the hypothalamus-hypophysis axis has been noted many years ago. It is now clear that other factors, and particularly molecules produced by the mammary gland itself and acting locally are of paramount importance, especially for the growth process.

Mammary gland is the subject of many biological studies for several reasons. It is a very good biological model to study the generation of an organ. Indeed, most of the organs are already formed at birth whereas mammary gland has to grow in each pregnancy-lactation cycle. Milk represents at least 20 % of the consumed proteins in rich countries. The mammary gland in humans in one of the organs in which tumors appear the most frequently. Recently, it has been demonstrated that milk from transgenic animals can be an abundant source of recombinant proteins for pharmaceutical use.

The study of mammary gland biology is thus being pursued with different and complementary approaches using modern techniques of cell biology and molecular biology. The present report aims at summarizing the major advances in this field of research.

II - THE DIFFERENT STEPS OF MAMMARY GLAND GROWTH

Mammary gland starts developping during the foetal life. It derives from ectoderm and the first mammry buds emerge from the skin. This process has been described in detail in the mouse (Sakakura, 1991). At birth and until puberty, the gland is restricted to poorly developped ducts growing at the same rate as the other organs of the female. After puberty an accelerated development of the duct network takes place. These ducts are ended by epithelial cells which are ready to multiply and to give rise to the generation of alveoli. In most species, the epithelial cells responsible for milk secretion do not appear until pregnancy. Significant differences can be observed however according to species. In rodents, the mammary gland is restricted to the ducts network before pregnancy and after weaning. In contrast, in human beings a significant proportion of the epithelial cells are already present after puberty. In all species, most of the secretory cells appear during pregnancy and the mammary gland growth and organization is achieved at the time of parturition. In species having short pregnancy, and particularly in rodents, a significant part of mammary gland growth occurs during the first week of lactation. In a simplified manner, it can thus be considered that mammary gland growth occurs during pregnancy whith no milk synthesis whereas milk

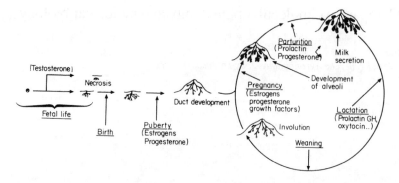

Fig. 1 : The different growing phases of the mammary gland. In rodent foetus, androgens induce a necrosis the mammary tissue. At puberty, the ovarian steroids, trigger a specific development of the duct network. During pregnancy, ovarian steroids prolactin and several locally produced growth factors support mammary gland growth. At parturition, the epithelial cells stop growing and start synthesizing milk after the drop of progesterone and the concomitent rise of prolactin. During the first week of lactation, the epithelial cells are hypertrophied. They become rich in Golgi apparatus, ribosomes, mitochondria, etc... to support milk synthesis and secretion. After weaning the epithelial tissue disappears until the next pregnancy.

secretion during lactation is accompanied by no additional development of the mammary tissue. After weaning, the epithelial secretory tissue is destroyed and the gland returns to its stable state, being restricted to a duct network (Fig. 1). The transient and cyclic existence of the mammary gland may be compared to that of other organs such as uterine endometrial tissue or corpus luteum. Evolution may have retained this rule for the sake of economy, from a metabolic point of view.

III - THE HORMONES WHICH CONTROL MAMMARY GLAND DEVELOPMENT

The physiological studies has long ago attributed to ovarian steroids, prolactin, growth hormone (GH) and glucocorticoids a major role in vivo in the development of the mammary gland. The exact action of these hormones is not yet completely elucidated but significant informations have emerged in the past years.

The first intervening hormones in the development of the mammary gland seem to be androgens. Indeed, in a certain number of species, and this is the case for rodents, a partial necrosis of the mammary tissue takes place during the foetal life. This necrosis is clearly due to foetal androgens. It occurs concomitently with the induction of androgens secretion and with the appearance of androgen receptors in the mammary buds. This necrosis does not occur in all species. In rodents, it is so marked that no teats are visible in adult males. The mechanism of action of androgens in mammary necrosis is not known in detail (Heubeger et al., 1982).

The secretion of androgens during foetal life has another essential role in all mammals. It modifies the sensitivity of the hypothalamus-hypophysis axis which becomes definitely unable to secrete large amounts of prolactin in males.

The onset of mammary gland growth during pregnancy is coincident with the emergence of oestrogens in blood of the mother. This is particularly striking in the ewe. In this species, a significant part of estrogens is synthetized by placenta. The development of this organ is accompanied by an increase of estrogens and progesterone after day 80 of pregnancy when the mammary gland starts growing. A more direct demonstration of the role of oestrogens has been given by the experiments leading

to an artificial induction of lactation. Indeed, repeated injections of estrogens with or without progesterone lead to rapid mammary gland growth and milk secretion in non pregnant females. Moreover, experiments carried out many years ago revealed that the mammary tissue explanted from virgin females cannot develop in vitro without a pretreatment of the animal by estrogens. Estrogens however have only a poor action in vitro on isolated mammary cells for growth (Edery et al., 1984). The exact mechanism of action of estrogens is not known. However, it is likely that part of its actions may be mediated by the stimulation of hypophysis which secretes more prolactin under oestrogens action (Fig. 2). An action of estrogens on local growth factors and on the extracellular matrix and which is described below is certainly of major importance.

Progesterone is known to favour mammary gland growth while preventing the induction of milk synthesis throughout pregnancy (Houdebine et al., 1983). The effect of progesterone on mammary gland growth can be observed in vivo (Assairy et al., 1974). A weak but significant capacity of progesterone to accelerate mammary cell division can also be obtained in vitro (Edery et al., 1984). The anti-lactogenic action of progesterone is experimentally obtained in vivo (Assairi et al., 1974 ; Houdebine and Gaye, 1975). The effect of progesterone effect during pregnancy may be mediated to a large extent through its capacity to reduce prolactin secretion (Fig. 2). Part of its action is however exerted independently of hypophysis since it counteracts the effect of prolactin injections on milk synthesis (Assairi et al., 1974 ; Houdebine and Gaye, 1975). Attempts to obtain the inhibitory effect of progesterone in vitro proved to be uneasy and disappointing. Such an effect can be obtained in certains conditions with rabbit mammary explants (Jahn et al., 1989) but surprisingly not with isolated rabbit mammary cells cultured on an extracelular matrix (Puissant et al., 1993). Hence, progesterone might act in part directly on the epithelial mammary cells for growth but not directly for its anti-lactogenic effect.

The mammogenic action prolactin in vivo has been observed long ago for the first time. This prolactin effect is probably the most visible in the rabbit. In this species, the mammary gland is particularly sensitive to prolactin and injections of the hormone to mid-pregnant rabbit induce a marked development of the mammary gland and an abundant milk synthesis (Houdebine

4

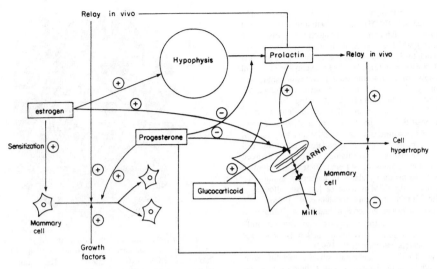

Fig. 2 : The major hormones controlling the development and the activity of the mammary gland. Some of these hormones act directly on the mammary gland whereas others act through unknown relays.

and Gaye, 1975). Similarly, in rats in which hypophysis has been grafted in kidney, the mammary gland grows under the action of the high level of prolactin. Surprisingly, prolactin *in vitro* has only a marginal effect, if any, on epithelial mammary cell multiplication (Edery et al., 1984). This clearly indicates that prolactin exerts its growth action on the mammary cells through a relay which remains to be found (Fig. 2). As opposed, the lactogenic effect of prolactin is fully obtained by a direct action on the epithelial cells.

Growth hormone is known to favour mammary gland development without being a key hormone (Cowie, 1970). Its effect is probably essential during the induction of lactation by estrogens. The growing phase of the gland is accompanied by a rise in IGF-I and it is significantly accelerated by injections of GH after the steroid treatment. A direct effect of GH on mammary gland development has been observed in mouse tissue cultured in the presence of insulin prolactin and glucocorticoids (Lyons et al., 1958). It is not know if GH acts by its direct contact with the epithelial cells or through the stimulation of IGF-I secretion. Glucocorticoids potentiate the effect of the other mammogenic hormones. In the lactating goat, hypophysectomy triggers an involution of the mammary gland. A new development of the mammary gland can be obtained by injections of prolactin, GH, and glucocorticoids (Cowie, 1970).

IV - THE GROWTH FACTORS WHICH CONTROL THE DEVELOPMENT OF THE MAMMARY GLAND

It is now well-established that cell multiplication is controlled by many factors often produced locally and not only by hormones. This is true as well for the mammary gland which synthesizes several growth factors.

In vitro and *in vivo*, EGF and its analogue TGF-α has a strong stimulatory effect on the multiplication of the epithelial mammary cells. EGF in blood is not significantly increased in the pregnant mouse but an ablation of the salivary gland which is the major source of EGF in the body, leads to an under-development of the mammary gland during pregnancy (Oka et al., 1991).

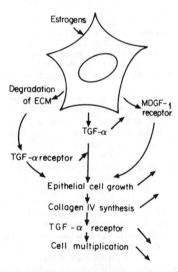

Fig. 3 : Effect of oestrogens on mammary gland growth. TGF-α, MDGF-I receptors are augmented while the extracellular matrix is locally degraded. These coordinated actions contribute to mammary cell division. The synthesis of collagen stimulated by the growth factors exerts a feed-back action on cell division.

Interestringly, the concentration TGF-α which uses the same cellular receptor as EGF is greatly increased in the mammary gland under the influence of estrogens which stimulate its secretion. Concomitently, the number the receptors for EGF-TGF-α is enhanced. Stimultaneously, estrogens induce the accumulation of MDGF-I receptors (mammary derived growth factor I) (Banco et al., 1992) in the mammary gland (Fig. 3). These effects of estrogens on mammary growth factors seem to

5

be related to the action of the extracellular matrix. The extracellular matrix (ECM) is a mixture of several macromolecules (laminin, fibronectin, collagens, proteoglycans,...) which are present in many tissues. In the mammary gland, the ECM surrounds the secretory cells and it is in close contact with them (Fig. 4). ECM prevents the epithelial cells to multiply while favouring their polarization and their differentiation. Under the action of estrogens, proteases are locally produced which partially degrade the ECM. This alleviates its inhibitory action and the concomitent effect of TGF-α and MDGF-I can be fully expressed. TGF-α and MDGF-I favour the synthesis of collagen IV and they tend in this way to attenuate their own stimulatory effect on cell division. In the normal mammary tissues, the balance between this contradictatory actions allows an efficient and limited development of the mammary gland. In mammary tumors, the feed-back action of the ECM is more or less lost, allowing a non-controlled cell multiplication (Monahan et al., 1988).

TNF-α may to some extent replace EGF and TGF-α, although it acts through its own receptor. TNF-α also inhibits milk synthesis. From this point of view, its action is somewhat simular to progesterone effect (Ip et al., 1992).

IGF-I is produced within the mammary gland. Prolactin seems to control synthesis of the IGF-I and IGF-II binding proteins. These effects most likely contribute to the control of mammary gland the development (Fielder et al., 1992).

cAMP in vitro or in vivo has a potent effect on mammary cell division and on the formation of the lobulo-alveolar structures (Silberstein et al., 1984). It is not known which physiological factors control cAMP concentration in the mammary gland but it is interesting to note that this nucleotide is at its highest level during pregnancy (Sapag-Hagaraud Greenbaum, 1974). Undoubtedly, other growth factors produced locally or else where in the body remain to be found. Such a factor found recently by Chomczynski et al. (1992) in hypophysis is a good candidate.

Several factors have been shown to limitate mammary gland development. This seems to be the case for TGF-β which is found at a lower level in the mammary area in rapid development. Interestingly, TGF-β stimulates the synthesis of collagen I and proteoglycans (Siberstein et al., 1990 ; Robinson et al., 1991). Its action might thus be at least in part, mediated through the accumulation of the components of ECM. TGF-β exists as several isoforms which seem to have somewhat different activity. TGF-β3 is elevated in the mammary gland throughout pregnancy and its concentration decreases after parturition. It has been shown to exert a potent inhibitory action on milk synthesis. This group of factors might therefore, as progesterone and TNF-α, allow or even favour the development of the mammary gland while inhibitory its differentiation (Meith et al., 1990 ; Daniel and Robinson, 1992).

Another inhibitor factor, MDGF-I (mammary derived growth factor inhibitor) has been found in cow mammary gland. Interestingly, this factor is present at a high level in the lactating animal and it is not so abundant during pregnancy (Politis et al., 1992).

Another inhibitor of mammary gland growth, mammostatin, has been identified in human mammary gland several years ago (Ervin et al., 1989). Little is known on this factor.

V - THE FACTORS CONTROLLING THE ONSET OF MILK SYNTHESIS AND SECRETION

Milk synthesis in most species starts during the last part of pregnancy but it remains at a very modest level. The real milk synthesis is triggered soon after parturition. It is clearly correlated with the progesterone drop. This drop is responsible

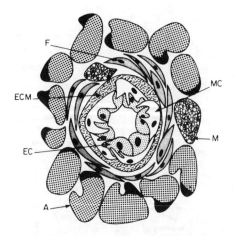

Fig. 4 : The organization of the various mammary cell types in the developped mammary gland (from Haslam, 1988). F : fibroblastes ; ECM : extracellular matrix ; EC : epithelial cells ; A : adipocytes ; M : mastocytes ; MC : myoepithelial cells.

for the strong release of prolactin at parturition. Two brakes are thus suppressed simultaneously when progesterone disappears : the inhibition of prolactin release and the direct inhibitory effect of progesterone on milk synthesis in the mammary gland. During lactation, progesterone is known not to be any more able to inhibit milk synthesis. This may be due to the strong prolactin signal during this period but also to the fact that progesterone receptors have become rare (Shyamala et al., 1990).

As mentioned above, TNF-α and TGF-β most likely contribute to maintain the mammary epithelial cells in a non-differentiated cells throughout pregnancy. Interestingly, TGF-β3 reduces milk synthesis at a post transcriptional level (Robinson et al., 1993). This may account for the fact that during the last part of pregnancy a relatively high level of milk protein mRNA are found although milk synthesis remains very low.

VI - THE ROLE OF THE EXTRACELLULAR MATRIX (ECM) ON THE ORGANIZATION OF THE MAMMARY TISSUE

Experiments carried out more than 15 years ago have clearly established that isolated epithelial mammary cells maintained on a plastic support are poorly sensitive to the lactogenic hormones (prolactin, insulin and cortisol) to synthesize milk. On the contrary, when cultured on floating but not on fixed collagen I in the presence of the hormones, these cells synthesize and secrete a relatively large quantity of milk proteins. A more detailed analysis has revealed that the cells layered on the collagen I gel synthesize several components of the ECM : collagen IV, laminin and proteoglycans. These molecules appeared to interact with the epithelial cells rather than collagen I per se. The role of collagen I was shown to stabilize the secreted components of the ECM which can form an active network in close contact with the epithelial cells. Mammary epithelial cells cultured on plastic support synthesize and secrete spontaneously a large amount of laminin, collagen IV and proteoglycans. These molecules cannot form an organized ECM network in these conditions and the cells permanently secrete them. When cultured on floating collagen I, the cells progressively stop secreting the ECM components which become accumulated in their vicinity. The ECM components thus exert a strong feed-back effect on their own biosynthesis, once stabilized (Streuli and Bissell, 1990). It is worth noting that the effect of collagen I on cell differentiation becomes effective only when this gel is floating (Barcellos-Hoff et al., 1989). The floating collagen allows polarisation of the cells to take place and it is considered as essential to favour their differentiation by the lactogenic hormones. Things may however be not so simple and the differentiation effect of ECM can be observed in some cases without any concommitent polarization of the epithelial mammary cells (Streuli et al., 1991).

The cellular and molecular mechanisms which direct the organization of cells in epithelium is not known. A substance named epimorphine (Gumbiner, 1992) seems to play an essential role. The exact role of the ECM in this process is not completely understood, but it is undoubtedly essential. As mentioned above, the ECM moderates the rate of cell division. Proteoglycans may sequester growth factors and reduce their effect on the cells. These factor may be released and favour cell division when ECM is degraded (Ruoslahti and Yamaguchi, 1991 ; Vukicevic et al., 1992).

The effect of ECM on the organization of the mammary tissue has been studied in detail in the past years and several important facts emerged. Isolated epithelial mammary cells layered on a gel of EHS matrix (Engelbreth, Holm, Swarn) extracted from a mouse tumor, rapidly become associated forming organoids and finally spheres ressembling strikingly to mammary alveoli. In these conditions, the cells are quite sensitive to lactogenic hormones and they secrete milk proteins preferentially in the inside compartment of the sphere. The EHS thus allowed an excellent reconstitution of well-formed and functional alveoli from isolated cells (Streuli et al., 1991). Unexpectedly, the mouse whey acid protein gene cannot be expressed even in the presence of hormones when the cells are cultured on floating collagen I. The more complex EHS matrix is required for this gene (Chen and Bissell, 1989 ; Schoenenberger et al., 1990). Laminin seems to be secreted by epithelial cells not only in the presence of collagen I but also in contact with the mammary fibroblasts. This is strongly suggested by experiments carried out with the cellular clone IM$_2$ which is a mixture of fibroblasts and epithelial cells. The only epithelial cells which are capable of synthesizing milk proteins in this cell line are those which are in close contact with the fibroblasts and which accumulate laminin (Reichmann, 1989). This experiment most likely reflects events really occuring in vivo and it emphasizes the importance of the interaction of the various cell types within the mammary gland.

Little is known on the composition of the ECM in the mammary gland during the normal pregnancy-lactation-weaning cycle. It is indeed concievable that subtle changes in the proportion of the various components of the ECM direct the organization of the mammary tissue during its development. In this respect, it is interesting to note that chondroitin sulfate is more abundant than dermatan sulfate in mouse mammary gland during pregnancy and that the reverse is true during lactation (Beck et al., 1993).

Interestingly, TGF-β$_1$ gene expression is strongly down-regulated by ECM in the mammary cells whereas the TGF-β$_2$ counterpart remains unchanged (Streuli et al., 1993). This strongly suggests that TGF-β$_1$ plays an important role in regulating ECM synthesis and cell-ECM interactions whereas TGF-β$_2$ might intervene rather in the morphogenetic processes.

All these experiments may explain some of the mechanisms leading to the tumorization of the mammary cells. Indeed, the mouse mammary cell line S-115 derived from a tumor multiplied much more slowly when it was transfected with a gene expressing a proteoglycan, syndecan (Leppä et al., 1992).

Proteoglycans are known to inhibit the expression of the cellular oncogenes c-fos and c-myc which are stimulated soon after addition of growth factors to quiescent cells (Bush et al., 1992).Tumorization might thus be due in part to the loss of the feed-back normally exerted by the accumulated ECM. Abnormally expressed proteases may be responsible for the loss of the extracellular matrix. One of this protease, stromelysin-3 has been identified. Unexpectedly, this protease is secreted by fibroblasts in some mammary tumors (Basset et al., 1990).

A comparison of different normal and tumor mammary cells has led to establish a correlation between the capacity of a line to form bona fide alveoli in the presence of EHS matrix and to divide slowly in the presence of the matrix. The most tumorized cells did not show arrested growth in the presence of EHS matrix and they form large cell aggregates rather than alveoli containing a limited number of cells (Petersen et al., 1992).

The mechanism of action of the ECM on the organization of the epithelial cells is only very partially known. Interestingly, the EHS matrix induces the accumulation of galactosyl transferase on the surface of the epithelial cells. This enzyme is not necessary for the adhesion of the cells to the support but it is required for the formation of the alveoli. Indeed, α-lactalbumin (which is a strong inhibitor of galactosyl transferase) added to the culture medium prevents the epithelial mammary cells layered on EHS matrix to form alveoli (Barcellos-Hoff, 1992). This impressive result may suggest that the reorganization of the mammary tissue has less chance to occur once milk synthesis has been triggered.

The ECM has also been shown to favour the synthesis and the secretion of mucin-1 by the mammary epithelial cells. This molecule accumulates on the apical side of the cells and it might thus contribute to maintain their polarization and their tight junctions (Parry et al., 1992).

On the other hand, glucocorticoids has recently been demonstrated to be a potent inducer of the formation of tight junctions in mouse mammary epithelial cells (Zett et al., 1992).

VII - THE MECHANISMS OF MAMMARY GLAND INHIBITION

The data reported above suggest that the organization of the mammary tissue is the result of a subtle balance between proteolytic and anti-proteolytic activities. Recent experiments indicate that the epithelial cells organized in alveoli by the EHS matrix secrete gelatinases in the outside compartment of the spheres. Several of these gelatinases are less abundant or less active during lactation than during pregnancy when the tissue in not being reorganized. They increase after weaning and they must participate to the involution of the gland (Talhouk et al., 1991 ; Talhouk et al., 1992). Interestingly, stromelysin-3 activity is also enhanced in normal mammary during apoptosis after weaning (Lefebvre et al., 1992).

VIII - THE FACTORS CONTROLLING MILK SYNTHESIS AND SECRETION DURING LACTATION

In most species, prolactin is required for the maintenance of milk secretion during lactation. Surprisingly however, it seems less and less necessary as lactation proceeds. Indeed, the withdrawal of prolactin secretion by bromocryptin injections prevents the onset of milk secretion at parturition in all species. One or two weeks later, bromocryptin reduces only by half milk secretion in rodents. In later stages of lactation, bromocryptin becomes poorly efficient. No clear explanation has been given to explain this fact. In ruminants, GH but not prolactin is required throughout lactation once milk secretion has been fully established. In rodents, GH seems to favour milk synthesis although to a moderate extent (Flint et al., 1992). The difference between rodents and ruminants in this respect is not easy to understand. A simple explanation might be that in ruminants and perhaps in late lactating rodents the mammary gland synthetizes prolactin acting through an autocrine or intacrine mechanism in sufficient amount to become more or less independant if the circulating hormone (Steinmetz et al., 1993).

It is generally admitted that bier and some plant extracts favour milk secretion in lactating women. Experiments carried out in the past years have revealed that the reputed active extracts do contain substances which can induce milk secretion. These substances stimulate prolactin and GH secretion when administered intraveinously in rodents and ruminants and also when administered orally in rodents. These substances have been identified. They are β-glucans in beer originating from malt (Sawadogo and Houdebine, 1988) and pectins in most of the plant extracts (Sawadogo et al., 1988).

Lactation becomes a priority after parturition and the metabolism of the female becomes reoriented in such a way as to prevent storage of energy in the body in favour of the mammary gland. This process which is rapidly reversible after weaning is under the dependency of the hormones which control metabolism. Experiments carried out about 50 years ago demonstrated that injections of GH to lactating cows increase milk secretion. This discovery was not used until the recombinant hormone becomes available. It is now well-established that injections of this hormone improve milk yield by 10 - 20 % without any significant adverse effect for the animals and no drawback for consummers (Juskevide and Guyer, 1990). It is admitted that the major mechanism of action of GH is to modify partition of body energy in favour of the mammary gland. Some local effect of the hormone and particularly on mammary blood flow are also possible (Mc Dowell, 1991).

The intensity of milk secretion becomes adapted to the efficiency of milking. This adaptory mechanisms seems not to be under the only control of hormones. In a recent study, Wilde et al. (1991) have suggested that milk contains substances which exert a feed-back inhibitory action on the mammary gland. These substances which are polypeptides might contribute to reduce the activity of the mammary cells when the gland becomes engorged with milk.

IX - THE MECHANISM OF ACTION OF LACTOGENIC HORMONES

After the growth of mammary gland and the formation of alveoli and before parturition, the epithelial cells remain small and they synthetize only small amounts of milk. After parturition, the concentration of the mRNAs coding for milk proteins and for enzymes responsible for the synthesis of lactose and lipids is considerably increased. During the first week of lactation, the epithelial cells become hypertrophied and polarized. They also become much richer in ribosomes, mitochondria, endoplasmic reticulum and Golgi membranes which are necessary for an efficient synthesis and secretion of milk.

The induction of milk protein gene expression by hormones can be easily obtained in vitro using mammary explants or isolated cells. Polarization of the epithelial cells is induced by extracellular matrix. In contrast, the accumulation of ribosomes cannot be obtained in vitro. In all species, prolactin is the essential inducer of milk synthesis and its effect is amplified by glucocorticoids, insulin or IGF-I and extracellular matrix. For this reason, the mechanism of action of prolactin is mainly studied. Its mechanism of action is still far from being understood (Houdebine, 1989). None of the classical

transduction mechanism seems to be involved in prolactin action on milk protein gene. In a recent work, it has been shown that several inhibitors of Ser/Thr kinase completely interrupt transmission of the prolaction signal to milk protein genes (Bayat-Sarmadi, 1993). In contrast, several inhibitors of Tyr kinase do not alter prolactin action, suggesting that a Ser/Thr kinase cascade plays an essential role in the transduction mechanism of the hormone. Prolactin receptor gene has been identified recently and this study revealed that it belongs to the cytokines receptor family (Kelly et al., 1991). Although the mechanism of action of cytokines is not known, it is generally admitted that the transduction of their message involves a Tyr kinase (Taga and Kishimove, 1992). This clear contrast with prolactin action may be not really surprising. Indeed, cytokines in most of their target cells induce both cell multiplication and differentiation. Prolactin is not mitogenic for mammary cells, in which it triggers only differentiation. Tyr kinase cascade might be involved in the initiation of the cell division whereas, a Ser/Thr kinase might rather activate a differentiation process. It is interesting to note that in Nb_2 cells which are strictly dependent on prolactin to multiply, the hormone can act only if Tyr kinases are active (Schechter et al., 1991 ; Rillema et al., 1992 ; Rui et al., 1992). Prolactin added to mammary explants from lactation rabbit stimulates rapidly milk secretion. This action of prolactin, which does not involve gene induction, is mediated through a phospholypase A_2-arachidonic acid-leukotriens cascade (Olliver-Bousquet, 1984). In contrast, phospholypase A_2 seems not to participate in the transfer of the prolactin message to milk protein genes (Devinoy et al., 1988). In a recent study, it has been shown that phospholipase A_2 is activated through a phosphorylation by MAP kinase and protein kinase C (Lin et al., 1993). The stimulation of milk secretion and the induction of milk protein gene (Bayat-Sarmadi et al., 1993) are both inhibited by staurosporine. It is concrevable that both prolactin actions are mediated through a kinase sensitive to staurosporine and which activate MAP kinase. MAP kinase might stimultaneously activates the phospholipase A_2 pathway to stimulate milk secretion and another pathway which remains to be found and which induces milk protein gene transcription.(Ollivier-Bousquet and Aubourg, 1992).

In mouse and rabbit (Puissant et al., 1993) transferrin gene is highly expressed in the mammary gland and the gene is stimulated essentially by the signal given to the mammary cell surface by the extracellular matrix but not, or only weakly, by prolactin. Milk protein genes appear therefore to be stimulated by at least three types of cellular signal (Fig. 5). The first which need not to be inducible may be mammary specific. The second is inducible by the extracellular matrix signal, most likely through integrin receptors which recognize matrix components. The transduction mechanism of this signal remains to be discovered. Preliminary results obtained in our laboratory do not suggest that a kinase cascade is involved in this mechanism. The third cellular signal is under prolactin dependency and it implies the action of a Ser/Thr kinase cascade.

Studies carried out in the last five years have led to the identification of the major milk protein genes in several species. The promoters of these genes are being studied using transfection into cells and transgenesis. This work was limited for long by the lack of appropriate cells for transfection. Several cellular systems are now available : mammary cells lines from mouse : HC11 (Ball et al., 1988) and CID9 (Schmidbauser et al., 1990) and from cow : MAC-T (Huynb et al., 1991). Primary mammary cells (Devinoy et al., 1991 ; Yoshimura et al., 1990) and CHO cells transfected by the prolactin receptor cDNA (Lesueur et al., 1990). The studies carried out with these tools permitted to define regions located in the upstream of several milk protein genes which are involved in prolactin and extracellular matrix action (Doppler et al., 1989 ; Yoshimura and Oka, 1990 ; Schmidbauser et al., 1990 ; Doppler et al.,

8

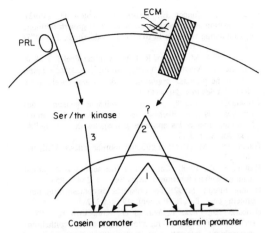

Fig. 5 : Schematic representation of the control mechanism of milk protein gene transcription. At least three signals are involved : 1 : mammary specific ; 2 : prolactin (PRL) ; 3 : extracellular matrix (ECM).

1991 ; Devinoy et al., 1991 ; Schmidbauser et al., 1992 ; Pierre et al., 1992). These experiments demonstrate with no ambiguity that milk protein genes are regulated to a large extent at the level of transcription. A DNA sequence which seems to play an essential role for the control of milk protein gene expression has been found in several genes. A nuclear transcription factor which binds this sequence is induced by the onset of lactation and deinduced by weaning (Watson et al., 1991 ; Schmitt-Ney et al., 1991 ; Schmitt-Ney et al, 1992 a ; Schmitt-Ney et al., 1992 b ; Wakao et al., 1992). Interestingly, this factor is inactivated by phosphatase are reactivated by caseine kinase II. The identification of the events which occurs between the binding of prolactin to its receptor and the activation of gene transcription through a kinase cascade can now be adressed much more easily. The exact role of this factor in the control of milk protein gene expression is however not yet clear. Indeed, experiments carried out with cow αs_2-casein gene indicated that the MGF is active in the mammary gland even in non-lactating animals. The authors concluded that the factor may be mammary specific but not lactation specific (Groenen et al., 1992). Moreover, with bovine β-casein, the mutation of the DNA sequence specific for MGF binding did not alter the capacity of the promoter to drive the expression of chloramphenicol acetyl transferase in transfected CID 9 cells (Schmidbauser et al., 1992).

A DNA region involved in the inhibition of casein gene expression by progesterone has been identified (Lee and Oka, 1992 a ; Lee and Oka, 1992 b). Interestingly, this sequence is not the consensus sequence which recognizes progesterone receptor. Progesterone therefore inhibits casein gene expression through a mechanism different of that involved in the induction of genes like ovalbumin. It remains unclear if progesterone acts directly on the epithelial cells to inhibit milk gene expression since this effect is easily obtained in vivo but not with isolated rabbit mammary cells (Puissant et al., 1993) or with CHO cells transfected with prolactin receptor (Bayat-Sarmadi et al., unpublished results).

Glucocorticoids are known to amplify milk protein gene expression. No glucocorticoids responsible elements have yet been found in the upstream region of milk protein genes. Such a sequence is not really expected to be present in casein gene

which are only slowly stimulated by glucocorticoids. In contrast, the whey acidic protein (WAP) gene is highly dependent on glucocorticoids in addition to prolactin, even in the rabbit and its induction by cortisol is very rapid (Puissant and Houdebine, 1991). The promoter region of WAP gene is therefore expected to contain a glucocorticoid responsive element.

Several groups of genes concentrated in the same locus on a chromosome are under the control of a strong common enhancer named locus control region. This is the case for the β-globin locus in higher vertebrates. Cow casein-genes are concentrated in a region not longer than 300 kb (Threadgill et al., 1990 ; Ferretti et al., 1990). The presence of a possible locus control region for casein genes has not been reported so far.

Several experiments suggest that milk protein genes are regulated not only at the transcriptional level but also post-transcriptionally. The extracellular matrix, prolactin and cortisol might contribute to the stabilization of milk protein mRNAs (Houdebine et al., 1978 ; Chomszynski et al., 1986 ; Eisenstein et al., 1988). The mechanism of this stabilization is totally unknown.

X - CONCLUSIONS

The use of the modern techniques of cellular and molecular biology has profoundly changed the study of the biology of lactation. These techniques have opened new avenues for research and they offer many new possibilities which just started being explored. One of the major problem which has been adressed with these new potent tools is mammary gland growth. It has become much easier to identify and to study new growth factors. Milk proteins exists in different forms according to the alleles from which they derive. Their property for milk industry are different (Grosclaude, 1988). The selection of progenitors harboring the most interesting alleles has been considerably facilitated and accelerated by using the RFLP technique (Leveziel et al., 1988). The possibility to transfer genes coding for factors controlling growth and organization of the mammary gland either in vitro or in vivo through transgenesis and gene therapy will certain lead to interesting observations in a near future. It has become possible to control the expression of foreign genes specifically in the mammary gland of different transgenic animals using promoters from milk protein genes (Hemighausen, 1992). This should lead to the modification of milk composition for human and offsprings consumption and also for cheese industry. This should contribute to reduce mastitis in lactating animals. There is little doubt that transgenic mammals will be used in a near future to produce various recombinant proteins in their milk. All these new approaches should facilitate the struggle against breast cancer and to improve genetic characteristics of animals.

REFERENCES

Assairi L., Delouis C., Gaye P., Houdebine L. M., Ollivier-Bousquet M., Denamur R. (1974). Inhibition by progesterone of the lactogenic effect of prolactin in the pseudopregnant rabbit. Biochem. J., 144, 245-252.

Ball R. K., Friis R. R., Schoenenberger C. A., Doppler W., Groner B. (1988). Prolactin regulation of β-casein gene expression and of a cytosolic 120-kd protein in a cloned mouse mammary epithelial cell line. EMBO J., 7, 2089-2095.

Bano M., Worland P., Kidwell W. R., Lippman M. E., Dickson R. B. (1992). Receptor-induced phosphorylation by mammary-derived growth factor 1 in mammary epithelial cell lines. J. Biol. Chem., 267, 10389-10392.

Barcellos-Hoff M. H. (1992). Mammary epithelial reorganization on extracellular matrix is mediated by cell surface galactosyltransferase. Exp. Cell. Res., 201, 225-234.

Barcellos-Hoff M. H., Aggeler J., Ram T. G., Bissell M. J. (1989). Functional differentiation and alveolar morphogenesis of primary mammary cultures on reconstituted basement membrane. Development, 105, 223-235.

Basset P., Bellocq J. P., Wolf C., Stoll C., Hutin P., Limacher J. M., Podhajcer O. L., Chenard M. P., Rio M. C., Chambon P. (1990). A novel metalloproteinase gene specifically expressed in stromal cells of breast carcinomas. Nature, 348, 699-704.

Bayat-Sarmadi M., Houdebine L. M. (1993). Effect of various protein kinase inhibitors on the induction of milk protein gene expression by prolactin. (1993) Mol. Cell. Endocrinol., 92, 127-134.

Beck J. M., Lekutis C., Couchman J., Parry G. (1993). Stage-specific remodeling of the mammary gland basement membrane during lactogenic development. Biochem. Biophys. Res. Comm., 190, 616-623.

Bush S. J., Martin G. A., Barnhart R. L., Mano M., Cardin A. D., Jackson R. L. (1992). Transrepressor activity of nuclear glycosaminoglycans on Fos and Jun/AP-1 oncoprotein-mediated transcription. J. Cell Biol., 116, 31-42.

Byatt J. C., Warren W. C., Eppard P. J., Staten N. R., Krivi G. G., Collier R. J. (1992). Ruminant placenta lactogens : structure and biology. J. Anim. Sci., 70, 2911-2923.

Chen L. H., Bissell M. J. (1989). A novel regulatory mechanism for whey acidic protein gene expression. Cell Regul., 1, 45-54.

Chomszynski P., Qasba P., Topper Y. J. (1986). Transcriptional and post-transcriptional roles of glucocorticoid in the expression of the rat 25,000 molecular weight casein gene. Biochem. Biophys. Res. Comm., 134, 812-818.

Cowie A. T. (1970). In Lactation Falconer IR, ed., Butterworths London.

Daniel C. W., Robinson S. D. (1992). Regulation of mammary growth and function by TGF-β. Mol. Reprod. Dev., 32, 145-151.

Doppler W., Groner B., Ball R. K. (1989). Prolactin and glucocorticoid hormones synergistically induce expression of transfected rat β-casein gene promoter constructs in a mammary epithelial cell line. Proc. Natl. Acad. Sci. USA, 86, 104-108.

Doppler W., Villunger A., Jennewein P., Brduscha K., Groner B., Ball R. K. (1991). Lactogenic hormone and cell type-specific control of the whey acidic protein gene promoter in transfected mouse cells. Mol. Endocrinol., 5, 1624-1632.

Edery M., McGrath M., Larson L., Nandi S. (1984). Correlation between in vitro growth and regulation of estrogen and progesterone receptors in rat mammary epithelial cells. Endocrinology, 115, 1691-1697.

Eisenstein R. S., Rosen J. M. (1988). Both cell substantrum regulation and hormonal regulation of milk protein gene expression are exerted primarily at the post-transcriptional level. Mol. Cell. Biol., 8, 3183-3190.

Ervin Jr. P. R., Kaminski M. S., Cody R. L., Wicha M. S. (1989). Production of mammastatin, a tissue-specific growth inhibitor, by normal human mammary cells. Science, 244, 1585-1587.

Ferretti L., Leone P., Sgaramella V. (1990). Long range restriction analysis of the bovine casein genes. Nucleic Acids Res., 18, 6829-6833.

Fielder P. J., Thordarson G., English A., Rosenfeld R. G., Talamantes F. (1992). Expression of a lactogen-dependent insulin-like growth factor-binding protein in cultured mouse mammary epithelial cells. Endocrinology, 131, 261-267.

Flint D. J., Tonner E., Beattie J., Panton D. (1992). Investigation of the mechanism of action of growth hormone in stimulating lactation in the rat. J. Endocrinol., 134, 377-383.

Groenen M. A. M., Dijkhof R. J. M., Van der Poel J. J., Van Diggelen R., Verstege E. (1992). Multiple octamer binding sites in the promoter region of the bovine αs_2-casein gene. Nucleic Acids Res., 20, 4311-4318.

Grosclaude F. (1988). Le polymorphisme génétique des principales lactoprotéines bovines. Relations avec la quantité, la composition et les aptitudes fromagères du lait. INRA, Prod. Anim., 1, 5-17.

Gumbiner B. M. (1992). Epithelial morphogenesis. Cell, 69, 385-387.

Haslam S. Z. (1988). Cell to cell interactions and normal mammary gland function. J. Dairy Sci., 71, 2843-2854.

Hennighausen L. (1992). The prospects for domesticating milk protein genes. J. Cell. Biochem., 49, 325-332.

Heuberger B., Fitzka I., Wasner G., Kratochwil K. (1982). Induction of androgen receptor formation by epithelium-mesenchyme interaction in embryonic mouse mammary gland. Proc. Natl. Acad. Sci. USA, 79, 2957-2961.

Houdebine L. M. (1989). Recent data on the mechanism of action of prolactin. Exp. Clin. Endocr. (Life Sci. Adv.), 8, 157-166.

Houdebine L. M., Gaye P. (1975). Regulation of casein synthesis in the rabbit mammary gland. Titration of mRNA activities for casein under prolactin and progesterone treatments. Mol. Cell. Endocr., 3, 37-55.

Houdebine L. M., Teyssot B., Devinoy E., Ollivier-Bousquet M., Djiane J., Kelly P. A., Delouis C., Kann G., Fevre J. (1983). Role of progesterone in the development and the activity of the mammary gland. Progesterone and Progestins, 297-319.

Huynh H. T., Robitaille G., Turner J. D. (1991). Establishment of bovine mammary epithelial cells (MAC-T) : an in vitro model for bovine lactation. Exp. Cell Res., 197, 191-199.

Ip M. M., Shoemaker S. F., Darcy K. M. (1992). Regulation of rat mammary epithelial cell proliferation and differentiation by tumor necrosis factor-a. Endocrinology, 130, 2833-2844.

Jahn G. A., Djiane J., Houdebine L. M. (1989). Inhibition of casein synthesis by progestagens in vitro. J. Steroid. Biochem., 32, 373-379.

Juskevich J. C., Guyer C. G. (1990). Bovine growth hormone : human food safety evaluation. Science, 249, 875-884.

Kelly P. A., Djiane J., Postel-Vinay M.-C., Edery M. (1991). The prolactin growth hormone receptor family. Endocrine Reviews, 12, 235-251.

Lee C. S., Oka T. (1991). A pregnancy-specific mammary nuclear factor involved in the repression of the mouse β-casein gene transcription by progesterone. J. Biol. Chem., 267, 5797-5801.

Lee C. S., Oka T. (1992). Progesterone regulation of a pregnancy-specific transcription repressor to β-casein gene promoter in mouse mammary gland. Endocrinol., 131, 2257-2262.

Lefebvre O., Wolf C., Limacher J.-M., Hutin P., Wendling C., LeMeur M., Basset P., Rio M.-C. (1992). The breast cancer-associated stromelysin-3 gene is expressed during mouse mammary gland apoptosis. J. Cell. Biol., 119, 997-1002.

Leppa S., Mali M., Miettinen H. M., Jalkanen M. (1992). Syndecan expression regulates cell morphology and growth of mouse mammary epithelial tumor cells. Proc. Natl. Acad. Sci. USA, 89, 932-936.

Lesueur L., Edery M., Paly J., Clark J., Kelly P. A., Djiane J. (1990). Prolactin stimulates milk protein promoter CHO cells cotransfected with prolactin receptor cDNA. Mol. Cell. Endocrinol., 71, R7-R12.

Levéziel H., Méténier L., Mahé M.-F., Choplain J., Furet J.-P., Paboeuf G., Mercier J.-C., Grosclaude F. (1988). Identification of the two common alleles of the bovine k-casein locus by the RFLP technique, using the enzyme hind III. Génét. Sél. Evol., 20, 247-254.

Lin L.-L., Wartmann M., Lin A. Y., Knopf J. L., Seth A., Davis R. J. (1993). cPLA$_2$ is phosphorylated and activated by MAP kinase. Cell, 72, 269-278.

Lyons W. R., Li C. H., Johnson R. E. (1958). The hormonal control of mammary growth and lactation. Recent Prog. Horm. Res., 14, 219.

McDowell G. H. (1991). Somatotropin and endocrine regulation of metabolism during lactation. J. Dairy Sci., 74, 44-62.

Mieth M., Boehmer F.-D., Ball R., Groner B., Grosse R. (1990). Transforming growth factor-β inhibits lactogenic hormone induction of β-casein expression in HC11 mouse mammary epithelial cells. Growth Factors, 4, 9-15.

Monahan S., Salomon D. S., Kidwell W. R. (1988). Substratum modulation of epidermal growth factor receptor expression by normal mammary cells. J. Dairy Sci., 71, 1507-1514.

Oka T., Yoshimura M., Lavandero S., Wasa K., Ohba Y. (1991). Control of growth and differentiation of the mammary gland by growth factors. J. Dairy Sci., 74, 2788-2800.

Ollivier-Bousquet M. (1984). Effet de la prolactine sur la sécrétion des caséines du lait : métabolisme de l'acide arachidonique. Biol. Cell., 51, 327-334.

Ollivier-Bousquet M., Aubourg A. (1992). The possible involvement of protein kinase C$_{(s)}$ and inositol phosphate metabolism in the basal but not in the prolactin stimulated casein release by the lactating rabbit mammary epithelial cell. Reprod. Nutr. Dev., 32, 441-451.

Parry G., Li J., Stubbs J., Bissell M. J., Schmidhauser C., Spicer A. M., Gendler S. J. (1992). Studies of Muc-1 mucin expression and polarity in the mouse mammary gland demonstrate developmental regulation of Muc-1 glycosylation and establish the hormonal basis for mRNA expression. J. Cell Sci., 101, 191-199.

Petersen O. W., Ronnov-Jessen L., Howlett A. R., Bissell M. J. (1992). Interaction with basement membrane serves to rapidly distinguish growth and differentiation pattern of normal and malignant human breast epithelial cells. Proc. Natl. Acad. Sci. USA, 89, 9064-9068.

Pierre S., Joliver G., Devinoy E., Theron M. C., Malienou N'Ghassa R., Puissant C., Houdebine L. M. (1992). A distal region enhances the prolactin induced promoter activity of the rabbit αs$_1$-casein gene. Mol. Cell. Endocr., 87, 147-156.

Politis I., Gorewit R. C., Muller T., Grosse R. (1992). Mammary-derived growth inhibitor protein and messenger ribonucleic acid concentrations in different physiological states of the gland. J. Dairy Sci., 75, 1423-1429.

Puissant C. et al. (submitted).

Puissant C., Houdebine L. M. (1991). Cortisol induces rapid accumulation of whey acidic protein mRNA but not αs$_1$- and β-casein mRNA in rabbit mammary explants. Cell. Biol. Int. Rep., 15, 121-129.

Reichmann E., Ball R., Groner B., Friis R. R. (1989). New mammary epithelial and fibroblastic cell clones in coculture form structures competent to differentiate functionally. J. Cell Biol., 108, 1127-1138.

Rillema J. A., Campbell G. S., Lawson D. M., Carter-Su C. (1992). Evidence for a rapid stimulation of tyrosine kinase activity by prolactin in Nb$_2$ rat lymphoma cells. Endocrinol., 131, 973-975.

Robinson S. D., Roberts A. B., Daniel C. W. (1993). TGF-β suppresses casein synthesis in mouse mammary explants and may play a role in controlling milk levels during pregnancy. J. Cell. Biol., 120, 245-251.

Robinson S. D., Silberstein G. B., Roberts A. B., Flanders K. C., Daniel C. W. (1991). Regulated expression and growth inhibitory effects of transforming growth factor-β isoforms in mouse mammary gland development. Development, 113, 867-878.

Rui H., Djeu J. Y., Evans G. A., Kelly P. A., Farrar W. L. (1992). Prolactin receptor triggering. Evidence for rapid tyrosine kinase activation. J. Biol. Chem., 267, 24076-24081.

Ruoslahti E., Yamaguchi Y. (1991). Proteoglycans as modulators of growth factor activities. Cell, 64, 867-869.

Sakakura T. (1991). New aspects of stroma-parenchyma relations in mammary gland differentiation. Int. Rev. Cytol., 125, 165-202.

Sapag-Hagar M., Greenbaum A. L. (1974). Adenosine 3' : 5'-monophosphate and hormone interrelationships in the mammary gland of the rat during pregnancy and lactation. Eur. J. Biochem., 47, 303-312.

Schmidhauser C., Bissell M. J., Myers C. A., Casperson G. F. (1990). Extracellular matrix and hormones transcriptionally regulate bovine β-casein 5' sequences in stably transfected mouse mammary cells. Proc. Natl. Acad. Sci. USA, 87, 9118-9122.

Schmidhauser C., Casperson G. F., Myers C. A., Sanzo K. T., Bolten S., Bissell M. (1992). A novel transcriptional enhancer is involved in the prolactin-and extracellular matrix-dependent regulation of β-casein gene expression. Mol. Biol. Cell, 3, 699-709.

Schmitt-Ney M., Doppler W., Ball R. K., Groner B. (1991). β-casein gene promoter activity is regulated by the hormone-mediated relief of transcriptional repression and a mammary-gland-specific nuclear factor. Mol. Cell Biol., 11, 3745-3755.

Schmitt-Ney M., Happ B., Ball R. K., Groner B. (1992). Developmental and environmental regulation of a mammary gland-specific nuclear factor essential for transcription of the gene encoding β-casein. Proc. Natl. Acad. Sci. USA, 89, 3130-3134.

Schmitt-Ney M., Happ B., Hofer P., Hynes N. E., Groner B. (1988). Mammary gland-specific nuclear factor activity is positively regulated by lactogenic hormones and negatively by milk stasis. Mol. Endocrinol., 6, 1988-1997.

Schoenenberger C. A., Zuk A., Groner B., Jones W., Andres A. C. (1990). Induction of the endogenous whey acidic protein (WAP) gene and a wap-myc hybrid gene in primary murine mammary organoids. Dev. Biol., 139, 327-337.

Shechter Y., Sakal E., Cohen R., Cohen-Chapnik N., Gertler A. (1991). Hydroxyphenyl acetate derivatives inhibit protein tyrosine kinase activity and proliferation in Nb$_2$ rat lymphoma cells and insulin-induced lipogenesis in rat adipocytes. Mol. Cell. Endocrinol., 80, 183-192.

Shyamala G., Schneider W., Schott D. (1990). Developmental regulation of murine mammary progesterone receptor gene expression. Endocrinol., 126, 2882-2889.

Silberstein G. B., Stricland P., Coleman S., Daniel C. W. (1990). Epithelium-dependent extracellular matrix synthesis in transforming growth factor-β$_1$-growth-inhibited mouse mammary gland. J. Cell. Biol., 110, 2209-2219.

Silberstein G. B., Stricland P., Trumpbour V., Coleman S., Daniel C. W. (1984). In vivo, cAMP stimulates growth and morphogenesis of mouse mammary ducts. Proc. Natl. Acad. Sci. USA, 81, 4950-4954.

Steinmetz R. W., Grant A. L., Malven P. V. (1993). Transcription of prolactin gene in milk secretory cells of the rat mammary gland. J. Endocrinol., 136, 271-276.

Streuli C. H., Bailey N., Bissell M. J. (1991). Control of mammary epithelial differentiation : basement membrane induces tissue-specific gene expression in the absence of cell-cell interaction and morphological polarity. J. Cell Biol., 115, 1383-1395.

Streuli C. H., Bissell M. J. (1990). Expression of extracellular matrix components is regulated by substratum. J. Cell Biol., 110, 1405-1415.

Streuli C. H., Schmidhauser C., Kobrin M., Bissell M. J., Derynck R. (1993). Extracellular matrix regulates expression of the TGF-β_1 gene. J. Cell. Biol., 120, 253-260.

Taga T., Kishimoto T. (1992). Cytokine receptors and signal transduction. FASEB J., 6, 3387-3396.

Threadgill D. W., Womack J. E. (1990). Genomic analysis of the major bovine milk protein genes. Nucleic Acids Res., 18, 6935-6942.

Vukicevic S., Kleinman H. K., Luyten F. P., Roberts A. R., Roche N. S., Reddi A. H. (1992). Identification of multiple active growth factors in basement membrane matrigel suggests caution in interpretation of cellular activity related to extracellular matrix components. Exp. Cell Res., 202, 1-8.

Wakao H., Schmitt-Ney M., Groner B. (1992). Mammary gland-specific nuclear factor is present in lactating rodent and bovine mammary tissue and composed of a single polypeptide of 89 kDa. J. Biol. Chem., 267, 16365-16370.

Watson C. J., Gordon K. E., Robertson M., Clark A. J. (1991). Interaction of DNA-binding proteins with a milk protein gene promoter in vitro : identification of a mammary gland-specific factor. Nucleic Acids Res., 19, 6603-6610.

Wilde C. J., Addey C. V. P., Knight C. H., Peaker M. (1991). Autocrine control in milk production and mammary development. Proceedings of the New Zealand Society of Anim. Prod., 51, 203-209.

Yoshimura M., Oka T. (1990). Transfection of β-casein chimeric gene and hormonal induction of its expression in primary murine mammary epithelial cells. Proc. Natl. Acad. Sci. USA, 87, 3670-3674.

Zettl K. S., Sjaastad M. D., Riskin P. M., Parry G., Machen T. E., Firestone G. L. (1992). Glucocorticoid-induced formation of tight junctions in mouse mammary epithelial cells. Proc. Natl. Acad. Sci. USA, 89, 9069-9073.

Dairy Products in Human Health and Nutrition, Serrano Ríos et al. (eds)© 1994 Balkema, Rotterdam, ISBN 90 5410 359 0

Milk composition in animals and humans: Nutritional aspects

L. Hambræus
Department of Nutrition, University of Uppsala, Sweden

ABSTRACT:

Teleologically there are reasons to assume that the composition of milk which varies considerably between mammals, reflects the specific nutritional and physiological needs of the newborn offspring. The present review deals with the nutritional aspects on the differences in the milk composition between human milk and other milks, with special reference to bovine milk, from a nutritional/physiological point of view.

There is a conflict between the strict nutritionally aspects which essentially take into account the macronutrient aspects to cover certain nutritional requirements, and a more specific physiological approach based on various specific more or less well-defined metabolic effects of certain components which occur in micro amounts. More studies are needed to evaluate the future for more specific nutritional and pharmacological use of milk components.

1. INTRODUCTION

The nutritional significance of milk components can essentially be divided into two sections: a macronutrient aspect, which essentially comprises the role of major components used as more or less non-specific nutrient sources, i.e. energy and protein, and a micronutrient or specific physiological aspect, in which the specific physiological functions of certain components which occur in smaller amounts are taken into consideration.

The macronutrient aspects comprise essentially the content of energy and essential nutrients which play essential roles in the anabolic processes, i.e. as sources of material for growth or repair of tissues during convalescence.

However there is a growing interest nowadays devoted to the specific physiological aspects of the micronutrients, i.e. trace elements, vitamins, hormones and growth factors and their roles for metabolic, endocrine and immunological functions in the body.

1.1 Why should milk be of specific nutritional interest?

One of the major characteristics of the nutritional situation during the neonatal period in mammals is

the fact that the offspring has to rely upon one single source of nutrients - milk, which means that there is no possibility to compensate for any lack of nutrients in the diet. On the same time there is a very pronounced growth of tissues during the neonatal period which creates an increased and specific demand for essential nutrients. A reduced tolerance for deviations in food intake due to the immaturity of the liver and kidneys, both of which play essential roles in the metabolism and excretion of metabolites, however, complicates the nutritional situation. Consequently it has rightly or wrongly been assumed that the composition of the milk of any mammalian species is the definitive indicator of the nutrition requirements of its offspring during the neonatal period.

The composition of milk obtained from various species shows great variations (Table 1). It has been reported that out of 4300 species of mammals, less than 200 milks have been analysed with respect to their content of protein, fat and carbohydrate and out of these only data regarding milk specimens obtained from about 50 species are considered to be reliable (Oftedahl, 1980, Widdowson, 1984).

As discussed above we may assume on a teleological basis that the composition of milks of different species

Table 1. Composition of milks obtained from different mammals

(from Jenness, 1974, Hambraeus, 1976, Oftedahl, 1980, Widdowson, 1984)

Species	Content in milk (per 100 ml)			
	protein g	fat g	lactose g	Kcal*
Primates				
Man	0.9	3.8	7.0	66
Rhesus	1.6	4	7	70
Ruminants				
Cow	3.4	3.7	4.8	66
Camel	3.7	4.2	4.1	69
Buffalo	3.8	7.5	4.9	102
Reindeer	10.3	16.9	2.8	205
Goat	2.9	4.5	4.1	69
Sheep	5.5	7.4	4.8	108
Rodents				
Rat	8.1	8.8	3.8	127
Marsupials				
Kangaroo	4-10	1-16	5-0	45-184
Perissodactyla				
Horse	1.9	1.3	6.9	47
Rhinoceros	1.4	0.2	6.6	34
Carnivorous				
Cat	10.6	10.8	3.7	154
Wolf	9.2	9.6	3.4	137
Lagomorpha				
Rabbit	10.3	15.2	1.8	185
Cetacea				
Dolphine	6.8	33	1.1	329
Blue whale	10.9	42.3	1.3	430
Marine carnivora				
Seal	10.2	49.4	0.1	486

* Energy calculated as follows: protein and carbohydrate: 4 kcal/g, fat: 9 kcal/g

represent the optimum composition of nutrients required during the neonatal period of that species. Several authors have anticipated that there would be a relationship between the rate of growth of the offspring and nutrient density, i.e. the amount of essential nutrients in relation to its energy content, e.g. g protein per 10 MJ or 1000 kcal (Jenness, 1970, 1974, Blanc, 1981).

There also seems to exist some similarities in the composition of milk within the same zoological group of animals. Thus rodents and carnivorous have a high protein content and moderately large amounts of fat and carbohydrates. Those feeding their offspring at long intervals have milks high in fat and energy. The ruminants have less protein and fat in the milk and more carbohydrate. Sea mammals have high protein content and very high percentage of fat. The high fat has been presumed to be necessary for animals who need to take in their meal in a very short time. The length of lactation period may also have an impact on milk composition, as well as the time alotted for the "meal". It is said that the dolphin only have a few seconds available as they must reach the surface every 30 seconds (Widdowson, 1984). The lactation period in man originally represents a relatively long period although it is arguable whether it represents the optimal single source of nutrients for infants for more than 4-6 months.

The milks of marsupials has been of great interest as it has been shown that milk composition changes drastically between the milk produced during the first part of lactation when the offspring is extremely immature to that in later phases of lactation. This is in addition to the well-known difference in composition between colostrum and mature milk. Interestingly, studies on milk composition in man have shown that mothers giving birth to preterm infants have another composition in their milk than those giving birth to full-term infants (Atkinson et al, 1981).

There are also certain interesting differences with respect to fat composition. rhinocerous milk only contains 0.2 % fat, rabbit milk is rich in MCT and capric acid is the major fatty acid in the elephant to give a few examples. Another difference which may have a metabolic relevance is that the cat's milk contains relatively large amounts of taurine which may compensate their inability to synthesize taurine from sulphur amino acids. The taurine in cow's milk is very low, and since taurine might also be of nutritional importance in the newborn infant proprietary milk formula are today enriched with taurine.

1.2 Grouping of nutrients in milk

Based on the observed differences in the composition of milk from various species Jenness (1974) divided milk components into the following groups based on whether they were specifically secreted in the mammary gland or not and whether they occurred only in certain species:

(1) organ and species specific;
(2) organ specific but not species specific;
(3) not organ specific but species specific; and
(4) neither organ nor species specific.

It can be assumed that milk components that are both organ and species specific or organ but not species specific are of greatest interest when nutritional and metabolic aspects of dairy products are discussed.

When discussing the nutritional significance of milk also a number of other questions arise which seem to be of relevance:

(1) Is there a difference with respect to various components, i.e. are some constituents more specific for the species than others? If so does this mean that they are also more essential for certain physiological/nutritional purposes than others?

(2) What evidence do we have that milk is the most relevant source of nutrients? During what age period does it seem to be the optimum food? Are milk products always valuable constituents of the human diet (even for adults)?

(3) What do we know about the stability of the composition of milk? What do the physiological variation in milk composition mean nutritionally?

(4) What do we know about the environmental factors and their impact on milk composition, i.e. maternal diet, drugs, contaminants, environmental pollution?

1.3 Effect of diet on milk composition

When comparisons are made between milk obtained from various species, it is of course most essential first to identify those due to the impact of environmental factors on milk composition from those of more or less genetic origin which might be of greater relevance when discussing the species characteristics of milk composition.

One of the most important environmental factors must be the dietary intake or effect of feeding the cattle. As a general role it seems that in those species where milk production has been "forced", i.e. intensive cattle feeding, the impact of feeding is more pronounced than in those who have a more normal production. But the effect of maternal diet may also be different in monogastric species versus

in ruminants. The two extreme situations might be represented by human lactation versus milk production in dairy cow farms with intensive feeding.

1.4 Changing milk composition by feeding trials or dairy technology?

Based on the assumption that there is an optimal composition regarding certain components in human milk it is thus a question to find out to what extent it is possible to change the composition in dairy milk products by changes in the feeding of the dairy cattle. Such examples seem most to have been discussed regarding the qualitative fat composition. May be also the content of certain vitamins and trace elements, or proteins with specific physiological or allergenic functions could be manipulated. However, with the advanced dairy technology of today it could be questionned whether a more realistic and effective way of changing milk composition could be by means of modern food technology. This might also mean a less stress on the cattle. The separation of the fat fraction in the dairy industry and substituting some fatty acids technologically might be an easier way to obtain the changes in fatty acid composition. Changes in the feeding pattern to obtain the same results may include losses in production yields as well as health risks for the dairy cow.

1.5 Nutritional aspects on milk composition not limited to the newborn period

Since this is a meeting on dairy products in human health and nutrition it is obvious that it could not be the purpose of this presentation only to discuss milk as a source of nutrients from the newborn's point of view. On the contrary, it can already from the beginning be said that since there are so definite differences in the milk composition when milk from various species are compared there is no real alternative to the species specific milk during the newborn period. Under normal conditions the species specific milk is the priority source of nutrients for the newborn.

However, the role milk and dairy products as a source of valuable nutrients in the diet of adults must be based on available data that certain components in human milk may exert specific physiological roles which might be relevant to a certain degree also during adulthood. Although it might be of interest to discuss all forms of milks I will concentrate the comments on a comparison between human and bovine milk since this seems to be the most relevant alternative from the practical point of view. There are also other milks which may have some dairy farm interest under certain circumstances, i.e. goat milk, sheep milk, buffalo milk and camel milk. However, as said before, as there are similarities in the milk composition within the ruminant group, bovine milk is used as a reference for these discussions.

1.6 Differ between nutritional and physiological/-metabolic roles of nutrients

Milk represents one of the most complete single food items within the diet no matter for which species it was originally adapted. The only other example of a complete food might be the egg.

In the diet of the adult however milk and dairy products are rarely used as a single food item but in combination with other food components. This means that we have essentially to look upon them as supplements of nutrients in the diet for man at all ages from the weaning period up to the old age. Thus most interest should be devoted to the components in which dairy products are especially rich or may have a specific nutritional or physiological implication as a supplement to a conventional diet.

The use of milk proteins in non-dairy products is of increasing interest as this is often based on the exploitation of the functional characteristics of certain milk components or due to their specific physiological impact on body function. There is reason to believe that such components are valid also in the diet of adults and may be dairy products will have an interesting role in the today increased interest for the development of "functional foods".

2. MILK AS SOURCE OF MACRO-NUTRIENTS

It is obvious that the dominating macronutrients where milk and dairy products may play an essential role are as source for energy, protein and calcium. On the other hand it is quite obvious that there are no problems to live on a milk-free diet, so there might be less reason to believe that milk and dairy products should be of any special concern with regard to its content of macro-nutrients.

2.1 Milk as energy source

From the energy point of view the nutritionally interesting aspect would essentially be to evaluate what the energy percentage distribution between the energy-yielding nutrients in human milk might indicate for future life. Interestingly human milk is

quite extreme versus not only cow's milk but also the characteristics of the diet in later life:

Table 2. Energy distribution in human and bovine milk versus adult western diet.

	Human milk	Cow's milk	Western diet
Energy% :			
Protein	6	21	12
Fat	52	50	38
Carbohydrate	42	29	50

The meaning of the extremely low protein energy% in human milk is not known. Interestingly, it is even less if one takes into consideration the protein fractions which are presumed to exert a physiological function and consequently not would be available as a conventional nutrient source (see below).

It is still not very clear what such a difference in the distribution of energy between the various energy yielding macronutrients will mean in practice for the future outcome and metabolic programming of the offspring. Especially with respect to the discussion on energy balance, fat quality and cardio-vascular diseases the low protein energy% as well as the high fat energy% are worth far more consideration.

2.2 Milk as protein source

Since milk contains a heterogeneous mixture of proteins, a variety of methods have been used to separate and characterize the various milk proteins. Milk proteins have been extensively studied throughout the year by protein chemists. Originally casein was assumed to be the only or major specific milk protein while most of the less abundant milk proteins found were thought to be derived from blood. The proteins of bovine milk has been more extensively studied than protein in other milks but during the last years also much interest has been devoted to comparative studies between human milk and bovine milk and its specific nutritional and metabolic implication (Hambræus, 1977, Blanc, 1981). Furthermore isolation and characterisation of milk proteins is complicated by their considerable tendency to associate and form complexes which makes the definition of their specific physiological, nutritional and immunological characteristics difficult.

From a strict macronutrient aspect, the nutritive value of milk as a source of dietary protein is related to its amino acid content as well as composition and availability of these amino acids. The protein and/or amino acid content has consequently two dimensions: qualitative and quantitative. The qualitative aspects might also lead to a question whether there is a difference between amino acid requirement for growth versus that for maintenance. The much discussed balance between the essential and non-essential amino acids as well as the balance between the individual essential amino acids is then of considerable scientific interest from the protein and amino acid metabolism point of view. In this respect it should be noted, however, that today the reference amino acid pattern for estimation of protein quality is close to that of of breast milk. The characteristics of this pattern is a relatively low content of sulphur amino acid methionine and higher content of the branched chain amino acids, leucine, isoleucine and valine.

Table 3. Proteins and non-protein nitrogen (NPN) in bovine and human milk (mg/ml).
(Ref Hambræus, 1977, Blanc, 1981, Lönnerdal, 1985)

	Human milk	Bovine milk
Protein (g/100 ml)	0.9	3.1
Caseins (g/100 ml)	0.25	3.73
Whey proteins (g/100 ml)	0.64	0.58
alfa-lactalbumin	0.26	0.11
lactoferrin	0.17	trace
Secretory IgA	0,05-0.1	
Immunoglobulins		
IgA	0.01	0.003
IgG	0.001	0.06
IgM	0.002	0.003
Enzymes		
Lysozyme	0.005	trace
Bile-salt stim lipase	0.01	
alfa-1-antitrypsin	0.001	
alfa-1-antichymotrypsin	0.001	
Binding proteins		
Folate binding	0.0007	
Corticosterol binding	0.01	
Others		
secretory component	0.02-0.03	
serum albumin	0.03	0.04
NPN (mg/100ml)	50	28
Urea N	25	13
Creatine N	3.7	0.9
Creatinine N	3.5	0.3
Uric acid N	0.5	0.8
Glucosamine	4.7	?
alfa-amino N	13	4.8

2.3 Calcium - the third macronutrient of concern

The third macronutrient of specific interest as it occurs in high concentration in milk is calcium. Obviously the calcium occurs essentially bound to casein, which is a very specific phosphoprotein. As calcium is essential as building material for bone tissues the intake of calcium and its relation to the future development of bone mass and occurrence of osteoporosis has been a matter of concern. Although there is still some confusion regarding the possibilities to prevent osteoporosis by increased dietary intake of calcium in the adult, most if not all scientists seem to agree that the calcium intake during infancy, childhood and adolescence is of importance (Andersson, 1990). In the western society dairy products constitute about 65-75% of calcium intake. It should however be noted that it is quite possible to obtain an acceptable calcium intake also on a milk free diet although this calls for a knowledge in practical nutrition.

As the calcium content is related to the casein content the mere fact that human milk has a low casein content indirectly means that there is also less calcium. Consequently the calcium intake during infancy and childhood is far higher in those given artificial products based on cow's milk when compared to those who are breastfed. Whether or not this is positive or negative in the longterm perspectives is impossible to say.

Table 4. Casein, calcium and phosphorous content in human and bovine milk

	Human milk	Cow's milk
Casein (g/L)	0.3	2.8
%of total prot	35	80
Calcium (mg/L)	340	1200
Phosphorous (mg/L)	140	950
Ca/P ratio	2.1-2.4	1.2-1.3

3. NUTRITIONAL VERSUS PHYSIOLOGICAL ROLES OF MILK PROTEINS

It could be said that the milk proteins have three roles to play:

(1) As a source of essential amino acids and nitrogen for protein synthesis;

(2) As a source of protein for specific physiological

functions, i.e. defence against microbial infections;

(3) As growth factors and modulators (essentially low-molecular proteins occurring in minor amounts).

Some of the proteins are considered to exert specific physiological roles and will withstand hydrolysis in the gastro-intestinal tract. This is especially valid with respect to human milk where proteins such as secretory IgA, lactoferrin and lysozyme are examples. They all constitute a considerable amount of the whey protein fraction, which is the dominating one in human milk. Thus the macronutrient aspects of milk protein must take into account the potential and specific physiological role of certain protein fractions. If specific proteins should exert their specific physiological role only if they are not digested and absorbed in the gastrointestinal tract, they should not be included in calculations of nutritionally available proteins in milk, i.e. as sources of amino acids for future protein synthesis. The practical implication of this is illustrated in the case of human milk, which may have a content of nutritionally available protein as low as 0.5 to 0.6 g per 100 ml constituting only 4% of less of the total energy content (Hambræus et al, 1984; Woelderen, 1987).

This statement has at least two dimensions:

1. A protein determination based only on nitrogen analysis might be greatly misleading when the nutritive value of various milk proteins is analyzed without compensation for proteins of specific physiological importance, which are not digested in the gastrointestinal tract.

2. All data regarding protein requirement in man during neonatal period may be overestimates since they are based on the assumption that human milk contains 1.1-1.2 g per 100 ml instead of 0.8-0.9 or even in the latter case 0.5-0.6. This in its turn will have an impact on the evaluation of the need for high valued protein in feeding the human being.

3.1 Specific characteristics of milk protein which may have an nutritional impact

Although obviously the protein intake quantitatively may represent a problem as it is so low in breast milk, much nutritional aspects on milk components from the protein point of view might also have to be related to the specific proteins.

The caseins represent the few naturally-occurring phosphoproteins which have a high content of ester-bound phosphate, a high proline content as well as a low content of cystine. There are also obvious differences in the composition of the casein moiety between bovine milk and human milk not only with regard to absolute amounts where the casein content in human milk is very low, but also that human casein is dominated by beta-casein while alfa-casein dominates in bovine milk. Furthermore human casein has a lower phosphorous content than bovine casein which might indicate that the phosphorous requirement is not as high as in other mammals. Although the primary nutritional role of casein is still not completely understood it might be to provide amino acids and calcium and inorganic phosphate. The curd formation has also been suggested to be of importance for the function of the digestive tract.

Among the physiologically functioning whey proteins lactoferrin, secretory IgA and alfa-lactalbumin are the dominating ones. In addition there are a number of proteins in minor amounts which also have significant physiological functions as transport proteins by binding vitamins or hormones, or comprise enzymatic functions, i.e. lysozyme.

Among the enzymes the peroxidase system is of interest in the defence against gastrointestinal infections. This can also be produced in larger amounts also from bovine milk and may thus constitute an interesting approach to future development of functional food items from dairy products. Lysozyme is another enzyme of great interest from human nutrition point of view due to its bactericidal effect. It does however not occur in such notable amounts in bovine milk that it is possible to isolate and concentrate in special preparations so far.

The role of lipases in human milk as well as bovine milk is of special interest and may not only be involved in the lipolysis of milk fat but also on bacterial lipids.

3.2 Lactoferrin - a functional protein of specific interest

Throughout the last years much interest has been devoted to the iron-binding protein in milk, lactoferrin. Although it is the dominating iron-binding protein in milk, lactoferrin is also produced in other fluids, such as tears, saliva and pancreatic juice. Human milk, however, is extremely rich in lactoferrin. Since lactoferrin also occurs in bovine milk, although in much less concentration, modern food technology has made it possible to isolate and concentrate lactoferrin making it available for pharmacological and other purposes.

The role of lactoferrin which originally was considered to be essentially an antimicrobial one, has throughout the years turned out to far more multifacetted and can be summarized under the following major headings:

(1) Antimicrobial effect;

(2) Nutritional aspects (bioavailability of iron, source of protein);

(3) Mitogenic and trophic activities on the intestinal mucosa.

With regard to the antimicrobial effect this has been proposed to be related to the binding capacity of lactoferrin to iron making it unavailable for the microorganisms. This has also been demonstrated in vitro although there is much less information regarding the bacteriostatic effect in vivo. Of specific interest from the comparative point of view is the fact that there seems to be a species specificity of lactoferrin which might indicate that the biological function is species specific. Of special interest is on the other hand the fashinating studies by the scientists at Morinaga Milk company (Hutchens et al, 1992) who recently described the bactericidal peptides, called lactoferricins, derived from N-terminal regions from bovine and human lactoferrin. This antimicrobial peptide is a 23 amino acid long strongly basic peptide. This opens up the possibilities to only use certain peptide fractions of the molecule for certain purposes.

Lactoferrin is a good example of the fact that if it exerts a specific physiological function it requires that it is kept intact more or less throughout the gastrointestinal tract. Thus its nutritional role as source of amino acids has to be questionned. The same is relevant for other whey proteins occurring in milk, i.e. secretory IgA and lysozyme and certain studies indicate that they in fact are identified more or less unaffected in the faeces.

Another funtion of lactoferrin is its role for the bioavailability of iron in milk. The extremely high bioavailability reported of iron in human milk (Saarinen et al, 1977) has been assumed to be due to the role of lactoferrin. Interesting recent studies illustrate the role of lactoferrin as a transporter and that there should be special lactoferrin receptors in the gut mucosa (Hutchens et al, 1992). Once more we are facing a practical problem of relevance when comparing various milks, as it seems as these receptors are rather species specific. Consequently bovine lactoferrin might not have the same beneficial effects as those characterising human lactoferrin.

Table 5. Fatty acid profile in bovine and human milk
(Ref. Gurr, 1981, Renner 1983)

	g/100 g total fatty acids	
	bovine	human
Saturated		
4:0	3.2	trace
6:0	2.0	< 0.1
8:0	1,2	< 0.1
10:0	2.8	1.5
12:0	3.5	6.7
14:0	11.2	7.7
16:0	26.0	21.8
18:0	11.2	7.4
20:0	0.2	0.2
	61.1	
Monounsaturated		
14:1	1.4	
16:1	2.7	3.2
18:1	27.8	33.5
	31.9	
Polyunsaturated		
18:2	1.4	10.2
18:2	1.5	
18:3		0.8
20.4	trace	0.3
	2.9	

Interestingly a growth modulator effect has also been discussed with regard to lactoferrin during the last years as well as a positive effect in the defence against free radicals (Hutchens et al, 1992).

4. FATTY ACIDS IN MILK

Lipids constitute about 3-5% of milk and 98% are triacylglycerols, thereby constituting 50-60% of the energy. In addition to providing essential fatty acids, precursors of prostaglandins, fat soluble vitamins sterols and phospholipids also the fatty acid composition is of great interest. Only 8-10 fatty acids constitute more than 1% each.

The mammary glands seem to be capable to synthesize saturated fatty acids essentially of 10-14 carbons in length, while increased carbohydrate intake seems to favour synthesis of medium chain triglycerides (MCT) in monogastric animals. Human milk contains a substantial amount of unsaturated fatty acids, i-e., oleic acid and linoleic acid, while the concentration of saturated fatty acids is low. This is in contrast to bovine milk where 62 % are saturated fatty acids. A relatively high proportion represent short chain (C4-C6) or medium chain (C8-C12) fatty acids. Monounsaturated constitute about 30% while polyunsaturated are less than 3%.

Interestingly the fat content seems to be influenced by the mothers diet and a marked elevation in the MCT fatty acids is reported to occur on a low-fat diet. The linoleic acid content is furthermore reported to show the most pronounced variation with maternal diet being extremely high in vegetarians and vegans. However this is in man and, may be, monogastric animals system.

During the last years interest has been devoted to changing the fatty acid composition by means of changes in the feeding. However efforts to increase the content of polyunsaturated fatty acids in cow's milk limits the storage life because of oxidative breakdown of unsaturated fatty acids leading to rancidity and taste problems. The essential reason for the very clear difference in fatty acid composition between human and bovine milk is probably due to the effect of microorganisms in the rumen which hydrogenate the polyunsaturated fatty acids in the cow's diet. The type of feed influences the pattern of fermentation of carbohydrates and proteins in the rumen and will result in changes in the proportions of fatty acids. Thus high fibre diets favour the production of short chain fatty acids, i.e. acetic acid, propionic acid and butyric acid.

The cholesterol content in milk has been a matter of great concern, and the physiological impact of the relatively high content of cholesterol and saturated fat in milk is still not fully understood.

Of special interest is also the fat globule membrane which not only stabilized the fat emulsion but also contains a number of interesting components, i.e. phospholipids, cholesterol, proteins, enzymes and various minerals.

Among the lipids should also carnitin be mentioned which plays an important role in energy metabolism in the neonate. Carnitin is requested for the transport of long-chain fatty acids for beta-oxidation in the mitochondria and reaches its maximum in human milk at 2 weeks of age.

5. VITAMINS IN MILK

There are considerable differences in the content of vitamins between human and bovine milk.

Table 6. Fat-soluble vitamins in human and bovine milk (Souci et al 1979)

	Human milk	Bovine milk
Vitamin A	54	30
Carotene	24	18
Vitamin D	0.05	0.06
Vitamin E	520	88
Vitamin K	3.4	17

With regard to fat soluble vitamins this is illustrated in table 6. It is seen that the main difference might be the higher content of vitamin E which might be due to but also needed due to the higher content of polyunsaturated fatty acids in human milk. The vitamin K content on the other hand is to the advantage of bovine milk. However, if we leave the specific aspects of the newborn infants which may call for the beneficial effect of vitamin K this is of very limited value in the adult when there is a normal intestinal flora. Consequently from the nutritional point of view the vitamin E-content might be of greatest interest.

With respect to the water-soluble vitamins the situation is somewhat different.

Most of the water-soluble vitamins are present in smaller amounts in human milk than in bovine milk, vitamin C and niacin however being exceptions. With respect to the bioavailability there is also the interesting situation that there are special binding proteins which may be of importance.

To what extent we can read anything of interest from the analyses of the content of various vitamins in various milk specimens for the physiological needs and function is still open for discussions and calls for more research.

Table 7. Water-soluble vitamins in human and bovine milk (Souci et al, 1979)

	Human milk	Bovine milk
Thiamin	15	37
Riboflavin	38	180
Pyridoxine	13	46
Cobalamine	0.05	0.42
Niacin	170	90
Folic acid	0.19	0.3-7
Pantothenic acid	210	350
Ascorbic acid	4400	1700
Biotin	0.58	3.5

Table 8. Mineral and trace elements in human and cow's milk

	Human milk	Cow's milk
Minerals (mg)		
Calcium	30	120
Magnesium	4	12
Sodium	15	45
Potassium	51	150
Chloride	41	106
Phosphorous	14	94
Sulphur	14	33
Trace elements (microg)		
Copper	42	11
Iron	74	60
Zinc	251	337
Selenium	2	3
Chromium	4	2
Cobalt	1	0.08
Manganese	3	5
Molybdenum	0.2	5.5
Iodine	20	8

(Ref Renner 1983)

6. MINERALS AND TRACE ELEMENTS

The mineral distribution in human milk and cow's milk is shown in table 8.

As seen human milk contains about 4 times less mineral salts than cow's milk which is essentially indicated by the differences in calcium, phosphorous, sodium and potassium content. With respect to trace elements this difference is less pronounced. Furthermore it should be noted that there are often substantial variations observed or reported regarding trace element content in various samples, possible partly due to methodological problems in collecting representative samples as well as analytical problems.

In addition to the absolute amounts also the bioavailability of the minerals and trace elements is of interest. This is especially notified regarding iron where lactoferrin may play en important role, which has been commented upon earlier. Also zinc seems to represent a special problem and it is not the zinc content per se but its bioavailability that is of interest. Thus diseases such as acrodermatitis enteropathica which is said to be due to zinc deficiency is not reported in breastfed infants but may arise after weaning. Interestingly mineral fractions are not only available in the water but

Table 9. Dairy products versus meat products as sources of minerals and trace elements in a Scandinavian diet (the figures refer to % of total intake)

Milk > meat		Meat > milk		Milk = Meat	
Ca	80 - 1	Fe	6 - 26	Zn	31 - 31
Ph	49 - 14	Cu	10 - 18	Al	13 - 10
Rb	39 - 14	Se	22 - 31	Cd	12 - 9
Mo	36 - 12			Hg	9 - 7
S	31 - 23			Si	7 - 6
K	31 - 11			As	5 - 3
Br	26 - 5			Ni	3 - 1
Mg	25 - 7			Mn	2 - 0,5
F	20 - 3				
Pg	18 - 7				
Co	11 - 4				
B	8 - 1				

often whey fraction but often bound to casein and/or the fat globule membrane.

Milk products have often been said to be deficient in minerals and trace elements when compared to meat products. This is not completely true as indicated in table 9. It is quite obvious that the iron content in milk is low, although this might be compensated for to some extent by its bioavailability. It is of course an open question whether this is a mere mistake by Nature or if there are any physiological advantages "hidden". The role of iron as enhancer of free radical formation have started a discussion whether the low iron content is physiologically desirable under certain circumstances.

With respect to a number of other trace elements it is obvious that milk and consequently dairy products are by no means much inferior to other products from the animal kingdom as indicatewd in table 9.

7. POTENTIAL HAZARDS WITH MILK

The nutritional aspects on various milk species is not only a question of the content of certain nutrients but also the presence of components which may represent potential hazards. Such examples are chemical contaminants, milkborn infections, naturally occurring toxicants, allergenic reactions and cardiovascular disease.

Since the potentially toxic chemical pollutants are concentrated in the food chain and subsequently stored in adipose tissue, as most of them are fat soluble, the chemical contamination of human milk is of great concern for at least two reasons. Firstly, there is a longer storage time in the human than in the cow, Secondly the relative milk production is higher in the dairy cow. This often leads to the fact that there is generally 5-10 times higher concentrations of pesticides in human milk when compared to that in cow's milk. Since the chemical pollutants are stored in maternal adipose tisue they will be mobilized when there is an increased breakdown of adipose tissue during energy deficit.

Milkborn infections on the other hand is a problem of formula-fed infants and the use of bovine milk and is essentially related to the hygienic situation in the food production and handling.

The milk intolerance problems may be related to reduced metabolic capacity to deal with certain components, e.g. lactose intolerance, or allergenic reactions to milk proteins. This could of course be dealt with by either using milk from animals producing low-lactose milk, i.e. milk from marine animals, or, which seems more realistic, by technologically reducing the lactose content in the dairy industry. The possibility to reduce the content of certain protein fractions, which are not occurring in human milk and may be potentially causing milk protein intolerance, i.e. beta-lactoglobulin, is of course also theoretically possible by means of modern biochemical techniques but probably a limited economic reality. Finally the discussion on diet-health relation with respect to saturated fatty acids has lead to the fact that dairy products due to their content of saturated fatty acids have been criticized. The potentials to manipulate the fatty acid pattern of dairy products by changes in the feed to dairy cows may be one way to overcome this problem.

In conclusion there are a lot of interesting differences both at the macro- and microlevel regarding composition of milk and we are still far from understanding the physiological backgrund for all these differences.

REFERENCES

Andersson, J.J.B. 1990. Dietary calcium and bone mass through the lifecycle. Nutrition today 9-14.

Atkinson, S.A., Andersson, G.H. & Bryan, M.H. 1981. Energy and macronutrient content of human milk during early lactation for mothers giving birth prematurely and at term. Am. J. Clin. Nutr. 34: 258-265.

Blanc, B. 1981. Biochemical aspects of human milk - comparison with bovine milk. Wld. Rev. Nutr. Diet.36: 1-89.

Gaull, G.E., Jensen, R.G., Rassin, D.K. & Malloy, M.H. 1982. Human milk as food. Adv. Perinatal. Med. 2: 47-120.

Hambræus, L. 1977. Proprietary milk versus human breast milk in infant feeding. A critical appraisal from the nutritional point of view. Ped. Clin. N. Am. 24: 17-36.

Hambræus, L. 1990. Human Milk: nutritional aspects. In O. Brunser, F., Carrazza, M. Gracey, B. Nichols & J. Senterre (eds.) Clinical Nutrition in the Young Child: 289-301. Nestec Ltd Vevey/Raven Press Ltd, New York.

Hambræus, L. 1992. Nutritional aspects of milk proteins. In P.F. Fox (ed) Advanced Dairy Chemistry 1: Proteins: 457-490. Elsevier Appl Sc, London.

Hambræus, L., Fransson, G.B. & Lönnerdal, B. 1984. Nutritional availability of breast milk protein. Lancet ii: 167-168.

Hutchens, T.W., Lönnerdal, B. & Rumball, S. (eds) 1992. Lactoferrin structure and function. Proc First Int Symp. Honolulu, Hawaii (in print)

Jenness, R. & Sloan, R.E. 1970. The composition of milk of various species: a review. Dairy Sci. Abstr. 32: 599-612.

Jenness, R. 1974. The composition of milk. In B. Larson & V.R. Smith (eds.), Lactation - A comprehensive treatise. Vol. 3: 3-105. Academic Press, New York.

Lönnerdal, B. 1985. Biochemistry and physiologi cal function of human milk proteins. Am. J. Clin. Nutr. 42: 1299-1317.

Oftedahl, O. 1980. In E.R. Maschgan, M.E. Allen, & L.E. Fischer (eds.) The Nutrition of captive wild animals: 67-83. First Annual Dr Scholl Nutrition Conference.

Renner, E. 1983. Milk and dairy products in human nutrition. W-GmbH, Volkswirthschaft licher Verlag, München.

Saarinen, U.M., Siimes, M.A. & Dallman, P.R. 1977. Iron absorption in infants: High bioavaila bility from human milk, simulated human milk and proprietary formulas. Pediatrics 60: 896-900.

Souci, S.Ww & Bosch, H. 1978. Lebensmittel-Tabellen für die Nährungswertberechnung 2 edt. Stuttgart. Wiss. Verl Ges.

Widdowson, E.M. 1984. Lactation and feeding
  patterns in different species. In Freed, D.L.J.
  (ed.) Health hazards of milk: 85-90. Baillière
  Tindall, W B Saunders Eastbourne, England
  1984.

Woelderen, B.F. van 1987. Changing insight into
  milk proteins: some implications. Nutr. Abstr.
  Rev. (ser A) 57: 129-134.

Dairy Products in Human Health and Nutrition, Serrano Ríos et al. (eds) © 1994 Balkema, Rotterdam, ISBN 90 5410 359 0

The milk gland as bioreactor for therapeutic and nutritional proteins

L. Hennighausen
Laboratory of Biochemistry and Metabolism, National Institutes of Health, Bethesda, Md., USA & Department of Molecular Cell Biology, Max-Planck-Institute of Biophysical Chemistry, Göttingen, Germany

ABSTRACT: It is possible to convert milk glands of transgenic animals into bioreactors, and produce human pharmaceuticals and proteins of nutrional value. Since the advent of transgenic mice in 1987 which secreted human tissue plasminogen activator (tPA) into their milk, the field of mammary transgenic biotechnology has expanded rapidly. Human pharmaceuticals such as α1-antitrypsin, tPA and protein C are being produced in large quantities in the milk of sheep, goat and swine, respectively. Once an animal is established which secretes large amounts of a pharmaceutical protein, high volumes of the product can be purified at reasonable costs.

Our information base on gene expression in the mammary gland is small, and no firm rules exist about vector design. In particular, juxtaposition of sequences in hybrid genes can lead to novel regulatory elements altering expression patterns. In addition there is evidence to suggest that the mode of gene activation in the mammary gland may differ between species. To predictably engineer the milk gland, we will need a thorough understanding of its physiology. Studies with transgenic animals have located mammary specific and hormone inducible transcription elements in the promoter/upstream regions of milk protein genes. However, it appears that in addition to individual promoter based transcription elements structural features of milk protein chromosomal loci may contribute to their tight regulation.

Here I will describe progress in the field of mammary biotechnology and present approaches which may cut lead time and costs of generating transgenic livestock. Given the speed with which molecular 'pharming' technology is being developed, barnyard biotechnology should soon find its place along side of conventional technologies for pharmaceutical production.

SUCCESS STORIES

The development of molecular 'pharming' included the generation of transgenic animals whose mammary glands produced human proteins. This was achieved with combined efforts by molecular biologists, embryologists and protein chemists. In particular, molecular biology provided the expertise for the isolation of genetic regulatory elements that target gene expression to mammary tissue, and embryology was critical for the generation of transgenic animals.

The introduction of cloning technologies in the early eighties facilitated the cloning of cDNAs from several milk proteins (Hobbs et al 1982; Hennighausen and Sippel 1982b). In addition to sequences for known caseins and whey proteins, novel proteins, such as the whey acidic protein (WAP), were identified (Hennighausen and Sippel 1982a). Using milk protein cDNAs as probes, genomic clones for WAP, α-lactalbumin and several caseins were isolated and extensively characterized (for review see Hennighausen 1992). Transgenic technologies established in the early eighties led to the introduction of a foreign gene into the germline of transgenic animals, and by that means a modified

physiology of the host (Palmiter et al 1982). However, only 1987 researchers could show that regulatory elements from the mouse WAP gene directed production of human proteins to mammary tissue of transgenic animals (Andres et al 1987). In the same year, a joint research venture between groups at the National Institutes of Health in Bethesda, and Integrated Genetics in Framingham, demonstrated that lactating transgenic mice carrying a human gene for tissue plasminogen activator (tPA) could secrete the active human protein into their milk (Gordon et al 1987). Also in the same year researchers at the AFRC in Edinburgh demonstrated that mammary regulatory elements could function across species boundaries (Simons et al 1987). The same group demonstrated the feasibility of producing human proteins in sheep milk (Clark et al 1989). In 1991, collaborative research between the NIH and the USDA demonstrated that gram quantities of a foreign protein could be produced in transgenic swine (Wall et al 1991). Researchers from Pharmaceutical Proteins Limited and the AFRC in Edinburgh generated transgenic sheep that produced gram quantities of human α1-antitrypsin in their milk (Wright et al 1991). Scientists from Tufts

University and Genzyme showed production of human tPA in goat milk (Ebert et al 1991; Denman et al 1991), while work from Genpharming in Leiden resulted in transgenic cows carrying a human lactoferrin gene under the control of a casein promoter (Krimpenfort et al 1991). Transgenic pigs generated in a joint effort by researchers from the American Red Cross and Virginia PolyTech secreted gram quantities of human ProteinC into their milk (Velander et al., 1992). Although all of this work is considered a major progress, problems occurring in the transgenic system have been reported. Aberrant expression of the mouse whey acidic protein (WAP) in pigs, which do not carry an obvious homologous gene, could interfere with mammary development and abrogate mammary function (Burdon et al 1991b; Shamay et al 1992b). In addition to the transgenic system, gene transfer systems have been developed that allow the introduction of DNA into mammary epithelium of pregnant and lactating animals in vivo and in vitro (Furth et al 1992).

ADVANTAGES OF THE MAMMARY BIOREACTOR

Although it possible to produce human proteins on a large scale in manipulated microorganisms, there are limitations to these systems since many proteins require extensive post-translational modification. Factor IX is a good example in that this essential component for blood coagulation is normally synthesized in liver and undergoes extensive posttranslational modifications that include glycosylation, β-hydroxylation and vitamin K-dependent γ-carboxylation (Di Scipio et al 1978). In contrast to microorganisms, mammalian tissue culture cells contain the enzymatic machinery for these types of modifications of proteins. Since it is both technically challenging and expensive to grow many cell types in tissue culture on a large enough scale to produce high yields of protein, current efforts are being directed toward alternative measures. One such system may be the mammary gland bioreactor. During lactation the mammary gland synthesizes large amounts of protein which is secreted into the milk in concentrations betwee 40 and 60 grams per liter. By targeting the expression of foreign genes to the mammary gland in transgenic animals it may be possible to produce human proteins on this scale in milk. This translates to about 20 kg or 100 kg for a goat or cow, respectively, per year. Although the expense of generating transgenic livestock are high, husbandary is relatively cheap and only low-tech facilities are needed. These assets of of transgenic technology can be contrasted to expensive fermenters for cells in culture and the cost of growth media for fastidious cell lines.

Production of high value human pharmaceuticals is not the only service of the mammary bioreactor. It should also be possible to produce food additives, such as human lactoferrin, to supplement infant formula.

Other long term goals are the generation of cows with an increased casein content in milk. Those aspects are under development by academic and industrial organizations.

MILK PROTEIN GENES

Several milk protein genes from a number of species have been isolated (for review see Hennighausen 1992). These include genes for α-lactalbumin, the whey acidic protein (WAP), β-lactoglobulin, β-casein, and α-casein. The mammary specificity of these genes is conveyed by promoter upstream sequences as shown in transgenic studies. Although many milk proteins are shared between species, some proteins are unique to the milk of certain species. WAP, for example, has only been found in mice, rats, rabbits and camels, and β-lactoglobulin is absent from mice, rats and camels. However, mammary regulatory elements have been conserved during evolution and between different species as shown by the expression of the mouse WAP gene in transgenic pigs (Wall et al 1991) and sheep which do not contain an obvious homologous WAP gene.

Developmental and hormonal regulation between milk protein genes can vary sharply (Hobbs et al 1982). For example, accumulation of WAP (Pittius et al 1988) RNA occurs just prior to parturition, but high levels of β-casein mRNA are detected in early pregnancy (Harris et al 1991; Hennighausen et al 1988; Shamay et al 1992a). Differences in regulation could be caused by a differential access of chromatin to individual signaling pathways. This hypothesis was supported by transgenic studies with the WAP gene in mice (Burdon et al 1991a and b; Pittius et al 1988) and pigs (Shamay et al 1992a). Developmental and hormonal regulation patterns seen with WAP transgenes differed dramatically with the integration site (Shamay et al 1992a). This suggests that chromatin features, such as matrix attachment regions (MAR), may be necessary for accurate regulation (McKnight et al 1992).

THE STEP FROM MICE TO FARM ANIMALS

Transgenic mice which produce human pharmaceuticals in their mammary glands and secrete the protein into milk have been established (Hennighausen 1990). However, the conclusions obtained with these model systems may not be transferable to farm animals. This has cleary been shown by extensive studies that have been conducted with the mouse WAP gene in transgenic mice, pigs and sheep. Whereas mice contain a WAP gene, pigs and sheep do not contain a recognizable WAP gene. Expression of the mouse WAP transgene in all three species was tightly restricted to the mammary gland, suggesting that the molecular basis of mammary-specific gene expression is conserved between species. Since pigs and sheep probably do not carry an endogenous WAP or related gene, it is likely that milk gene regulation is also conserved between different milk protein genes. Interestingly, the frequency of expressors and expression levels between these species varied dramatically. While only about 50% of the transgenic mice express integrated WAP transgenes, high levels of expression were found in all transgenic pigs and sheep. Similarly, expression levels of a hybrid gene containing WAP regulatory elements and human proteinC sequences were dramatically higher in pigs than in mice (Velander et al 1992). Regualtory conservation was also observed with the sheep β-lactoglobulin gene. Although mice do not carry this gene, a transgene was expressed at high levels in mice (Simons et al 1987). It is not known whether the increased expression levels observed in heterologous species will be a general phenomena.

DESIGNER GENES

Promoter/upstream sequences from the WAP, α-casein, α-lactalbumin, β-lactoglobulin, and the β-casein gene have been used to direct the synthesis of foreign proteins to mammary tissue of transgenic mice, rabbits, sheep and pigs (for references see Wilmut et al 1991; Ebert et al 1991; Wright et al 1991; Hennighausen, 1990 and 1992). In general, genomic clones appear to be expressed at higher levels than cDNAs. Whereas expression of cDNA sequences encoding non-milk proteins under the control of milk protein gene specific regulatory elements has been overall poor, genomic sequences linked to milk protein promoter elements showed greatly improved expression levels (Archibald et al., 1990). Increased activity of intron containing transgenes may be the result of splicing (Brinster et al 1988; Palmiter et al 1991; Choi et al 1991), or to the presence of regulatory elements located in specific introns. The particular reporter gene used can also influence expression levels and expression of recombinant genes can greatly vary between different species.

In many cases transgenes are not expressed because they are subject to position effects imposed by the site of integration. Matrix attachment regions (MARs) are sequences which help to functionally separate genes from surrounding chromatin/regulatory regions, possibly by anchoring genetic domains to the nuclear matrix (Bonifer et al 1991). When WAP transgenes were coinjected with MAR elements, accurate expression was found in almost all lines suggesting that such 'insulator' sequences may be helpful in obtaining more expressing transgenic lines for any given transgene McKnight et al 1991). Since DNA fragments coinjected into fertilized oozytes will in many cases integrate into the same transgene locus (Burdon et al 1991a; Overbeek et al 1991; McKnight et al 1992), this strategy should allow the generation of transgenic animals that carry several different hybrid genes and therefore secrete several different proteins into their milk.

FUTURE DEVELOPMENTS

Additional developments should speed up integration of the mammary bioreactor into the industrial complex. It is conceivable that the availability of elements that build genetic chromatin domains will help to reliably generate 'expressing' transgenic animals. In addition, in vivo gene transfer systems will be used as screenng systems to rapidly evaluate the functionality of hybrid genes.

Overall, expression of a given transgene is seen in about 50% of transgenic lines, and expression is highly variable and position dependent. Moreover, expression levels between animals from a defined genetic line may vary considerably. It is now possible to shield transgenes from integration site dependent position effects using chromatin domain organizers. This should permit the reproducible establishment of transgenic lines which reliably produce proteins at high levels. Matrix attachment regions (MARs) and locus control regions (LCRs) are experimental systems which may help us to consistently express transgenes at high levels. MARs may define genetic units, and their presence 'cross-talk' of genetic regulatory units in neighboring chromatin domains (Bonifer et al 1991). Without MAR sequences, expression and regulation of mammary directed transgenes was highly position dependent, but more reliable expression patterns were observed in the presence of MARs from the chicken lysozyme locus (McKnight et al 1992). Whereas MARs appear to be to shield genetic domains, locus control regions (LCR) are cis-acting enhancers, that confer position independent expression to genes in transgenic loci (Grosveld et al 1987). The introduction MAR or LCR like sequences into genetic vectors systems may be necessary to reach the biotechnological goal. However, it is probably not necessary to integrate such elements into expression vectors, because the cointegration of MARs with hybrid genes can be achieved through coinjection into the zygotes (McKnight et al 1992). The introduction of MAR sequences into transgenic loci may facilitate appropriate transgene regulation (McKnight et al 1992) which is of particular importance in the light of potential cytotoxic effects caused by some proteins. For example, precocious expression of WAP in both transgenic mice (Burdon et al 1991b) and swine (Shamay et al 1992b) resulted in impaired mammary development. From a pragmatic point of view, significant benefits maybe realized by including either homologous or heterologous MARs with transgene constructs in transgenic livestock. The proportion of transgenic large animals that express their transgene is approximately 60%. Given that the cost of producing transgenic sheep and pigs is in the tens of thousands of dollars, and production of transgenic cattle may be an order of magnitude higher, the use of MARs could substantially reduce transgenic animal production costs.

Most mammary transgenes analyzed to date yielded suboptimal expression levels, suggesting that important genetic control elements, such as transcription factor binding sites, RNA processing or mRNA stabilization signals were not present in the hybrid gene. Since the evaluation of hybrid genes encoding valuable proteins in transgenic mice is time consuming, expensive, and in the light that the results may not be transferable to farm animal species under consideration, it is necessary to devise fast and reliable assay systems. The physical introduction of DNA into mammary epithelial cells of living animals represents such a screening method (Furth et al 1992). Jet injection into mammary tissue appears to be a rather efficient and non-toxic means to evaluate the quality of hybrid genes. Therefore this technology allows the analysis of mammary vector systems in the context of the dairy animal species which has been chosen for the production of particular proteins. This technology should also facilitate the introduction of DNA into mammary epithelial stem cells, and thus should result in somatic transgenic cows. Bypassing the germline would speed up the introduction of the mammary bioreactor by several years.

References

Andres A-C, Schönenberger C-A, Groner B, Hennighausen L, LeMeur M, Gerlinger P 1987 Ha-ras oncogene expression directed by a milk protein gene promoter: tissue specificity, hormonal regulation, and tumor induction in transgenic mice. Proc. Natl. Sci. U.S.A. 84,1299-1303.

Archibald AL, McClenaghan M, Hornsey V, Simons JP, Clark AJ 1990 High-level expression of biologically active human α_1-antitrypsin in the milk of transgenic mice. Proc. Natl. Acad. Sci. 87, 5178-5182.

Bonifer, C., Hecht, A., Saueressig, H., Winter, D.M. and Sippel, A.E. (1991) Dynamic Chromatin: The regulatory domain organization of eukaryotic gene loci. J. Cell. Biochem. 47, 99-108.

Brinster, R.L., Allen, J.M., Behringer, R.R., Gelinas, R.E. and Palmiter, R.D. (1988) Introns increase transcriptional efficiency in transgenic mice. Proc. Natl. Acad. Sci. U.S.A. 85, 836-840.

Burdon, T., Sankaran, L., Wall, R.J., Spencer, M., and Hennighausen, L. (1991a) Expression of a whey acidic protein transgene during mammary development: Evidence for different mechanisms of regulation during pregnancy and lactation. J. Biol. Chem. 266, 6909-6914.

Burdon, T., Wall, R.J., Shamay, A., Smith, G.H. and Hennighausen, L. (1991b) Overexpression of an endogeous milk protein gene in transgenic mice is associated with impaired mammary development and a milchlos phenotype. Mech. of Dev. 36, 67-74.

Choi, T., Huang, M., Gorman, C., and Jaenisch, R. (1991) A generic intron increases gene expression in trangenic mice. Mol. and Cell Biol.11, 3070-3074

Clark, A.J., Bessos, H., Bishop, J.O., Brown, P., Harris, S., Lathe, R., McClenaghan, M., Prowse, C., Simons, J.P., Whitelaw, C.B.A., and Wilmut, I. (1989) Expression of human anti-hemophilic factor IX in the milk of transgenic sheep. Bio/technology 7, 487-492.

Denman, J., Hayes, M., O'Day, C., Edmunds, T., Barlett, C., Hirani, S., Ebert, K.M., Gordon, K., McPherson, J.M. (1991) Transgenic expression of a variant of human tissue-type plasminogen activator in goat milk: purification and characterization of the recombinant enzyme. Bio/Technology 9: 839-843.

Ebert, K.M., Selgrath, J.P., DiTullio, P., Denman, J., Smith, T.E., Memon, M.A., Schindler, J.E., Monastersky, G.M., Vitale, J.A., and Gordon, K. (1991) Transgenic production of a variant of human tissue-type plasminogen activator in goat milk: Generation of transgenic goats and analysis of expression. Biotechnology 9, 835-838.

Furth, P.A., Shamay, A., Wall, R.J., Hennighausen, L. (1992) Gene transfer into somatic tissues by jet injection. Anal. Biochem. 205, 365-368.

Gordon, K., Lee, E., Vitale, J.A., Smith, A.E., Westphal, H. and Hennighausen, L. (1987) Production of human tissue plasminogen activator in mouse milk Bio/technology 5, 1183-1187.

Grosveld, F., van Assendelft, B.G., Greaves, D.R., and Kollias, G. (1987) Position-independent, high level expression of the human β-globin gene in transgenic mice. Cell 51, 975-985.

Hennighausen, L. (1990) The mammary gland as a bioreactor: Production of foreign proteins in milk. Protein Expression and Purification 1, 3-8.

Hennighausen, L., Westphal, C., Sankaran, L., and Pittius, C.W. (1988). Regulation of expression of milk protein genes. In First and Haseltine (eds.), Transgenic Technology in Medicine and Agriculture, Butterworth, 61-70.

Hennighausen, L.G. and Sippel, A.E. (1982) Characterization and cloning of the mRNAs specific for the lactating mouse mammary gland. Eur. J. Biochem. 125, 131-141.

Hennighausen, L.G. and Sippel, A.E. (1982) The mouse whey acidic protein is a novel member of the family of 'four-disulfide core' proteins. Nucleic Acids Res. 10, 2677- 2684.

Hobbs, A.A., Richards, D.A., Kessler, D.J. and Rosen, J.M. (1982) Complex hormonal regulation of rat casein gene expression. J. Biol. Chem. 257, 3598-3605.

Krimpenfort, P., Rademakers, A., Eyestone, W., van der Schans, A., van den Broek, S., Kooiman, P., Kootwijk, E., Platenburg, G., pieper, F., Srijker, R. and de Boer, H. (1991) Generation of transgenic dairy cattle using 'in vitro' embryo production. Bio/Technology **9**, 844-847.

McKnight, R.A., Shamay, A., Sankaran, L., Wall, R.J. and Hennighausen, L. (1992) Matrix attachment regions impart position independent regulation of a tissue specific gene in transgenic mice. Proc. Natl. Acad. Sci. U.S.A. **89**, 6943-6947.

Overbeek, P.A., Aguilar-Cordova, E., Hanten, G., Schaffner, D.L., Patel, P., Lebovitz, R.M., Lieberman, M.W. (1991) Coinjection strategy for visual identification of transgenic mice. Transgenic Res. **1**, 31-37.

Palmiter, R., Sandren, E., Avarbock, M., Allen, D., Brinster, R. (1991) Heterologous introns can enhance expression of transgenes in mice. Proc. Natl. Acad. Sci. **88**, 478-482.

Palmiter RD, Brinster RL, Hammer RE, Trumbauer ME, Rosenfeld MG, Birnberg NC, Evans RM (1982) Dramatic growth of mice that develop from eggs microinjected with metallothionein-growth hormone fusion genes. Nature **300**, 611-615.

Pittius, C.W., Sankaran, S., Topper, Y. and Hennighausen, L. (1988) Comparison of the regulation of the whey acidic protein gene to a hybrid gene containing the whey acidic protein gene promoter in transgenic mice. Mol. Endocrinol. **2**, 1027-1032.

Shamay, A., Pursel, V., Wall, R., and Hennighausen, L. (1992a) Induction of lactogenesis in transgenic virgin pigs: evidence for gene and integration site-specific hormonal regulation. Molecular Endo. in press.

Shamay, A., Pursel, V.G., Wilkinson, E., Wall, R.J. and Hennighausen, L. (1992b) Expression of the mouse whey acidic protein gene in transgenic pigs is associated with agalactia and deregulated gene expression. Transgenic Research, in press.

Shamay, A., Pursel, V.G., McKnight, R.A., Alexander, L., Beattie, C., Hennighausen, L., and Wall, R.J. (1991) Production of the mouse whey acidic protein in transgenic pigs during lactation. Journal of Animal Science, **69**, 4552-5562.

Simons, J.P., McClenaghan, M., and Clark, A.J. (1987) Alteration of the quality of milk by expression of sheep β-lactoglobulin in transgenic mice. Nature **328**, 530-532.

Velander, W.H. (1992a) Production of biologically active human protein C in the milk of transgenic mice. Biochemical Engineering VII, in press.

Velander, W.H., Johnson, J.L., Page, R. L., Russell, C.G., Morcol, T., Subramanian, A., Wilkins, T.D., Canseco, R., Williams, B.L., Gwazdauskas, F., Knight, J.W., Pittius, C., Young, J.M., and Drohan, W.N. (1992b) High level expression in the milk of transgenic swine using the cDNA encoding human protein C. Proc. Natl. Acad. Sci. U.S.A., in press.

Wall, R.J., Pursel, V.G., Shamay, A., McKnight, R.A., Pittius, C.W. and Hennighausen, L. (1991) High-level synthesis of a heterologous milk protein in the mammary gland of transgenic swine. Proc. Natl. Acad. Sci. U.S.A. **88**, 1696-1700.

Wilmut, I., Archibald, A.L., McClenaghan, M., Simons, J.P., Whitelaw, C.B.A. and Clark, A.J. (1991) Production of pharmaceutical proteins in milk. Experientia **47**, 905-912.

Wright, G., Carver, A., Cottom, D., Reeves, D., Scott, A., Simons, P., Wilmut, I., Garner, and Colman, A. (1991) High level expression of active human alpha-1-antitrypsin in the milk of transgenic sheep. Biotechnology **9**, 830-834.

Dairy Products in Human Health and Nutrition, Serrano Rios et al. (eds) © 1994 Balkema, Rotterdam, ISBN 90 5410 359 0

Technological evolution in dairy products from craftsmanship to bio-technology

F.-M. Luquet
CIRDC/Danone, Paris, France

It is no easy matter to present the evolution of the Dairy Industry and its technologies in thirty minutes - if I succeed, it will be a record.

I would therefore ask you to forgive me if I leave anything out.

Our presentation can be broken down into four parts.

1) The history of milk throughout the ages.

2) The major events of the last decades.

3) The bio-technology of a modern product : yoghurt.

4) One or two points concerning the future.

1) THE HISTORY OF MILK AND DAIRY PRODUCTS

About 10 million years ago, the glaciers finally melted. Reindeer, horses and mammoths were replaced by animals that were better adapted to life in a temperate zone. Man who, up to then, had been a hunter and a berry picker, started to farm and to husband animals. He caught, enclosed and bred sheep, goats, pigs and later, bovines, and he drank their milk every day.

Cheeses

The milk sometimes coagulated and became curds. The caveman tasted these and found them to be good. What a stroke of luck! He had found himself a healthy and ever available food supply. From that moment on he concentrated on mastering this natural procedure caused by the acidification of the milk. By the end of the stone age, the Neolithic man had had the ingenious idea of putting the milk into the stomach of young ruminants. These original water jars with their active rennet, helped to make the curds. The resulting curds were then kept in wooden containers and churned with sticks of pine.

As man became more sedentary, societies became organised and animals were enclosed and the procedures of cheese-making became more precise. The Hebrews fermented milk with fresh herbs and, according to Aristotle, the Greeks used the flowers of the Bed Straw plant (gallium mollugo) known as "milk curdler".

Was Jupiter fed on goat's milk? We are entitled to think so as, on the Island of Crete, his mother's companion was that mythical goat Amaltheia.

Aristaeus, the son of Apollo and Cyrene, was brought up by the centaur, Chiron, who, among other things, is supposed to have taught him the art of making curds and cheese. As Virgil calls him the divine soothsayer and mediator and, as such, he surely passed on his cheese-making skills to man.

Ancient Rome set up the first industrial cheese-making industry that acted, in some way, as a prelude to the Common Market. In round about the third century A.D., Roman cheese found its way across the Valais and became implanted in Switzerland and, later, in Gaul.

Later on the Vikings took over the pasture lands of Normandy and its russet cows with their rich milk. The abbeys went in for animal husbandry in a big way. Pilgrims and crusaders compared the "know how" and the produce of these veritable "experimental farms". The monks, restricted to a meagre diet by their vows, kept the whey for themselves and sold the butter which was no longer considered to be a sacred food but which remained rare and hard to come by.

Monks perfected such cheeses as Munsters, Maroilles, Livarot, Epoisses and the ancestor of the Port-Salut cheese. Each century contributed to the development of cheese. The thirteenth century saw the flourishing of farm cheeses and cheese-making co-operatives which enabled peasants to face the lean season of the year with an adequate stock of Tomes, Vacherin, Beaufort, Gruyère or Comté . They took the excess to the towns and ports as part of a sales circuit and thereby provided a more balanced diet for town-dwellers and sailors.

These cheese-making dairies "Fruitières" were an intelligent form of co-operative which enabled its members to pool the milk collected daily from their little herds and flocks. The cheese was made in each farm in turn and the farm concerned provided help, fuel and fed the cheese-makers. The individual shares were worked out in accordance to the quantity of milk provided. The use of a special cheese-making area with its own dairy, production room and cellar has, in no way, put an end to the tradition of the individual share.

In the twelfth century, the Mongol Society introduced Koumis produced by fermenting whey from mare's milk with its nutritive and diuretic values as well as GRUT which is sour milk, boiled, curdled and then dried in leather bags : the forerunner of powdered milk perhaps?.......

Medicine and Epicurean Tastes

Travelling, exchanges and battles introduced people to new products that came from civilisations that were virtually entirely pastoral.

Caucasian Kefir, inoculated milk under various names followed the Turks as they conquered lands round the Mediterranean.

What was this mysterious brew? Koumis, fermented milk used, as we have already seen, in Mongolia or Kefir, the same sort of drink as is produced by the mountain people of the Caucasians from inoculated milk made by associating bacteria (Diaspora Caucasian) and yeast (saccharomyces kefir).

Cream/Butter

As from the 18th century, the rapid expansion of towns provided a market. Peasants from the neighbouring villages delivered milk in time for breakfast. Cheese was always popular because it stayed fresh. Gradually heavy, very filling food gave way to more refined gastronomy. Thus "Crème Chantilly" or whipped cream presented by Vatel to Louis XIV became, and still is, very popular.

Butter is a more recent invention. It is only a little more than three thousand years old. And even then, only if one accepts the Indian "ghee" as being "clarified butter".

And then? This product "melts" into history. Practically no mention remains from classical history. According to Pline butter did exist, but only with the "Barbarians" and even it was a rare and very expensive product.

A thousand years later it appeared in the West perhaps due to the Vikings who had a great liking for it.

In the Middle Ages butter was highly appreciated, butter from Brittany for example. It arrived, salted, on Epicurean Parisian plates (the first known price was an ecu per pound in 1590).

Later on, other regions proved to be good producers as well. The East of France as well the mountainous zones and, especially, the Poitou Charentes region where, at the end of the last century the vineyards, devastated by phyloxera, were replaced by pastures in which, from that day to this, large dairy herds have flourished.

With the 20th Century, we entered into the era of industrial production. Wooden butter churns and moulds can now only be found in folk museums.

The evolution and improvement of dairy farming : XVIII century

Simple cattle husbandry was transformed into different intensive cattle rearing systems.

JETHRO TULL, Shalbourne called Mount Prosperous. In order to increase his grain-producing efficiency, he improved the quality of his cattle, suppliers of fertilisers. To this end he started to grow cattle fodder and invented a mechanical seed drill. He was thus able to sow his sainfoin and white turnips intended as cattle fodder in spaced lines that were hoed several times during vegetation in order to improve water penetration and to remove weeds. After, in 1725, ROBERT BAKEWELL introduced the idea of cattle selection by crossing quality animals in order to develop dairy or meat specifications.

At the same time, the first industrialised cheeses manufactured by abbeys appeared on the market: Cheshire, Shropshire, Suffolk, Essex, Cheddar and lastly Stilton.

Then came the factories :

- Dairy co-operatives

- Cheese Factories and Butter Factories.

In every country, the dairy industry became one of capital importance ......but this national economy has to conform to the other EEC countries as the following facts will show you :

The dairy economy : ten years of evolution

1976 :

FRANCE had 780,000 farms exploiting bovines. It produced 28.7 million tons of milk, 20.6 million of which was collected by dairies.

1977:

The EEC brought in a 'co-responsibility tax' for producers.

1978:

French cheese production reached a million tons.

1980:

The world butter and powdered milk prices that had been rising over the three previous reached its ceiling.

1981:

The Community stocks were at their lowest : 10,000 tons of butter and 2 million tons of powdered milk.

1983:

World stocks were replenished (butter: 1.3 million tons, powdered skimmed milk 2 million tons) and prices fell.

1984:

The year of the milk quotas - over 40,000 farmers gave up dairy production in France.

1985:

A second programme was introduced in France to encourage farmers to stop producing. The European Community had a butter mountain of over 1 million tons. The G.A.T.T. lowered the minimum prices.

<u>What is the position of the Dairy Industry in Europe and in the world as a whole?</u>

Number of Dairy Cows		Milk Yield (Kg / Cow / Year	
World	**225.000.000**	**Monde**	**2115**
E.E.C. (12)	23.730.000	E.C.	4510
Asia	54.820.000	Asia	945
C.I.S	41.700.000	C.I.S.	2615
North America	19.760.000	North America	4303
		Africa	485

NUMBER OF DAIRY FARMS
(thousands)

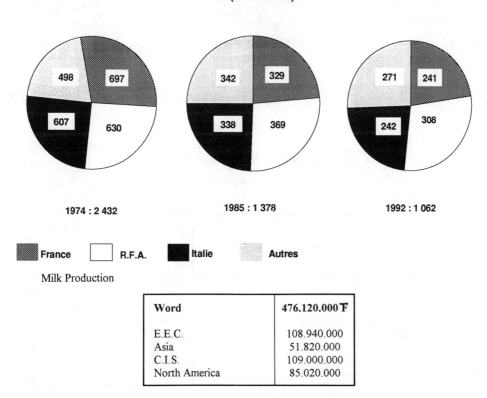

| 1974 : 2 432 | 1985 : 1 378 | 1992 : 1 062 |

France   R.F.A.   Italie   Autres

Milk Production

Word	476.120.000 **F**
E.E.C.	108.940.000
Asia	51.820.000
C.I.S.	109.000.000
North America	85.020.000

PROCESSED PRODUCTS WITHIN THE EUROPEAN COMMUNITY OF TWELVE

Butter	1.780.000 T
Cheeses	5.273.000 T
Skimmed milk powder	1.400.000 T
Whole milk powder	823.000 T
Concentrated milk	1.256.000 T
Casein	104.000 T

NUMBER OF DAIRY COMPAGNIES
(Buying directly from dairy farmers)

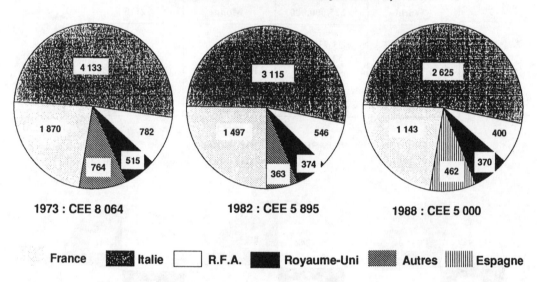

| 1973 : CEE 8 064 | 1982 : CEE 5 895 | 1988 : CEE 5 000 |

France   Italie   R.F.A.   Royaume-Uni   Autres   Espagne

Consumption per kilo / product / capita

	Liquid milk		Butter		Cheeses
Iceland	197.5	New Zealand	9.9	France	22.8
Spain	101.0	France	8.3	Italy	18.6
Italy	78.6	Germany	6.5	Germany	18.5
France	77.1			Spain	5.6
Germany	70.8				-

1) Purifying : Thermal Treatment

The need to preserve food became apparent when people undertook long journeys by sea as well as military expeditions. The problem became serious in the 18th century with the development of inter-continental sea travel.

During the 19th century different heating methods were proposed for the preservation of farm produce. Two very different people led this evolution : Nicolas APPERT (1749 - 1841), confectioner and Louis PASTEUR (1822 - 1895) chemist.

In 1810, Nicolas APPERT had his new process approved by the Society for the Encouragement of National Industry. He combined the blanching of vegetables with storing them in air-tight glass jars.

In 1860, PASTEUR realised that the deterioration of wine was due to the multiplication of micro-organisms. Lack of oxygen of oxygen was not enough to stabilise the product. It also had to be heated in order to destroy these micro-organisms. He presented the pasteurisation of wine as an extension of APPERT's preservation process.

In 1895, Emile DUCLAUX, Director of the Pasteur Institute, tried to find out how to preserve milk at the same time as pleasing consumer tastes. Pasteur had observed that it was only necessary to heat milk to 107°/108°C for it to be sterilised, but that it had a disagreeable "cooked" taste and some substances, necessary to man, had deteriorated.

DUCLAUX favoured using the wine-pasteurisation technique to keep milk fresher, longer, but it had to be cooled very quickly otherwise the toughest germs multiplied even faster.

Research was also carried out to find the best shape for the container.

The 'magic' figures   63.5°C for 30 minutes
                                            ☞ destruction of the tuberculosis bacillus
(continuous holder process) 72°C for 15 seconds

This principle is behind a whole range of processes which today allows us to enjoy a wide variety of high quality, long-life milks.

Low Pasteurisation   ->   Parabolic pasteurizer
High Pasteurisation   ->   Stassanizator using hot water or low pressure steam

then
specialists developed   -> Drum Pasteurises, Plate pasteurisers and Tubular pasteurisers

Then followed a mixture of pasteurisation and rapid cooling in various types of stainless steel exchangers.

And finally, we now have HTST pasteurisation which has been very largely developed throughout the world.

An improvement to the quality of pasteurised milk came with the homogenisation of the milk fat through the breaking down of the butterfat globules to a diameter of $\emptyset.2/0.3\mu$.

The production of sterilised milk both in bulk and in single unit packs developed along side the development of high pasteurisation. Some of the numerous systems tried out still exist today, others have disappeared.

The sterilisation temperatures used to destroy the spores were 115°C for 10 to 15 minutes but, unfortunately, this turned the milk brown and gave it an unpleasant taste. After this, the UHT or uperization techniques were developed in Switzerland (135°-150°C for a few seconds) by the injection of steam and by aseptic storage in different kinds of one-way package...plastic, carton........

These techniques do not change the initial colour of the milk nor do they interfere with the taste. Furthermore, they do not destroy, or hardly destroy, such vitamins as thiamin, cobalamin or pyridoxin as well as the biological protein value (a little lysine is lost).

Today new technologies are being introduced.

* Micro-wave Pasteurisation which instantly heats right through and in a selective and homogenous way. The most common frequencies are between 300MHz and 30GHz and the wave lengths between 1m and 1cm.

   Used a great deal for dry and granular products (flour, sliced bread, fresh pasta, packaged meats) this technique is still not used for liquid milks despite the fact that it only involves a single thermic effect.

* Electrical Pasteurisation
   The tubular heater with its direct electrical current is a development of the use of electricity as a source of heat (thermal induction generator)

   Strong, low-tension currents pass through the exchanger tubes in such a way that the electricity can be compared to a thermic fluid containing steam or hot water.

   Currently commercialised under the name "Actijoule" this machine is used to pasteurise milk, mayonnaise and viscous liquids.

   It presents the following advantages

      - easy to run (low inertia)
      - surfaces remain clean
      - regularity during the process
      - precision in the temperature regulation.

* Ohmic Heating

This system involves direct conduction. Heat is generated by joule effect within the product itself. This technique looks to be promising for the treatment of highly thermo-sensitive liquids and reduces the risk of soiling or scratching as there are no heating surfaces. It insures the homogeneity of the heating of low pH heterogeneous liquids containing bits such as fruit and meat without pollution (no water vapour).

* The use of accelerated high energy electrons

This technique is used for processing packaged solids (meat, vegetables) and is very flexible to use and also very practical because it is integrated into the process itself contrary to rays which have to be specially installed.

Up to now we have not heard of any industrial applications of this technique for fresh dairy products, with the exception of the Isigny plant, where it is used to treat the surface of soft bodied cheeses.

* Very High Pressure

This technique inactivates micro-organisms and enzymes by a global action on the cells at an ambient or low temperature which makes it very interesting as it guarantees but the sensory and nutritional values of the foodstuffs thus treated (vitamin C for example). The pressure used varies from 6 to 10 thousand bars applied for about 10 minutes and the effect varies from product to product.

Both discontinuous and continuous material is being developed for industrial use both in Japan and in Europe.

The current applications are

- the tenderising of meats
- the compression of powders
- to increase the thickness of milk and decrease its turbidity and to free the calcium in the casein micelle
- the sterilisation of fruit and fruit juices.

This process is of interest because it permits the cold-sterilisation of packed foodstuffs.

2) Milk collection/milking and refrigeration on the farm

Various systems for the stabling and the rational feeding of dairy herd were perfected during this century.

However, the major event was the generalisation of milking machines, the refrigeration of milk on the farm itself and its transport in tanker lorries to the processing centres.

The reason why milk is kept refrigerated is to stop the initial qualities from being lost (bacteriological, physico-chemical and sensory). But the quality of milk can never be improved if it comes from stressed, sick or badly nourished animals or if it is collected in an unhygenic way. This is why in modern countries where both human and animal hygiene is considered to be important, milk is refrigerated at + 4° C and is of excellent quality (low in somatic cells, total amount of germs in the flora between 10 and 30 thousand, absence of pathogenic flora and, of course, absence of any residual antibiotics, antiseptics or phytosanitary products). The storage and transport of refrigerated milk is generally done using tanks made from material that is both inert (stainless steel) and insulated.

3) **Separation techniques**

The performances achieved by the semi-permeable membranes, the progress made in their development, the possibilities opened up by their use are such that the resulting technologies, inversed osmosis, ultra-filtration and micro-filtration....represent a real technological revolution.

The membrane techniques used in the dairy industry are resumed in the following table:

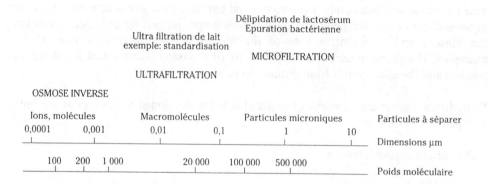

(Ions, molecules, macromolecules, micron particles, particles to be separated, dimensions µm, molecular weight)

*   Separation Techniques : new raw materials

The fractionation of the component elements of natural raw materials such as milk, wheys results in a multitude of products certain of which can undergo, among other things, chemical, biological, enzymatic and microbial conversions.

The fractionation of biological components on an industrial scale depends on their characteristic physico-chemical principals, that is to say the hydrophilic character on which their solubility depends as well as their steric size and their weight.

The main applications are related to casein preparation through pHi (isoelectric point) precipitation, the delipidation of the whey and the preparation of phospholipids by the interaction of phosphorylated groups and calcium under defined conditions of both pH and temperature.

The exploitation of the difference in the molecular size of the components for their separation was made possible by the development of tangential micro-filtration techniques.

Tangential ultra-filtration and microfiltration on mineral or organic membranes that are either flat, tubular or made of hollow fibre have developed rapidly over the last few years in all areas of the agricultural food products sector.

* Membrane Techniques : New Dairy techniques

The microbial cleaning of milk can be carried out by tangential microfiltration as well as by separating phases which is sometimes difficult by centrifugation (delipidation of caseins....). This physical process that cleanses but does not destroy, eliminates between 99.5 and 99.9% of the contamination flora in skimmed milks and whey.

* Protein standardisation of milking

Membrane ultrafiltration means you can regulate as required the protein value, the consumer milks, the cheese milk with the same degree of flexibility as creaming which enables the standardisation of the butterfat level.

* New cheese-making techniques

Ultrafiltration helps in
1)   the preparation of pre-cheese liquids
2)   the preparation of the retentates for the regularisation of cheese factories and in order to adjust the required protein levels (the casein/total protein ratio).

We are also entitled to think that within a few years these techniques will allow the continuous inoculation of milk with lactic bacteria (starter tank membrane).

*   **The breaking-up of milk components**

Delipidation of whey   **casein separation**

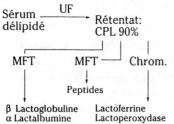
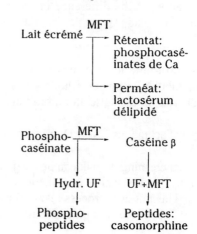

Filtration techniques separate the different milk molecules (2000) in order to use them for specific ends (baby foods, delicatessen products, dietary products, functional property elements, foaming and gelifying agents, bactericidal property proteins such as lactoferrin, lactoperoxydase) and to concentrate biological activity molecules (morphinomimetic activity peptides, immunostimulant activity peptides etc...).

4. Industrial automation

When the Verona architect, Vitruvius, in the first century BC dreamed up the word "automation" for posterity (from the Greek word 'automates': which can move on its own) as he admired the animated statues in the Temple of Daedalus, he had no idea that machines, carefully conceived to imitate human behaviour, could replace man in the carrying out of tedious or unpleasant tasks.
The automation of industrial manufacturing or laboratory work has led to a more or less complete overhaul of the processes and technologies introduced beforehand and were often merely a mechanisation of manual operations.

This development or rather revolution is the result of research carried out by multi-discipline groups or teams made up of technologists, managers, ergonomists, sociologists, electro-mechanical engineers, computer specialists, automation specialists, etc., who, before introducing automation have to make models hence the mechanical research and the creation of multi-parametric captors capable of closely analysing the raw material.

The Dairy Industry can be seen to be an innovator in this field. Examples of this are:

- the Camembert moulding robot
- the automated procedure for bacterial fermentation

-the automated control of milk elements
-the continuous cheese production line
-the automated Gruyere curing factories
-the aseptic processing and packing of UHT milk

and, finally, the concept of a factory combining safety, efficiency and flexibility - a manufacturer's dream.

5.   The ultra-sterile factory

The cheese-making and dairy industries have proved to be pioneers among the farm-produce industries when it comes to the cleaning, disinfection, sterilisation and air treatment of the work place.

Factories must be designed to prevent the development of micro-organisms. The air filtered by over-pressure must protect sensitive and fresh products and the double airjet technique should isolate the packing machine from the rest of the workshop by means of air expulsion.

Stainless steel material, cutting by waterjet and packing machines designed to be cleaned by CIP (cleaning in place).

CIP systems adapted to the different kinds of soiling (CIP raw milk, CIP packing line, CIP preparation and mix thermalisation line), ultra-sterile clothing, the correct training of the work force - all this helps to create a concept of total quality pursued by dynamic companies who wish to meet customer requirements

- with regard to perceived needs
  . satisfaction (taste, smell, colour, etc.)
  . service (protective wrapping, preserving, preparation, rapid use....)

with regard to implicit needs
   . SAFETY (hygienic products)
   . LOYALTY (informative labelling)
   . HEALTHY (nutritional value)

Thanks to this, the quality assurance system for company certification, in compliance with ISO standards, have been put in place.

3 THE BIOTECHNOLOGY OF DAIRY PRODUCTS : YOGHURT

1)   Its history according to RASIC and KURMANN

The use of fermented milks dates back many centuries, although there is no precise record of the date when they were first made. One legend tells that an angel descends with the pot which contained the first yoghurt or leben, while another claims that the ancient Turks, who were Buddhists, used to offer yoghurt to the angels and stars who protected them (KRÜNITZ, 1803; YAYGIN, 1969a).

In the Bible it is recorded that when the Patriarch Abraham entertained three angels, he put before them soured and sweet milk (Genesis VIII,8). And Moses, having considered the foods given by Jehovah to his people, mentions the soured milk of cows and goats (Deuteronomy, XXXII, 14)(Davis, 1952).

The ancient Greeks and Romans were also acquainted with the preparation of soured milks. The biography of the Roman Emperor Elagabalum (A.D.218-222) mentions two recipes of soured milk preparations.

The first written mention of the Turkish word "Yoghurt" goes back to 1071 to the TSING-KIANG where it appears in Mahmoud Al Kachgari's first Arabic-Turkish dictionary under the name of YOGURUT.

In 1712 E. KAEMPFER on his travels to Asia described the palace of the Emperor of Persia, which had a special room denominated as "Yoghurt choneh". Yoghurt or maast was used in the preparation of human food and in the feeding of birds.

In France yoghurt first appeared in the reign of François I who was cured of an intestinal infection by eating yoghurt prescribed by a doctor sent to him by a Turkish dignitary.

Finally, METCHNIKOFF, a Ukrainian scientist who became naturalised French, noted how the beneficial effects of yoghurt contributed to the longevity of the mountain peoples of the Caucasus and the Balkans.

METCHNIKOFF, who won the Nobel prize in 1908 for his work on the relation behind longevity and a healthy gut, was behind the development of yoghurt in Western Europe. This development was slow to start with.

In 1917, in Barcelona, ISAAC CARASSO started to produce yoghurt by industrial means - This was the origin of Danone.

In 1922, a Georgian General who was a refugee living in Chatou, France, produced small quantities of yoghurt for experts.

In 1925 the word "yaourt" or "yoghurt" figured in the Petit Larousse. This was the consecration that DANIEL CARASSO, Isaac's son, had been waiting for in order to set up the first French yoghurt factory in LEVALLOIS. This factory was soon followed by others, some industrial and some more like dairy co-operatives, and this throughout the world.

Yoghurt became industrialised but remained true to itself, that is to say, a LIVING FOOD.

Such is the long history of yoghurt, the living food:

in Turkish : Yoghurt　　　　　　　　in Persian : Maast
in Egyptian : leben　　　　　　　　 in Arabic : Rhaib
in Indian : Dadhi　　　　　　　　　 in Italian : Gioddu
in Russian : Matzun

. 3000 years to come to Western Europe
. 30 years to conquer Europe
. and now a world wide boom.

3,950,000 tons of yoghurt is sold in Europe in various forms (natural, vegetable and fruit flavoured), stirred or set which is to say, on average, 16.3kg per person per year in the European Community with the Dutch taking the lead at 32kg/person.

2)   Controlled Fermentation:

Since Metchnikoff, yoghurt and fermented milks have become more to the consumer than a nutritive source of food with a nice taste which brings variety to the table. From the pure natural product called milk which is first collected and transported under hygienic conditions and then fermented using selected lactic bacteria with the production of metabolites and bio-active, anti-microbial substances with antitumoral growths we finish with a product that is said to be beneficial to the health.

When used ALIVE these bacteria have a pro-biotic effect. The development of yoghurt may be considered to have gone through four phases.
1)   up to 1910 :   home or local production with undefined floral, natural
2)   1910 - 1930 :   semi-industrial with undefined micro-flora
3)   1930 - 1980 :   industrial production with semi-defined microflora
4)   1980 - present : Industrial production both regulated and controlled using selected bacteria with defined probiotic, technological and sensory properties. Diversification of fresh dairy products.

A great deal of research has been carried out on

a)   the different racemized forms L+ and D- of lactic acid and their consumption in both their forms

b)   the production of peptides by lactic bacteria

c)   the increase in the proportions of alanine, glycine, methionine,

d)   the proteolytic action of <u>Lactobacillus debrueckii</u> subsp. <u>bulgaricus</u> and peptidasic action of <u>Streptococcus</u> - <u>thermophilus</u>, bacteria which are typical in yoghurt,

e)   a better assimilation of calcium and phosphorus both in yoghurt and in milk.

3) Mastering the procedures

1) Preparation of fermentation cultures

*   Selection and identification of the strains........,

New products have been developed taking into consideration health claims as well as good flavour and texture characteristics. From this point of view new strains must be selected using criteria other than those for traditional fermented milks.

Selected intestinal strains can be applied so that they:

.   meet health claims, for example to enhance the possible prophylactic health properties of fermented milks, and

.   improve biotechnical properties.

Many strains can be identified according to their biochemical reactions, that is, the fermentation pattern of carbohydrates and enzymatic reactions.

Genetic methods, for example plasmid analysis or DNA restriction mapping may prove useful for ultimate identification.

Health claims:

Specific health-related subjects are the reduction of cholesterol and the release of active β-galactosidase in fermented milk, which might be responsible for the more complete hydrolysis of lactose in the gastro-intestinal tract of lactose-intolerant individuals. A further criterion for the selection of intestinal bacteria is their detrimental influence on pathogenic micro-organisms in the gut.

*   Use of cultures : controlled fermentation

The bacterial cultures are inoculated into the maturing tanks (stirred yoghurts) or into the potted milk (set yoghurt) using different procedures. At the present time concentrated, frozen or lyophilised techniques are the most commonly used.

This Direct Innoculation technique (freeze dried) has numerous advantages :

*   each strain can be produced under optimal conditions with respect to oxygen, nutrients and pH. Since the cells are concentrated, most growth additives are removed and not transferred to the milk

*   each strain can be controlled for purity and activity before use

*   the amount of culture to be used is more easily controlled and cultures which are difficult to grow together can be mixed in the milk in differing proportions.

46

The industrial techniques vary according to what is required :

Liquid, stirred and set fermented milks.

Each company has its own industrialisation practices.

The manufacture of fermented milks can be considered as a two-stage process (the first stage consists of the pre-fermentation of the milk ; bacteria are produced). In the second stage further acidification causes the milk to coagulate. To avoid syneresis the coagulating milk should not be disturbed. At the end of this stage the fermented milk is stirred, cooled and packed.

The main technologies are resumed in the following diagram :

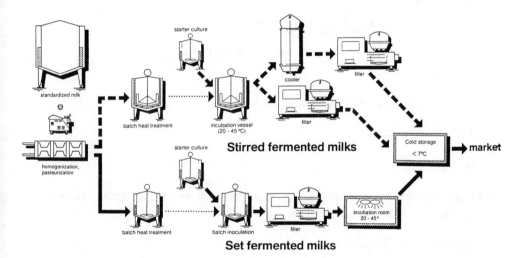

In the case of set yoghurt, the milk is inoculated and then put into pots and incubated at a regulated temperature.

Numerous studies are being carried out to improve the stability of the required quality : stable acidity, defined texture, specific smell, etc. This research work is essentially based on the knowledge :

- of the bacteria used and their characteristics

- of the way the mix is prepared

- of the fermentation process

Although, of course, true yoghurt is a living product without any additives or preserving agents.

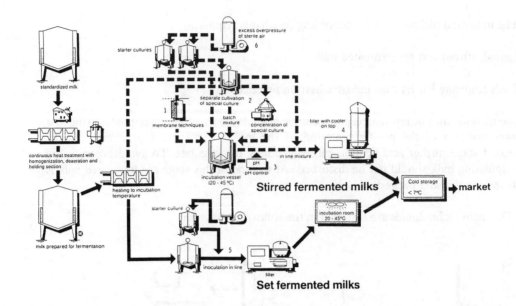

Stirred fermented milks

Set fermented milks

4) The nutritional and health attributes of yoghurt

Yoghurt has two kinds of action:

* improved digestibility........

The living yoghurt bacteria pre-digest milk through enzymatic action thereby providing the body with nutrients.

- the digestibility of carbohydrates

Lactose, a natural element of milk, is digested by the beta-galactosidase or lactase to be found in the fringed edges of the intestinal epithelium cells and becomes easily absorbed glucose and galactose.

Some populations have a genetic deficiency or a loss of lactasic activity which can lead to the poor digestion or intolerance of lactose. Numerous authors have shown that yoghurts reduce the clinical signs of intolerance.

- the digestibility of proteins

Lactobacillus delbrueckii sup. bulgaricus proteolyses the milk casein thereby freeing low molecular weight peptides. This action is completed by that of Streptococcus Thermophilus which attacks these peptides.

By producing lactic acid, the yoghurt bacteria induce the precipitation of the protein factions into more easily digested particles (gastric emptying is faster when yoghurt rather than milk is consumed).

- Calcium bio-availability

Thanks to its acid pH which favors the ionised form of calcium, yoghurt supplies the body with a bio-available calcium of particular interest to those who cannot tolerate milk.

- Other minerals : vitamins and oligo-elements

Phosphorus, magnesium, iron, zinc are more easily dissolved and therefore more bio-available. Certain bacteria-synthesised vitamins increase in a noticeable way, but this is very strain-dependent.

Vitamins	Milk (UHT)	Yoghourt ppm	15 % RDI for Europe
B1 (Thiamine) mg/100 g	0,05	0,04	0,21
B2 (Riboflavin) mg/100 g	0,17	0,25	0,24
B9 (Total folates) µ g/100 g	0,38	15,0	30,00

For riboflavin (vitamin B2) yoghurt contains over 15% of the recommended daily input.

In conclusion, the mineral and vitamin content of yoghurt makes it particularly useful in physiological situations such as growth, pregnancy, breast feeding, menopause and ageing.

* Improving the Body's immunisation capacities

A lot of research has shown the beneficial effect of yoghurt bacteria on infectious germs in animals (the fight against diarrhoea, E-coli infections, Salmonella) or in man (clinical studies on under-nourished children and those with diarrhoea).

- Yoghurt would appear to have an immuno-modulating effect which is manifest in the production of immunoglobin G and a stimulation of the intestinal glands, an effect which disappears with pasteurized yoghurts.

- In vitro, yoghurt bacteria induce the production of γ-interferon by human blood cells in the presence of an activator, as well as a "natural killer" activity.

- Experiments carried out on human beings have shown a non specific stimulation of the defence mechanisms (increase of lymphocyte B, increase of certain immunoglobulins G, increased γ-interferon activity within four hours after eating yoghurt).

On the other hand, it has not been proven that the lactic bacteria become implanted in the body. They are transiting, influencing the correct balance of the intestinal flora (pro biotic effect) and are part of a protective food pattern to fight cancer (breast and bowel cancer).

4) THE NEAR OR DISTANT FUTURE

1) Obtaining quality at Factory Level : the use of artificial intelligence

An expert system also known as artificial intelligence is a unit comprising software, an inference engine and rules formalised by experts.

A certain number of these exist throughout the world and, by way of an example, let me just mention that of the Institute Technique du Gruyere (France). This institute works for 1000 cheese-making factories and curing workshops.

To develop this expert system, 62 analysts describe and define Emmental catalogued under different headings : presentation, texture, smell, taste......

Then a list was drawn up of all the parameters that have an effect of the faults or the required quality, for example, the milk used, the bacteria, the curing........there are 110 variables. An analysis was then made of all the different technologies used to achieve a defined quality.

The technologists, with the held of a cognitician, have established the parametric relationship between production and describers.

The users, that is to say the technicians working in the cheese-making factories, consult this expert service in three ways :

-   the Fault approach

    How can we get rid of it?

-   The Constatational Approach

    How can we correct an existing anomaly?

-   The preventional approach

    Such a fault may occur - how can we prevent it?

The results achieved in this present case are

-   a computer library

-   an increase in quality of around 20%.

2   Biotechnologies : The efficiency of the Dairy Sector

The milk producer of the coming years will have new obligations. His responsibilities in product safety, environment, nature and animal welfare will increase. Bio-technology will help him meet these challenges by :

-    the use of BST

-    embryo transplants on a worthwhile economic scale,

-    in vitro-fertilisation

-    animals modified genetically to produce milk with specific proteins or with less butterfat or saturated fatty acid

-    the use of enzymes produced by genetic manipulation and encapsulated (lyposomes)

-    attenuated starters obtained by cellular lysis , thermal shock or genetic recombining (low acid production level, low proteolysis level....).

     Of course, these new starters will have to conform to existing regulations.

-    The industrial metabolisms regulated by the use of programmed micro-organisms.

CONCLUSIONS

This wide panorama of the evolution of the Dairy Industry has shown the enormous progress made in

- milk production and collection

- the permanent innovation in terms of the means, technologies and procedures employed

- the search for products that increasingly meet consumers' needs, but what will tomorrow hold?

We think that the Dairy Industry Sector will have to face six challenges :

1)   THE QUALITY CHALLENGE :

      The growth in production is not a priority as much as the choice of raw materials.

2)   THE ENVIRONMENTAL PROTECTION CHALLENGE

      Industrial waste should be even more restricted and means of production optimised.

3) THE FOOD AND HEALTH CHALLENGE

Consumers will be more and more particular in this field (the health and nutritional properties of foodstuffs).

4) THE INNOVATION CHALLENGE

Variety, the speed taken in replying will be what consumers expect from us

5) OPTIMIZATION of the size of companies, the flexibility and the increased appreciation of the intrinsic value of man .

6) GENERALISATION of the principle of transmitting the bio-technological results of production to the consumer.

REFERENCES

Adria Normandie 1991. - Bactéries Lactiques, Université de Caen France.

Alais, Ch.. Science du lait, éd. Sepaic Paris

Bhan M.K., Sazawal S., Behatnagar, B.L., Jailkhani, N.K. Arora (India). Efficacy of yoghurt in comparison to milk in malnourished children with acute diarrhea. Congrès sur les laits fermentés - Décembre 1989.

Bourlioux, P. and POCHARD P. 1988. Nutritional and health properties of yogurt. Wld Rev.Nutr. Diet. 56 : 217.

Brulé, G. Pression des progrès techniques et scientifiques dans le fonctionnement de nouveaux produits. ENSA Rennes.

Bull. IDF. New Technologies for fermented milks n° 277/92.

Cidil/Cniel. L'histoire au fil du lait Doc. 1-2-3-4.

Desmazeaud, M. 1983. L'état des connaissances en matière de nutrition des bactéries lactiques. Le lait, 63, 267 : 316.

Driessen, FM et Loones, A. Bulletin FIL/IDF n° 277.

Gilliland, S.E. 1979. Beneficial interrelationships between certain microorganisms ans humans : Candidats microorganisms for use as dietary adjuncts. J. Food Prot. 42, 164-167.

Goldin, B.R., Gorbach SL. 1984. The effect of milk and Lactobacillus feeding on human intestinal bacterial enzyme activity. Am J. Clin. Nutr. : 39,756 - 61.

Hewitt, D. and Bancroft H.J. 1985. Nutritional value of yogurt. J. of Dairy research, 52, 197 : 207.

Hunger W. et Peitersen N. 1992. New technical aspects of the préparation of starter cultures 277 17-21, bulletin IDF 277.

Kurmann, J.A. 1986. The future of market milk. Northern European Dairy Journal (Copenhagen)

Kurmann, J.A. 1988. Starters vith selected intestinal bacteria. Bulletin of the IDF/FIL n° 227: 41-55.

Libbey, J. 1989. Eurotext, les laits fermentés Syndifrais.

Luquet, FM 1985. Laits et Produits Laitiers (vache, brebis, chèvre) Les laits de la mamelle à la laiterie - vol. 1 Les produits laitiers - Transformation et technologie (1990) - vol. 2 Tables de composition par Coordinateur - Tec et Doc Lavoisier PARIS . Qualité énergie vol. 3

Maubois, J.L. 1990. Nouvelles applications des techniques à membranes dans l'industrie laitière. Congrès FIL Montréal (vol. 2) n° 9-10, 309-310.

Perdigon, G. 1990. Prevention of gastrointestinal infection using immunobiological methods vith milk fermented with L. Casei and L. acidophilus.

Piaia, M. 1991. J. Dairy Science 74-409-413

Ramesh, C., Chandan, Ph.D. Yogurt : Nutritional and health properties. National Yogurt Association. Mc Lean, Virginia,USA.

Rasic, JY et Kurmann, JA. 1978 . Yoghurt Technical Dairy Pub. House, Copenhague

Reddy, G.V., Friend B.A., Shalani and R.E. 01/083. Farmer Antitumor of yogurt components. J. of Food Protection.

Rochard Ph., Lemonnier D., Huland D. 1989. Yaourt et Santé, journées de nutrition pratique DIETECOM Paris.

Scriban R. 1982. Biotechnologie - Tec et Doc Lavoisier Paris.

Touhami M., Boudraa G., Mort J.Y., Soltania R., Desjeur J.F. Conséquences cliniques du remplacement du lait par le yoghourt dans les diarrhées persistantes du nourrisson Ann : Pédiatrie 1992 : 39 : 79 - 86.

Underdahl, N., Torres Medina, A. and Doster, A. 1982. Effect of Steptococcus faecium C-68 in control of Escherichia coli induced diarrhoea in gnotobiotic pigs. American J. of Veterinary Research 43 : 2227 - 2232.

Dairy Products in Human Health and Nutrition, Serrano Ríos et al. (eds) © 1994 Balkema, Rotterdam, ISBN 90 5410 359 0

Dairy products and milk production tendencies and strategies in the world

R.Gemperle
Nestlé World Trade Corporation, Vevey, Switzerland

ABSTRACT: World milk production is unevenly spread between regions. Its evolution is different per continent. Growing production in developing countries is encouraging. However, their share is still small. Milk production and dairy products manufacture is influenced by climatic conditions, agricultural policies, industrial structures, consumption and prices. This paper analyses the interaction for all these factors and makes some long term assessments.

1 WORLD MILK PRODUCTION

According to data published by the FAO, milk production (including about 10 % of sheep, goat and buffalo milk) reached 516 mio. tonnes in 1992. This volume is in constant progression since 1980 (460 mio. tonnes) with the exception of the two last periods 1991 - 1992.

As shown in table 1, production has also increased in developing countries. However, their share of the world total is only about 30 %.

World Milk Production

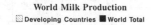

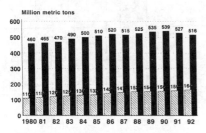

Figure 1

2 DISTRIBUTION PER CONTINENT AND EVOLUTION

As indicated in table 1, the distribution between continents is very pronounced; very high level of production in Europe and in the former Soviet Republics (strong decrease however during the past years) as well as in Northern America (increases); the production is relatively low but increasing in Oceania (New Zealand and Australia). As far as developing countries are concerned, the evolution is positive, in particular in Latin America and Asia.

PRODUCTION DE LAIT / MILK PRODUCTION

	1990	1991 estim.	1992 prévis.
	(.. millions de tonnes ..)		
WORLD TOTAL TOTAL MONDIAL	539	527	516
Pays en déve- loppement	156	159	164
DEVELOPPING COUNTRIES Amérique latine	42	43	45
Afrique	13	13	13
Asie	101	103	106
Pays déve- loppés	383	368	352
DEVELOPPED COUNTRIES Amérique du Nord	75	75	76
Europe	174	167	160
(CEE)	(121)	(118)	(116)
Ex-URSS	109	100	90
Océanie	14	14	15

SOURCE: FAO   DÉC 1992

Figure 2

3 ANALYSIS PER REGION

The current decrease of production in Eastern Europe is due to a reduction in the number of dairy cows and their yields; generally as a consequence of the drought and in particular because of the substantial decrease in profitability following marked cost increases of animal food. These countries also suffer from a decrease in demand due to strong rises in prices following the elimination of subsidies as well as deficient internal distribution networks.

The reduction of production in Western European countries is especially due to the introduction of quota systems, these countries having had to take measures to diminish surplus production (EEC since 1984).

In the USA increased yields largely compensate reductions in the number of cows. In Canada, however, production remains limited by national quotas.

In Australia and New Zealand climatic conditions were favourable during the past three years. Furthermore, international quotations, which play an important role in these export orientated countries, have encouraged the improvement of production.

In Asia and particularly in India, main producer among developing countries, production increased by 4 % in 1992, as a result of an improvement of pastures and animal feeding.

The expansion in China continues with about + 7 % in 1992 due to government support for the development of local production. In Latin America, price increases at production level (elimination of state controls in some cases) as well as favourable climatic conditions stimulated production generally in 1992, with the exception of Peru and Venezuela.

No increase can be noted in Africa where deficient feeding caused by drought has been the main cause.

4 DISPARITY IN YIELDS PER COW

Figure 3 provides a good idea of the variability of yields per cow and per continent/country. The world average yield amounts to 2'100 kg of milk/cow/year. It varies between 485 kg in Africa and 6'600 kg in the USA. It has to be noted that yields are relatively low in Oceania (3'600 kg). Here, a production structure based on grass feeding without addition of concentrates for animal diet constitutes the limiting factor.

5 DISPARITY OF MILK AVAILABILITIES PER CAPITA AND IN THE WORLD

The projection of milk availabilities per capita expressed in milk equivalent shows that the gap in present availability, and

le rendement laitier / MILK YIELD

Unité : kg/vache/an
KG/COW/YEAR

Régions Années	Moyenne 1979-1981	1988	1989	1990
MONDE dont :	1.957	2.092	2.104	2.114
Europe dont :	3.384	3.725	3.745	3.745
C.E.E. à 12 (1) dont :	4.050	4.504	4.561	4.510
France (1)	3.635	4.662	4.701	4.928
Asie dont :	698	874	889	945
Inde	530	718	746	831
Israël	6.817	8.709	8.552	8.519
U.R.S.S.	2.095	2.531	2.586	2.614
Amérique du Sud	954	1.048	1.041	1.036
Amérique du Nord dont :	3.638	4.073	4.248	4.303
U.S.A.	5.371	6.416	6.461	6.673
Canada	4.404	5.761	5.694	5.780
Afrique	483	489	486	485
Océanie dont :	3.128	3.596	3.615	3.646
Australie	2.989	3.758	3.885	3.879
Nouvelle-Zélande	3.306	3.530	3.471	3.528

Figure 3

also that of the long term (year 2000), remains very important : from 42 kg in developing countries to 290 kg in industrial countries, i.e. a factor of 1 to 7 (see table 4). This takes into account the level of production, birth rates and export movements from developed to developing countries.

WORLD DAIRY SITUATION AT A GLANCE - PAST AND PROJECTED

	Milk production	Net Imports	Availability	
			Total	Per caput
	million tons			kg
WORLD TOTAL 1974-76	422	...	422	106
1986-88	521	...	521	104
2000	585	...	585	95
DEVELOPED COUNTRIES 1974-76	335	-8	327	292
1986-88	388	-20	368	300
2000	400	-15	385	290
DEVELOPING COUNTRIES 1974-76	87	8	95	32
1986-88	136	20	156	41
2000	185	15	200	42

Figure 4   Source : FAO

Here we observe the conjunction of two limiting factors : climatic and economic. Nevertheless, potential demand exists.

6 FACTORS WHICH INFLUENCE MILK PRODUCTION

Considering the above data, we perceive the principal factors which influence milk production and its evolution.

6.1 Firstly the climatic factor : Europe, Oceania and part of the American continent have ideal climates for milk production. It is, therefore, natural to find the most important production concentration in these zones. In certain areas, there exists no alternative but grazing. Seasonal production variations, however, are important when complements of feeding concentrates are restricted or non-existent and rearing oriented towards "natural" methods (grass in New Zealand and Australia). These variations are less significant in countries with more sophisticated breeding and feeding methods (CEE, USA). In certain developing countries there are zones where the climatic conditions will never allow significant milk production.

6.2 Agricultural policies

They constitute an important element for inciting or discouraging production on a long term basis. Different systems of support are in force (internal prices, internal and external aids for the disposal of production (quotas). A decisive element will finally be the effect on the remuneration of milk at producers' level and at the level of the processing industry. For export markets, it is evident that the monetary variations will have an important influence on the different origins which now enter into competition on the world market (namely USD vs ECU). A relatively simple table shows all the aspects mentioned above, i.e. the comparison of prices at production level in the main dairy producing countries in the world.

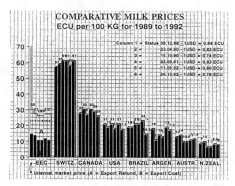

Figure 5

Internal price levels reflect the agricultural and milk policies of different countries : Switzerland with a massive support system, New Zealand where the support is at a minimum and the EEC in an intermediate situation.

This table is also interesting when comparing local prices with international market levels.

The world price follows the trends set by the big players in the world market and is obviously interacting for New Zealand exporting the main part of its production. In order to remain competitive, other countries are obliged to subsidize exports in one way or the other through compensation, bringing their internal price to the international level. Systems are different.

The EEC introduced the export refund system. These remarks apply to the whole agricultural sector. Various studies related to the GATT negotiations, on which we shall come back later, prove that practically all countries subsidize their agriculture as can be seen in the following table (Producer subsidy equivalent).

PRODUCER SUBSIDY EQUIVALENTS (PSE)

INTERNATIONAL COMPARISON

PSE IN % OF PRODUCTION VALUE	1984	1985	1986	1987	1988	1989
CANADA	31	39	49	46	43	35
AUSTRALIA	10	14	16	11	10	10
AUSTRIA	33	39	50	53	48	44
EEC	32	43	51	51	49	38
FINLAND	60	67	70	71	70	72
JAPAN	67	69	76	77	74	72
NEW ZEALAND	18	23	33	14	8	6
SWEDEN	38	40	54	61	58	47
U.S.A.	28	32	43	41	34	27
AVERAGE	34	41	51	50	45	39

PSE = AMOUNT TO BE GIVEN TO THE FARMERS TO COMPENSATE FOR INCOME LOSSES DUE TO ELIMINATION OF ALL SUPPORTS.

Figure 6

6.3 Interaction of support policies and milk production

On the one hand milk production meets the requirements of local markets and, on the other, exports. These latter represent in fresh milk equivalent about 30 mio. tonnes or about 5 to 6 % of world production.

In table 7 we can see that the part of the EEC in these exports is prominent (more than 50 %).

The small size of the segment represented by the international market and its cost for the major exporting countries are factors tending to reduce motivation towards a production increase, except for countries like New Zealand and Australia where exports are a vital element in their foreign trade. In these two countries the limiting factors are, however, due to the production structure with, as we have seen, relatively low production yields.

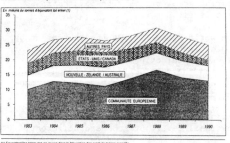

EEC IN WORLD DAIRY EXPORTS
la C.E.E. dans les exportations mondiales de produits laitiers

(1) Equivalent lait entier mis en œuvre dans la fabrication des produits laitiers exportés

Source : C.E.E.

Figure 7   International milk market

As far as local markets are concerned, the major volumes are concentrated in industrialized countries where consumption in general is high and the market relatively saturated. Even there the cost of support schemes represents a limiting factor for the authorities and production quota is one means to set these limits. In these cases, the potential for production development will depend on reforms of agricultural policies and the capacity for innovation in new products in order to give additional stimulus to the demand which fluctuates widely by product and by country.

In the long term, a positive expectation for a potential production growth lies in the Eastern European countries once they have solved their political, economic and structural problems. Developing countries where climatic conditions and milk "culture" are already present(i.e. India, China, Latin America), have a potential for growth in consumption.

6.4   Milk processing

The evolution of fresh milk production is closely linked to different product groups processed basically in line with the demand.

The following tables summarize the main production trends for butter, cheese, skimmed and full cream milk powders, concentrated milk and casein.

CONSUMPTION
PER CAPITA CONSUMPTION (KG/CAP)

La consommation

la consommation humaine par habitant
des principaux produits laitiers dans le Monde

Année 1990   Unité : kg de produit

· LAITS LIQUIDES (1) LIQUID MILKS		CRÈME (2) CREAM	
Islande	197,5	Suède	2,88
Irlande	184,1	Danemark	2,75
Finlande	178,7	Luxembourg	2,58
Norvège	158,8	Islande	2,48
Suède	135,9	Norvège	2,45
U.R.S.S. (5)	133,1	Suisse	2,28
Nouvelle-Zélande (3)	123,3	Finlande	2,05
Royaume-Uni	121,2	R.F.A.	1,98
Danemark	120,6	U.R.S.S. (5)	1,58
U.S.A. (3) (5)	107,5	Hongrie	1,46
Suisse	105,9	Autriche	1,32
Tchécoslovaquie	104,7	Belgique	1,25
Australie (4)	103,6	Tchécoslovaquie (5)	1,11
Espagne	101,0	Royaume-Uni	1,08
Autriche	94,0	Australie (5)	1,02
Canada	92,0	Pays-Bas	0,97
Pays-Bas	90,0	France	0,92
Portugal (5)	79,2	Israël (5)	0,91
Luxembourg	79,1	Italie	0,81
Italie	78,6	Grèce	0,80
France	77,1	Irlande	0,75
Hongrie	75,5	Canada	0,66
R.F.A.	70,8	Espagne	0,35
Belgique	69,8	Afrique du Sud	0,27
Israël (5)	68,5	Chili	0,20
Grèce	66,9	Japon	0,16
Inde	53,9	Portugal	0,10
Japon	41,9		
Afrique du Sud	40,8		

(1) Non compris les laits aromatisés
(2) La crème est exprimée en équivalent M.G. butyrique
(3) Y compris la crème, en équivalent lait
(4) Y compris les laits aromatisés
(5) Résultats 1989

Source : F.I.L., O.S.C.E.

BEURRE (1) BUTTER		FROMAGES (2) CHEESES	
Nouvelle-Zélande	9,9	France	22,8
Danemark	9,3	Italie	18,6
France	8,3	R.F.A.	18,5
Belgique	7,7	Grèce	18,0
Tchécoslovaquie	7,7	Belgique	17,7
Finlande	6,6	Luxembourg	17,1
R.F.A.	6,5	Islande	16,4
Luxembourg	6,3	Suède	16,4
Irlande	5,8	Israël	16,2
Suisse	5,6	Suisse	16,2
Suède	5,4	Pays-Bas	15,0
U.R.S.S. (3)	5,4	Danemark	14,8
Islande	4,9	Canada	14,0
Autriche	4,5	Finlande	13,6
Royaume-Uni	3,8	Norvège	12,7
Canada	3,6	U.S.A. (3)	12,3
Pays-Bas	3,5	Tchécoslovaquie	12,1
Norvège	3,1	Autriche	11,0
Australie	2,9	Australie	8,9
Italie	2,0	Royaume-Uni	8,6
U.S.A. (3)	1,9	Nouvelle-Zélande	7,7
Hongrie	1,6	U.R.S.S. (3)	6,6
Inde	1,4	Hongrie	6,3
Portugal	1,4	Espagne	5,6
Grèce	1,0	Irlande	5,5
Japon	0,7	Portugal	5,1
Israël	0,6	Chili	3,8
Afrique du Sud	0,5	Afrique du Sud	1,6
Espagne	0,5	Japon	1,2
Chili	0,5	Inde	0,2

(1) Beurre + M.G. butyrique, en équivalent beurre
(2) Y compris les fromages frais
(3) Résultats 1989

Figure 8   Consumption

la production de beurre
Butter production

Unité : 1.000 tonnes

Régions Années	1988	1990	1991 (p)	1992 (1)
Europe Occidentale	1.913	1.990	2.026	1.997
dont :				
C.E.E. à 12 (2)	1.690	1.752	1.807	1.780
dont :				
France (2)	523	541	480	460
Finlande	61	63	54	52
Suède	61	76	65	60
Suisse	36	38	37	37
Europe Orientale	834	816	513	520
U.R.S.S. (3)	1.724	1.730	1.600	1.550
Amérique du Sud	104	118	111	118
Amérique du Nord	684	722	754	695
dont :				
U.S.A.	547	591	620	560
Canada	105	97	100	100
Afrique du Sud	15	21	18	18
Inde	850	970	1.040	1.020
Japon	68	76	70	76
Océanie	374	387	383	378
dont :				
Australie	98	111	114	111
Nouvelle-Zélande	276	276	269	267
TOTAL	6.566	6.830	6.515	6.372

(p) Résultats provisoires
(1) Prévision
(2) Production totale : laitière (beurre, M.G.L.A.) + fabrications fermières ; incluant à partir de 1991, les données des territoires de l'ex-R.D.A. dans le total C.E.E.
(3) Les chiffres 1991 et 1992 se rapportent aux territoires de l'ex-U.R.S.S.

Source : U.S.D.A.

56

la production de fromages
Cheese production

Unité : 1.000 tonnes

Régions Années	1988	1990	1991 (p)	1992 (1)
Europe Occidentale	5.240	5.501	5.648	5.754
dont :				
C.E.E. à 12 (2)	4.758	5.011	5.168	5.273
dont :				
France (2)	1.383	1.471	1.494	1.530
Finlande	75	81	73	72
Suède	115	108	107	109
Suisse	134	138	139	140
Europe Orientale	604	613	465	466
U.R.S.S. (3)	894	881	800	770
Amérique du Sud	561	566	592	590
Amérique du Nord	3.149	3.383	3.345	3.535
dont :				
U.S.A.	2.527	2.749	2.695	2.885
Canada	252	250	255	250
Afrique du Sud	43	48	46	47
Japon	26	28	29	30
Océanie	304	297	301	309
dont :				
Australie	176	175	176	180
Nouvelle-Zélande	128	122	125	129
TOTAL	10.821	11.317	11.226	11.501

(p) Résultats provisoires
(1) Prévision
(2) Toutes catégories (exceptés les fromages fondus), tous laits, y compris les productions fermières ; incluant à partir de 1991, les données des territoires de l'ex-R.D.A. dans le total C.E.E. .
(3) Les chiffres 1991 et 1992 se rapportent aux territoires de l'ex-U.R.S.S.
Source : U.S.D.A.

la production de lait écrémé en poudre
Skimmed milk powder

Unité : 1.000 tonnes

Régions Années	1988	1990	1991 (p)	1992 (1)
Europe Occidentale	1.473	1.794	1.610	1.491
dont :				
C.E.E. à 12 (2)	1.350	1.665	1.509	1.400
dont :				
France (2)	480	580	452	450
Finlande	28	22	15	15
Suède	36	51	29	20
Suisse	36	32	31	31
Europe Orientale	169	185	168	159
U.R.S.S. (3)	350	300	280	260
Amérique du Sud	70	101	88	94
Amérique du Nord	559	502	512	450
dont :				
U.S.A.	444	398	410	350
Canada	110	95	93	91
Afrique du Sud	19	26	21	20
Inde	80	72	65	75
Japon	159	179	170	176
Océanie	318	352	326	316
dont :				
Australie	120	144	155	151
Nouvelle-Zélande	198	208	171	165
TOTAL	3.197	3.511	3.240	3.041

(p) Résultats provisoires
(1) Prévision
(2) Vrac et conditionné, y compris babeurre en poudre
(3) Les chiffres 1991 et 1992 se rapportent aux territoires de l'ex-U.R.S.S.
Source : U.S.D.A.

la production de lait entier en poudre
Whole milk powder production

Unité : 1.000 tonnes

Régions Années	1987	1988	1989	1990
C.E.E. à 12	893	925	890	823
U.R.S.S.	310	303	300	287
Brésil	150	130	130	135
Nouvelle-Zélande	170	184	174	234
U.S.A.	66	78	81	72
Argentine	93	87	115	84
Australie	65	68	67	49

la production de laits concentrés
Concentrated milk production

Unité : 1.000 tonnes

Régions Années	1987	1988	1989	1990
C.E.E. à 12	1.285	1.333	1.307	1.256
U.S.A.	260	268	232	264
U.R.S.S.	595	673	670	695
Canada	100	84	15	4
Australie	60	82	80	44

la production de caséines
Casein production

Unité : 1.000 tonnes

Régions Années	1987	1988	1989	1990
C.E.E. à 12	176	183	151	104
Nouvelle-Zélande	62	66	56	64
Pologne	22	24	33	38
Australie	8	9	7	5

Summarizing, we note a worldwide tendency towards decrease in production of butter, skimmed milk powder, whilst there is an increase foreseen for cheeses, full cream milk powders and also for liquid milks and fresh milk products. The latest indications we have been able to obtain for all these products are as follows :

Butter and butter oil :
  further decline of 2.5 % in 1992 and 2 % foreseen for 1993

Cheeses :
  1 % increase in 1992 and 1 % increase foreseen for 1993.

Skimmed milk powder :
  8 % production decrease in 1992. Further decrease in 1993.

Full cream milk powder :
  the production has globally increased in 1991. This trend slowed down in 1992 as a result of a decrease in the EEC, compensated by an important increase in New Zealand.

Sweetened condensed milk and evaporated milk:
  the relative decrease of production noted during the eighties has been compensated by a switch of certain big markets to full cream milk powder.

Casein :
  the level of production of casein depends on the one hand on the regular and constant requirements of the product and, on the other, on the relative returns obtained from other milk based products. Internal aids are granted in some countries. Concretely, in the EEC it has been reduced in 1992. After an increasing world production by 13 % in 1992, the European production will certainly be lower in 1993, leading to a slight reduction of total output.

Lactoserum :
  This production is linked to the manu-

facture of cheese with increased volumes. Environmental measures prohibit now certain countries to dispose of this ingredient as waste. This will probably stimulate production in future.

6.5. Consumption and prices

Finally, the basic element which is at the origin of all production : consumption which is in turn closely related to price levels.

In 1992, world consumption of liquid and fresh milk products increased by 1 %, very strongly in Asia but diminished in Eastern Europe. The tendency of an increased demand for products with low fat content continues.

Simultaneously, we note a decrease of consumption of butter by 2% between 1991 and 1992. The decrease in Eastern countries continues, mainly for economic reasons. This same tendency is also reflected for skimmed milk powder. However, the consumption of cheese increased by about 2 % p.a. in the eighties and particularly in speciality cheeses. This tendency is to continue in 1993. The consumption of lactoserum has also increased, mainly for usage in dietetic and pharmaceutical products. The same is true for concentrated milks and casein in 1992.

World prices of milk products in the beginning of the eighties remained relatively levelled, as shown in the following table covering 13 years since the creation of the International Dairy Agreement (sort of GATT for dairy sector). In 1982 an important increase of production, not followed by demand, led to decreases in prices due to a strong building up of stocks. In 1986 and 1987 an upward price movement for powders and cheese took place and later on for fat. Prices reached a record level in 1988.

The different tendencies for milk components are clear : proteins (skimmed milk powder) with firm prices and in competition with vegetable proteins (mainly soya) in opposition to butter and butter-oil with prices lowering in spite of the strong decreases of world stocks. The reduction of imports by Eastern Europe (Russia) partly explains this movement. Fluctuations of world prices also depend on fluctuations of exchange rates (mainly USD against European currencies).

7 MILK POLICIES

For some time, and this tendency can be extrapolated on a long-term basis, there has been a marked intention to liberalize the milk market and diminish state interventions. The object is to reduce the costly export mea-

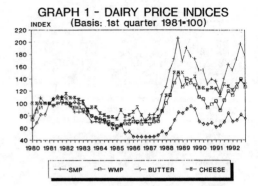

Figure 10   Price indexes for milk products

sures (including stocks) and to re-organize production as well as a better control of milk processing in particular in Europe.

The most important producer countries have tried to reduce their expenses for the dairy sector during the last two years and several of them have maintained or even reduced their production quotas.

Additional efforts are orientated towards quality products and the diversification towards more added value, and this tendency will continue.

It is also important to note that one of the priorities of the milk sector in developing countries consists in the import of high yielding breeding livestock and the improvement of animal feeding practises.

The dramatic situation in Central Europe and in the East will unfortunately still require some time before a real development in these regions can be expected.

In general, the potential for the increase of productivity certainly exists in many parts of the world and depends on genetic improvements, feeding and technological progress.

The milk sector will remain in competition with imitation products, all the more since the dairy prices will be firmer. Nevertheless, the consumer easily perceives the differences with milk (taste, usage) which makes this competition relative. Furthermore, they still generally contain important quantities of milk components (casein, lactoserum and skimmed milk powder).

CONCLUSION

An encouraging future for the milk sector may

be predicted in spite of the difficult stages
it has currently to face. An important factor
for its success and the rapidity with which
such success will be reached is conditioned
by the signature of the GATT agreement where
negotiations have been dragging along for the
last seven years. An agreement favouring
exchanges and restating, at least in part,
the laws of supply and demand would give a
new impulse to the world economy of which
the milk sector is a component. This would
also revitalize the International Dairy
Agreement which, for the moment, still remains imperfect and non representative (only
16 members).

A failure of GATT would create new pro-
tectionist measures and a general lack of
confidence. This would represent a break or
even a stop of the process of development
which we all would like to continue to be
more and more liberalized.

REFERENCES

FAO, Perspectives de l'alimentation, De-
    cember 1992
IDF, International Dairy situation and out-
    look, W. Krostitz, Oct. 1991
CNIEL (Centre National Interprofessionnel de
    l'Economie laitière), L'Economie laitière
    en chiffres, mai 1992
EEC Commission
OSCE (Office de statistique de la Communauté
    Européenne)
USDA
GATT - Status report on the World Market for
    dairy products, March 1993

Dairy Products in Human Health and Nutrition, Serrano Ríos et al. (eds) © 1994 Balkema, Rotterdam, ISBN 90 5410 359 0

The economy of milk production: A worldwide overview

H. Schelhaas
Commodity Board for Dairy Produce, Netherlands

ABSTRACT: The economic problems in dairying in the three principal milk producing regions are completely different: from reorientation in dairy policy in the Western countries, arisis in Eastern Europe to undersupply in developing countries. Causes are assessed and future developments are analysed. It is concluded that much will depend on the final outcome of the GATT Negotiations.

1 INTRODUCTION

The origin of dairying lies in the Middle East. To be precise: the start of keeping milk cows for human purposes lies in Mesopotamia, about 6,000-7,000 years B.C. From this region dairying spreads to other regions, to Asia, Europe, North and East Africa.

For not more than about a hundred years, the greater part of world dairying has taken place in the Western countries (Western Europe and North America). But the percentage of milk production taking place in the Western countries has been decreasing again since the beginning of the eighties and will most probably decrease further in the coming decades.

Percentage of world milk production

	1970	1980	1990	2000*
Western countries (including Oceania)	50	49	44	40
Eastern Europe	29	28	28	24
Developing countries	21	23	28	36

* Forecast

The economic problems in dairying in the above mentioned three principal milkproducing regions are completely different. In the developed countries the major problem is how to create an acceptable balance between supply and demand while maintaining reasonable farm incomes and the habitability of the country-side.

In Eastern Europe the principal problem is how to solve the serious crisis in dairying - which has led to a substantial decrease in production and sales - caused by the transition from a command economy to a market economy.

In the developing countries the principal problem is how to stimulate milk production as much as possible, in order to supply more food and to create employment.

2 THE ECONOMIC PROBLEMS OF THE WESTERN COUNTRIES

2.1 *Introduction*

The Western dairy industry has been characterized by rapid changes in recent decades. These changes will, it is expected, gather pace even further in the coming years. Of Western society as a whole it may be said that "a whirlwind of change" is taking place; this also applies to the dairy sector. These changes will now be described below.

2.2 *The three determining factors*

The factors which have determined developments in the Western dairy industry in the recent past were the strong level of protection enjoyed by that industry, the strong growth of production technology, and the generally stagnating demand. It may be stated that, since the Second World War, the dairy industry was one of the industrial sectors that was most sheltered from the effects of the free market. Government protection enables the market to act to a very limited extent against

61

undesirable developments, especially in terms of the balance between output and sales (i.e., supply and demand). And though that protection has been reduced in recent years, the dairy industry is still one of the sectors where government exerts the greatest influence on the market process.

This relatively strong protection of the dairy sector against market influences led to a price level that, even today, is still well above the world market price level, and it was also one of the factors responsible for the creation of surpluses. The strong growth of production technology led to a strong reduction in the number of dairy farmers in the developed countries, namely from 2.5 million in 1980 to 1.6 million in 1990; a further decline to 750,000 by the year 2000 cannot be ruled out.

It may be noted that this strong reduction occurred in spite of the strong level of dairy market protection which has just been mentioned.

The stagnating demand for milk and dairy products is a feature which is common to food demand in Western countries. As incomes continue to rise, demand for food tends as a general rule to go up little if at all. There are, course, exceptions to this general rule. For example, the demand for cheese is still rising in almost all Western countries. On the other hand, demand for butter is falling while demand for liquid milk is stable.

2.3 *Changes in dairy policy*

The sharply rising dairy surpluses which featured the 1970s and the early 1980s led in many countries to the introduction of a quota system for milk production (EC, Switzerland, Canada, Finland, Sweden, Austria). At the present date, almost 70% of milk production in Western countries comes under a quota system. The principal exeptions are the United States of North America; the sharply rising demand for dairy products in that country mean that (mostly) there has been a reasonably balanced supply and demand situation. On the other hand, in recent years the level of protection has fallen in the USA and with it the milk price.

Because of the quota systems introduced in many countries, the dairy industry differs substantially from almost all other socio-economic sectors. Both inside and outside agriculture, there has since the early 1980s been a strong tendency towards a highly market-oriented policy. "Less government, more market" was - and remains - an almost universally accepted principle.

In the dairy industry, too, we see government moving into the background; this trend, however, is overshadowed by the quota systems introduced. In this situation, the scale of production is determined by means of the political decision process, and thereupon enforced by government measures.

Whether and how the dairy industry will be able to sustain this exceptional position is uncertain at this moment in time. What is certain is that the milk quota system will operate in the EC at least until the year 2000.

2.4 *Changed priorities: less attention for food production and more for the environment, landscape and nature*

Important changes are taking place in the priorities of western society. In the EC, there is no longer a shortage of food, on the contrary: too much food is being produced. According to the study entitled "Rural Areas in Europe", made on behalf of the EC and performed by the Netherlands Scientific Council for Government Policy, EC agriculture production could theoretically take place on one third of the present land area. Between 70 to 90 million hectares of farmland can be potentially earmarked for building villages and towns, recreation or nature. Food remains necessary, indeed very necessary, but it is no longer in short supply. The environment, landscape and nature, on the other hand, are in short supply. Also, animal welfare and protection of meadow birds ranks high on the list of priorities.

This means among others that the pollution caused by dairy farming to the soil, water and atmosphere must be zero or minimal. In concrete terms, in areas with environment problems this may mean a reduction of ammonia, nitrate and phosphate emissions. Possible remedies are:
- development of new manure storage systems;
- modifications of new manure storage systems;
- development of new techniques for using manure;
- limitations on the use of pesticides;
- limitations on the use of energy, detergents and packaging.

2.5 *Developments in European dairy farming*

The strong decrease of the number of milk producers in the past decades has been mentioned before.

There are at least three factors which cause us to expect these developments to accelerate, namely,
- the more market-oriented policy;
- the GATT negotiations, leading to a lower milk price in many developed countries;
- the considerable acceleration of the technological and economic progress.

Statements by experts in the Netherlands indicate that - based on the technical and economic possibilities for specialized dairy farms - by the year 2000 we must expect an average milk production per cow of between 9,000 and 10,000 kg and an average dairy herd per farm of at least 100 cows. Of course, such figures must be treated with due caution. Even the average EC dairy farm still falls short of this standard. The average milk production in the EC is about 4,600 kg and the average number of milk cows per farmer is about 20. However, there is another important trend taking place, namely the occurrence of mixed dairy farms with a secondary operation in addition to dairy (keeping different animals, recreation, landscape management, farming systems focused on nature conservation, protection of meadow birds, part-time farming, etc.).

It may be advisable, for environmental reasons or in order to improve the habitability of the country side, to stimulate this trend by government measures.

The conclusions may be:

- for specialized dairy farms within the EC, an accelerating trend seems very likely towards more cows per farm, larger milk production per cow and fewer dairy farmers;

- alongside the specialized dairy farms, an ever-growing group of mixed farms will appear, for which the requirements will be less high.

2.6 *Strong concentration in the milk processing industry*

The strong concentration everywhere in the Western industry is also taking place in the dairy processing industry, albeit in a less strong way.

The following figure showing the 10 biggest dairy manufacturers illustrates this point.

The Dairy Millionaires in the Community (1991)

No.	Name of the dairy	Country	Quantity (1,000 tonnes)
1	Campina-Melkunie Comelco	NL	4,160
2	Besnier-Bridel-Valmont	F	3,950
3	Dairy Crest	UK	3,621
4	MD Foods	DK	3,025
5	Sodiaal	F	2,600
6	Coberco-Ormet-Heino	NL	2,597
7	Northern Dairies-Express	UK	2,509
8	ULN-Souli-Corman-Sudlait	F	2,460
9	Unigate	UK	2,134
10	Noord-Nederland-Friesland	NL	1,920

It is expected that the trend towards scale enlargement will increase. There are expectations that by the year 2000 the 10 biggest dairy enterprises will be processing between 50% and 70% of all the EC milk. However, during the last year the concentration process in the dairy industry is weakening, maybe temporarily. Regarding the food market in general, it is virtually certain that by the year 2000 the 10 biggest food enterprises will account for around 80% of total turnover. As a matter of fact, the above-mentioned turnover of the present 10 biggest dairy enterprises is not extremely large bearing in mind the concentration taking place elsewhere in the food industry. In 1988, the three biggest enterprises in the food industry, namely Unilever, Nestlé and Philip Morris, each had a total turnover of more than 25 billion dollars, whereas the biggest dairy enterprise did not achieve more than about 1.5 billion dollars. Our present "giants" in the dairy processing industry are, in fact, compared with this developments, medium sized enterprises.

2.7 *The GATT negotiations*

The GATT negotiations are extremely important for the Western agriculture in general and also for the Western dairy sector. The GATT negotiations are a direct consequence of the increasing internationalization of the world. Although many countries are involved in the GATT negotiations, these remain above all a duel between the United States and the European Community. The GATT negotiations represent a substantial curb on the scope available for the national agriculture policy.

The so-called Blairhouse Agreement of the end of last year between the EC and the Common contains the following:

- freer imports into the EC: 36% reduction of import restrictions, and a minimum market access of 5% of the internal consumption,

- less subsidies on exports: 36% reduction of support to exports,

- reduction of the volumes exported: 21% volume reduction, itemized by product,

- reduction of the level of national support: by 20%, possibly compensated by means of income supplements.

No agreement has yet been reached on these proposals between the 108 partners to a GATT agreement.

At this moment the expectations regarding the conclusion of a GATT agreement in the short term are not very optimistic. Maybe not before the end of this year, a GATT agreement between 108 participants will be reached.

An agreement along the lines of the deal between the EC and the USA can have the following consequences:

- there will be a reduction in the EC

milk price in the coming years (up to 1999) and a further limitation of milk production;
- there may be major price rises on the world market for dairy products;
- even by the year 2000 - in spite of the GATT negotiations - European agriculture and the US dairy sector will still be a long way from being left at the mercy of free play between supply and demand. An important - albeit considerably reduced - support will remain for agriculture in the EC. With regard to the dairy sector, I expect that in the year 2000 there will still be intervention systems for butter and skimmed milk powder, and the EC milk quota system (known as the superlevy) will still be in operation. Income supplements will provide compensation for at any rate part of the price reduction.

The conclusion is that, even by the year 2000, neither the EC nor the USA will have a completely free dairy market. Also, by the year 2000 the dairy markets in the EC and in the USA will be more free than at the moment but nevertheless will remain organised markets.

2.8 Structural changes in the food market; purity as the symbol of the 1990s

2.8.1 Present developments

The food market is in constant motion. In recent years major changes have taken place, such as socio-demographic changes (many more single person households, small families), disappearance of traditional eating habits, a more multiracial society, more eating out, more priority for themes such as health, naturalness and freshness and more demand for food produced in an environment- and nature-friendly way.
For modern consumers, there are six key issues: Quality, Variation, Convenience, Enjoyment, Health and Distinctiveness.

Another important aspect is the increase in market segmentation. In the various market segments, the consumers require the products to satisfy different wishes. The following wishes can be distinguished:
  a. health, slimness and fitness (the healthconscious consumer, the modern woman);
  b. strength and energy (the sporting consumer);
  c. flavour and variation (the fashionable consumer);
  d. convenience, fast food (two-income families with little time to spare);
  e. long store life (the efficient consumer).

2.8.2 Future developments: purity develops to become the symbol of the 1993

New developments in the 1990s may be as follows:
- health will become an even more important factor, subdivided into the following elements: ingredients, freshness appreciation, nutritional value, purity and naturalness; light is out, organic is in; the health claim will be assessed for its true value;
- consumers will probably maintain or even intensify their efforts to reduce fat consumption;
- across the board there will be a growing aversion to things synthetic; purity develops to become the symbol of the 1990s;
- there is a (further) increase in willingness to try out new products; the life cycle of products becomes shorter and shorter, also due to the further individualization of society;
- the convenience trend will continue even more strongly, helped by the fact that deepfreezers and microwaves become commonplace; there is a future for ready-to-prepare products;
- the coming years show a shift away from choosing for appearance towards choosing for quality, for inner motivation, and for the essential. For food, this will mean that special attention will be given to its composition.
Growth in sales will have to be achieved by satisfying specific needs in the various segments, by developing new possible applications and by reacting adequately on the structural changes in the food market.

2.9 Conclusions

- The dairy industry in the developed countries has reached the limits of growth. Generally speaking, in the Western countries we see the government moving into the background. However, in the dairy industry especially in countries with a quota system of milk production, the role of government is still important.
- Also via measures intended to protect the environment, landscape and nature, the role of government is substantial in the dairy sector.
- The dairy industry in the Western countries has to meet more and more the requirements of a durable society; this without doubt will lead to higher costs.
- By adapting itself to the developments on the food market, a (further) reduction of consumption may be prevented; profitability can be improved by producing products with a high added value.

3 THE ECONOMIC PROBLEMS IN EASTERN EUROPE

3.1 *Introduction*

The changes in Eastern Europe are spectacular and dramatic. They comprise the following enormous changes: the transfer from centrally planned economics to a market economy, the introduction of democracy, the disappearance of communism and the break-up of the Soviet Union.
The introduction of a market economy surely can stimulate production in the long run. In the short term however the transitional problems have caused a serious economic crisis in nearly all Central and Eastern European countries.

3.2 *Crisis in the dairy industry: a substantial decrease in milk production*

The livestock sector as a whole and the milk sector in particular is severely affected by the transfer from centrally-planned to market-oriented economy. That the situation must be described as a crisis is by no means remarkable. The change in ownership status (the so-called privatization process), the introduction of a radical by different dairy policy, the building of a totally new infrastructure and the sudden substantial decrease in demand for dairy products are extremely drastic and time-consuming processes, the seriousness of which was underestimated at the beginning of the revolution.

The clearest sign of the crisis in the dairy sector is the substantial decrease in milk production since the revolution began. The following table illustrates the development of milk deliveries to the dairy industry since 1989, the last year before the revolution made itself felt. However, it must be remarked that the milk production has fallen less sharply than milk deliveries. This is because in many countries there has been an increase in direct supplies to consumers. A substantial direct farmer to consumer market is more or less traditional in many East European countries and has already existed for years in many countries.
Taking into account the larger direct supplies to consumers, it may be stated that total milk production in Eastern

Milk deliveries		1989	1990	1991	1992 (1,000 tons)
Poland		11,400	10,120	8,000	6,900 1)
	Index	100	89	70	61
Czechoslovakia		6,392	6,060	4,730	4,000 2)
	Index	100	95	74	63
Hungary		2,514	2,500	1,971	1,860 3)
	Index	100	99	78	74
Bulgaria		1,778	1,738	1,450	1,140 4)
	Index	100	98	82	64
Ukraine		17,836	17,940	15,480	11,400 5)
	Index	100	101	87	65
Latvia		1,977	1,770	1,540	n.a.
	Index	100	90	78	-
Estonia		1,258	1,180	920	790 6)
	Index	100	94	73	63
Lithuania		2,964	2,890	2,560	2.100
	Index	100	98	86	65
Russian Federation		40,463	37,400	30,700	22,500 7)
	Index	100	92	76	56

1) Figures based on the first eight months of 1992.
2) Figures based on the first seven months of 1992.
3) Expectation of the Hungarian government.
4) Figures based on the first six months of 1992.
5) Figures based on the first nine months of 1992.
6) IDF forecast (IDF Bulletin No. 274/1992).
7) Figures based on the first six months of 1992.

Europe fell by at least 20% in 1991 compared to 1989, and that it fell by at least 30% in 1992 compared to 1989. The largest decreases have taken place in Russia and Poland.

3.3 *Causes of the fall in milk production*

The causes of the decreases differ from country to country. However, the following factors are involved almost everywhere.
- The difficulties around privatization, which will be explained in a separate section.
- The radical change in dairy policy: the usually abrupt abolition of government support to agricultural enterprises, abolition of subsidies on use of cereals, fuel and artificial fertilizer, and abolition of interest subsidies. As a result, the prices of artificial fertilizer and other inputs soared.
- The lack of a good working new infrastructure: transition to a market economy requires more than just liberalizing prices, privatizing all former state farms and companies, and abolishing trade barriers. What is needed is an adequate infrastructure. Governments are realizing that even in the Western countries no economy is totally liberal and without government intervention.
- The generally very uncertain and unstable economic situation, which means that the risks of investments intended to improve production are very great; it would seem more advisable to wait until the climate has improved sufficiently before making those investments.
- The poor cattle feed situation, caused by rising cereal prices and by the loss of import possibilities (the collapse of the USSR, which eliminated traditional import flows, and also the lack of foreign currency); in 1992 this situation was aggravated in a number of Eastern European countries by drought, in particular in Poland.
- The lack of money for the urgently needed new investments.
- The declining productivity on the large state enterprises due to demotivation and the uncertain economic situation; in many cases the employees started in business for themselves and usually took the best cows with them.

In view of these causes, which are complicated and complex it does not seem probable that production will already recover substantially in the coming years; possibly it may even fall further, for example in Russia and the Ukraine. In the earlier mentioned study, the World Bank has expressed the expectation that production will stabilize at the present level during the coming five years.

According to a recent forecast of USDA milk production will fall by 3,5% in Eastern European countries in 1993, after a drop of 10% in 1992.

3.4 *The development of consumption*

The fall in consumption was caused by the abrupt abolition of the consumer subsidies and the decline in purchasing power. At first, especially in 1990 and the first half of 1991, the decline in consumption was larger than the decline in production. This resulted in export surpluses, which disrupted the international markets. Later, in 1991 and 1992, the fall in production exceeded the fall in consumption, and the export surpluses disappeared. According to very provisional indications, consumption levels in Poland, Hungary and Czechoslovakia even stabilized in 1992. A World Bank study refers - perhaps somewhat over-optimistically - to consolidation of consumption at 80% of the pre-1990 level, while for the coming years an annual increase in consumption might be expected in the region of 1%. If the conclusion should be correct that the decrease of consumption has already reached its deepest point, then the basis for a recovery also of milk production may be founded.

3.5 *The way to privatize is unclear*

Privatization of the large state enterprises, both in agriculture and in the dairy sector, is a very important step for successful transition from a centrally planned economy to a more market-oriented economy. So far, however, the privatization process has not managed to get going properly. The problems are largest in the privatization of the large agricultural enterprises. There are reports which indicate a strong increase in the number of private farms. For example, the number of peasant farms in Russia now totals almost 134,000, compared with just 4,400 less than two years ago.
Further analysis of these reports, however, shows them to be very small businesses which are often intended to supply the family and nothing more. In almost all countries, the greater part of agricultural production was still taking place on the large, collective enterprises. Setting up family farms, which are a feature of Western Europe and the United States, is also difficult in Eastern Europe for the following reasons:
- There are not many experienced all-round farmers on the state farms and large cooperatives, although there are for example specialized dairy cattle handlers, tractor drivers, etc.
- The real entrepreneurial mentality has still to develop after the many years of communist regime.
- There is little capital available to start a business. Similarly, not enough modernized technical equipment is available.

- Furthermore, there is a climate of great uncertainty, both financial, social and political, and this uncertain climate is certainly no incentive to accept the risk of starting an own business.

Even in East Germany, the privatization process is still in a very early stage. Since mid 1991, it has even been stagnant, among other things due to the uncertain ownership status. The number of family farms is no more than a few hundred, and some of these originate from other countries. This is all the more striking in the light of the drastic reorganisation of the dairy processing industry in East Germany. Of the 264 original dairy factories, only 56 remain; this number will continue to decrease to 26; the number of employees has fallen from 26,000 to 8,000 and will go on falling to 5,000-6,000.
In many Eastern European countries the division of large state enterprises into many small family farms has no longer been at the top of the agenda.
At present, thoughts in many countries do not extend beyond dividing up the huge mammoth enterprises into farms with several hundred dairy cows. A kind of limited liability form is then possible, for example with the employees of the farm as shareholders.

3.6 Conclusions

The entire Eastern European economy is in a deep crisis and the same applies to the dairy sector. The following conclusions are possible:
- The transition to a market economy is only in its first stage. The initial conditions were unfavourable and it is becoming clear that changing the entire institutional foundation of an economy is creating major transitional problems. This is why the initial big-bangapproach in many countries is being replaced by a more gradual approach in a growing number of countries.
- The most urgent and complicated problems are:
- how to privatize;
- how to formulate and implement a dairy policy;
- how to create the necessary infrastructure.
Uncertainty regarding the solution of these problems is the major cause of the present decline in milk production. In particular the privatization problem is crucial here. As long as the privatization problem has not been sufficiently resolved, no substantial recovery of the production may be expected. Only then can a start be made on modernizing the dairy farming sector and the dairy industry.

4 THE ECONOMIC PROBLEMS IN THE DEVELOPING COUNTRIES

4.1 Introduction

Food shortages continue to be the principal feature of the food situation in the developing countries; nevertheless in recent decades there has been a substantial growth in the world's food production. The production growth rate (2.3% a year) has even exceeded the population growth rate (1.8%). This enabled the numbers of under-nourished persons to decrease by around 100 million to around 500 million. Since 1986, however, we have seen the per capita food production stagnate at the world level. In the period 1985-1989 food production per caput decreased in not less than 94 countries. Even today, the world food situation can still be described as hunger in the midst of abundance. The problem of hunger is only solved for the majority of world's population. Projections for the coming years, amongst others as regards demographic trends and income trends, indicate that over the next 25 years the world food production will have to be doubled, that is 0.5% per year more than in the past 20 years and mainly to be realised in the developing countries. From a technological point of view it is a difficult but not impossible task.

4.2 The structure of dairying

The developing countries can be divided into traditional and non-traditional milk consuming countries. Traditionally milk producing regions are - roughly - the countries in the Mediterranean and in the Middle East, the Indian subcontinent, the Savannah regions in Western Africa and the Highlands in Eastern Africa and to a certain extent South and Central America. The consumption of milk and dairy products played an important role among the nomads in Africa and Asia.
The majority of the humid tropical regions, South East Asia, China, Korea and Japan belong to the non-traditionally milk consuming and producing countries. Nevertheless for example, in China milk was seen as very beneficial to ill and elderly people.
In the traditionally milk producing regions in Asia and also partly in Africa the structure of milk production is characterized by the small farmer with not more than 3 or 4 animals. Dairying there is nearly always part of a mixed farming system. Cattle are often also used as draught animals. Livestock are fed principally on agricultural residues, waste and on natural pastures from non-arable land. Cattle keeping and milk production is largely supported on the by-products of agriculture.
In Central and South America the size and

setup of dairying is medium-scale with mixed beef/dairy operations. Average milk production per cow is higher than in the above mentioned regions. The average here is about 1,000 kg per year but ranges from 1,400 kg to 1,900 kg in the temperate zone which covers the central part of Chile and eastern part of the Argentine, the whole of Uruguay and the southern part of Brazil.

Countries with a large milk producing capacity in the long run are the Argentine, Uruguay and Southern Chile where milk production costs, at about $ 100 per ton, are among the lowest in the world.

In the non-traditionally milk producing countries the structure of dairying is more varied. In these regions there are – besides small farms – also large scale specialized dairy farms, mostly founded in colonial times or after the Second World War.

Centrally-planned economies often opt for large scale capital-intensive and specialized state farms e.g. in Cuba, China, Ethiopia and Tanzania.

4.3 A substantial growth of milk production is possible

In the period 1983/85 to 2000, milk production in the developing countries will probably rise sharply. The FAO estimates the following annual increases in milk production on an extrapolation of past trends:

Africa (Sub-Saharan)	3.1%
North East + North Africa	3.2%
Asia (excl. China)	2.8%
Latin America	3.4%
93 developing countries	3.1%

The growth rates are roughly in line with those in the period 1970-1985. It should be noted that these countries in most cases feature a high population growth.

4.4 The demand for dairy products

In the developing countries, there is a large potential demand for milk and dairy products. At present consumption of milk and dairy products in developing countries mostly is concentrated among middle and high income groups, just as in the Western countries in the 19th century. Given increasing incomes, demand for food will rise very sharply. The income elasticity of the demand for milk and dairy products is high. The FAO estimates the income elasticity in many countries at between 0.5 and 0.8; recent studies in India even find an income elasticity of 1.2 for milk and dairy products.

The traditionally milk-consuming and milk-producing countries have experienced rising demand in dairy products, but also

the regions such as tropical Western Africa and South-East Asia, where there is little tradition for consumption of milk & milk products.

4.5 Arguments in favour of a stimulation of milk production

Provided that the conditions for milk production are favourable, the development of milk production has a number of distinct advantages, such as:
- Milk production is labour-intensive and creates employment;
- Milk production is particularly important for small farmers;
- Milk is a source of regular income;
- Employment is created in the development of dairy processing and marketing;
- The country's food situation is improved by the production of high-grade foodstuffs;
- By means of dairy cattle is often possible to convert otherwise useless agricultural residues into a high-grade food. Failure to develop dairying in vast areas of the Third World would be to lose the potential of otherwise unutilizable natural resources.

To conclude, it may be stated that the development of milk production makes it possible to improve the nutritional standard of the country and to raise rural incomes and living standards of small farmers.

4.6 Conclusions

- In the next 25 years world food production will have to be doubled, that is 0.5% per year more than in the past 20 years, mainly to be realised in the developing countries.
- In the period 1983/1985 to 2000, the FAO expects an annual increase in milk production of about 3%.
- There is a large potential demand for dairy products in the developing countries.
- Simulation of milk production is advisable for reasons of creating employment and increasing the supply of high grade food.

5 CONCLUDING REMARKS

Essential for the future developments above all is the conclusion of a GATT agreement. An important effect will most probably be a substantial improvement of world market prices.

In the Western countries the priorities in society are changing; there is less attention for food production and more for the environment, landscape and nature.

In the Eastern European countries, the essential issue is to solve the present crisis, caused by the switch from a command economy to a market oriented policy, but this surely will take time.
In the developing countries, the slogan for the coming decades is continuing growth.

2 Dairy products and human health in the world

Dairy Products in Human Health and Nutrition, Serrano Ríos et al. (eds) © 1994 Balkema, Rotterdam, ISBN 90 5410 359 0

Dairy products in human nutrition: Present and future

F. Mayor Zaragoza
U.N.E.S.C.O., Paris, France

Mr President,

These remarks are about dairy products and human nutrition, in the present and in the future. You have mentioned that I am here as a Professor in Biochemistry, as the specialist I used to be in innate metabolic errors. One of the reasons which might justify my presence here is having received from farmers and manufacturers, in the same way as my colleagues who so suitably directed the Congenital Metabolic Errors Research Team, those dairy products which would better adapt to the diet of identified pathological cases. I am here, as I have mentioned with a certain amount of flattery, as an addict consumer of milk. Dr Segovia de Arana who is present here, knows well that, for certain reasons, years ago I was, forced at first, and then with great enthusiasm, to consume a great amount of milk.

But I am also here, as our President mentioned, as General Director for UNESCO who knows and appreciates the important role that milk and dairy products play both in ordinary circumstances in school-children care and in humanitarian aid – I will come back to this later – in social emergency situations. I would also like to mention that Professor Ugarte's early suggestion has much to do with my presence here today and, above all, Dr Ana Sastre's influence in my decisions, with her efficiency, her tremendous diligence and also, why not, her perseverance.

Mr President,

Ladies and gentlemen,

This is a polyfacetic subject in which so many different aspects concur: anthropologic, chemical, bromatologic, industrial, commercial, nutritional, sociologic, economic, etc. It also has local, regional, national and international dimensions. What I find of the utmost importance is its undoubted significance in the quality of life on a world scale, particularly in the less developed countries. In exceptional circumstances, as I have already mentioned, it also interests me as one of the leading characters in all kinds of humanitarian aid programs. As befits its status of basic food for the human species, the amount of research and information accumulated on this subject is extraordinary. Therefore, without trying to view the subject exhaustively, let us make the following query: on what does the present situation of dairy products in human nutrition depend and which are its reasonable future projections?

I will try to present very quickly some of the features of its chemical composition, different dairy products, origins, feeding and cooking habits, and will briefly stop at the biological aspects, before concluding with my point of view about the future.

First of all, the chemical composition of milk and its modifications – which should always be born in mind – through physical, chemical and/or biological processes used to obtain the different dairy products or for its presentation, transport and, above all, for its preservation. It is a well-known fact that milk has a high protein content, as well as a high sugar and oligoelement content, especially calcium, with, as you all know, more than one gram per liter, but also iron, magnesium, zinc and vitamins, up to the point that one of the vitamins normally studied in General Biology, Vitamin B_2, used to be called lactoflavin, and when its composition became more fully known it started being called riboflavin. Milk is also very rich in retinol or Vitamin A, in nyacin, folic acid and Vitamin B. In fact, as might be expected being the primary food for the human species, as a mammal, and of all those species sharing this characteristic, all those elements which are necessary for growth are present in milk. Using the adequate additives and treatments, milk is adapted, transformed in new-born infant formula, made to resemble more the physical and chemical characteristics of the mother's milk. Or it can be adapted according to medical and dietetical objectives. Thus, for example, non-fat dairy products represent a way to establish a decreasing gradient of fats and all liposoluble components. Maintaining a chemical composition adapted to different situations calls for very sophisticated processes. Here, the quality of hygiene is essential. Milk is a true rawstuff from which an extremely wide range of dairy products emerge, besides its direct utilization. Some of the most outstanding dairy products are butter, cheese, cream, yoghurt, kefir and all fermented milks. In my travels around the world I have been able to verify just how far, in many countries, tradition has deep scientifical roots, especially as regards the transformation of milk by means of fermentation.

Liquid milk consumption in all its forms represents between 200 and 500 grams per person/day in the European Community, 45 times the consumption of powdered, condensed or evaporated milk, 22 times the consumption of all types of cheese and 15 times the consumption of yoghurt, in spite of the spectacular increase there has been, in yoghurt consumption in the past ten years. We find cows', goats', sheeps', camels' and other animals' milk, depending on its place of *origin*. Cows' milk, with an annual figure of 462 tons/year (1988 figures) represents 57 times the figure of goats' milk (between 8 and 9 tons). Nevertheless, both goats' and sheep's milk are very much appreciated in the Mediterranean area, especially because of the cheese made from those kinds of milk. As regards sheep's milk, we are not to forget its importance in Asia. The world is 'large and wide' and therefore we should not only consider Spanish or EC figures but also those figures from countries who are important producers of milk and dairy products.

Therefore, both from a scientific and from a strategic point of view we should have an open vision of the production of milk, its origins and different dairy products in the whole world. There is an evident influence here – that of *feeding habits* – so very different according to place, condition and age. Nutritional tradition evolves following culinary practices and according to certain recommendations of dietetic patterns, some of a scientific nature, some not, spreading all over the world. In the last 30 years, the influence of audiovisual media has been extraordinary in this sense. We have seen how traditions – some of them very deeply-set – in many countries, concerning the consumption of milk and dairy products have been substantially modified. Consumption, as I said before, is universal for the human species, characterized, just as all other mammals, by having milk as its primary nutritional source.

Thus, it is obvious that milk must contain all the necessary elements for an adequate development, especially in the first months of life. It provides aminoacids, energetic substrata, sugar and lipids, vitamins and mineral elements, especially calcium, necessary for cellular proliferation and osteogenesis. Milk is a complete and essential food, easily adaptable to the characteristics of each period in life, not only childhood but also adolescence and pregnancy. Thus in adults and the aged, those components which were essential for tissue and bone development are now essential to compensate demineralization, osteoporosis and other complaints arriving precisely at life's decline, when processes have different patterns and rhythms from those of the first years of life.

Fortunately, much research has been carried out in Spain about chemical composition resulting from the application of different cooking recipes and obtention of dairy products which can provide specialists with the exact information of the composition of the ingesta. I would like to insist in this point. Generally speaking, the information available is very general and often we do not realize that cooking treatments and the preparation of dairy products can modify considerably the properties of the original foodstuff. All this is of great importance to establish diets with scientifical rigueur and not following advertising interests or amateur or charlatan recommendations. I will come back to this in a few moments.

I will now mention *physiopathological aspects* of milk. The metabolism of milk has been studied in great depth, as well as that of some of the best-known dairy products such as yoghurt and fermented milk. Nevertheless, when we consider that the present situation is exceptionally dynamic, with a tremendous amount of innovation, research should also evolve very quickly. Concerning pathologies, galactosemia and lactase intolerance are today known in great detail. We have a tremendous amount of information which allows us to know not only the disease as a whole, but also the means for early detection, which is so advisable. Fenilcetanuria and organoaciduria are metabolic alterations of post-natal manifestation whose treatment requires a specific diet and dairy products which do not contain certain milk components. Therefore, supplying infant formulae devoid of some of these aminoacids – fenilalanine for example – is basic for the treatment of these cases (numerically very few in Spain, as only one in every ten thousand babies presents fenilcetanuria at birth, but very important from the sanitary point of view of quality of life at a national scale). The prevention of infant subnormality today is not merely a possibility, but an ethical exigence.

In this field, as well as in others (those of fatty acids and sweeteners and other food compounds), conclusions with no scientific value and insufficient perspective have been widely divulged. These rash divulgations have probably been made in good faith. Thus, the role of cholesterol, its levels and how it can be regulated have become so popular that arteriosclerosis, ischemia, osteoporosis, have become commonplace topics. And nevertheless, few foodstuffs allow such a wide range of possibilities of adaptation, of modulation, as milk, which offers this great versatility allowing the addition or suppression of different elements, remaking it according to our specific needs. The composition of milk cannot be judged, on the other hand, without considering the rest of the diet; how much its composition – and consequently the nature of its variants and by-products – can adapt to global ranges recommended for different situations and disfunctions, depends on the diet as a whole, and in some infrequent cases, it also depends on digestive peculiarities either acquired or congenital. It likewise depends, as I have already mentioned, on the cooking method and treatment of food.

On the other hand, cholesterol is by no means the only cause of arterovenous functional decline which is also influenced by a series of risk factors (vehicular proteins, circulating lipids, thrombogenic elements, etc.) and personal habits such as smoking or an excessively sedentary life. Age also intervenes, as well as place of residence and cooking habits and other concomitant pathologies such as diabetes, without forgetting, in this case, the individual's gender and, not only because of biological factors but also because of social factors, as is evidenced by a higher incidence in men than women in similar geographico-social and ingesta conditions.

Thus, most Europeans, less accustomed to olive and other vegetable oils than their Mediterranean neighbours, consume ten times more butter and three times more cheese than people in Spain. It is the influence of what could be called 'product of the land' and tradition. It is therefore quite clear that, scientifically speaking one cannot make generalizations with respect to feeding and cooking habits nor with respect to age, gender and lifestyle. The simplicity of some current recipes, greatly defended and fervently followed by some otherwise cultured people does not consider that living creatures, with the wisdom of metabolic balance, possess mechanisms which transform glucids into lipids and proteins. This is well evidenced by obesity in people who eat great quantities of carbohydrates.

It is quite clear then that ingesta is modulated by our endogenous transformation capacity and prescriptions should be personalized, appealing when necessary to the specialist physician, but that it is very dangerous to follow, because of advertising patterns or widespread recipes, any dietetical pattern which is not based in scientific rigueur.

The future, ladies and gentlemen, depends, just like the present, on three main issues: production, industrialization and consumption. Production depends in turn on genetic quality, an issue where an extraordinary field is currently being developed, with all the opportunities that the knowledge of transgenic beings and the skills offered by genetic engineering to improve the quality of cattle, which, in turn depends on environmental and feeding conditions and extraction techniques.

In the second place we have industrialization. Progressive and competitive diversification has led in the last years, especially in the EC, to an extraordinary degree of technification both in preservation processes and obtention of dairy products and in presentation and transport formulae. But in all this, as in any other market, the most important part is consumption, from the product's point of view, the industrial point of view, and, especially, the consumer himself. The consumer's perspective is essential in any type of market. The important thing, in my opinion, is to consolidate the number of already existing consumers and to extend their number with a wider view of the international market for milk and dairy products. In this respect we have to point out the importance of extraction and preservation techniques, milking and refrigeration, thermic treatments. EC rules and regulations and, in general, those directives concerning procedures, additives, etc. should be strict, as I said before, but they should adapt, and adapt very quickly, to a very exacting market in all its aspects: quality, economy, competence, etc.

In spite of the tremendous increase in consumption of the last decades, in the EC there are still large quantities of surplus butter, cheese and milk. Supply is still higher than demand. Therefore, and I am now speaking as the General Director of an Organization which, together with the United Nations Refugee High Commission, The World Food Program, the OMS and UNICEF, is in charge of humanitarian aid programs, which occur immediately after help programs – in exceptional circumstances we could imagine *a huge world-wide food agreement* which would be part of the *new security measures* which will soon have to be adopted all over the world. It is true that extreme poverty leads to radicalization and violence and also leads, and Spain knows this well, to massive emigrations. If there has been something positive about Somalia, this collective shame, it is that it has reminded us of the most important of the Commandments – Thou shalt not kill. And, nevertheless, every day and day after day, thousands of human beings, our brothers, die of hunger...

It is a question of security at an international scale. The United Nations was emerged almost fifty years ago when different nations got together to face the dangers of a nuclear conflagration. At that time, security was threatened by nuclear war. Fifty years later, international security is threatened by other reasons: extreme poverty, ignorance, inability for interethnic co-existence and intercultural dialogue and degradation of the environment. Against these new threats we need new strategies, and one of them is to avoid poverty in the world. To avoid it we must learn how to invest, just as we invest in armament, armies and other sections of defense, in this new mode for defense, that is to say, provide, at an international scale, the possibility, for all human beings, of surviving with dignity.

Planetary markets are, in my opinion, within a very reasonable vision of the future. Milk and dairy products are an essential part of these large new international markets and should be financed just as the defense of international security and of frontiers is financed.

As an example I would like to remind you that the cost of United Nations military presence in Cambodia is currently 1,500 million dollars, while the sum allotted to alleviate hunger, provide a better quality of life or to provide education for Cambodians is, at present, less than 30 million dollars. If I quote these figures it is just to show that the capacity exists to make this change of relative weight in the kind of investments that should be made at an international scale to face the new threats of our age.

Spain knows how many illegal immigrants arrived in our country last year and knows all about the problems posed by this issue with regard to human rights. The sphere of democracy is not only national; there is also an international sphere for democracy. We cannot apply a set of rights to the inhabitants of the country in question and a different set of rights to those people coming from outside just because the circumstances existing in their homeland are such that they have been forced to leave. We have to remember every day that the Declaration of Human Rights is a *universal* declaration and that these rights are for all people and each person in particular. I am saying this because, in my opinion, the myopic vision of local markets, national or regional, such as European markets, will soon have to transform itself into a much more global vision of markets and of the competencies which will have to be exercised to be able to stay in them.

In my opinion, the improvements that are applicable to the different sources can be divided in three groups, namely, genetic improvement, improvement in production and improvement in industrial procedures. Concerning genetics, it is possible to improve by means of the race, or in the same race, the composition and quantity. When I speak of composition I am also referring to physical characteristics. We could even consider such important details as better biological characteristics for the improvement of mechanical extraction.

In the second place, production, with the fundamental aspect of veterinary health care, hygiene, as well as the conditions of the premises where the animals are housed, the way animals are handled, milking procedures and, above all, the food they are given.

Finally, although I shall not linger on this subject, as all of you know much more about it than I do, manipulations and transformations of all kinds at an industrial scale, to which can be added an extraordinarily important aspect of our days: transport systems. The importance, already emphasized, of feeding habits, has a very good example, in my opinion in yoghurt. Between 1964 and 1980, the general consumption of milk and dairy products increased by 73%. It is a really important increase for a consumer product, especially if we bear in mind the evolution of the population during the same period. And in this figure, the most spectacular increase is found in the consumption of yoghurt, together with infant formulae and dairy products adapted to the feeding possibilities of children, sick people and the aged. All of them are good examples of expansion in the already existing markets but, as I mentioned before, their use can still be promoted, just as in many other countries in which milk and dairy products are present in a large quantity of local dishes and not exclusively breakfast or tea-time, but also in stews and desserts and as a conveyance for ice-cream, milk-shakes, cereal, etc.

For all this, Mr President, to improve the present products, expand their number in the national market and their competitivity in the European market, to start, as from now, thinking and designing nutrition plans on a world scale so that the principle of solidarity which today is fundamental for world security can be put into practice, the best ally is, in spite of all, science. Only scientific rigueur can temper at a short term the purely economic interests and provide a solid base for a projection for the future which contributes to increase the quality of human life in the whole planet.

Thank you very much.

Dairy Products in Human Health and Nutrition, Serrano Ríos et al. (eds) © 1994 Balkema, Rotterdam, ISBN 90 5410 359 0

Meeting dietary nutrient requirements with cow's milk and milk products

D.J.Bissonnette & K.N.Jeejeebhoy
University of Toronto, Ont., Canada

ABSTRACT: The high nutrient density of milk makes it a valuable food in human nutrition. It is often an important component of school breakfast programs and was part of the Montreal Diet Dispensary program for the nutritional management of the underprivileged since 1879 and of specifically pregnant women since 1948. Similarly the National Health Service in Chile, introduced in 1970 a milk distribution program that provided 500 ml to each Chilean child, pregnant and nursing mother. The high biological value and digestibility of milk protein has risen it to prominence as an effective supplement to the normal diet. This is of particular interest to children, pregnant women and the elderly. The wide spectrum of micronutrients available in many milk products ensures a significant contribution towards meeting the RNI (recommended nutrient intake) for calcium, phosphorus, potassium, chromium, riboflavin, pantothenic acid, niacin, zinc and cobalamin.

1 INTRODUCTION

The role of milk in the human diet stems back to the domestication of the cow by nomadic populations as far back as 9000 B.C.. Soon after, butter and cheese were produced and became an important staple of the diet because of the relative stability and ease of transportation. Milk has endured as one of the main components of the human diet because of the diversity of by-products that were produced from it and from which are associated a wide spectrum of aromas and flavors. Hence, it is no wonder that cheese became one of the great delicacies of Roman imperial dining. The Greek Olympians recognized cheese as a food of unusual sustaining power and included it as part of their training diet along with dried fruits.

The high nutrient density of milk and its by-products gives it a role of prominence amidts the fast pace life-styles of industrialized countries, where eating habits are often rushed and where concern for fat intake may cause unnecessary food restrictions. Its importance is also evident among the poor of these nations as well as among the people of developing countries requiring protein of greater biological value.

It is important and timely to put this food group into perspective and critically examine its features, using our current understanding of human nutrient requirements. We propose, in the following discussion on nutrient needs, to first explore the basis for our energy, protein, carbohydrate and fat requirements as well as briefly outline the rational behind determining our micronutrient needs. In a second step, we will discuss the composition of milk as it relates to these needs and to disease.

2 ENERGY AND NUTRIENT REQUIREMENTS

The recommended energy and nutrient intakes (RNI) for each generalized age group is displayed in Table 1 and are based on means and ranges determined by the findings of the Bureau of Nutritional Sciences of the Health Protection Branch of Health and Welfare Canada. The values were obtained using guidelines established by the 1985 report of the FAO/WHO/UNU.

Several requirements are calculated using mean weights found in Table 2.

TABLE 1. Nutrient requirements

	Children 1-12 y	Adolescents 13-18 y	Men 19 - 74 y	Women	Preg+ Lactn	+75 y
E° (Kcal/kg)	61-101	40-57	36	32	+300-500Kcal	26
Macronutrients						
CHO (g)	207-343	294-419	366	273	327	238
Protein (g/kg)	1.1-1.7	0.8-1.0	0.82	0.75	+5-24	0.78
Fat Total (g)	50-83	71-101	91	66	+13	58
n-6 (g)	4-8	7-11	8-10	7	+0.9	7
n-3 (g)	0.6-1.4	1.2-1.8	1.45	1.15	+0.16	1.05
Minerals						
Ca (mg)	500-1100	700-1100	800	750	+500	800
P (mg)	300-800	850-1000	1000	850	+200	925
Mg (mg)	40-135	180-230	247	203	+42.5	220
K (mg)	234-312	500	624	546	39-468	546
Na (mg)	138-230	80-230	80	80	+69-230	80
Trace Elements						
Fe (mg)	6-8	10-13	9	8-13	+5-10	8.5
Zn (mg)	4-9	9-12	12	9	+6	9-12
Cu (mg)	0.05-0.1mg/kg	2	2	2	**	2
Cr (μg)	**	**	20	30	+0.15	25
Se (μg)	**	**	50	50	**	50
Mn (mg)	**	**	3.5	3.5	**	3.5
Mo (μg)	**	**	48-96	48-96	**	**
Vitamins (Fat Soluble)						
A (RE)	400-800	800-1000	800	1000	100-400	900
D (μg)	2.5-10	2.5-5	2.5-5	2.5-5	+2.5	5
E (mg)	3-8	7-10	8.7	6.3	+2.25	5.5
vK(μg)	**	**	10-25	10-25	**	17.5
Vitamins (Water Soluble)						
B1 (mg)	0.43-1.2	0.80-1.3	1.05	0.8	same	0.8
B2 (mg)	0.53-1.5	1.0-1.6	1.31	1.0	+0.35	.9
Niacin (NE)	7.6-21.3	14.3-23.0	18.92	14.28	+2-3	12.9
B6 (mg)	0.27-0.77	0.55-0.9	0.93	0.70	+0.22	0.80
Panth (mg)	2.4-6.8	4.5-7.4	5-7	5-7	**	6
Folate (μg)	40-126	168-217	226	192	+100-300	206
C (mg)	20-25	30-40	40	30	+10-25	35
B12 (μg)	0.3-1.0	1.5-1.9	2.0	2.0	+0.5-1	2.0

References: Adapted from Murray et al., 1990; FAO/WHO/UNU., 1985.
** (Requirements are not known)

2.1 Energy requirements .

The energy requirement of an individual is based on the total energy expenditure of the body . In normal persons, this will depend upon the mean activity factor of the individual, and the REE (resting energy expenditure) which is dependent on BMI (Body Mass Index). The aim is to adjust intake to meet expenditure and in so doing, obtain energy balance. From a public health standpoint, recommended energy intakes for adults 19 years of age and up, are based on the ability to successfully maintain males and females of various age groupings within a desirable BMI range, which is associated with the lowest health risks.

Energy is derived from all three macronutrients; namely proteins, carbohydrates, and fats. These nutrients act as sources of energy after transformations by hydrolysis into amino acids, monosaccharides and fatty acids and glycerol respectively. The gross energy value of carbohydrates, proteins and fats are 4, 4, and 9 kcal/g of weight respectively.

2.2 Protein requirements.

Dietary protein requirements are based on factorial and N balance studies that establish nitrogen needs for maintenance and growth. 2 SD have been added as a safety margin. The protein requirements are also altered by the energy intake. The more abundant the non-protein energy, the more efficient is the utilization of protein for tissue building and N balance. Based on the FAO/WHO/UNU (1985) report, average requirements for maintenance are approximated at 0.6g/kg/day for normal adults. This value is then adjusted by 2 SD using a coefficient of variability of 12.5%. For growth, the CV is 32% (Beaton & Chery, 1988). The amount of dietary protein required to meet these needs is close to our RNI in Canada, when the quality of the protein is taken into account (Murray, 1990). The quality is based on an amino acid composition, which permits the most efficient nitrogen retention. High quality proteins usually have a larger proportion of essential amino acids (EAA). Egg and milk proteins are used as the gold standards for quality. Children need more essential amino acids during periods of active growth (Jansen 1978). The elderly who take less energy, need a higher quality animal protein for N balance. It has also been speculated that higher quality protein in the aged could prevent metabolic disorders related to the liver (Gersovitz, 1982)

2.3 Carbohydrate requirements

Carbohydrates are seen as a valuable source of readily available energy. Complex carbohydrate in the form of starch is more slowly digested than the simpler disaccharides and are often associated with a wide variety of B complex vitamins which are key components in energy metabolism.

A total of about 400 g of carbohydrate is eaten per day in a normal diet; 50-60 percent as starch; 30 per cent as sucrose; and 10 per cent as lactose. Starch is made up of 80 per cent amylopectin and 20 per cent amylose. Amylose is a straight-chain molecule with alpha(1--4) linkages. In contrast amylopectin, in addition to these linkages, has brancl points with alpha(1-- 6) linkages. Sucrose and lactose are disaccharides composed of glucose and fructose (sucrose) and glucose and galactose (lactose) respectively.

2.4 Fat requirements

Our dependency on dietary fat is seen from three perspectives. First, the caloric density of fat is such that it contains more than double the calories per gram than either protein or carbohydrate and is therefore a rich caloric contributor to the diet. Second, fat is the medium by which fat soluble vitamins are taken in the diet. Third, 95 % of dietary fat is in the form of triglycerides and is composed of long chain fatty acids that are either saturated, monounsaturated or polyunsaturated. More importantly the diet will provide fatty acids which cannot be produced by the body and on which the body relies on for essential activity. Both linoleic and linolenic acids are called essential fatty acids (EFA) because they cannot be synthesized in vivo from non-dietary sources. The FAO (1977) report suggest that at least 3% of energy intake be in the form of EFA.

2.5 Electrolyte requirements

The requirements for electrolytes in the diet are primarily based the body's need for maintaining extra-cellular ionic concentrations of Ca^+, Na^+ and Cl^- constant as well as preserving the stability of the intra-cellular K^+, Mg^+ and phosphorus levels. This is essential as it is evident that the acid-base and osmotic balances of the body are influenced by the Na^+, Cl^- and K^+ concentrations. The Na^+ and Cl^- requirement are not well known, however obligatory losses are used as an estimate of physiological needs. Phosphorus is a part of bone and tooth structure but more importantly it is also an integral part of proteins, nucleic acids and phospholipids.

The importance of fluid and electrolyte replacement for promoting tissue perfusion and ionic equilibrium is self-evident. In addition, the processes of malnutrition and refeeding are both associated with major changes in electrolyte balance. With protein-caloric malnutrition there is loss of the intracellular ions potassium (K^+) (Mann et al., 1975), magnesium (Mg^{2+}) (Montgomery, 1960), together with a gain in sodium (Na^+) (Garrow et al., 1968) and water (Brinkman, 1965). On refeeding it is necessary to give potassium (Rudman et al., 1975), magnesium (Freeman, 1977), phosphorus (as monovalent or divalent phosphate) (Rudman et al., 1975), and zinc (Zn^{2+}) (Wolman et al., 1979) to ensure optimum nitrogen retention. Initially the sodium balance may become markedly positive and cause water retention during refeeding, particularly with carbohydrate (Ververbrants & Arky, 1979)).

This rapid gain in weight, seen during the early phases of resumption of food intake, has been noted clinically - the so-called refeeding edema.

Diuresis occurs as the nutritional status improves, and the edema disappears. In emaciated patients refeeding has to be undertaken with caution since pulmonary edema may occur if the attempts are too vigorous. Furthermore, these patients may have hyponatremia (Waterlow et al., 1978) due to an inability to excrete free water, perhaps as a result of Mg^{2+} and K^+ deficiencies (Magnitius & Epstein, 1963).

2.6 Micronutrient needs

The major part of our dietary intake is composed of water, proteins, carbohydrates, fats, and electrolytes. However, for the utilization of these nutrients it is essential to absorb other substances, called micronutrients, in relatively smaller and in some instances minute amounts. These micronutrients belong to two main groups of substances called trace elements and vitamins. The former are inorganic elements, while the latter are complex organic compounds. Both are essential because they regulate metabolic processes as constituents of enzyme complexes required for the utilization of carbohydrates, proteins, and fats.

The requirement for minerals and micronutrients are displayed in table 1. The RNI's are based on established absorption rates; balance studies; the ability to prevent deficiency symptoms and depletion of body reserves; ensure maintenance of specified pool sizes and normal growth. Requirements may also be dependent on the concomitant intake of other nutrients. For example vitamin E requirements are altered by the polyunsaturated fatty acid (PUFA) intake. However these guidelines may vary by as much as 12 to 30% in individuals.

a- Trace elements. Cotzias (1967) defined an essential trace element as one that has the following

characteristics: (1) present in the healthy tissues of all living things; (2) constant tissue concentration from one animal to the next; (3) withdrawal leads to a reproducible functional and/or structural abnormality; (4) addition of the element prevents the abnormality; (5) the abnormality is associated with a specific biochemical change; and (6) the biochemical change is prevented and/or cured along with the observed clinical abnormality by giving the nutrient.

In animal studies, 15 elements have been found to be essential for health. They are iron, zinc, copper, chromium, selenium, iodine, cobalt, manganese, nickel, molybdenum, fluorine, tin, silicon, vanadium, and arsenic. However, using the strict criteria suggested by Cotzias (1967), only the first seven have been shown to be necessary for health in humans. Of these cobalt is essential only insofar as it is part of the corrin ring in vitamin B_{12}.

Trace elements are absorbed as inorganic substances and as organic compounds. In natural foods the latter often predominate.
Vitamins are essential nutrients which are active in minute quantities. The current available studies and the recommendations based on them have been simple observations of plasma or blood levels during a given regimen (Lowry et al., 1978). They are classified as either fat-soluble or water-soluble.

The former are soluble in fat and require for the most part pancreatic secretions and bile for absorption (MacMahon & Thompson, 1970). They are transported by chylomicrons and usually stored in the liver or adipose tissue. In the circulation vitamin A is bound to a circulating protein - retinol binding protein (RBP) - and 25-OH-D3 is bound to an a2-globulin. Vitamin toxicity may occur if excessive amounts are consumed because these vitamins are stored.

The latter are distinguished by the fact that most contain nitrogen (unlike fat-soluble vitamins) and are components of coenzymes catalyzing biochemical reactions. Five of these vitamins are especially concerned with energy metabolism: thiamine, riboflavin, niacin, biotin, and pantothenate.

3 COMPOSITION OF MILK

The full impact of milk on the

TABLE 2. Milk intake and the RNI's for macronutrients in women

Age Group	MILK 3.3% RDA(ml)	MEAN WEIGHT Kg	Prot %RNI	CHO %RNI	Fat %RNI	n-6 %RNI	n-3 %RNI
Children	500-750	23.0	56	9	29	6	32
Adolescents	750-1000	56.0	54	10	30	6	32
Men	500	73.0	30	7	20	4	32
Women	500	62.0	39	9	27	5	22
Lactation	750	--	44	11	34	7	37
Elderly	500	66.5	35	10	31	5	31

References: Hamill, 1979; Health & Welfare Canada 1992; Murray et al., 1990. (RDA is the recommended daily allowance.)

nutritional status of all age groups can be seen in Table 2 which outlines the extent to which the macronutrient needs of various age groups can be met. To facilitate however the discussion of the role of milk in human nutrition, the woman will be used as the reference person for meeting RNI's because women have higher requirements for certain nutrients such as iron (Fe), chromium (Cr) and vitamin A, making them more vulnerable to micronutrient deficiency. This difficulty is accentuated by the lower food intake in women because of their lower mean weight. Thus, if milk is limiting in a micronutrient then it will be especially observed in women.

3.1 Milk proteins

The protein, carbohydrate and fat content of milk is in fact what makes it a unique food. The protein is composed of 80% casein and 20% whey protein and includes all 8 essential amino acids (EAA) in addition to a variety of non-essentials. This makes it a protein of high quality. The casein is made up of 4 fractions (α,β,gamma,k) all of which have various concentrations of amino acids. The whey protein is likewise formed by 3 different globulin fractions identified as albumin, ß-lactoglobulin, α-lactal-albumin (Gordon & Kalan, 1974). The biological value of cow's milk is 91% using whole egg as a referent. The net protein value (NPV) - this takes into account the biological value, digestibility and protein concentration of the food - is 82%, indicating the ease with which milk protein is assimilated and

metabolized. It may be surprising to most that the NPV of beef is 73% (Renner, 1983). It becomes clear by referring to Figure 3, the extent to which milk protein is utilized by the body in comparison to other foods. There are however two major concerns related to milk proteins that are clinical in nature. One is long-standing and is related to protein hypersensitivity and the other is more recent and pertains to the link between bovine alpha-lactoglobulin and insulin-dependent diabetes (IDDM).

a- Protein hypersensitivity. The hypersensitivity to milk protein is a relatively rare condition, as it occurs 1 in 5000 (Whitington & Gibson 1977). Therapy classically involves cow's milk restriction. This is not regarded as necessary since heat treatment will first denature the whey protein - the main allergen - and often permit consumption of some milk without deleterious effects. (Jost & Monti, 1991).

In extremely rare instances, prenatal sensitization to cow's milk by the mother has resulted in colitis (Wilson & Self 1990).

b- Type I diabetes. The suspicion that cow's milk protein could mimic a pancreatic islet-cell antigen stems from work by Elliot & Martin (1984). Around that same time an inverse relationship between the incidence of IDDM and the duration of breast feeding in Norway and Sweden had been proposed (Borch-johnsen et al., 1984). More recently in a case-control design study Karjalainen (et al. 1992) suggest that the antibodies produced in response to bovine serum albumin (BSA) and to an albumin peptide (ABBOS), react with a beta-cell surface protein called p69 which in fact maintains the response of the

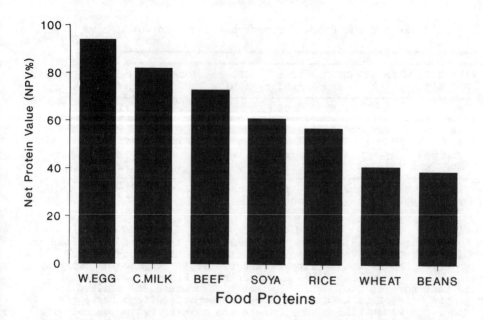

Figure 3. The net protein value (NPV) of milk in comparison to other protein foods. (Renner, 1983)

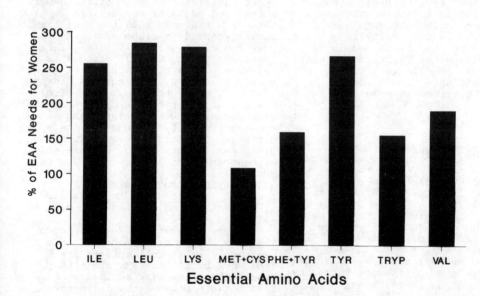

Figure 4. Percent of minimum EEA requirements for women met with 500 ml of 3.3% milk. (Adapted from, Leverton 1959; Food & Nutrition Board Committee on amino acids 1959 and Orr & Watt, 1968)

antibodies until the β-cells are totally destroyed. This finding is still controversial and needs to be supported by a cohort design. Ultimately, if proven true, the consumption of cow's milk before the age of one year would be discouraged. This would further give credence to the argument that breast milk is uniquely adapted to meet infant needs

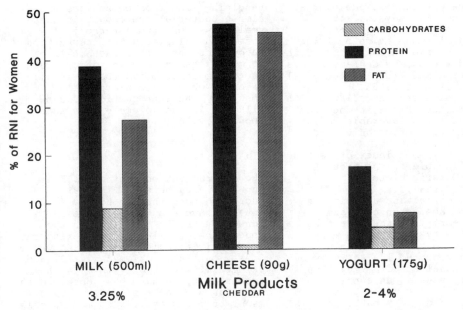

Figure. 5 The percent of macronutrient needs met with milk, cheese and yogurt. (Adapted from Murray et al., 1990; Health & Welfare Canada, 1988).

especially in light of the lower electrolyte content as well as types of proteins that are present (Raiha, 1989; & Renner, 1983).

The degree to which the availability of vegetable protein can be heightened with the inclusion of milk is based on the surplus of EAA in milk. This is illustrated in Figure 4 as the percentage of minimum EAA needs met with 500 ml of milk. The high biological value of milk proteins can in fact complement the lower chemical score of vegetable and cereal proteins. Combining milk powder with low cost foods like maize, rice, millet and wheat, raises the biological value of the mixture considerably and allows protein requirements to be met cheaply in developing countries. (Becker et al. 1971).

It has also been suggested that whey protein - making up 20% of milk protein, containing more sulfur based amino acids and characterized by a higher EAA score than egg (1.07%) - if added to milk or to vegetable proteins, increases the BV of both.

Dairy products as a rule, are mostly noted for their protein and fat contribution to the human diet. Cheese and milk given in portions outlined in Figure 5, can provide

between 38 to 46% of the RNI for protein. Within this context, milk's role in human nutrition reaches far beyond the realm of industrialized nations, known for their abundance of protein, to developing countries with primarily vegetable and cereal based diets.

A further appreciation of the contribution of milk protein to human nutrition can be reached using the economic food value index, which essentially compares the cost of a protein unit for various foods in relation to their nutritive value. (Traver et al., 1981).

3.2 Milk carbohydrate

The carbohydrate or sugar component is mostly lactose and represents 4.8% of cow's milk (Nickerson, 1974). The ability to absorb lactose is dependent on the activity of the lactase enzyme which hydrolyses the disaccharide lactose into galactose and glucose. Both monosaccharides are then actively transported into the cell. This is in contrast to the diffusion of most other hexoses. This translates into lactose being more slowly absorbed compared with sucrose. The supply of energy therefore takes place over a longer period. It may in fact contribute to a more efficient utilization of amino acids by first increasing the biological value of the protein and second, by decreasing its true digestibility. (Turlington et al. 1989; Sewell & West, 1965). Lactose has also been associated with decreased caries, since it does not produce plaque - a favorable medium for the formation of organic acids (Andlaw, 1977).

The lower glycemic index of lactose makes it allowable in the diet of diabetics (Ontario Dietetic Association, 1989), .

The level of lactase activity is dependent on age, ethnicity and mucosal integrity of the intestine. Lactase activity declines in many cultures during the post-weaning period with reported low activity by age 5 (Lebenthal et al. 1975). This is typically seen as an ethnic specific trait that takes place independent of dietary patterns. Malabsorption of lactose, in this instance, will clinically present itself as primary lactase nonpersistence. Many studies have in fact shown that prolonged exposure to lactose did not improve the lactase activity nor did it enhance lactose absorption (Cuatrecasa 1965, Gilat 1972). While the mechanism behind the observed decline in activity is yet unknown, ethnic differences in tolerance are clearly documented (Barr 1977, Cuatrecasa 1965). It has been postulated, based on work in Finland (Sahi et al.1973), Nigeria (Ransome-Kuti 1975), and on the American Pima indian (Johnson 1977) that primary lactase nonpersistence is the result of an autosomal recessive gene. The ability to absorb is a completely penetrant autosomal dominant gene. The clinical importance of this reported intolerance in many cultures, has been questioned in light of the ability of many of these individuals to consume between 300-500 ml of milk without gastrointestinal problems (Yap et al. 1989, Wittenberg & Moosa 1990, O'Keefe et al. 1990, Tadesse et al. 1992).

Loss of mucosal integrity will manifest itself as secondary lactase deficiency. This is often precipitated by surgery, or any conditions that destroy the brush border of the intestine. Hence, it is often seen in many diarrheal diseases, originating from acute or chronic gastroenteritis, infectious organisms resulting from food poisonings or simple bacterial overgrowth in the small bowel or from a retroviral infection. Therapeutic intervention recommends the use of lactose-free formulas for infants who demonstrate lactose malabsorption (Dagan 1980). Cases in which mild diarrhea is observed, the introduction of some milk may in fact promote tolerance (Donovan, 1987) .

3.3 Milk fat

The natural fat content of milk is known to vary between 2 and 8%. The increased concern that higher fat intakes have a number of adverse consequences, has resulted in the appearance of milk with different fat contents; including homogenized whole 3.3%., partially skimmed milk 2% and skimmed milk with 0.1% fat. In the recent past, we have even observed the appearance of a 1% fat milk. The manufacturer's ability to mechanically manipulate fat content has provided the consumer with the opportunity to make low fat choices. Moreover, milk fat is highly digestible, owing this trait first to the natural dispersion of milk fat, a state that can be further increased by homogenization, thereby greatly reducing the size of the fat globules (Mulder & Wastra, 1974). The trend towards decreasing fat has reached the full spectrum of milk & milk products to include cheeses, yogurts, frozen yogurts, and ice cream. The marketing approach is primarily aimed at the consumer's anti-fat outcry which is largely the result of recommendations to lower dietary cholesterol intake, as the latter has often been regarded as a risk factor for atherosclerosis and coronary artery disease. Consequently, animal fats, which also includes milk fat, have attempted to be reduced in the diet.

The link however, between dietary cholesterol intake and heart disease is very weak. Atherosclerosis is in fact a multifactorial disease influenced by the interaction of the environment, genetics and characteristics of the arterial wall (Davignon et al., 1983). While there is direct evidence that lowering plasma cholesterol levels can slow the progression of atherosclerosis and decrease mortality (Grundy et al. 1988), 40% of myocardial infarcts (MI) and coronary artery disease (CAD) occur in the absence of hyperlipidemia

(Davignon et al. 1977). Still, the general consensus is to reduce total fat (Denke & Breslow 1988) with special emphasis placed on saturated fat (Hegsted & Ausman 1988). The negative impact of these guidelines on milk consumption is however unwarranted, since milk and dairy products in Canada only contribute 16.2% of the total fat intake and 30% of saturated fats (Kakis & Anderson, 1991). Nevertheless, to address this issue, work is currently being done to alter the fatty acid composition of the milk and butter by increasing the unsaturated dietary fat content of the cow feed. Stegeman at al., (1992) have recently shown that adding fat in the form of safflower, sunflower and bovine somatotropin, resulted in a lower concentration of short chain fatty acids (SCFA), medium chain fatty acids (MCFA) and higher long chain fatty acids (LCFA) in milk fat and butter. Furthermore, higher concentrations of unsaturated fatty acids (UNFA) were observed in the butter of sunflower and safflower treated animals. The actual impact of these changes in fat composition on improvement in human health awaits further studies.

Some studies (Newbern et al. 1990.; Birt, 1990; Van't Veer et al., 1990 and Palmer et al., 1990), have also found a correlation between elevated dietary fats and the risk of breast, colorectal, and pancreatic cancers. The committee on diet, nutrition and cancer of the National Research Council (1982), had qualified the association between dietary fat and breast cancer to be "causative". The types of fats implicated in the induction of tumorigenesis have been identified by several studies (Carroll et al. 1971., Carter et al. 1985.) to be linoleic acid. The consumption of milk and its by-products do not contravene any prudent dietary guidelines aimed at reducing the incidence of cancer. These products can easily fit into currently accepted restrictions in fat intake, which are of the order of 30% of calories. Equally importantly, is the fatty acid make up of milk. Linoleic (2.5%) and arachidonic (0.23%) acids represent a small proportion of total milk fat, whereas 26% is oleic acid - a fatty acid recognized to have no tumor promotion properties (Carroll, 1987).

3.4 Electrolytes in cow's milk

Guéguen (1971) reported a range of 7-10 g of minerals per liter of milk. Table 6 provides a breakdown of percentages of the RNIs met with the ingestion of the lower limit of recommended milk intake per age group. The concentrations of these minerals can vary depending on the stage of lactation. The beginning (colostrum) and end of lactation are particularly high in Calcium (Ca), phosphorus(P) sodium(Na) and chloride(Cl). Generally, however, these concentrations are not altered by either the feed or the season (Guéguen, 1971). This is because of the stability related to their colloidal inorganic form or as they bind with casein and lipids found in the milk (Renner, 1983).
a- Calcium. While calcium is abundant in vegetables, it is less available because the high oxalates and phytates found in vegetables and cereals bind calcium and prevent absorption (Krause & Mahan 1979).
Milk and milk products by contrast are sources of readily absorbable calcium because of the abundance of calcium in these foods as well as an optimal calcium:phosphate ratio necessary for maximal absorption.

TABLE 6. Mineral contribution of milk in the diet of women

Age Group	MILK 3.3% RDA(ml)	Ca %RNI	P %RNI	K %RNI	Na %RNI	Mg %RNI
Children	500-750	77	87	286	229	79
Adolescents	750-100	103	78	235	244	51
Men	500	77	48	125	315	28
Women	500	82	56	143	440	34
Lactation	750	74	69	147	165	42
Elderly	500	77	52	143	315	31

Reference: Health & Welfare Canada, 1992 & 1988; Murray, 1990 and Renner, 1983. (RDA is the recommended daily allowance)

Vitamin D added to milk also promotes calcium absorption through activation of a vitamin D-dependent calcium-binding protein.

b- Phosphorus. The absorption of phosphorus is remarkably efficient, favoring a 70 to 90 percent absorption. The high content of phosphorus in milk ensures that at least 50% of the requirements are met by a regular consumption of milk.

c- Potassium. Potassium is present in a variety of foods and is especially abundant in milk, meat, potatoes, and fruits. Traditionally, orange juice and bananas are given as rich sources of potassium. Although milk is not popularly considered a good source of potassium, it is surprising to note that only 2 glasses of milk will supply 140% of the K^+ requirements.

d- Sodium. Milk, cheese, bread, and cereals are rich sources of sodium. Fruits and potatoes on the other hand, are relatively low in sodium. Foods high in sodium are often high in chloride. Chloride is also high in foods which are low in sodium and high in potassium such as bananas, tomatoes and sweet potatoes.

Processing and preserving foods introduce large amounts of sodium and chloride in the form of sodium chloride. Certain medical conditions, such a hypertension, cardiovascular, renal and liver diseases in addition to adrenocortical steroid therapy, will dictate the need to prescribe a sodium restricted diet that can vary from 22 mmol to 217 mmol/day. The consumption of 500 ml of 3.3% milk will surpass the basic need for sodium by 294%. Using our current knowledge of what constitutes a safe intake (2.3 g/day), a half liter of whole milk would represent only 11% of that guideline. Sodium restricted diets, in the range of 130-217 mmol, can therefore accommodate liberal servings of milk. Limitations are usually placed on processed cheese, because of the use of emulsifying salts in its manufacturing process as well as other processed goods. In severe restrictions the number of milk servings allowed per day can be limited to one, but is almost never eliminated from the diet because of its nutrient density (Ontario Dietetic Association, 1989).

e- Magnesium. Milk, meat, cheese, leafy vegetables and wheat are rich in magnesium. The processing of food, however, particularly diminishes the magnesium content. Refining whole grain wheat or polishing rice for example can eliminate 80% of the magnesium from the food. Likewise, the home preparation of vegetables, which often involves boiling, will reduce magnesium content by 50%. (Wester, 1987). Milk emerges as a good source of magnesium allowing women to meet close to 30% of their requirements. Furthermore, it is doubtful that the pasteurization process, particularly "flash pasteurization", would greatly reduce the mineral content or availability of these nutrients in milk. (Renner, 1983)

In summary milk is a good and reliable source of calcium, phosphorus, potassium, magnesium and sodium.

3.5 Trace elements in cow's milk

Many of the trace elements are in the form of organic compounds. This means that they are associated either with the fat globule membrane (Cu,Zn,Mn,Fe), casein micelles (65% Fe), casein (80% Zn) and immunoglobulins (20% Zn). Only selenium is in the free inorganic from, as are zinc and iodine (Allen & Miller, 1980 Flynn, 1992). Molybdenum (Mo), Zn and Mg are also combined with enzymes such as xanthine oxidase - in the case of Mo - and alkaline phosphatase - in the case of Zn and Mg (Krause & Mahan, 1979). For the most part, the content of many of the elements can vary again with period of lactation, season and feed (Johnson, 1974). Extreme variances, as shown in Figure 6, are the consequence of mistakes in analysis and external contamination from containers for example (Murthy et al., 1972).

The infiltration of heavy metals such as lead, mercury and cadmium into the milk as a result of feed contamination, was thought to be minimal (Renner, 1983), since the body burden from contaminants like lead are essentially found in the bones, kidneys and liver of the animal (Donovan et al. 1969; Mitchell & Aldous, 1974.). This notion has recently been challenged by Krelowska-Kulas (1990), who studied led and cadmium levels in cow's milk in the vicinity of "Lenin's" iron and steel works in Nowa Huta. Concentrations were ten times greater than controls.

It is apparent, based on Figure 6, that milk is a consistent source of

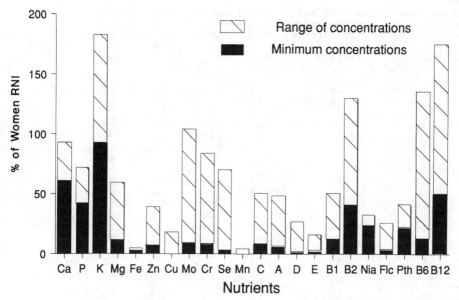

Figure. 6 Meeting the RNI for electrolytes and micronutrients in women with 500 ml of 3.3% milk. (Adapted from Murray, 1990; Renner, 1983 and Health & Welfare Canada 1988)

calcium, phosphorus and potassium. It also has the potential to meet, in an important way, the needs for molybdenum, chromium, and selenium, depending on the feed and degree of external contamination. What is most interesting, is the even greater importance of milk in children and adolescent diets, in terms of the supply of calcium, phosphorus and magnesium, as shown in Table 5 and zinc in Table 7.

The significance of this contribution is especially relevant to the very rapid bone formation and protein synthesis associated with the growth patterns typical of these ages.

a- Zinc. In addition to milk and cheese, zinc is a widely distributed element in foodstuffs (shellfish, liver, and wheat,bran) and in the human body. It has been identified as part of about 120 enzymes (Valee & Falchuk, 1981) and is also an integral constituent of DNA polymerase, reverse transcriptase, RNA polymerase, tRNA synthetase, and the protein chain elongation factor (Valee & Falchuk, 1981). Thus, zinc deficiency can alter protein synthesis at a number of different points. It is not surprising that in the absence of zinc, growth arrest occurs (Prasad, 1979). The interrelation between zinc

and nucleic acids are also interesting, in view of the clinical observation that a number of functions, dependent on protein synthesis, are suppressed by zinc deficiency. These include cellular immunity, (Golden et al., 1978), growth, fertility, hair growth (Prasad, 1979), wound healing (Golden et al., 1980), and plasma protein levels. Within this context, milk and its by-products may play a vital role in providing important quantities of zinc. Children between the ages of 1 and 3, who consume a minimum of 500 ml of milk /day, can meet 50% of their requirements for zinc. Pregnant and lactating women can meet 25% of their RNI by drinking 4 cups of milk (1000 ml) per day.

b- Chromium. In addition to milk, other dietary sources of chromium are brewer's yeast, corn oil, vegetables, whole grains and cheese. Chromium (Cr) is therefore a nutrient not normally deficient in a well balanced diet. It appears that Cr is best absorbed in the organic form - the form in which it is naturally occurring in food. The chromium in yeast for example, is absorbed to the extent of 10 to 25 per cent of the oral dose (WHO, 1973). Three percent of inorganic chromium, on the other

TABLE 7. Milk consumption and RNI's for micronutrients in women

Age Group 3.3% RDA Milk(ml)	Children 500-750	Adolescents 750-1000	Men 500	Women 500	Preg+ Lact 750-1000	+75 500
T.Elements						
Fe %RNI	4	3	3	2½	2	3
Zn %RNI	28	26	16	22	20	17
Cu %RNI	3	4½	3	3	--	3
Cr %RNI	24	--	42	28	42	34
Se %RNI	--	--	25	25	--	25
Mn %RNI	--	--	0.7	0.7	--	0.7
Mo %RNI	--	--	38	38	--	38
Vitamins						
A %RNI	41	41	31	24½	29	27
D %RNI	6	16	11	11	10	8
E %RNI	10	10	6	9	10	10
VK %RNI	--	--	13	16	--	86
B1 %RNI	24	29	21	25	37	25
B2 %RNI	83	97	60	84	93	93
Niacin %RNI	30	35	23	31	39	34
B6 %RNI	41	45	23	31	35	27
Panthn %RNI	35	41	27	27	--	27
Folic %RNI	35	24	11	14	10	13
B12 %RNI	283	162	92	92	100	92
C %RNI	18	17	10	13	13	11

Reference: Adapted from Murray, 1990; Renner, 1983 and Canadian Nutrient File, 1985. (RDA is the recommended daily allowance)

hand, is absorbed (Donaldson & Barreras, 1966). The contribution of milk and most notably cheese in Cr, is significant. Eating 45g of cheese can supply more than 100% of the RNI for this nutrient in women.

c- Selenium. Selenium is generally quite abundant in cereals depending on the richness of the soil. More stable sources are meat, poultry and milk. The ingestion of 500 ml of milk can supply close to 30% of the RNI for women. Deficiencies are not usually a concern except in infants living in areas with selenium impoverished soil (Yang et al., 1984).

Selenium is interrelated with other antioxidants such as vitamin E (Diplock & Lucy, 1973). Deficiency of one can be partially corrected by giving the other. Selenium is part of glutathione peroxidase, a selenoenzyme whose activity in association with superoxide dismutase (SOD), controls levels of superoxide anion radical and peroxide (Hunt & Groff, 1990).

d- Molybdenum. Legumes, organ meats, milk, cheese and yeast are relatively good food sources of this element. Close to 40% of a woman's RNI can be met with 500 ml milk per day. Molybdenum is an essential component of xanthine oxidase (de Renzo et al.,

1953), sulfite oxidase (Cohen et al., 1971), and aldehyde oxidase (Mahler et al., 1954). Xanthine oxidase catalyzes the conversion of oxypurines to uric acid. In its absence the levels of oxypurines will rise and those of uric acid fall. Sulfite oxidase similarly influences the conversion of sulfite to sulfate. The lack of sulfite oxidase has been shown to be responsible for neurological abnormalities (Cohen et al., 1973), and it is of interest that Abumrad et al. (1981) described a TPN patient who developed coma when infused with amino acid solutions containing sulfite. The coma was reversible by supplementing the TPN solutions with 300 µg of molybdenum per day.

Milk is very poor in iron, copper and manganese. The consumption of other foods is needed to prevent deficiency of these elements.

3.6 Fat-soluble vitamins

a- Vitamin A. Milk is not regarded as a major source of vitamin A. The wide range as shown in Figure 6 means that in some cases a woman may only meet 5% of her RNI. Liver and vegetables like carrots and spinach on the other hand,

90

will meet a major portion of the RNI. A 110 g baked sweet potato will provide 89% of the requirement. Deficiency of this vitamin is rarely a concern in industrialized nations today, because of the widespread distribution of a variety of food and the degree of fortification in foods. In Canada, fortification of milk allows a woman to meet about 16% of the RNI. Milk can be a steady source of this vitamin in the diet, which will help maintain liver reserves. Cheese, with no fortification, can supply up to 20% of her needs.

Clinically, vitamin A deficiency results in night blindness due to decreased rod function (Wald, 1933). In addition, because glycoprotein synthesis is reduced, there is drying of the conjunctiva (xerophthalmia), hyperkeratosis of the skin, and an increased susceptibility to infection. The xerosis of the eye is manifested as shiny gray foamy triangular areas called Bitot's spots and may cause corneal ulceration and blindness. This is observed in certain developing countries and represents a major public health concern which has been addressed by international aide (W.H.O., 1982).

b- Vitamin D. The fortification of milk in Canada has been a decisive factor in the virtual eradication of rickets. Overt cases of rickets are still reported among children drinking unfortified milk (1μg vit.D /500ml) or among strict vegetarians who have eliminated milk altogether or children who have been solely breast fed for over a year. Risks of osteomalacia have been reported to be high among Britain's elderly population, who has little exposure to sunlight or fortified foods (Parfitt et al. 1982). In contrast, a Canadian woman drinking 500 ml of fortified milk in Canada, may meet between 88 and 176 percent of her RNI depending on her age. Although sun light represent the major source of vitamin D, it is generally felt that the diet must supply a minimal amount for those with limited exposure to the sun. Within this context, 12.5 μg (500 I.U) of dietary vitamin D has been recommended as a safety guideline. Because of the normally occurring mixed influence of diet and sun light, it has been found that less than 5 μg/day influences the serum 25-OHD levels minimally (Fraser, 1983) providing the body reserves are not subnormal.

The concern over the fortification of both milk and infant formula has recently been raised by Holick, et al. (1992). They conclude that these products rarely contain the degree of fortification stated and that under and over-fortification, to the degree found in their investigation, must be avoided because of the danger of toxicity.

c- Vitamin K. Green vegetables are the chief source, while meat dairy and milk represent intermediate to low sources of vitamin K (Olson, 1988). Deficiency is not an issue in the general healthy population because of the content in the food supply and since endogenous gut bacteria synthesize vitamin K (Pyke & Brown, 1975). Two exceptions are noted: the neonate, characterized by minimal storage and a reduced intestinal synthesis of this vitamin and term infants, strictly dependent on breast milk - known to be low in vitamin K. (Haroon et al., 1982). Vitamin K concentrations in milk vary greatly because of environmental contamination and consequently cannot be considered a reliable source. Concentrations have been found to vary from trace amounts to 485 % of the RNI for a woman. (Renner, 1983)

3.7 Water soluble vitamins

a- Riboflavin. Milk, milk products, and vegetables are the main sources of dietary riboflavin. Consumption of the Canada Food Guide's lower recommended limit of milk intake, ensures that at least 80% of the RNI is met for the average woman with only 16 percent of the daily energy requirements. Breakfast cereals and enriched bread are also good sources of this vitamin and when combined with milk, become in themselves valuable dietary sources of riboflavin, thiamine and niacin (Health & Welfare Canada, 1988). Milk should however be kept in opaque containers to avoid any riboflavin photodegradation.

b- Pantothenic Acid. Pantothenic acid is found in all foods except fruit, especially in liver, eggs, mushrooms, milk, and milk products. Five hundred milliliters of whole milk will meet about 27% of the RNI for women while, 175 g of plain yogurt will supply 16% of requirements (Health & Welfare Canada, 1988).

c- Pyridoxine. Animal products such as liver, meat, fish and dairy products are good sources of pyridoxine. As illustrated in Figure 1, 31% of the RNI can be met with milk

(Health & Welfare Canada, 1988). Bananas and avocados are also rich sources, but other fruits do not contain as much. Grains and legumes are are also valuable sources of pyridoxine. In animal products B6 is present as pyridoxal phosphate and pyridoxamine phosphate, which are very bioavailable forms of the vitamin. In contrast, the plant form of pyridoxine, although well absorbed, is poorly metabolized (Kabir et al. 1983). The heat treatment used in the processing of animal foods can reduce the content by 25-30%. This is not so much a concern with milk, since the pasteurization process is short enough, especially the 15 second treatment used in "flash-pasteurization", that most of the B complex vitamins suffer less than a 10% loss. UHT treatment and particularly sterilization can however heighten the loss to anywhere between 10 and 50%. This range can be as great as 20 to 100% in the case of cobalamin (Ford & Thompson, 1981)

The losses that do occur in the processing of milk are much smaller than what might take place in household preparations of food. Milk becomes within this scenario a reliable and good source of the vitamin.

d- Cobalamin. Meat and meat products, dairy products and eggs constitute the main sources of vitamin B_{12}. (Herbert & Coleman 1988). Vegetable sources are devoid of this vitamin. Possible deficiency has been raised with regards to strict vegetarians who exclude all milk and milk products from their diet. The lasting effect of liver storage however, makes deficiency reports very rare. This is because most of the body reserve forms a rapid equilibria within the body pool (Adams et al., 1968). The minimal losses that do occur are mostly in urine, feces and skin and amount to a 0.05 to 0.2% from the body pool per day. It would take around 5 years for the pool size to get depleted if bacterial and dietary intake amounted to zero. Armstrong et al. (1974) have estimated that vegetarians consume anywhere between 0.25 to 0.5 μg/day depending on the the strictness of the diet. This would prevent depletion of reserves from taking place and any ensuing signs of deficiency.

While it is clear that milk significantly helps meet the RNI for vitamins in women, as has been clearly outlined in Figures 6, vitamins A, D, E and C are not naturally present in sufficient amounts to meet nutritional needs. Fortification greatly enhances the completeness of this food and heightens its role as a vehicle for public health.

4 CONCLUSION

The value of milk in human nutrition is vital and necessary as it completes the diet of the young and the elderly in particular, from the perspective of protein quality. Diets dominated by grains and cereals would greatly benefit from the inclusion of milk with respect to increasing the amino acid score and consequently the biological value of the protein. The nutrient density of this food brings it to prominence with respect to calcium and phosphorus - key players in bone formation. In addition, cobalamin, pyridoxine, niacin, pantothenic acid and riboflavin are consistently elevated in milk and therefore represent a reliable source for these nutrients. Noteworthy is the minimal loss of nutrients from milk before consumption, since it is mostly ingested directly from the container without heating. This is contrasted with other foods that require baking, frying and boiling, processes during which nutrients are lost. As well, naturally occurring phytates, frequently found in cereals and seeds, bind certain nutrients in food and make them unavailable. Painted against this background, milk surfaces as a nutrient dense food from which minimal losses occur. It is apparent however, that significant ranges in concentration of nutrients can be observed. In some instances for example, molybdenum, chromium, and selenium levels in milk can be elevated to the extent that 100, 80 and 70 percent of the respective RNI's can be met with 500 ml of whole milk. These extreme ranges are often attributed to measurement errors and environmental contamination.

Milk does not contribute in any important way towards meeting women's requirements for iron, copper, manganese, vitamin E, and folic acid. Many of these micronutrients are however found in cereals and vegetables and can, when combined with milk, complete the consumption pattern of many of these nutrients. With vitamin D fortification, requirements at all ages can be easily met.

The concern over the widespread

incidence of lactose intolerance is highly overrated. In many cases, while the lactose tolerance test may have been positive, it is still possible to tolerate a certain quantity of milk in the diet. Furthermore, the introduction of commercially available lactase, in the form of yeast β-galactosidases, can significantly improve tolerance.

Dairy products now come in a wide variety of fat contents, thereby offering the consumer many possible ways of fitting into prudent health guidelines for decreasing the risk of cardiovascular disease and cancer.

REFERENCES

Abumrad NN, Schneider AJ, Steel D, et al. 1981. Amino acid intolerance during prolonged total parenteral nutrition reversed by molybdate therapy. Am. J. Clin. Nutr. 34: 2551-2559.

Adams, J.F., Hume, R., Kennedy, E.H., Pirriew, T.G., Whitelaw, J.M. and White, A.M. 1968. Metabolic res-ponses to low doses of cyanocobala-min in patients with megaloblastic anaemia. Br.J.Nutr. 22:575-582

Allen, J.C., Miller, W.J. 1980. Selenium binding and distribution in goat and cow's milk. J.Dairy Sci 63:526-531

Andlaw, R.J. 1977. Diet and dental caries - a review. J.Human Nutrition 31:45-52

Armstrong, B.K., Davis, R.E., Nico, D.J., Van Merwyk, A.J. and Larwood, C.J. 1974. Hematological vitamin B12 and folate studies on Seventh Day Adventist vegetarians. Am.J. Clin.Nutr. 27: 712-718

Barr, R.G., Becker, M.C., Heymann, P.W., Watkins, J.B. 1978. Lactose malabsorption, abdominal pain and lactose ingestion in a multiethnic school population. Gastroenterology 74:1006

Beaton, G.H. and Chery, A. 1988. Protein requirements of infants: a reexamination of concepts and approaches. Am.J.Clin.Nutr. 48:1403 -1412

Becker, D.J., Pimstone, B.L., Hansen, J.D.L., Hendricks J. 1971. Serum albumin and growth hormone relationship in kwashiorkor and nephrotic syndrome J.Lab.Clin.Med. 78:865-871

Birt, D.F. 1990. The influence of dietary fat on carcinogenesis: Lessons from experimental models. Nutrition Reviews. 48(1):1-5

Borch-Johnsen, K., Mandrup-Poulsen, T., Zachau-Christiansen, B., et al. 1984. Relation between breast-feeding and incidence of insulin-dependent diabetes mellitus. Lancet 2:1083-6

Brinkman GL, Bowie MD, Frus-Hansen B, et al. 1965. Body water composition in kwashiorkor before and after loss of edema. Pediatrics 36:94-103.

Carroll, K.K., Khor, T.T. 1971. Effect of level and type of dietary fat on incidence of mammary tumors induced in female Spague-Dawley rats by 7.12-dimethylbenz(a)anthracene. Lipids 6:415-420

Carroll, K.K. 1987. Summation:which fat/how much fat-animal. Prev.Med. 16:510-515

Carter, C.A., Ip, C., Ip, M.M. 1985. Requirement of essential fatty acid for mammary tumorigenesis in rats. Cancer Res. 45:1997-2001

Cohen H.J, Fridovich I, Rajagopalan, KV. 1971. Hepatic sulfite oxidase. A functional role for molybdenum. J. Biol. Chem. 246:374-382.

Cotzias G.C. 1967. Role and importance of trace substances in environ-mental health. In DD Hemphill (ed). Proc First Ann.Conf. on Trace Subst. Environ. Health. Columbia, MO, University of Missouri. 1:5-19.

Cuatrecasas, P., Lockwood, D.H., Caldwell, J.R. 1965. Lactase defi-ciency in the adult. Lancet 1:14-18

Dagan, R., Gorodischer, R., Moses, S., Margolis, C. 1980. Lactose-free formula for infantile diarrhea. Lancet 1:207

Davignon, J., Lussier-Cacan, S., Ortin-George, M., Lelievre, M., Bertagna, C., Gattereau, A. and Fontaine, A. 1977. Plasma lipids and lipoprotein patterns in angio-graphically graded atherosclerosis of the legs and in coronary heart disease. Can. Med. Assoc. 116: 1245-1250

Davignon, J., Dufour, R. and Cantin, M. 1983. Atherosclerosis and hyper-tension. In Hypertension: physio-pathology and treatment. 2nd ed. Genest, J., Kuchel, O., Hamet, P. and Cantin, M. eds. McGraw-Hill, New York: 810-852

Denke, M.A. and Breslow, J.L. 1988. Effects of a low fat diet with and without intermittent saturated fat and cholesterol ingestion on plasma lipid, lipoprotein, and apolipo-protein levels in normal volunteers. J.Lipid Res. 29:963-969

de Renzo EC, Kaleita E, Heytler P, et al. 1953. Identification of the xanthine oxidase factor as molybdenum. Arch.Biochem.Biophys. 45:247-253.

Diplock AT, Lucy JA. 1973. The biochemical modes of action of vitamin E and selenium: a hypothesis. FEBS. Lett. 29:205-210

Donaldson RM, Barreras RF. 1966. Intestinal absorption of trace quantities of chromium. J.Lab. Clin.Med. 68:484-493.

Donovan, G.K., Torres-Pinedo, R. 1987. Chronic diarrhea and soy formulas:Inhibition of diarrhea by lactose. Am.J.Dis.child. 141:1069-71

Donovan, P.P., Feeley, D.T. and Canavan, P.P. 1969. Lead contamination in mining areas in western Ireland. II. Survey of animal pastures, foods and waters. J.Sci.Food.Agr.20(1):43-45

Elliot, R.B. and Martin, J.M. 1984. Dietary protein: a trigger of insulin-dependent diabetes in the BB rat? Diabetologia 26:297-9

FAO/WHO. 1977. Dietary fats and oils in human nutrition: report of an expert consultation. Rome.

FAO/WHO/UNU. 1985. Energy and protein requirements. Report of a joint FAO/WHO/UNU Expert Consultation. W.H.O. Tech. Rep. Ser. 724

Flynn, A. 1992. Mineral and trace elements in milk. Adv.Food & Nutr. Research. 36;209-252

Food and Nutrition Board Committee on Amino Acids. 1959. Evaluation of protein nutrition. Publication 711. Washington, D.C. National Academy of Sciences- National Research Council.

Fraser, D.R. 1983. The physiological economy of vitamin D. Lancet 1:969-972

Freeman JB. 1977. Magnesium requirements are increased during total parenteral nutrition. Surg.Forum 28:61-62.

Garrow JS. 1965. body potassium in kwashiorkor and marasmus. Lancet 2: 455-458.

Garrow JS, Smith R, Ward EE. 1968. Electrolyte Metabolism in Severe Infantile Malnutrition. Oxford, Pergamon Press, :56.

Gersovitz, M., Motil, K., Munro, H.N., Scrimshaw, N.S., Young, V.R. 1982. Human protein requirements: assessement of the adequacy of the current RDA for dietary protein in elderly men and womenAm.J.Clin.Nutr. 35:6-14

Gilat, T, Russo, S., Gelman-Malachi, E., Aldor, T.A.M. 1972. Lactase in amn: A non-adaptable enzyme. Gastroenterology 62:1125-27

Golden MHN, Golden, BE., Harland PSEG, et al. 1978. Zinc and immunocompetence in protein-energy malnutrition. Lancet 1:1226-1227.

Golden MHN, Golden BE, Jackson AA. 1980. Skin breakdown in kwashiorkor responds to zinc. (Letter.) Lancet 1:1256.

Gordon, W.G. & Kalan, E.B, 1974. Proteins of milk. In: Fundamentals of dairy chemistry. 2nd ed., Eds. Webb, B.H. Johnson, A.H. and Alford, J.A. Avi Publ. Co. Westport. CT

Grundy, S.M., Barrett-Connor, E., Rudel, L.L., Miettinen, T. and Spector, A.A. 1988. Workshop on the impact of dietary cholesterol on plasma lipoproteins and atherogenesis. Arteriosclerosis 8:95-101

Gueguen, L. 1971. La composition mineral du lait et son adaptation aux besoins mineraux du jeune. Ann. Nutr.Alim. 25:A335-381

Hamill, P.V.V., Drizd, T.A., Johnson, C.L., Reed, R.B., Roche, A.F. and Moore, W.M. 1979. Physical growth: National Center for Health Statistics percentiles. Am.J.Clin. Nutr. 32:607-629

Haroon, Y., Shearer, M.J., Rahim, S., Gunn, W.C., McEnery, G. and Barkham, P. 1982. The content of phylloquinone (vitamin K1) in human milk, cow's milk and infant informula foods determined by high performance liquid chromatography. J.Nutr. 112: 1105-1117

Health & Welfare Canada. 1988. Canadian nutrient file.

Health & Welfare Canada. 1992. The Canada food guide. Ministry of Supply and Services. Ottawa, Canada.

Hegsted, D.M. and Ausman, L.M. 1988. Diet, alcohol and coronary heart disease in men. J.Nutr. 118:1184-1189

Herbert, V.D. and Colman, N. 1988. Folic acid and vitamin B12. In Modern Nutritiion in Health and Disease. 7th Ed. Shils, M.E. and Young, V.R., eds. Lea & Febiger, Philadelphia: 388-416

Holick, M.F., Shao, Q., Liu, W.W. and Chen, T.C. 1992. The vitamin D content of fortified milk and infant formula. New.Engl.J.Med. 326(18)1178-817.

Hunt, S.M. & Groff, J.L. 1990. Advanced Nutrition And Human Metabolism. West Publishing Company. New York.

Jansen, G.R. 1978. Biological evaluation of protein quality. Food Technol. 32(12):52-56

Johnson, A.H. 1974. the composition of milk. In: Fundamentals of dairy chemistry. 2nd ed., Eds. Webb, B.H. Johnson, A.H. and Alford, J.A. Avi Publ. Co. Westport. CT

Johnson, J.D., Simoons, F.J., Hurwitz R., Grange, A., Mitchell, C.H. et al., 1977. Lactose malabsorption among Pima Indians in Arizona. Gastroenterology 73:1299-1304

Jost, R., Monti, J.C. and Pahud, J.J. 1991. Reduction of whey protein allergenicity by processing. Adv. Exp.Med.Biol. 289:309-320

Kabir, H., Leklem, J. and Miller, L.T. 1983. Measurements of glycosylated vitamin B6 in foods. J.Food Sci. 48: 1422-1425

Kakis, G. and Anderson, G.H. Proceedings of the symposium, Optimizing heart health: the diet connection. Depart.Nutr.Sci. University of Toronto, Canada.

Karjalainen, J., Martin, J.M., Knip, M. et al. 1992. A bovine albumin peptide as a possible trigger of insulin-dependent diabetes mellitus. N.Engl.J.Med. 327:302-7

Krause, M.V. and Mahan K.L. 1979. Food nutrition and diet therapy. 6th Ed. W.B. Saunders. Philadelphia.

Krelowska-Kulas, M. 1990. Lead, cadmium, iron, copper and zinc in fresh milk rom selected areas of the Cracow region. Nahrung 34(3):213-7

Lebenthal, E., Antonowicz, I., Shwachman, H. 1975. Correlation of lactase activity, lactose tolerance and milk consumption in different age groups. Am.J.Clin.Nutr. 28:595-600

Leverton, R.M. 1959. Amino acid requirements of young adults. In: Protein and amino acid nutrition, A. A. Albanese, ed, Academic Press

Lowry SF, Goodgame JT, Maher MM, et al. 1978. Parenteral vitamin requirements during feeding. Am.J. Clin.Nutr. 31:2149-2158.

MacMahon, M.T. and Thompson G.R. 1970. Comparison of the absorption of a polar lipid, oleic acid, and a non-polar lipid, α-tocopherol from mixed micellar solutions and emulsions. Europ.J.Clin.Ivest. 1:161-166

Mahler, HR., Mackler, B., Green, DE., et al. 1954. Studies on metalloflavo protein. J.Biol.Chem. 210:465-480.

Manitius A, Epstein FH. 1963. Some observations on the influence of a magnesium-deficient diet on rats, with special reference to renal concentrating ability. J.Clin. Invest. 42:208-215.

Mann MD, Bowie MD, Hansen JDL. 1975. Total body potassium and serum electrolyte concentrations in protein energy malnutrition. S.Afr. Med.J. 49:76-78.

Mitchell, D.G. and Aldous, D.G. 1974. Lead content of foodstuffs. Environ. Health Persp.7:59-64

Montgomery RD. 1960. Magnesium meta-bolism in infantile protein mal-nutrition. Lancet 2:74-76.

Mulder, H. and Walstra, P. 1974. The milk fat globule. Emulsion science applied to milk products and comparable foods. Commonwealth Bureaux, Farnham Royal, Bucks, England.

Murray, T.K. 1990. Nutrition recommendations: report of the scientific review committee. Health & Welfare Canada.

Murthy, G.K., Rhea, U.S. and Peeler, J.T. 1972. Copper, iron, manganese, strontium and zinc content of market milk. J.Dairy Sci. 55(12):1666-74

National Research Council. 1982. National Academy of Sciences. Diet, Nutrition and Cancer. Washington, D. C.:National Academic Press.

Newberne, P.M., Bueche, D., Riengropitak, S., Schrager, T.F. 1990. The influence of dietary levels of vitamin A and fat on colon cancer. Nutrition and Cancer 13(4): 235-242

Nikerson, T.A. 1974. Lactose. In: Fundamentals of dairy chemistry. 2nd ed., Eds. Webb, B.H., Johnson, A.H. and Alford, J.A. Avi Publ. Co. Westport, CT.

O'Keefe, S.J.D., Young, G.O. and Rund, J. 1990. Milk tolerance and the malnourished African. European J.Clin.Nutr. 44:499-504

Olson, R.E. Vitamin K. 1988. In Modern Nutrition in Health & Disease. 7th Ed. Shils, M.E. and Young, V.R., Eds. Lea & Febiger, Philadelphia: 328-339

Ontario Dietetic Association. 1989. Nutritional care manual. 6th Ed. O.H.A. Don Mills, Ontario, Canada

Orr, M.L. and Watt, B.K. 1968. In: Amino acid content of foods. Home Economics Research Report. No.4. U.S Dept. of Agriculture. Washington, D.C.

Palmer, S., Kramer, J., Bagheri, S. Effects of a high fat diet and L364,718 on growth of human pancreatic cancer. Digest.Dis.Sci. 1990;35(6):726-732

Parfitt, A.M., Gallagher, J.C., Heaney, R.P., Johnston, C.C., Neer, R. and Whedon, G.D. 1982. Vitamin D and bne health in the elderly. Am.J. Clin.Nutr. 36:1014-1031

Pike, R.L. & Brown, M.L. 1975. Nutrition: An Integrated Approach.

2nd Ed. John Wiley & Sons. New York.

Prasad AS. 1979. Zinc in Human Nutrition. Boca Raton, FL, CRC Press: 1-80.

Raiha, N.C.R. 1989. Milk protein quantity and quality requirements during development. Adv.Pediatr. 36:347-368

Ransome-Kuti, O., Kretchmer, N., Johnson, J.D., Gribble, J.T. 1975. A genetic study of lactose digestion in Nigerian families. Gastroenterology 68:431-36

Renner, E. 1983. Milk and dairy products in human nutrition. W-Gmbh, Volkswirtschaftlecher Verlag, München

Rudman D, Millikan WJ, Richardson, TJ, et al. 1975. Elemental balances during intravenous hyperalimentation of underweight adult subjects. J. Clin. Invest 33:94-104.

Sewell, R.F. and West, J.P. 1965. Some effects of lactose on protein utilization in the baby pig. J. Animal Sci. 24:239

Sahi, T., Isokoski, M., Jussila, J., Launiala, K. and Pyorala, K. 1973. Recessive inheritance of adult type lactase malabsorption. Lancet 2:823-826

Stegeman, G.A., Baer, R.J., Schingoethe, D.J., and Casper, D.P. 1992. The composition and flavor of milk and butter from cows fed unsaturated dietary fat and receiving bovine somatotropin. J.Dairy Science 75(4):962-70

Tadesse, K., Leung, DTY and Yuen, RCF. 1992. The status of lactose absorption in Hong Kong children. Acta Paediatr. 81:596-600

Traver, L.E., Bookwalter, G.N., Kwolek, W.F. 1981. A computer-based graphical method for evaluating protein quality of food blends relative to cost. Food Technol. 35 (6):72-78

Turlington, W.H. Allee, G.L. and Nelssen, J.L. 1989. Effect of protein & carbohydrate sources on digestibility. J.Animal Sci. 67(9): 2333-40

Vallee, BL., Falchuk, KH. 1981. Zinc and gene expression. Phil.Trans.R. Soc.Lond.B. 294:185-197.

Van t Veer, P., Kok, K.J., Brants, H.A.M., Ockhuizen, T., Sturmans, F. and Hermus, R.J.J. dietary fat and the risk of breast cancer. Inter.J. Epidemiol. 1990;19(1):12-18

Veverbrants E, Arky PA. 1969. Effects of fasting and refeeding. I. Studies on sodium, potassium and water excretion on a constant electrolyte and fluid intake. J Clin Endocrinol. 29:55-62.

Wald, G. 1933. Vitamin A in the retina Nature. 132:316-317

Waterlow, JC., Golden, MHN., Patrick, J. 1978. Protein-energy malnutrition :treatment. In Dickerson JWT, Lee HA (eds). Nutrition in the Clinical Management of Disease. London, Edward Arnold Ltd.: 49-71.

Wester, P.O. 1987. Magnesium. Am.J. Clin.Nutr. (suppl)45(5):1305-12

Whitington, P.F., Gibson R. 1977. Soy protein intolerance: four patients with concomitant cow's milk intolerance. Pediatrics 59:730-732

Wilson, N.W., Self, T.W., and Hamburger, R.N. 1990. Severe cow's milk induced colitis in an exclusively breast-fed neonate. Case report and clinical review of cow's milk allergy. Clinical Pediatrics 29(2):77-80

Wittenberg, D.F., and Moosa, A. 1990. Lactose maldigestion:increased age-related prevalence in institution-alized children. J.Ped.Gastr.Nutr. 11:489-495

World Health Organization, 1973. WHO. Tech.Rep.Ser. No.532:20-24.

World Health Organization. 1982. Report of the joint WHO/UNICEF/USAID /HKI/IVACG meeting. Control of vitamin A deficiency. Tech.Rep.Ser. no.672.

Wolman SL., Anderson GH., Marliss EB., et al. 1979. Zinc in total parenteral nutrition. Requirements and metabolic effects. Gastroenterology 76:458-467.

Yang, G. Chen, J., Wen, Z., Ge, K., Zhu, L., Chen, X. and Chen, X. 1984 The role of selenium in Keshan disease. Adv.Nutr.Res. 6:203-231

Yap, I., B. Berry, J. Kang, M. Math, M. Chu, D. Miller and A. Pollard. 1989. Lactase deficiency in Singapore-born and Canadian-born Chinese. Digest.Dis.Sci. 34(7):1085-1088

Dairy Products in Human Health and Nutrition, Serrano Ríos et al. (eds) © 1994 Balkema, Rotterdam, ISBN 90 5410 359 0

Biological properties of milk proteins

P.F. Fox & A. Flynn
Department of Food Chemistry and Nutrition, University College, Cork, Ireland

Milks are the characteristic secretion of mammals designed to meet the complete nutritional requirements of the neonate of the species. However, milk serves several functions in addition to strictly nutritional. Most of the non-nutritional functions of milk are served by proteins and peptides which include immunoglobulins, enzymes and enzyme inhibitors, binding or carrier proteins, growth factors and antibacterial agents. Because the nutritional and physiological requirements of the neonate of each species are more or less unique, so is the milk of each species (see Widdowson, 1984). Of the > 4,000 mammalian species, the milks of only ~ 180 have been analyzed and the data for only ~ 50 of these are considered to be reliable.

In this review, we will consider primarily bovine and human milks, which are well characterized. The proteins of bovine milk are probably the best characterized food protein system (see Fox, 1982, 1989, 1992). However, they are normally considered from the chemical, physical or functional/technological viewpoints. Food scientists have learned to exploit many of the unique functional properties of milk proteins, but these are not their natural functions. Nutritionists normally consider milk proteins as a source of essential amino acids, but many proteins can serve this function. Many of the unique nutritional, physiological, biochemical, immunological and other biological properties of these proteins are usually ignored.

Human milk has been studied more thoroughly in this regard than bovine or other milks, mainly by paediatricians. Generally, when they have been sought, similar biologically active proteins/peptides have been found in human and bovine milks, although usually at different, sometimes very marked, concentrations. Presumably, biologically active proteins are common to the milks of most species. Books and reviews on human milk and lactation include: Jensen & Neville (1985), Atkinson & Lonnerdal (1989), Goldman et al. (1985,

1987), Blanc (1981), Koldovsky (1989), Schaub (1985), Walker (1985) and Goldman (1988).

The objective of this presentation is to review the literature on the principal biologically active proteins in milk.

Enzymes and enzyme inhibitors

Milk contains up to 60 indigenous enzymes, many of which, because of their technological significance, have been studied extensively. The literature on the indigenous enzymes in bovine milk has been reviewed by Andrews et al. (1992) and in human milk by Hamos et al. (1985) and Hernell & Lonnerdal (1989).

Most, if not all, the indigenous enzymes in milk are probably adventitious. Many occur in the fat globule membrane which is derived from the apical membrane of the mammocyte which envelopes the fat globules during excretion from the secretory cells. The apical membrane lost on excretion of fat globules is replaced by Golgi membrane during excretion of milk proteins, lactose and salts and hence many milk enzymes are of intracellular origin. Some indigenous enzymes, e.g. lipoprotein lipase, plasmin, xanthine oxidase, phosphatases, superoxidase dimutase and lactoperoxidase, are technologically significant, others are indicators of animal health, e.g. catalase, N-acetyl glucosamidase. A few enzymes are physiologically or nutritionally significant to the neonate. In addition to the lipoprotein lipase, which occurs in the milks of all species examined, human milk and those of some other primates contain a bile salts-activated lipase which contributes to the digestion of lipids by the human baby whose pancreatic function is immature and in whom lipases from 4 sources contribute to lipid digestion - pancreatic lipase, lingual lipase, milk lipoprotein lipase and milk bile salts-activated lipase. Human milk, in contrast to bovine milk, is very rich in lysozyme which is believed to play a bacteriocidal role in the intestine. Milk lysozyme is significantly different from egg white lysozyme; it survives passage through the intestine and is excreted in active form in the faeces. Bovine milk is rich in lactoperoxidase, in contrast to human milk. Although the biological function of indigenous lactoperoxidase is unclear, it is a very potent bacteriocidal agent in the presence of H_2O_2 and ^-SCN. Addition of lactoperoxidase/H_2O_2/^-SCN to calf or piglet milk replacers effectively prevents enteritis and it is probable that the indigenous enzyme plays a similar role. Lactoperoxidase may also play a bacteriocidal role in the mammary gland during the dry (non-lactating) period.

α-Lactalbumin, one of the principal whey proteins in most milks, is an enzyme modifier in lactose synthetase (see Brew & Grobler, 1992) but has no enzymatic function in milk.

Binding proteins

Most, perhaps all, milk proteins exhibit some form of binding property, ranging from non-specific metal-binding by the caseins to highly specific binding of vitamins.

Metal binding

Casein
All the caseins are phosphoproteins; bovine α_{s1}-, α_{s2}-, ß- and κ-caseins contain 8-9, 10-13, 4-5 and 1-2 mole P/mole protein, respectively. The phosphate groups, which occur mainly as clusters of phosphoseryl residues, bind metal ions strongly, resulting in charge neutralization, and in the case of α_{s1}-, α_{s2}- and ß-caseins, in precipitation or, as in milk, in micelle formation. Calcium is the principal metal involved but a substantial portion of the zinc in milk is also chelated by the phosphate residues. Additional calcium and zinc are associated with the inorganic colloidal calcium phosphate (CCP) in the casein micelles.

Both the casein-bound calcium and the CCP are highly significant in many technologically important properties of milk, e.g. rennet coagulation, heat stability, alcohol stability, and are probably nutritionally significant also. It is generally believed that casein phospho-peptides facilitate the absorption of metal ions and are being promoted as nutritionally-desirable supplements. However, although bovine milk contains more Zn than human milk, it is commonly reported that Zn is less readily available from the former, a feature commonly attributed to the higher degree of phosphorylation of the former. However, Zn

is almost fully absorbed by suckling rats from both bovine and human milks, although somewhat faster from the latter (Brennan, 1990). In bovine milk, ~ 95% of total Zn is associated with the casein micelles, ~ 40% of which is bound by the casein, presumably via phosphoserine residues, with 60% being a constituent of CCP (Singh et al., 1989). In human milk, casein binds only ~ 14% of total Zn while the whey proteins and citrate each bind ~ 35% (Lonnerdal et al., 1982). The reduced bioavailability of Zn from bovine milk may be due to its high content of CCP, which is absent, or nearly so, from human milk. Reduction of the CCP content of bovine milk, e.g. by acidification/dialysis, increases the bioavailability of its Zn (Kiely et al., 1988).

Casein-derived phosphopeptides stimulate the absorption of Ca (Sato et al., 1986), proportional to the degree of phosphorylation; however, the situatio is ambiguous (Kitts & Yuan, 1992). These highly negatively charged peptides are resistant to proteolysis; they have been detected in the small intestine of the rat and may pass intact through the intestinal wall.

Iron is also bound by phosphoserine residues; casein phosphopeptide - Fe complexes have been proposed as useful sources of dietary Fe and methods for their production have been developed (see Maubois & Lonil, 1989).

The serine phosphate groups of casein may have a specific metabolic function, e.g. one of the phosphate groups of ß-casein is released faster than the others and may be transferred to ADP by a specific AMP-independent casein kinase to form ATP, suggesting that it may be a type of high-energy phosphate (Cochet et al., 1983). The structure and function of the phosphorylated residues of casein were reviewed by West (1986).

α-Lactalbumin and serum albumin

α-Lactalbumin and blood serum albumin bind metal ions strongly but this is probably not nutritionally significant.

Lactotransferrin

The most significant of the specific metal-binding proteins in milk are the transferrins, especially lactotransferrin. Various aspects of the transferrins and related iron-binding proteins are reviewed in the text edited by Spik et al. (1985).

Human colostrum and milk contain 6-8 mg/ml and 2-4 mg/ml lactotransferrin, respectively; concentrations in bovine colostrum and milk are ~ 1 and 0.02-0.35 mg/ml (Reiter, 1985). Lactotransferrins of several species, including human and cow, have been isolated and well characterized (see Fox & Flynn, 1992). Because of their apparent physiological and nutritional significance, several improved methods for the isolation of lactotransferrins, including various forms of affinity chromatography, have been published; some are designed for commercial-scale operation (see Fox & Flynn, 1992).

Lactotransferrin binds iron very strongly, indicating two roles for this protein: iron absorption and protection against enteric infection in the neonate (see Arnold et al., 1977; Spik et al., 1985; Reiter, 1985; Lonnerdal, 1985). Because the concentration of lactotransferrin in human milk is considerably higher than that in bovine milk, there is considerable interest in supplementing bovine milk-based infant formulae with lactotransferrin. The concentration of lactotransferrin in milk increases markedly during mastitic infections, suggesting that it may have a protective role in the mammary gland (Harmon et al., 1976).

Milks of various species studied also contain serotransferrin (see Williams, 1985). The heterogeneity of bovine sero-transferrin was studied by Maeda et al. (1980).

Vitamin-binding proteins

Milks of several species contain proteins that bind retinol, folic acid, riboflavin or Vitamin B_{12}. These proteins probably facilitate the absorption of the appropriate vitamin and may have bacteriocidal effects.

ß-Lactoglobulin

ß-Lactoglobulin is the principal whey protein in bovine, ovine and caprine milks; a similar protein occurs in the milks of several species but is absent from human and rodent milks. The extensive literature on this very well characterized protein was reviewed by Hambling et al. (1992).

ß-Lg is capable of binding hydrophobic molecules, including retinol, and may function in vivo to protect retinol against oxidation and to transport it through the stomach to the small intestine; its resistance to peptic hydrolysis is probably significant in this regard. ß-Lg also binds fatty acids and consequently stimulates the activity of pregastric (and probably other) lipase (Perez et al., 1992); it may play such a role in vivo.

Vitamin B_{12}-binding protein

Gregory (1954) showed that Vitamin B_{12} in the milks of cow, goat, sheep, sow, woman and rat was almost entirely bound to a whey protein; the porcine protein was partially purified and characterized by Gregory & Holdsworth (1955a, b). The B_{12}-binding protein was isolated from human milk by Burger & Allen (1974) and Sandberg et al. (1981), who identified 2 Vit B_{12} binding proteins in human milk. The principal B_{12}-binding protein had a molecular weight of 61-63,000 and contained ~ 35% carbohydrate. Porcine milk is rich in Vit B_{12}-binding protein which has been isolated (affinity chromatography on B_{12}-Sepharose) and characterized with respect to Mr (~ 62,000), carbohydrate content (24%), amino acid profile and binding affinity for B_{12} (Trugo, 1988). The Vit B_{12}-binding protein of rat milk was partly purified and characterized by Raaberg et al. (1989).

The B_{12}-binding protein in milk probably plays 2 roles: absorption of Vit B_{12} and bacteriocidal. Animal experiments indicate that protein-bound Vit B_{12} is efficiently absorbed from the intestine (Ford et al., 1975; Trugo et al., 1985). However, Sandberg et al. (1981) suggest that cobalamin must be released from its binding protein by proteolysis and then combined with an intrinsic factor for absorption. Vit B_{12}-binding protein attaches to the brush border membrane where it stimulates absorption of vitamin B_{12} (Trugo & Turvey, 1987). Human milk can bind ~ 43 ng cyanocobalamin/ml but in milk most of the protein is unsaturated (Ford et al., 1977); its binding capacity is reduced by heat treatments to a minimum at 75°C x 15 min. Human milk inhibits the uptake of cyanoco-balamin by intestinal bacteria but this inhibitory effect is progressively lost on heating (Ford et al., 1977). It therefore appears that this protein protects Vit B_{12} against bacterial uptake in the gut and may strongly influence the ecology of the intestinal microflora and the vitamin nutrition of the suckling infant (Ford, 1974). However, Cole et al. (1983) could not confirm this hypothesis for Vit B_{12}-binding protein, folate-binding protein and lactotransferrin in rabbits.

Ford et al. (1977) suggested that the minimum stability of Vit B_{12}-binding protein at ~ 75°C may be due to the action of an enzyme [presumably plasmin, which is activated by mild heat treatments] which is denatured at higher temperatures. They argue that if this is so, refrigerated storage should also cause considerable loss of Vit B_{12}-binding activity.

Folate-binding proteins

Folate-binding proteins (FBP) from a variety of tissues have been characterized. They fall into 2 molecular weight ranges: 100,000-200,000 and 25,000-40,000, and may be extracellular, i.e. in fluids such as milk, blood serum, cerebrospinal fluid, or intracellular which may be sub-divided into those that are membrane-bound and those that are soluble. General reviews on FBPs include Waxman (1975), Colman & Herbert (1980) and Wagner (1982); FBPs in milk have been reviewed by Fox & Flynn (1992) which should be consulted for references.

Low MW FBPs have been isolated from bovine, caprine and human milks; the latter also contains a high MW FBP. Commercial preparations of bovine ß-lg contain FBP. ELISA methods have been developed for the FBPs of bovine and human milks; these FBPs show no cross-reactivity.

The complete amino acid sequence (222 residues) of FBP from bovine milk has been determined. The protein contains ~ 10% carbohydrate, attached to Arg residues, probably 49 and 141, and has a molecular weight of ~ 30,000, including carbohydrate. The amino acid composition of human milk FBP has been reported and the sequence of 60 residues from the N-terminal determined; the 5 N-terminal residues of the bovine protein appear to be missing from the human protein but otherwise the 2 proteins showed a high degree of homology. The high and low molecular FBPs may be the consequence of gene duplication; alternatively, the low MW form may result from proteolytic cleavage of the larger protein. FBP associate extensively up to 30 monomers, depending on pH and protein concentration. The mechanism of folate binding by milk FBP has been studied; the FBP-folate complex dissociates at acidic pH values and reforms on neutralization.

The physiological significance of FBP in milk was reviewed by Salter & Mowlem (1983). Protein-bound folate is efficiently absorbed from the intestine. Breast-fed babies have higher plasma and red blood cell folate concentrations than their mothers or adult references, suggesting that milk contains a factor that facilitates folate uptake by intestinal cells. In vitro studies on intestinal cells showed that FBP-bound folate was absorbed more effectively than free folate; the beneficial effect of FBP on folate absorption increased throughout the length of the small intestine while absorption of free folate was independent of intestinal segment. Absorption of folate from FBP was not influenced by glucose, dilantin, Ca or EDTA, in contrast to free folate. Colman & Herbert (1980) reported that the intestine contains FBP receptor sites but Said et al. (1986) claimed that free folate was absorbed faster than FBP-bound folate in the jejunum and at about the same rate in the ileum; they suggested that FBP regulates the nutritional bioavailability of folate rather than promotes its absorption. Tani et al. (1983) also reported that FBP reduces the rate of absorption of folate in perfused rat intestine while Swiatlo & Picciano (1988) claimed that FBP reduced the bioavailability of folate to the rat.

FBP reduces the availability of folate to intestinal bacteria and thus may have an antibacterial effect (Ford, 1974; Ford et al., 1977) although Cole et al. (1983) could not confirm this in rabbits. The folate binding properties of FBP are reduced by heat treatment, although only slightly by commercial pasteurization.

Riboflavin binding

Egg white and yolk contain almost identical riboflavin-binding proteins (RfBP) which are required for the transport of riboflavin across the vitellin membrane from the blood serum, which contains a similar protein, into the white and yolk. These proteins have 8 phosphoseryl residues, analogous to casein, which are essential for the transport function of RfBP, apparently serving as recognitions site for binding of the protein at the membrane (Miller et al., 1982, 1984). Riboflavin-binding proteins were reviewed by White & Merrill (1988).

Raw bovine milk contains a RfBP which was partially purified by Toyosaki et al. (1987); its molecular weight was estimated to be 38,000. Based on amino acid, carbohydrate and phosphate composition, the M_r of egg white RfBP is 29,200, although higher values (30-36,000) were found using sedimentation equilibrium and SDS-PAGE (see White & Merrill, 1988). Since the RfBP of egg white and yolk are derived from blood plasma, it is likely that RfBP in milk is also of blood origin. Riboflavin bound to RfBP of milk or egg white has good antioxidant properties (Toyosaki et al., 1987; Toyosaki & Mineshita, 1988). RfBP plays a major nutritional role in the egg; a similar role for RfBP in milk has not been demonstrated.

West (1986) argues that although the caseins do not function as riboflavin-binding proteins, the similarity of the clustered serine phosphates in these two unrelated proteins suggests the possibility that the casein serine phosphates may act as a membrane recognition signal.

Immunoglobulins

Immunoglobulins (Igs), one of the principal defence mechanisms of the body, are present in the mammary secretions, especially colostrum, of all species studied. Bovine colostrum contains ~ 10% Ig but this level decreases to ~ 0.1% within about a week post-partum.

There are large inter-species differences with respect to the concentration and type of Ig in milk which are largely a reflection of the two mechanisms, in utero or via colostrum, by which passive immunity via maternal Igs is transferred to the neonate. In general, the milks and colostra of those mammalian species (e.g. human, rabbit) that transfer passive immunity to the foetus in utero contain lower amounts and different ratios of the Ig classes than those species, e.g. cow, goat, horse and pig, that transfer passive immunity via colostrum and in which ingestion of Ig from colostrum is essential for the health of the neonate. Members of a third group, e.g. mouse, rat, dog, transfer Igs both in utero and via colostrum. The milks and colostra of those animals that transfer Ig principally in utero contain mainly IgA while those that transfer immunity via colostrum are especially rich in IgG1. The mammary secretions of those species that transfer Ig both in utero and via colostrum contain high levels of both IgA and IgG.

IgG1 is the principal Ig class in bovine milk and colostrum, representing ~ 80 and 73% of total Ig, respectively, in contrast to ~ 50% in blood serum. It is believed that, except during inflammation, Ig is transported transcellularly (i.e. through the mammary cells) rather than paracellularly (i.e. through leaky junctions between the cells). However, Ig is selectively transferred from the blood to milk since the proportions of the various classes differ in the two fluids; some Igs, especially IgA and IgM, are also synthesised with the mammary gland.

It is not intended to review the chemistry of the Igs in general or the Igs in milk. Readers referred to (Butler, 1969; Eigel et al., 1984; Larson, 1992) for general reviews on the Igs, earlier reviews on the Igs in milk and the ingestion of Igs.

Large molecules such as Igs can be absorbed from the intestine of young ruminants and some other species for about 3 days post-partum. Since ruminants are born devoid of blood antibodies, they are very susceptible to infection and it is highly desirable, probably essential, that they receive colostrum by suckling or pail-feeding within 6 h post-partum. Maternal Igs appear in the blood of the neonate within hours of suckling and can be detected in its blood for about 4 months thereafter. In situations where it is not possible to feed colostrum, an alternative source of Ig is necessary and for this purpose, calf and piglet milk replacers enriched with Ig are available.

The classical method for preparing Igs is by salting out, usually with $(NH_4)_2SO_4$. While this method is effective, it is too expensive for commercial operation and most commercial methods for the preparation of Ig, exploit ultrafiltration of colostrum or milk from hyperimmunized cows, e.g. Kothe et al. (1986), Scott and Lucas (1987), Taniguchi et al. (1990) or a combination of UF and ion exchange chromatography, e.g. Dubois (1986), Bottomley (1989). Other methods include a monoclonal antibody system (Gani et al., 1982), gel filtration (Al-Mashikhi and Nakai, 1987) and metal chelate interaction chromatography (Al-Mashikhi and Nakai, 1988; Al-Mashikhi et al., 1988).

A number of colostrum substitutes for calves, lambs or piglets are commercially available, e.g. Calf Volostrum (Volac), Immuno-Bac (Alltech) and Colostrx (Protein Technology Inc.), which appear to be essentially UF retentates of bovine colostral whey.

Although the human infant in unable to absorb Ig from its intestine, Ig still plays an important defensive role by reducing the incidence of intestinal infection. There is general agreement on the superiority of breast feeding in the nutrition of healthy full-term infants but it is frequently impossible to breast-feed pre-term or very-low-birth-weight infants, who are frequently be fed on banked human milk. However, low-birth-weight pre-term infants have high protein and energy requirements which may not be met by bulked human milk; for these, special formulae have been developed. The preparation of "milk immunological concentrate" (MIC) by diafiltration of the acid whey from colostrum and early lactation (< 30 days) milk from immunized cows for addition to in such formulae was described by Hilpert (1984). The final product contained ca. 75% protein, 50% of which was Ig, mainly IgG1 and not IgA, which is predominant in human milk. The immuno-logical supplementation of cows' milk formulations was discussed by Goldman (1989).

Bifidus factors

It has been recognized for many years that breast-fed babies are more resistant to gastroenteritis than bottle-fed babies [see Bullen & Willis (1971) and Rasic & Kurmann (1983) for references]. This is undoubtably a multi-factorial phenomenon, including better hygiene, more appropriate milk composition, several antibacterial systems, especially immunoglobulins, lysozyme, lactotransferrin, vitamin-binding proteins, lactoperoxidase, and a lower intestinal pH. Bullen & Willis (1971) attributed the lower pH of the faeces of breast-fed compared with bottle-fed babies, 5.1 and 6.4, respectively, to the lower buffering capacity of human milk compared to formulae, due to the lower protein and phosphate content of the former. While buffering capacity is undoubtably important, differences in the intestinal microflora of breast-fed and bottle-fed infants are of major significance.

Bifidobacteria represent about 99% of the faecal microflora of breast-fed infants (see Rasic & Kurmann, 1983). These bacteria are also present at high numbers in the faeces of bottle-fed infants but several other genera, e.g. Bacteroides, Clostridium, Coliforms, also occur at high numbers. Furthermore, the predominant species of Bifidobacterium in breast-fed infants is B. bifidum, with lesser numbers of B. longum; the principal Bifidobacterium in the faeces of bottle-fed infants is B. longum with lower numbers of B. bifidum, B. infantis, B. adolescentis and B. breve (Beerens et al., 1980).

The preponderance of B. bifidum in the faecal microflora of breast-fed infants is due to stimulatory factors in human milk. Bifidobacteria are festidious and are stimulated by several factors (see Rasic & Kurmann, 1983), including lactulose and N-acetylglucosamine-containing saccharides (bifidus factor 1).

Lactulose stimulates the growth of Bifidobacteria, Lactobacillus and several other genera. It is an unnatural sugar but is produced from lactose by relatively mild heat treatments, such as used in the manufacture of UHT milks and sterilized infant formulae. The inclusion of lactulose in feed for calves and piglets is recommended (see Modler et al., 1990).

György (1953) and György et al. (1954 a, b, c) reported that N-acetylglucosamine-containing saccharides are essential for the growth of B. bifidum. This factor is present at high concentrations in human milk and colostrum and in bovine colostrum but at very low levels in bovine, ovine and caprine milks. Beerens et al. (1980) reported that bovine, ovine and porcine milks did not stimulate the growth of B. bifidum but did contain factors, which were not studied, that stimulated B. infantis and B. longum.

Most (40-75%) of the bifidus-promoting factors in human milk are non-dialyzable and appear to be a mixture of glycoproteins and oligosaccharides. The glycoproteins contained N-acetylneuraminic acid (NANA) and had no bifidus activity unless the NANA residue(s) was removed by treatment with neuraminidase (György et al., 1974).

Bovine and human colostra and milks contain several glycoproteins, in both the casein and especially in the whey fractions, that contain N-acetylglucosamine. These proteins, which have been described by Flynn & Fox (1992), stimulate the growth of Bifido bacteria following acid or enzymatic hydrolysis.

Growth Factors

"Growth factor" is a term applied to a group of highly potent hormone-like polypeptides which play a critical role in regulation and differentiation of a variety of cells, acting through cell-membrane receptors. Milks of several species have been found to stimulate in vivo growth of gastrointestinal tissues, to promote in vitro replication of cultured cells and to contain assayable growth factors. In general, such growth-promoting characteristics are more pronounced in colostrum than in mature milk.

At least 16 distinct growth factors have been detected in the milk of human and other species. These include epidermal growth factor, insulin, insulin-like growth factors 1 and 2 (IGF 1, 2), three human milk growth factors ($TGF_{\alpha 1}$, $TGF_{\alpha 2}$ and TGF_a), two mammary-derived growth factors (MDGF I, II), colony stimulating factor, nerve growth factor, platlet-derived growth factor (PDGF) and bombesin. Some of these can be grouped together on the basis of similarity of biological activity (Kidwell & Salomon, 1989).

The source of these polypeptides may be blood plasma, mammary gland or both. The biological significance of these growth-promoting activities in colostrum and mature milks is not yet clear. In terms of possible physiological significance, two potential targets may be considered, i.e. the mammary gland or the neonate. In general, most attention has focussed on the latter. It is not known whether the factors in milk that possess the capacity to promote cell proliferation, (a) influence growth of mammary tissue, (b) promote growth of cells within the intestine of the recipient noenate, or (c) are absorbed in a biologically active form and exert an effect on enteric or other target organs.

The original work in this area was undertaken by Widdowson and her colleagues who observed striking increases in the mass of intestinal mucosa of suckled newborn piglets (Widdowson et al., 1976) and rabbits (Hall & Widdowson, 1979) compared to litter-mates that were fasted for the first 24 h after birth. Subsequently, Heird et al. (1984) showed that small intestinal mucosal mass was increased by 75%, and mucosal DNA and protein contents by 65% and 93%, respectively, in beagle puppies suckled for the first 24 h after birth compared with litter-mates fed an artificial formula.

Berseth et al. (1983) reported similar findings in rats and Mirand et al. (1990) showed that feeding newborn lambs with cow or ewe colostrum stimulated intestinal protein synthesis more than cow's milk over the first 18 h of life.

Human milk contains growth factor activity and is capable of stimulating the growth of fibroblasts in culture (Klagsbrun, 1978). Bovine milk contains growth-promoting factors that stimulate DNA synthesis and cell division in cultured Balb/c 3T3 cells (Klagsbrun & Neumann, 1979). The mitogenic activity of colostrum is higher than that of mature milk from several species, including human, cow, sheep and goat (Klagsbrun, 1978; Klagsbrun & Neumann, 1979; Brown & Blakeley, 1983).

Epidermal growth factor (EGF) belongs to a family of growth factors that act through the EGF receptors on the cell membrane. Five such factors have been detected in human milk - EGF, MDGFII, $TGF_{\alpha 1}$, $TGF_{\alpha 2}$ and HMGIII.

EGF contains 53 amino acids (M_r: 6045, pI: 4.4) and is derived from a precursor of M_r 130,000 (Scott et al., 1983) that is synthesized in the salivary glands and other tissues (Cohen, 1962). Human milk and colostrum contain considerable amounts of EGF (Carpenter, 1980). The concentration is highest in colostrum (23 to 125 nmol/1) (Read et al., 1984) and falls shortly after delivery to about 5 nmol/1. About 70% of the growth factor activity of human milk can be neutralized by antibodies against human EGF (Carpenter, 1980), suggesting that EGF is the major growth factor in human milk. EGF has been purified to homogeneity from human milk and sequenced (Petrides et al, 1985).

EGF is present in the milk of the mouse (Beardmore & Richards, 1983) and rat (Thornburg et al., 1984) and EGF-like activity has been detected in bovine colostrum (Klagsbrun & Neumann, 1979) and milk (Yagi et al., 1986), but not in bovine milk-based formulae (Carpenter, 1980; Yagi et al., 1986). Klagsbrun & Neumann (1979) showed that the EGF-like activity of bovine colostrum decreases abruptly after parturition, e.g. activity 50 h after parturition, with only 1% that after 8 h. Fractionation of colostrum by gel filtration gives one major active peak with M_r 30,000-45,000. Isoelectric focusing of this peak indicated two active components with pIs of 6.5 and 9.0, suggesting that these EGF-like factors are molecularly distinct from EGF.

Klagsbrun (1978) and Shing & Klagsbrun (1984) isolated and characterized three polypeptides from human colostrum and milk which stimulate DNA synthesis and proliferation of cultured fibroblasts in vitro; these were named human milk growth factor (HMGF) I, II and III. HMGF III,

which constituted 75-95% of HMGF activity, had a M_r of 5,000-6,000 and a pI of 4.4-4.7, suggesting that it may be identical to EGF. HMGF I (M_r 34,000-38,000, pI 4.2-4.5) and HMGF II (M_r 10,000-20,000; pI, 3.2-4.8) represent about 5% and 20%, respectively, of the fibroblast growth factor activity in human milk.

Zwiebel et al. (1986) isolated a factor from human milk with EGF-like activity which they called mammary-derived growth factor II (MDGF II). It has a M_r of 17,000 and a pI of 4.0, which suggests that it is molecularly distinct from EGF.

Human milk contains growth factor activity that resembles transforming growth factor α (TGF_α), a factor which can transform anchorage-dependent into anchorage-independent cells (Zwiebel et al., 1986). The TGF_α activity of human milk can be resolved by isoelectric focusing into two components with pIs of 6.5 ($TGF_{\alpha 1}$) and 7.0 ($TGF_{\alpha 2}$).

Members of the insulin family include insulin itself and two insulin-like growth factors, IGF1 and IGF2. Insulin and IGF1 have been detected in human milk (Read et al., 1984; Baxter et al., 1984). IGF2 has been detected, but not quantified, in human milk (Read et al., 1983).

The concentration (3.75 nmol/1) of insulin (M_r 5,796; pI 5.7) in human colostrum is 30 times that in blood serum but decreases 5-6 fold within a few days (Read et al., 1984). While these authors reported that the concentration of insulin in human colostrum and milk was less than that required to stimulate significant increases in protein and DNA synthesis in several cell lines in vitro, Ballard et al. (1982) claimed that insulin accounts for a substantial amount of the mitogenic activity of human colostrum, as shown by the selective removal of insulin by immunoaffinity chromatography. The discrepancy may be due to the different cell lines used by the two groups. Ballard et al. (1982) reported that the concentration of insulin in bovine colostrum (2-3 nmol/1) was about 100-fold that in blood serum.

IGF1 (M_r 7,649; pI 8.4; Rindernecht & Humbel, 1976) is largely bound to a carrier protein in human milk (Baxter et al., 1984) and in bovine milk most of the IGF1 is associated with a 45 kDa binding protein, which is unsaturated, and from which it is readily dissociated by acidification (Campbell & Baumrucker, 1989). Suikkari (1989) reported that the concentration of IGF1 in human milk decreased from 49 µg/l at 4 h post-partum to 29 µg/l at 92 h post-partum. Frankenne et al. (1989) purified IGF1 from bovine colostrum and showed it to have the same molecular weight as IGF1 from human milk.

Treatment of cows at 35-47 weeks of lactation with recombinantly-derived bovine growth hormone (rbGH) for 7 days increased the concentration of IGF1 in milk from 0.44 to 1.6 nmol/l (Prosser et al., 1989). However, maximum IGF1 concentration during rbGH treatment was lower than that in early lactation milk and equivalent to that in mature human milk. They showed that about 80% of IGF1 in bovine milk is associated with proteins of molecular mass 40,000-150,000.

Mammary-derived growth factor I (MDGF I) is a polypeptide which stimulates mouse mammary cells and rat kidney cells in vitro to synthesize extracellular proteins, including collagen. It was purified from human milk by Bano et al. (1985) and shown to be a polypeptide with a M_r of 62,000 and a pI of 4.8.

Platlet-derived growth factor (PDGF), a polypeptide of M_r 28,000-35,000 and a pI of 9.9, is present in colostrum and mature milk from cows, sheep and goats (Brown & Blakeley, 1984). Transforming growth factor ß (TGF$_a$), which acts synergistically with TGF$_\alpha$ and IGF1 in promoting cell growth in culture, has been detected in colostrum and milk from human (Noda et al., 1984) and goat (Brown & Blakeley, 1984). Sinha & Yunis (1983) partially purified a protein from human milk with colony stimulating factor (CSF) activity; it had a M_r of 240-250,000 and a pI of 4.4-4.9. Jahnke & Lazarus (1984) detected a bombesin immunoactive peptide of M_r 3,200 in bovine milk while Ekman et al. (1985) showed that human milk contains 60-430 µg/ml of bombesin-immunoactive material.

Nerve growth factor (NGF), which plays a role in the survival and differentiation of selected neurons of the nervous system, has been identified in mouse (Grueters et al., 1985) and human (Wright & Gaull, 1983) milks.

It is not known if the gastrointestinal mucosal proliferation observed on feeding colostrum to newborn animals is attributable to any of the growth factors described above. To date, most attention has focussed on EGF which appears to be the major growth factor in human milk. Feeding EGF in pharmacological doses to neonatal rats (Berseth, 1985) or rabbits (O'Loughlin et al., 1985) resulted in increased DNA in intestinal tissues. Stomach growth during the first 24 h after birth was faster in neonatal rats fed formula containing EGF than in suckled neonates (Falconer, 1987). Feeding EGF at physiological levels to neonatal rats also resulted in increased intestinal length (Moore et al., 1986) while neonatal rats fed artificial formula containing EGF for 39 h had greater intestinal DNA synthesis and content than rats fed an EGF-free formula (Berseth, 1987). Rats given pooled milk with antibodies to EGF for 39 h had lower intestinal weight and less DNA in the intestine than animals fed rat milk without antibodies.

There is also evidence that orally-administered EGF can affect tissues other than the intestine. Berseth & Go (1988) showed that ingestion of a formula containing added EGF by newborn rats for five days increased liver DNA and RNA and heart and kidney weight compared to formula-fed controls. These results suggest that oral ingestion of EGF is associated with growth of non-intestinal organs. For EGF consumed orally to exert such effects requires absorption of intact EGF, or of one of its metabolites, and distribution to target tissues. Little degradation of EGF occurred in the rat stomach during the suckling and weanling periods, and degradation by luminal fluid from the small intestine of 12 day-old rats was lower than in weanling (31 day old) rats (Britton et al., 1988). Absorption of intact EGF has been demonstrated in suckling, weanling and adult rats (Thornburg et al., 1984, 1987). Gale et al. (1989) reported that urinary excretion of EGF was higher in breast-fed infants than in infants receiving cow's milk-based formula or total parenteral nutrition. They suggested that these results were consistent with the hypothesis that EGF ingested in human milk crosses the gastrointestinal wall to enter the general circulation in the suckling infant.

Biologically active peptides from casein hydrolyzates

Peptides with various types of biological activity have been isolated from the hydrolyzates of casein and whey proteins (Meisel et al., 1989; Maubois & Lenoil, 1989). At least some of these peptides are produced in vivo and may have physiological effects. The presence of these latent peptides led Migliore-Samour & Jolles (1988) to refer to casein as a "prohormone".

Caseinomorphins

Peptides with opioid activity have been identified in enzymatic digests of food proteins and are called exorphins. Several such peptides have been isolated from digests of milk proteins; the literature has been reviewed by Chiba & Yoshikawa (1986), Meisel & Schlimme (1990) and Fox & Flynn (1992).

Brantl & Teschemacher (1979) detected peptides with opioid activity in some batches of baby foods, casein digests and cows' milk. These peptides were isolated from enzymatic digests of casein and characterized as a family of peptides containing 4-7 amino acids with a common N-terminal sequence, H-Tyr-Pro-Phe-Pro-, and 0-3 additional residues (Gly, Pro, Ile) (see Fox & Flynn, 1992). The peptides represent residues 60-63/6 of ß-casein and are called ß-caseinomorphins 4 to 7, respectively; they possess μ-type opiate receptor activity. ß-CM-5 was the most effective of the ß-CMs which are 300-4,000 times less effective than morphine; the amide of ß-CM-4 is more active than ß-CM-5. Various physiological effects of ß-CMs have been investigated (see Fox & Flynn, 1992, for references). ß-CM's are very resistant to enzymes of the GIT and appear in the contents of the small intestine following ingestion of milk. Meisel (1986) isolated a new ß-caseinomorphin, ß-CM-11 (ß-CN f 60-70), from the duodenal chyme of minipigs. ß-CM-11 is less effective than ß-CM-5 but may be hydrolyzed to smaller, more active ß-CMs by the action of intestinal peptidases. Certain proteolytic bacteria growing in milk produce ß-casomorphins (Hamel et al., 1985).

Teschemacher et al. (1986) found no evidence for ß-CM in human plasma after ingestion of cows' milk and milk products but Teschemacher (1987) reported that ß-CM precursors occur in the plasma of new born calves and infants and of pregnant, lactating and non-lactating females. While ß-casomorphins appear to have physiological effects in the intestine (Tome et al., 1987), rather high concentrations are required to affect sleep patterns and concentrations reaching the plasma or brain are probably not sufficiently high (Taira et al., 1990).

The sequence 51-57 of human ß-casein, Tyr-Pro-Phe-Val-Glu-Pro-Ile, corresponds to bovine ß-casein 60-66 (i.e. Tyr-Pro-Phe-Pro-Gly-Pro-Ile). The opioid activity of synthetic hß-CM-4 and -5 was considerably less than that of bovine ß-CM-4 and ß-CM-5 (Brantl, 1984). Several synthetic peptides with sequences corresponding to segments of human ß-casein 51-57 had opioid activity (Yoshikawa et al., 1986). Peptides corresponding to human ß-casein 41-44 and 59-63 were also synthesized and had weak opioid activity, as did the peptides Tyr-Gly-Leu-Phe, which occurs in α-lactalbumin, and Tyr-Leu-Leu-Phe, which occurs in bovine ß-lactoglobulin. The latter peptides were isolated from tryptic-peptic hydrolyzates of α-la and ß-lg (Antila et al., 1991).

Exorphins have also been isolated from peptic hydrolyzates of α-casein and shown to be α-casein f 90-95 and f 90-96 [Arg-Tyr-Leu-Gly-Tyr-Leu (Glu)] (Zioudrou et al., 1979; Loukas et al., 1983). Several sequences, especially 35-41, 57-60 and 25-34, of bovine and human κ-caseins were found to have opioid activity and were called casoxins A, B and C, respectively (Yoshikawa et al., 1986b; Chiba et al., 1989).

Three peptides with opioid properties were also isolated from peptic digests of lactotransferrin: Tyr-Leu-Gly-Ser-Gly-Tyr (lactoferroxin A), Arg-Tyr-Tyr-Gly-Tyr (lactoferroxin B), Lys-Tyr-Leu-Gly-Pro-Gln-Tyr (lactoferroxin C) (Chiba et al., 1989). The activity of the 3 peptides was markedly increased by methylation of the α-carboxyl group.

Thus, all the major milk proteins contain sequences which, when liberated by gastro-intestinal proteinases, possess opioid activity. These peptides are very resistant to proteolysis by gastrointestinal proteinases and because of their high hydrophobicity can be absorbed intact from the intestine. They have been shown to have physiological activity in vitro but their activity in vivo is as yet uncertain.

Immunomodulating Peptides

Gattegno et al. (1988) reported that enzymatic digests of human caseins contained immunomodulating peptides which stimulate the phagocytic activity of human macrophages in vitro and exert a protective effect in vivo in mice against Klebsiella preumoniae infection (see Migliore-Samour et al., 1989). Two of the peptides were characterized as Val-Glu-Pro-Ile-Pro-Tyr (ß-CN f54-59) and Gly-Leu-Phe (origin not identified).

Platelet-modifying peptide

The undecapeptide, Met-Ala-Ile-Pro-Pro-Lys-Lys-Asn-Gln-Asp-Lys (κ-CN f106-116) inhibits the aggregation of ADP-treated platelets, a property also exhibited by the structurally-related C-terminal dodecapeptide (residues 400-411) of human fibrinogen γ-chain (Jolles et al., 1986). This peptide is produced from the caseino(glyco)macropeptide, κ-CN f106-169, produced by the action of chymosin; κ-CN f106-112 and 113-116 have similar but lower activity. A peptide with similar properties was isolated from a hydrolyzate of lactotransferrin (Mazoyer et al., 1990).

Angiotensin Converting Enzyme (ACE) Inhibitor

ACE is a peptidyl-dipeptidase (EC 3.4.15.1) which cleaves dipeptides from the carboxyl terminal of peptides. It converts angiotensin I to the potent vasoconstrictor, angiotensin II, and inactivates the vasodilator bradykinin. Maruyama & Suzuki (1982) isolated the dodecapeptide, Phe-Phe-Val-Ala-Pro-Phe-Pro-Glu-Val-Phe-Gly-Lys, from tryptic hydrolyzates of casein; this corresponds to α_{s1}-CN f23-34. Other inhibitory peptides were isolated later, e.g. Thr-Thr-Met-Pro-Leu-Trp, the C-terminal sequence of α_{s1}-casein (Maruyama et al., 1987). Kohmura et al. (1989) synthesized 69 peptides corresponding to sequences of human ß-casein; several peptides had ACE inhibitory activity, especially those with sequences corresponding to peptides from the region 39-52 of ß-CN the most active being Ser-Phe-Gln-Pro-Gln-Pro-Leu-Ile-Try-Pro (ß-CN f43-52).

REFERENCES

Al-Mashikhi, S.A., E. Li-Chan & S. Nakai 1988. Separation of immunoglobulins and lactoferrin from cheese whey by chelating chromatography. J. Dairy Sci. 71: 1747-1755.

Al-Mashikhi, S.A. & S. Nakai 1987. Isolation of bovine immunoglobulins and lactoferrin from whey proteins by gel filtration techniques. J. Dairy Sci. 70: 2486-2492.

Al-Mashikhi, S.A. & S. Nakai 1988. Separation of immunoglobulin and trans-ferrin from blood serum and plasma by metal chelate interaction chromatography. J. Dairy Sci. 71: 1756-1763.

Andrews, A.T., S.V. Olivecrona, G. Bengtsson-Olivecrona, P.F. Fox, L. Bjorck & N.Y. Farkye. 1992. Indigenous enzymes in milk. In P.F. Fox (ed.), Advanced Dairy Chemistry - 1 - Proteins: 285-367. London: Elsevier Science Publishers.

Antila, P., I. Paakkari, A. Järvinen, M.J. Mattila, M. Laukkanen, A. Pihlanto-Leppälä, P. Mantsälä & J. Hellman 1991. Opioid peptides derived from in vitro proteolysis of whey proteins. Intern. Dairy J. 1: 215-229.

Arnold, R.R., M.F. Cole & J.R. McGhee 1977. A bactericidal effect for human lacto-ferrin. Science 197: 263-265.

Atkinson, S.A. & B. Lonnerdal 1989. Protein and Non-Protein Nitrogen in Human Milk. Boca Raton, FL: CRC Press.

Ballard, F.J., M.K. Nield, G.L. Francis, G.W. Dahlenberg & J.C. Wallace 1982. The relationship between the insulin content and inhibitory effects of bovine colostrom on protein breakdown in cultured cells. J. Cell Physiol. 110: 249-254.

Bano, M., D.S. Salomon & W.R. Kidwell. 1985. Purification of a mammary derived growth factor from human milk and human mammary tumors. J. Biol. Chem. 260: 5745-5752.

Baxter, R.C., Z. Zaltsman & J. Turtle 1984. Immunoreactive somatomedin C/IGF1 and its binding protein in human milk. J. Clin. Endocrinol. Metab. 58: 955-959.

Beardmore, J.M. & R.C. Richards 1983. Concentrations of epidermal growth factor in mouse milk throughout lactation. J. Endocrinol. 96: 287-292.

Beerens, H., C. Romond & C. Neut 1980. Influence of breast-feeding on the bifid flora of the newborn intestine. Am. J. Clin. Nutr. 33: 2434-2439.

Berseth, C.L. 1985. EGF-mediated breast milk-enhanced intestinal growth in neonatal rats. Pediatr. Res. 19: 213A.

Berseth, C.L. 1987. Enhancement of intestinal growth in neonatal rats by epidermal growth factor in milk. Am. J. Physiol. 253: G662-G665.

Berseth, C.L. & V.L.W. Go 1988. Enhancement of neonatal somatic and hepatic growth by orally administered epidermal growth factor. J. Pediatr. Gastroenterol. Nutr. 7: 889-893.

Berseth, C.L., L.M. Lichtenberger & F.H. Morriss 1983. Comparison of the intestinal growth promoting effects of rat colostrum and mature rat milk in newborn rats in vivo. Am. J. Clin. Nutr. 37: 52-60.

Blanc, B. 1981. Biochemical aspects of human milk - comparison with bovine milk. Wld. Rev. Nutr. Diet. 36: 1-89.

Bottonley, R.C. 1989. Isolation of an immunoglobulin rich fraction from whey. Eur. Pat. Appl. 0 320 152 A2.

Brantl, V. & H. Teschemacher 1979. A material with opioid activity in bovine milk and milk products. Naunyn-Schmildeberg's Arch. Pharmacol. 306: 301-304.

Brennan, M. 1990. Absorption of iron and zinc from milks and infant formulae in suckling rats. M.Sc. Thesis, Dublin: National University of Ireland.

Brew, K. & J.A. Grobler 1992. α-Lactalbumin. In P.F. Fox (ed.), Advanced Dairy Chemistry - 1 - Proteins: 191-229. London: Elsevier Science Publishers.

Britton, J.R., C. George-Nasciento & O. Koldovsky 1988. Luminal hydrolysis of recombinant human epidermal growth factor in the rat gastrointestinal tract: segmental and developmental differences. Life Sci. 43: 1339-1347.

Brown, K.D. & D.M. Blakely 1983. Cell growth - promoting activity in mammary secretions of the goat, cow and sheep. Br. Vet. J. 139: 68-78.

Brown, K.D. & D.M. Blakely 1984. Partial purification and characterization of a growth factor from goat colostrum. Biochem. J. 219: 609-617.

Bullen, C.L. & A.T. Willis 1971. Resistance of the breast-fed infant to gastroenteritis. Br. Med. J. 3: 338-343.

Burger, R.L. & R.H. Allen 1974. Character-ization of Vitamin B_{12}-binding proteins isolated from human milk and saliva by affinity chromatography. J. Biol. Chem. 249: 7220-7227.

Butler, J.E. 1969. Bovine immunoglobulins: A review. J. Dairy Sci. 52: 1895-1909.

Campbell, P.G. & C.R. Baumrucker 1989.
Insulin-like growth factor-1 and its
association with binding proteins in
bovine milk. J. Endocrinol. 120: 21-29.

Carpenter, G. 1980. Epidermal growth factor
is the major growth promoting agent in
human milk. Science 210: 198-199.

Chiba, H. & M. Yoshikawa 1986. Biologically
functional peptides from food proteins:
new opioid peptides from milk proteins.
In R.E. Feeney & J.R. Whitaker (eds.),
Protein Tailoring for Food and Medical
Uses: 123-153. New York: Marcel Dekker.

Chiba, H., F. Tani & M. Yoshikawa 1989.
Opioid antagonist peptides derived from
κ-casein. J. Dairy Res. 56: 363-366.

Cochet, C., J.-J. Feige & E.M. Chambaz 1983.
Reversibility of the phosphate transfer
between ATP and phosphoproteins catalysed
by a cyclic nucleotide independent
(G type) casein kinase. Biochim. Biophys.
Acta 744: 147-154.

Cohen, S. 1962. Isolation of a mouse
submaxillary gland protein accelerating
incisor eruption and eyelid opening in the
newborn animal. J. Biol. Chem. 237: 1555-
1562.

Cole, C.B., K.J. Scott, M.J. Henschel, M.E.
Coates, J.E. Ford & R. Fuller 1983.
Trace-nutrient-binding proteins in milk
and the growth of bacteria in the gut of
infant rabbits. Br. J. Nutr. 49: 231-240.

Colman, N. & V. Herbert 1980. Folate
binding proteins. Ann. Rev. Med. 31: 433-
439.

Dubois, E. 1986. Procede de separation de
certaines proteines du lactoserum et du
lait. Fr. Pat. 2 605 322.

Eigel, J.E., J.E. Butler, C.A. Ernstrom,
H.M. Jr. Farrell, V.R. Harwalkar, R.
Jenness & R.McL. Whitney 1984.
Nomenclature of proteis of cow's milk:
Fifth revision. J. Dairy Sci. 67: 1599-
1631.

Ekman, R., S. Ivarsson & L. Jansson 1985.
Bombesin, neurotensin and pro-gamma-
melatotropin immunoreactants in human
milk. Regul. Peptides 10: 99-105.

Falconer, J. 1987. Oral epidermal growth
factor in trophic for the stomach in the
neonatal rat. Biol. Neonate. 52: 347-350.

Ford, J.E. 1974. Some observations on the
possible nutritional significance of
vitamin B_{12} and folate-binding proteins in
milk. Br. J. Nutr. 31: 243-257.

Ford, J.E., B.A. Law, M.E. Marshall & B.
Reiter 1977. Influence of the heat
treatment of human milk on some of its
protective constituents. J. Pediatrics
90: 29-35.

Ford, J.E., K.J. Scott, B.F. Sansom & P.J.
Taylor 1975. Some obsrevations on the
possible nutritional significance of
Vitamin B_{12}- and folate-binding proteins
in milk. Absorption of [^{58}Co]
cyanocobalamin by suckling piglets. Br.
J. Nutr. 34: 469-492.

Fox, P.F. 1982. Developments in Dairy
Chemistry - 1. London: Applied Science
Publishers.

Fox, P.F. 1982. Developments in Dairy
Chemistry - 4. London: Elsevier Applied
Science Publishers.

Fox, P.F. 1992. Advanced Dairy Chemistry -
1 - Proteins. London: Elsevier Science
Publishers.

Fox, P.F. & A. Flynn. 1992. Biological
properties of milk proteins. In P.F. Fox
(ed.), Advanced Dairy Chemistry - 1 -
Proteins: 255-284. London: Elsevier
Science Publishers.

Frankenne, F., C. Marcotty, A. Duyckaerts,
J. Beeumen & G. Maghuin-Rogister 1989.
Purification and characterization of
insulin-like growth factor - 1 from cow
colostrum. Biochem. Soc. Trans. 17: 602.

Gale, S.M., L.C. Read, C. George-Nasciento,
J.C. Wallace & F.J. Ballard 1989. Is
dietary epidermal growth factor absorbed
in premature human infants? Biol. Neonate
55: 104-110.

Gani, M.M., K. May & K. Porter 1982. A
process and apparatus for the recovery of
immunoglobulines. Eur. Pat. 0 059 598 A1.

Gattegno, L., D. Migliore-Samour, L. Saffar
& P. Jolles 1988. Enhancement of phagocytic activity of human monocytic-
macrophagic cells by immunostimulating
peptides from human casein. Immunol.
Lett. 18: 27-32.

Goldman, A.S. 1988. Immunologic supple-
mentation of cow's milk formulations.
Special Address, Budapest: International
Dairy Federation, Annual Sessions.

Goldman, A.S. 1989. Immunologic supple-
mentation of cow's milk formulations.
Bulletin 244, 38-43. Brussels:
International Dairy Federation.

Goldman, A.S., S.A. Atkinson & L.A. Hanson
1987. Human Lactation. 3. The Effects
of Human Milk on the Recipient Infant.
New York: Plenum Press.

Goldman, A.S., A.J. Ham Pong & R.M. Goldblum
1985. Host defences: development and
maternal contribution. Adv. Pediatrics
32: 71-100.

Gregory, M.E. 1954. The microbiological
assay of Vitamin B_{12} in the milk of
different animal species. Br. J. Nutr. 8:
340-347.

Gregory, M.E. & E.S. Holdsworth 1955a. The
occurrence of a cyanobalamin-binding
protein in milk and the isolation of a
cyanobalamin-protein complex from sow's
milk. Biochem. J. 59: 329-334.

Gregory, M.E. & E.S. Holdsworth 1955b. Some
properties of the cyanobalamin-protein
complex from sow's milk, and the mode of
linkage of cyanobalamin with protein.
Biochem. J. 59: 335-340.

Grueters, A., J. Lakshmanan, R. Tarris, J.
Alm & D.A. Fisher 1985. Nerve growth
factor in mouse milk during early
lactation: lack of dependency on

submandibular glands. Pediatr. Res. 19: 934-937.

György, P. 1953. A hitherto unrecognized biochemical difference between human milk and cow's milk. Pediatrics 11: 98-108.

György, P., R.F. Norris & C.S. Rose 1954a. Bifidus factor. I. A variant of Lactobacillus bifidus requiring a special growth factor. Arch. Biochem. Biophys. 48: 193-201.

György, P., R. Kuhn, C.S. Rose & F. Zilliken 1954b. Bifidus factor, II. Its occurrence in milk from different species and in other natural products. Arch. Biochem. Biophys. 48: 202-208.

György, P., J.R.E. Hoover, R. Kuhn & C.S. Rose 1954c. Bifidus factor. III. The rate of dialysis. Arch. Biochem. Biophys. 48: 209-213.

György, P., R.W. Jeanloz, H. von Nicolai & F. Zilliken 1974. Undialyzable growth factor for Lactobacillus bifidus var. pennsylvanicus. Eur. J. Biochem. 43: 29-33.

Hall, R.A. E.M. Widdowson 1979. Response of the organs of rabbits to feeding during their first days after birth. Biol. Neonate 35: 131-139.

Hambling, S.G., A.S. McAlpine & L. Sawyer 1992. ß-Lactoglogulin. In P.F. Fox (ed.), Advanced Dairy Chemistry - 1 - Proteins: 141-190. London: Elsevier Science Publishers.

Hamel, U., G. Killwein & H. Teschemacher 1985. ß-Casomorphin immunoreactive materials in cows' milk incubated with various bacterial species. J. Dairy Res. 52: 139-148.

Hamos, M., L.M. Freed, J.B. Jones, S.E. Berkow, J. Bitman, N.R. Mehta, B. Happ & P. Hamos 1985. Enzymes in human milk. In R.G. Jensen & M.C. Neville (eds.), Human Lactation: Milk Components and Methodologies: 251-266. New York: Plenum Press.

Harmon, R.J., F.L. Schanbacher, L.C. Ferguson & K.L. Smith 1976. Changes in lactoferrin, immunoglobulin G, bovine serum albumin, and α-lactalbumin during acute experimental and natural coliform mastitis in cows. Infect. Immun. 13: 533-542.

Heird, W.C., S.M. Schwarz & I.H. Hansen 1984. Colostrum induced enteric mucosal growth in beagle puppies. Pediatr. Res. 18: 512-515.

Hernell, O. & B. Lonnerdal 1989. Enzymes in Human Milk. In S.A. Atkinson & B. Lonnerdal (eds.), Protein and Non-protein Nitrogen in Human Milk: 67-75. Boca Raton, FL: CRC Press.

Hilpert, H. 1984. Preparation of a milk immuoglobulin concentrate from cow's milk. In A.F. Williams & J.B. Baum (eds.), Human Milk Banking: 17-28. New York: Raven Press.

Jahnke, G.D. & L.H. Lazarus 1984. A bombesin immunoreactive peptide in milk. Proc. Natl. Acad. Sci. 81: 578-582.

Jensen, R.G. & M.C. Neville 1985. Human Lactation: Milk Components and Methologies. New York: Plenum Press.

Jolles, P., S. Levy-Toledano, A.-M. Fiat, C. Soria, D. Gillessen, A. Thomaidis, F.W. Dunn & J.P. Caen 1986. Analogy between fibrinogen and casein. Effect of an undecapeptide isolated from κ-casein on platelet function. Eur. J. Biochem. 158: 379-382.

Kidwell, W.R. & D.S. Solomon 1989. Growth factors in human milk: sources and potential physiological roles. In S.A. Atkinson & B. Lonnerdal (eds.), Protein and Non-Protein Nitrogen in Human Milk: 77-91. Boca Raton, FL: CRC Press,

Kiely, J., A. Flynn, H. Singh & P.F. Fox 1988. Improved zinc bioavailability from colloidal calcium phosphate-free cow's milk. In L.S. Hurley, C.L. Keen, B. Lonnerdal & R.B. Rucker (eds.), Trace Elements in Man and Animals - 6: 499-500. New York: Plenum Press,

Kitts, D.D. & Y.V. Yuan 1992. Caseinophos-phopeptides and calcium bioavailability. Trends Food Sci. Technol. 3: 31-35.

Klagsbrun, M. 1978. Human milk stimulates DNA synthesis in cultural fibroblasts. Proc. Natl. Acad. Sci. 75: 5057-5061.

Klagsbrun, M. & J. Neumann 1979. The serum-free growth of Balb/C 3T3 cells in medium supplemented with bovine colostrum. J. Supramol. Struct. 11: 349-359.

Kohmura, M., N. Nio, K. Kubo, Y. Minoshima, E. Munekata & Y. Ariyoshi 1989. Inhibition of angiotensin-converting enzyme by synthetic peptides of human ß-casein. Agric. Biol. Chem. 53: 2107-2114.

Koldovsky, O. 1989. Search for role of milk-borne biologically active peptides for the suckling. J. Nutr. 119: 1543-1551.

Kothe N., H. Dichtelmuller, W. Stephan & B. Eichentopf 1986. Method for the production of a solution of milk and/or colostrum immunoglobulins and their uses. Eur. Pat. Appl. 0 173 999 A2.

Larson, B.L. 1992. Immunoglobulins of the mammary secretions. In P.F. Fox (ed.), Advanced Dairy Chemistry - 1 - Proteins: 285-367. London: Elsevier Science Publishers.

Lonnerdal, B. 1985. Biochemistry and physiological function of human milk proteins. Am. J. Clin. Nutr. 42: 1299-1317.

Lonnerdal, B., B. Hoffman & L.S. Hurley 1982. Zinc and copper binding proteins in human milk. Am. J. Clin. Nutr. 36: 1170-1176.

Loukas, S., D. Varoucha, C. Zioudrou, R.A. Streaty & W.A. Klee 1983. Opioid activities and structures of α-casein derived exorphins. Biochemistry 22: 4567-4573.

Maeda, K., H.A. McKenzie & D.C. Shaw 1980. Nature of the heterogeneity within genetic variants of bovine serum transferrin. Anim. Blood Grps. Biochim. Genet. 11: 63-75.

Maruyama, S. & H. Suzuki 1982. A peptide inhibitor of angiotensin I-converting enzyme in the tryptic hydrolyzate of casein. Agric. Biol. Chem. 46: 1393-1394.

Maruyama, S., H. Mitachi, J. Awaya, M. Kurono, N. Tonizuka & H. Suzuki 1987. Angiotensin I-converting enzyme inhibitory activity of the C-terminal hexapeptide of α_{s1}-casein. Agric. Biol. Chem. 51: 2557-2561.

Maubois, J.L. & J. Leonil 1989. Peptides du lait à activité biologique. Lait 69: 245-269.

Mazoyer, E., S. Levy-Toledano, F. Rendu, L. Hermant, H. Lu, A.-M. Fiat, P. Jolles & J. Caen 1990. KRDS, a new peptide derived from lactotransferrin, inhibits platelet aggregation and release reaction. Eur. J. Biochem. 194: 43-49.

Meisel, H. 1986. Chemical characterization and opioid activity of an exorphin isolated fron in vivo digests. FEBS Lett. 196: 223-227.

Meisel, H. & E. Schlimme 1990. Milk proteins: precursors of bioactive peptides. Trends Food Sci. Technol. 1: 41-43.

Meisel, H., H. Frister & E. Schlimme 1989. Biologically active peptides in milk proteins. Z. Ernährungswiss. 28: 267-278.

Migliore-Samour, D. & P. Jolles 1988. Casein, a prohormone with an immunomodulating role for the newborn? Experientia 44: 188-193.

Migliore-Samour, D., F. Floc'h & P. Jolles, 1989. Biologically active casein peptides implicated in immunomodulation. J. Dairy Res. 56: 357-362.

Miller, M.S., M. Benore-Parsons & H.B. White 1982. Dephosphorylation of chicken riboflavin-binding protein and phosvitin decreases their uptake by oocytes. J. Biol. Chem. 257: 6818-6824.

Miller, M.S., M.T. Mas & M.S. White 1984. Highly phosphorylated region of chicken riboflavin-binding protein: chemical characterization and ^{31}P NMR-studies. Biochem. 23: 569-576.

Mirand, P.P., L. Mosini, D. Levieux, D. Attaix, G. Bayle & Y. Bonnet 1990. Effect of colostrum on protein metabolism in small intestine of newborn lambs. Biol. Neonate 57: 30-36.

Modler, H.W., R.C. McKellar & M. Yaguchi 1990. Bifidobacteria and bifidogenic factors. Can. Inst. Food Sci. Technol. J. 23: 29-41.

Moore, M.C., H.L. Greene, H.M. Said, F.K. Ghishan & D.N. Orth 1986. Effect of epidermal growth factor and artificial feeding in suckling rats. Pediatr. Res. 20: 1248-1251.

Noda, K., M. Umeda & T. Ono 1984. Transforming growth factor activity in human colostrum. Gann 75: 109-112.

O'Loughlin, E.V., M. Chung, M. Hollenberg, J. Hayden, I. Zahavi & D.G. Gall 1985. Effect of epidermal growth factor on ontogeny of the gastrointestinal tract. Am. J. Physiol. 249: G674-G678.

Perez, M.D., L. Sanchez, P. Aranada, J.M. Ena, R. Oria & M. Calvo 1992. Biochim. Biophys. Acta 1123: 151-155.

Petrides, P.E., M. Hosang, E. Shooter, F. Esch & P. Bohlen 1985. Isolation and characterisation of epidermal growth factor from human milk. FEBS Lett. 187: 89-95.

Prosser, C.G., I.R. Fleet & A. Corps 1989. Increased secretion of insulin-like growth factor I into milk of cows treated with recombinantly derived bovine growth hormone. J. Dairy Res. 56: 17-26.

Raaberg, L., E. Nexo, S.S. Poulsen & L. Tollund 1989. Cobalamin and its binding protein in rat milk. Scand. J. Lab. Invest. 49: 529-535.

Rasic, J.L. & J.A. Kurmann 1983. Bifidobacteria and their Role. Basel: Birkhauser Verlag,

Read, L.C., G.L. Francis, J.C. Wallace & F.J. Ballard 1983. Characterisation of growth factors in milk. Proc. Aust. Biochem. Soc. 15: 38.

Read, L.C., F.M. Upton, G.L. Francis, J.C. Wallace, G.W. Dahlenberg & F.J. Ballard 1984. Growth promoting activity of human milk during lactation. Pediatr. Res. 18: 133-139.

Reiter, B. 1985. The biological significance of the non-immunoglobulin protective proteins in milk: lysozyme, lactoferrin, lactoperoxidase. In P.F. Fox (ed.), Developments in Dairy Chemistry - 3: 281-336. London: Elsevier Applied Science Publishers.

Rindernecht, E. & R.E. Humbel 1976. The amino acid sequence of human insulin-like growth factor I and its structural homology with proinsulin. J. Biol. Chem. 253: 2769-2776.

Said, H.M., D.W. Horne & C. Wagner 1986. Effect of human milk folate binding protein on folate intestinal transport. Arch. Biochem. Biophys. 251: 114-120.

Salter, D.N. & A. Mowlem 1983. Neonatal role of milk folate-binding protein: studies on the course of digesion of goat's milk folate binder in the 6-d-old kid. Br. J. Nutr. 50: 589-596.

Sandberg, D.P., J.A. Begley & C.A. Hall 1981. The content, binding, and forms of

Vitamin B_{12} in milk. Am. J. Clin. Nutr. 34: 1717-1724.

Sato, R., T. Noguchi & H. Naito 1986. Casein phosphopeptide (CPP) enhances calcium absorption from the ligated setment of rat small intestine. J. Nutr. Sci. Vitaminol. 32: 67-76.

Schaub, J. 1985. Composition and Physiological Properties of Human Milk. Amsterdam: Elsevier Science Publishers (Biomedical Division).

Scott, G.H. & D.O. Lucas 1987. Immunologically active whey fraction and recovery process. Eur. Pat. Appl. 0 239 722 A1.

Scott, J., M. Urdea, M. Quiroga, R. Sanchez-Pescador, N. Fong, M. Selby, W. Rutter & G.I. Bell 1983. Structure of a mouse submaxillary gland mRNA coding for EGF and seven other related peptides. Science 221: 236-240.

Shing, V.W. & M. Klagsbrun 1984. Human and bovine milk contain different sets of growth factors. Endocrinol. 115: 273-282.

Singh, H., A. Flynn & P.F. Fox 1989. Zinc binding in bovine milk. J. Dairy Res. 56: 249-263.

Sinha, S.K. & A.A. Yunis 1983. Isolation of a colony stimulating factor from human milk. Biochem. Biophys. Res. Commun. 114: 797-803.

Spik, G., J. Montreuil, R.R. Crichton & J. Mazurier 1985. Proteins of Iron Storage and Transport. Amsterdam: Elsevier Science Publishers,

Suikkari, A.M. 1989. Insulin-like growth factor (IGF-1) and its low molecular weight binding protein in human milk. Eur. J. Obstet. Gynecol. Reprod. Biol. 30: 19-25.

Swiatlo, N.L. & M.F. Picciano 1988. Relative folate bioavailability from human, bovine and goat milk containing diets. FASEB J. 2: 4600 (Abstr.).

Taira, T., L.A. Hilakivi, J. Aalto & I. Hilakivi 1990. Effect of Beta-casomorphin on neonatal sleep in rats. Peptides 11: 1-4.

Tani, M., T. Fushiki & K. Iwai 1983. Influence of folate-binding protein from bovine milk on the absorption of folate in gastrointestinal tract of rat. Biochim. Biophys. Acta 757: 274-281.

Taniguchi H., M. Goto, T. Okamoto, I. Sakauchi, T. Ando, O. Kirihara & K. Ando. 1990. Process for preparing a therapeutic agent for rotavirus infection. Eur. Pat. Appl. 0 391 416 A1.

Teschemacher, H. 1987. ß-Casomorphins: do they have physiological significance? In A.S. Goldman, S.A. Atkinson & L.A. Hanson (eds.), Human Lactation. 3. The Effects of Human Milk on the Recipient Infant: 213-225. New York: Plenum Press.

Teschemacher, H., M. Umbach, U. Hamel, K. Prectorius, G. Ahnert-Hilger, V. Brantl, F. Lottspeich & A. Henschen 1986. No evidence for the presence of ß-casomorphins in human plasma after ingestion of cows' milk or milk products. J. Dairy Res. 53: 135-138.

Thornburg, W., L. Matrisian, B. Magun & O. Koldosisky 1984. Gastrointestinal absorption of epidermal growth factor in suckling rats. Am. J. Physiol. 246: G80-G85.

Thornburg, W., R.K. Rao, L.M. Matrisian, B.E. Magun & O. Koldovsky 1987. Effects of maturation on gastrointestinal absorption of epidermal growth factor in rats. Am. J. Physiol. 253: G68-G71.

Tome, D., A.-M. Dumontier, M. Hautefeuille & J.-F. Desjeux 1987. Opiate activity and transepithelial passage of intact ß-casomorphins in rabbit ileum. Am. J. Physiol. 253: G737-G744.

Toyosaki, T. & T. Mineshita 1988. Antioxidant effects of protein-bound riboflavin and free riboflavin. J. Food Sci. 53: 1851-1853.

Toyosaki, T., A. Yamamoto & T. Mineshita 1987. Partial purification of an antioxidizing component in raw cow milk. J. Food Sci. 52: 88-90.

Trugo, N.M.F. 1988. Characterization of the Vitamin B_{12}-binding protein isolated from sow's milk and its affinity for cyanocobalamin and other corrinoids. Brazilian J. Med. Biol. Res. 21: 883-894.

Trugo, N.M.F. & A. Turvey 1987. Immunofluorescent localization of Vitamin B_{12}-binding protein from sow's milk in the ileal mucosa of piglets. Brazilian J. Med. Biol. Res. 20: 285-288.

Trugo, N.M.F., J.E. Ford & D.N. Salter 1985. Vitamin B_{12} absorption in the neonatal piglet. 3. Influence of Vitamin B_{12}-binding protein from sows' milk on uptake of Vitamin B_{12} by microvillus membrane visicles prepared from small intestine of the piglet. Br. J. Nutr. 54: 269-283.

Wagner, C. 1982. Cellular folate binding proteins; function and significance. Ann. Rev. Nutr. 2: 229-248.

Walker, W.A. 1985. Nutrition in Pediatrics - Basic Sciences and Clinical Application, Boston: J.B. Watkins, Littler, Brown & Co.

Waxman, S. 1975. Folate binding proteins. Br. J. Haematol. 29: 23-29.

West, D.W. 1986. Structure and function of the phosphorylated residues of casein. J. Dairy Res. 53: 333-352.

White, H.B. & A.H. Merrill 1988. Riboflavin-binding proteins. Ann. Rev. Nutr. 8: 279-299.

Widdowson, E.M. 1984. Milk and the newborn animal. Proc. Nutr. Soc. 43: 87-100.

Widdowson, E.M., V.E. Colombo & C.A. Artavanis 1976. Changes in the organs of pigs in response to feeding for the first 24 h after birth. II. The digestive tract. Biol. Neonate 28: 272-281.

Williams, J. 1985. The structure of
transferrins. In G. Spik, J. Montreuil,
R.R. Crichton & J. Mazurier (eds.),
Proteins of Iron Storage and Transport:
13-23. Amsterdam: Elsevier Science
Publishers,

Wright, C.E. & G.E. Gaull 1983. Nerve
growth factor is present in human milk.
Pediatr. Res. 17: 144A.

Yagi, H., S. Suzuki, T. Noji, K. Nagashima &
T. Kurouma 1986. Epidermal growth factor
in cow's milk and milk formulae. Acta
Paediatr. Scand. 75: 233-235.

Yoshikawa, M., F. Tani, T. Yoshimura & H.
Chiba 1986. Opioid peptides from milk
proteins. Agric. Biol. Chem. 50: 2419-
2421.

Zioudrou, C., R.A. Streaty & W.A. Klee 1979.
J. Biol. Chem. 254: 2446-2449.

Zwiebel, J.A., M. Bano, E. Nexo, D.S.
Salomon & W.R. Kidwell 1986. Partial
purification of transforming growth
factors from human milk. Cancer Res. 46:
933-939.

Dairy Products in Human Health and Nutrition, Serrano Ríos et al. (eds) © 1994 Balkema, Rotterdam, ISBN 90 5410 359 0

Positive health benefits of consuming dairy products

M.I.Gurr
Maypole Scientific Services, UK

ABSTRACT: Important nutritional qualities of milk are the wide range of nutrients it contains (of the important trace elements, only iron is in short supply) and the good balance of its major nutrients: protein, fat and carbohydrate. Milk is also a very flexible food: thus a wide range of fat-reduced products can be obtained leaving the distribution of most vitamins and minerals unchanged. Milk enhances the nutritional quality of other foods when eaten together with them. Milk and milk products have 'protective' properties in relation to the gastrointestinal tract, bone disease, dental caries, hypertension, some cancers and coronary heart disease and these are subjects of active research.

1 BACKGROUND: THE RISE AND FALL OF MILK

As knowledge develops, nutritional advice tends to change over a period of time and this may be a source of confusion to laymen. Thus, a few decades ago milk and milk products were regarded as cornerstones of nutrition and actively recommended as 'body building', 'protective' and 'energy' foods. Then, during the 1970s and 80s, recommendations to reduce consumption of milk fat because of its alleged contribution to high plasma cholesterol concentrations and risk of coronary heart disease (CHD) influenced the consumption of dairy products in several important ways. There was increased demand, first for liquid milks, then for other dairy products with lower fat contents. The industry's response was such that about half of liquid milk sales are now low fat varieties and many other types of reduced fat dairy products are now available. Butter consumption has fallen precipitately, partly as a result of health concerns, partly from considerations of cost and poor spreadability.

There has also been a tendency for milk to have a less wholesome image than formerly as a result of widespread concern about allergies and lactose intolerance. More recently, some nutritionists have questioned the liberal consumption of dairy products on the grounds that too much dietary calcium may compromise iron nutrition or cause duodenal ulcers. Research attention has also focused on the possible role of a milk protein in the development of insulin dependent diabetes mellitus. Yet at the same time,

the need for ample calcium from milk and milk products is also being stressed, further reinforcing public confusion.

The aim of this review is to highlight current knowledge of the nutritional and health benefits of milk and milk products, indicating where such knowledge is substantial as distinct from aspects where more research is clearly required.

2 TRADITIONAL ROLES OF MILK IN NUTRIENT PROVISION

Three important aspects of the nutrient contribution of milk are:
* *Wide range of nutrients.* Of the important trace elements, only iron is in short supply. There is a good balance between the protein, fat and carbohydrate components, each being present in similar amounts. In northern European countries, milk supplies more than one-fifth of the daily intake of several very important nutrients: protein, calcium, riboflavin, zinc and vitamin A and high proportions of the WHO recommended daily amounts of many other vitamins (Gurr, 1992).
* *High nutrient density.* The supply of nutrients is high in relation to the calorie content of the food. Nutrient-dense foods are particularly valuable for people who cannot eat very bulky foods, for example, small children and the elderly and for people trying to reduce weight.
* *Milk is a very flexible food.* Milk products can be

obtained that vary widely in their water, fat, lactose, protein, vitamin and mineral contents. They can, therefore, contribute to a wide variety of eating patterns and fulfil many nutritional uses.

Milk and milk products are not eaten alone but in the context of a mixed diet. This is important as the nutrients in foods complement and interact with each other. Thus, when milk products are eaten in conjunction with other foods, the milk protein is able to raise the value of poorer quality cereal proteins. The habit of eating cheese with bread, for example, is nutritionally advantageous. Inclusion of a certain amount of 'fibre' in diets is regarded as being important for health. However, high fibre products are often not particularly palatable when eaten alone, but when eaten with milk can become very pleasant indeed. Milk also enhances the bioavailability of calcium from vegetable sources that normally have poor bioavailability (Weaver and Heaney, 1991).

To these traditional roles, can be added certain 'protective' roles, by which is meant an ability to protect against ill health and positively to promote good health. Some of these aspects have long been part of folklore and have only comparatively recently been subjected to careful research scrutiny. The degree of confidence that may be placed on current understanding will be indicated.

3 DENTAL HEALTH

The evidence for a role for milk products, especially cheese, in protection against dental caries, even in the presence of sucrose, is now substantial and is consistent from animal experiments, human intervention and observational studies (Herod, 1991). The effect is due, in part, to the buffering capacity of the milk product, reducing the influence of acid production by cariogenic bacteria but other research suggests that milk minerals may protect the enamel independently of an effect on pH (Harper et al, 1987). New techniques confirm that eating cheese in the presence of sucrose can significantly increase oral pH and salivary flow, and decrease plaque formation in human beings (Silva et al, 1986, 1987). The fatty acids in cheese have antimicrobial properties against cariogenic bacteria. Casein and whey proteins also form a surface layer on the enamel, restricting ionic diffusion at the surface and preventing demineralization. The mechanism may involve specifically casein phosphopeptides.

Research is needed to clarify and elucidate the many different modes in which milk or cheese may be effective and a clinical trial on the effect of cheese on the incidence of dental caries is a research priority.

4 BONE HEALTH AND OSTEOPOROSIS

A major health problem in developed countries is that of osteoporosis: brittle bones, leading to increased risk of fracture as a result of an abnormal loss of bone in later life. The question of how much calcium is normally required is vigorously debated. It is undeniable that average Ca intakes in Europe are much higher than in many developing countries where osteoporosis is virtually unknown, but other lifestyle factors such as exercise, as well as heredity, may interact with diet. In developed countries, certain individuals or sub-groups may have much lower than average intakes. This may be particularly true of the elderly and adolescent girls. The latter may substitute milk as a drink by various soft drinks (Chan, 1991).

There have also been reports of childhood rickets induced by replacing formulas based on cow's milk with soya-based formulas after diagnosis of allergy (Ahmad et al, 1990).

Scientists and doctors have been preoccupied with two main questions: (1) Can extra dietary calcium help to build up a greater "peak bone mass", so that bones are bigger and stronger and better able to withstand the inevitable losses later in life? (2) Can extra calcium help to prevent the loss of bone later in life, both normal physiological losses and the more severe losses of osteoporosis?

The importance of dietary Ca in the early years of life in helping to establish optimal peak bone mass seems well established. Several recent studies have provided evidence that calcium intakes in young people (2-18 years) are significantly and positively associated with bone mineral density (Chan, 1991; Renner et al, 1991; Sentipal et al, 1991; Johnston et al, 1992).

Calcium alone is not enough for healthy bones. When poorly nourished children in India were given calcium supplements, their growth did not improve but when milk was given, growth improved enormously because the milk supplied not only calcium but calories, proteins and other minerals important in bone structure (British Nutrition Foundation, 1989). In other published studies trace element supplements containing Cu, Zn and Mn enhanced the beneficial effect of Ca supplementation on bone mineral density in post-menopausal women. Magnesium, zinc, copper, manganese and boron, present in milk, all contribute to bone health (Beattie and Avenell, 1992).

The role of diet in preventing excessive bone loss in later life is still controversial but there appears to be a consensus that extra Ca given to people with rather poor Ca intakes, can reduce the rate of bone mineral loss, the dosage of hormone needed to achieve a given effect in post menopausal women and the

114

tendency for bones to fracture (British Nutrition Foundation, 1989). Exercise enhances the effect of calcium in the mineralization of bone (Prince et al, 1991).

Debilitating bone disease may be caused by excessive intakes of toxic elements such as cadmium, an effect that can be counteracted by high intakes of Ca and other minerals found in milk (Beattie and Avenell, 1992).

The dairy industry has perhaps been inclined to focus on Ca in its promotion of milk. Future strategy might emphasize the importance of milk as a "cocktail" of most of the important nutrients needed for good health. Further research is needed to clarify the complex interactions between dietary minerals in relation to bone health.

5 LACTOSE DIGESTION

While most of the world's population loses the ability to digest lactose efficiently after the first or second decade of life, many such people can tolerate moderate amounts of milk products in a mixed diet (Katz and Speckmann, 1978). For those who develop adverse symptoms even with moderate amounts of milk, the now well established finding that the lactose in yoghurt is better digested than the same quantity in unfermented milk is a positive nutritional benefit (Kim and Gilliland, 1983; Kolars et al, 1984; Lerebours et al, 1989).

In explanation, the lactase in the starter culture hydrolyses some lactose in the gut. (Heat-treatment of yoghurt destroys the beneficial effect on lactose digestion in parallel with loss of lactase in some but not all experiments.) Moreover, the transit time of yoghurt lactose from mouth to large intestine can be considerably slower than that of milk lactose resulting in an increased time available for lactose to be digested, either by the yoghurt bacteria or by the small amount of residual lactase remaining in the person's gut.

There are, however, considerable differences between the effectiveness of products made with different strains of yoghurt bacteria (Martini et al, 1991). Current research aims to identify those strains of culture bacteria that are active in lactose digestion in the gut (since not all are equally effective) , so that claims for the efficacy of specific products can be given better scientific foundation.

Lactase treated milks provide another product alternative for people with lactose intolerance. In one study, milks with only 50% of the lactose removed were almost as well tolerated as those in which 80% had been removed (Brand and Holt, 1991).

6 ULCERATION

Drinking milk has been a common recommendation for those with stomach ulcers for generations but whether there has been any scientific basis for this observation is obscure. A recent line of research has demonstrated a protective action of milk against gastric ulcers in experimental animals, which was attributed to the phospholipid fraction of the milk (Dial and Lichtenberger, 1987). The mucosa may have been protected by the coating of a layer of phospholipids over the surface, similar to the action of the lung surfactant, which is a combination of specific phospholipid and protein. The possibility that phospholipids associated with a particular milk protein may give mucosal protection needs further research.

Contrary to these animal experiments, a human case-control study suggested that calcium in milk may in fact aggravate ulceration (Katschinski et al, 1992). Although there was a graded increase in the relative risk of ulceration in patients compared with controls as calcium intake increased, the effect was only significant at Ca intakes over 1000mg/day, implying that in the general population, consuming on average 800mg/day, there is minimal risk. The authors suggested that the increase in gastric acid secretion stimulated by Ca provokes ulceration.

7 DIARRHOEA

Despite long-standing assertions that cultured products have therapeutic properties for diarrhoea and constipation, the results of most studies are not convincing. However, a recent well designed study of children with persistent diarrhoea compared the clinical outcomes when the diet contained unfermented milk or yoghurt and found that it was significantly better in the presence of yoghurt (Boudraa et al, 1990).

Applications of cultured or culture-containing milk products to human health are worth pursuing since quite effective bacterial preparations ("probiotics") for improving animal health have been commercially available for some time. Culture organisms augment the benign effects of the natural flora by competing successfully with invading pathogens and denying them access to sites of adhesion on the gut wall where they could colonize and grow; or by secreting compounds (including acids) that either kill the pathogens or prevent their proliferation (International Dairy Federation, 1983, 1991). Milk contains whey proteins capable of stimulating the growth of culture bacteria (Petschow and Talbott, 1991). Well designed experiments with well characterized specific strains of *lactobacilli* and *bifidobacteria* derived from human gut microflora are required.

8 IMMUNITY

A mechanism by which organisms present in cultured products may benefit gastrointestinal health is by stimulating the immune system (International Dairy Federation, 1991). Research, mainly conducted with small laboratory animals, is still at an early stage, however, and its relevance to human health is by no means clear. Much research interest is now being devoted to the biological effects of so-called 'immune milks', especially in Japan. 'Immune milk' is a product that contains raised levels of antibodies to specific gut microorganisms after immunization of cows with killed pathogens. Several studies with laboratory rodents have demonstrated improvements in gut physiology including an increased ratio of *Lactobacilli* to *Enterobacteriaceae*, higher levels of IgA, and higher activity of cells involved in bacterial killing (Kobayashi *et al*, 1991). Culture microorganisms, *Lactobacillus* spp and *Bifidobacterium* spp, are also reported to reduce the translocation of pathogens across the gut wall (Murosaki *et al*, 1990). Inclusion of yoghurt containing *L.acidophilus* in the diet was able to inhibit *Candida* infection of the vagina (Hilton *et al*, 1992).

Until recently, little regard has been paid to the metabolic profile of the strains of organisms used in culture-containing products. This has led to much confusion and inconsistency in the scientific literature and the marketing of products with dubious effectiveness. Different therapeutic applications of culture organisms require different strains with distinct characteristics: adherence to the gut wall, resistance to bile, production of effective antibacterial agents, ability to stimulate the immune system and ability to digest lactose in the gut. These strains must be able to survive the manufacturing process and retain their activity on storage. It is unlikely that all these desirable properties will be found in the same strains.

9 HYPERTENSION

Individually, evidence available from animal studies, epidemiology and intervention studies that dietary Ca reduces existing hypertension or prevents the age-related rise in blood pressure is weak. However, as more research is reported, there is a consistency in the results which gives some confidence that there is a real effect. Calcium intake from dairy products was inversely related to diastolic blood pressure in adult men after controlling for age, alcohol intake and body mass index (Ackley *et al*, 1983) and in a study of children after adjusting for age, sex, body mass index, and Na and K intakes, there was a significant 2mm decrease in systolic blood pressure for each increment of 100mg Ca/1000kcal/day (Gillman *et al*, 1992).

The best evidence for real effects of additional Ca intake in reducing hypertension comes from studies undertaken in pregnancy. Thus, it has been observed that women with high calcium intakes, specifically from dairy products, are less prone to pregnancy-induced hypertension that those with low intakes (Marcoux *et al*, 1991). Intervention studies have also provided supportive evidence that supplementation of the diet with calcium reduces the incidence of hypertensive disorders during pregnancy (Belizan *et al*, 1991). However, the evidence is not firm enough yet for strong promotional claims for milk products in this regard because effects were obtained with large doses of non-milk Ca.

As in the case of bone health, the evidence is for the importance of interactions between calcium and many other essential minerals, suggesting an important role for milk. It is likely that effects will only be seen in individuals who have high blood pressure and have habitually consumed very low calcium diets.

10 CANCER

As long ago as 1933, medical research workers in London demonstrated a very striking protective effect of milk against several types of cancer (Stocks and Karn, 1933). Amongst cancer patients there was a much higher percentage of people who never drank milk and a much smaller percentage of people who drank milk daily than among the healthy control subjects. Similar effects have also been observed in relation to specific cancers such as cancer of the bladder (Mettlin and Graham, 1979). Epidemiological evidence for a protective effect of milk products is thus suggestive but inconclusive without firm experimental backing.

The most promising area of current research in regard to a protective effect of Ca is in relation to colon cancer. For example, a 19-year prospective study of 1954 men in Chicago found that a dietary intake of >3.75 microgram vitamin D per day was associated with a 50% reduction in the incidence of colon cancer and an intake of >1200mg/d Ca was associated with a 75% reduction (Garland *et al*, 1985). Protective effects of milk may involve Ca phosphopeptides, which bind to bile acids, preventing their toxic effects (van der Meer and Lapre, 1991). Another mechanism may involve the suppression by

Ca of abnormally high rates of cell division in colonic mucosa, which may be a forerunner of cancerous growth (Wargovitch *et al*, 1991).

In experiments with mice harbouring cancers induced by chemical carcinogens, diets containing most of their protein as cow's milk whey proteins reduced tumour numbers five-fold and the area occupied by tumours four-fold compared with standard laboratory diets (Papenberg *et al*, 1990). The multiplication of human cancer cells in culture was inhibited by whey proteins (Bourtouralt *et al*, 1991).

A case-control study in The Netherlands observed a significantly lower consumption of fermented milk products (predominantly yoghurt, buttermilk and Gouda cheese) among 133 incident breast cancer cases than in 289 population controls (van't Veer *et al*, 1989). In explanation, it was suggested that some lactobacilli produce anticarcinogenic or antimutagenic compounds but proof of their existence has been elusive. Alternatively, bacteria may metabolize and destroy known carcinogens such as nitrosamines or they may reduce the activity of enzymes that convert procarcinogens into carcinogens. Finally, dietary cultures may act by stimulating the immune system as discussed above (International Dairy Federation, 1991).

A recent report summarized work on the effects of 'conjugated linoleic acid' (CLA), present in milk, as a cancer inhibitor. CLA is mixture of isomers of linoleic acid (*cis*-9, *cis*-12-octadecadienoic acid) the main component being *cis*-9,*trans*-11-octadecadienoic acid. Evidence for involvement in cancer development has so far been confined to small laboratory animals and tests *in vitro* (Pariza, 1991).

In summary, evidence for protective effects of milk constituents against cancer is accumulating and is persuasive. However, following on from the epidemiological and laboratory animal work on which this evidence is based, direct observations on specific human cancers are now needed.

11 HYPERLIPIDAEMIA AND CORONARY HEART DISEASE

There is now sufficient evidence from epidemiology (Micheli *et al*, 1982; Staehelin *et al*, 1992), from human intervention studies and animal experiments (Gurr, 1989) taken together that consumption of milk products, even those containing milk fat, does not result in hyperlipidaemia. This knowledge is largely unheeded. There are some interesting indications that a lifestyle characteristic of people who also happen to be milk drinkers is associated with a low risk of CHD (Medical Research Council, 1991). This is consistent with a strategy to promote milk as part of an integrated healthy lifestyle in which diet and other factors play a part.

REFERENCES

Ackley, S., Barrett-Connor, E. & Suaraz, L. 1983. Dairy products, calcium and blood pressure. *American Journal of Clinical Nutrition* 38: 457-461.

Ahmad, T., Watson, S. & Eastham, E.J. 1990. Soy milk induced nutritional rickets: a case report. *Journal of Nutritional Medicine* 1: 227-229.

Beattie, J.H. & Avenell, A. 1992. Trace element nutrition and bone metabolism. *Nutrition Research Reviews* 5: 167-188.

Belizan, J.M., Villar, J. Gonzalez, L., Campodonico, L. & Bergel, E. 1991. Calcium supplementation to prevent hypertensive disorders of pregnancy. *New England Journal of Medicine* 325: 1399-1405.

Boudraa, G., Touhami, M., Pochart, P., Soltana, R., Mary, J-Y. & DesJeux, J-F. 1990. Effect of feeding yoghurt versus milk in children with persistent diarrhoea. *Journal of Pediatric Gastroenterology and Nutrition* 11: 509-512.

Bourtouralt, M., Buleon, R., Samperez, S. & Jouon, P. 1991. Effet des proteines du lactoserum bovin sur la multiplication de cellules cancereuses humaines. *Comptes Rendus de la Societe de Biologie* 185: 319-323.

Brand, J.C. & Holt, S. 1991. Relative effectiveness of milks with reduced amounts of lactose in alleviating milk intolerance. *American Journal of Clinical Nutrition* 54: 148-151.

British Nutrition Foundation. 1989. Calcium: Report of the British Nutrition Foundation Task Force. British Nutrition Foundation, London.

Chan, G.M. 1991. Dietary calcium and bone mineral status of children and adolescents. *American Journal of Diseases of Children* 145: 631-634.

Dial, E.J. & Lichtenberger, L.M. 1987. Milk protection against experimental ulcerogenesis in rats. *Digestive Diseases and Sciences* 32: 1145-1150.

Garland, C.F., Shekelle, R.B., Barrett-Connor, E. *et al*. 1985. Dietary calcium, vitamin D and risk of colorectal cancer: a 19-year prospective study in men. *Lancet* i: 307-309.

Gillman, M.W., Oliveria, S.A., Moore, L.L. & Ellison, R.C. 1992. Inverse association of dietary calcium with systolic blood pressure in young children. *Journal of the American Medical Association* 267: 2340-2343.

Gurr, M.I. 1989. Effects of fermented milks on cholesterolaemia: a critical review of the literature. In: Fermented Milks and Health, Proceedings of a workshop in Arnhem, The Netherlands, 1989, pp 77-87. NIZO, Ede, The Netherlands.

Gurr, M.I. 1992. Milk products: contribution to nutrition and health. *Journal of the Society of Dairy Technology* 45: 61-67.

Harper, D.S., Osborn, J.C., Clayton, R. & Hefferren, J.J. 1987. Modification of food cariogenicity in rats by mineral-rich concentrates from milk. *Journal of Dental Research* 66: 42-45.

Herod, E.L. 1991. The effect of cheese on dental caries: a review of the literature. *Australian Dental Journal* 36: 120-125.

Hilton, E., Isenberg, H.D., Alperstein, P., France, K., Borenstein, M.T. 1992. Ingestion of yogurt containing *Lactobacillus acidophilus* as prophylaxis for candidal vaginitis. *Annals of Internal Medicine* 116: 353-357.

International Dairy Federation. 1983. Cultured Dairy Foods in Human Nutrition. Document 159, International Dairy Federation, Brussels.

International Dairy Federation. 1991. Cultured Dairy Products in Human Nutrition. Document 255, International Dairy Federation, Brussels.

Johnstone, C.C., Miller, J.Z., Slemenda, C.W., Reister, T.K., Hui, S., Christian, J.C. & Peacock, M. 1992. Calcium supplementation and increases in bone mineral density in children. *New England Journal of Medicine* 327: 82-87.

Katschinski, B.D., Logan, R.F.A., Edmond, M. & Langman, M.J.S. 1992. Duodenal ulcer and calcium intake: a case-control study. *European Journal of Gastroenterology and Hepatology* 4: 897-901.

Katz, R.S. & Speckmann, E.W. 1978. A perspective on milk intolerance. *Journal of Food Protection* 41: 220-225.

Kim, H.S. & Gilliland, S.E. 1983. *Lactobacillus acidophilus* as a dietary adjunct for milk to aid lactose digestion in humans. *Journal of Dairy Science* 66: 956-966.

Kobayashi, T., Ohmori, T., Yanai, M., Kawanishi, G., Yoshikai Y. & Nomoto, K. 1991. Protective effect of orally administering immune milk on endogenous infection in X-irradiated mice. *Agricultural and Biological Chemistry* 55: 2265-2272.

Kolars, J.C., Levitt, M.D., Aouji, M. & Savaiano, D.A. 1984. Yogurt: an autodigesting source of lactose. *New England Journal of Medicine* 310: 1-3.

Lerebours, E., N'Djitoyap Ndam, C., Lavoine, A., Hellot, M.F., Antoine, J.M. & Colin R. 1989. Yogurt and fermented-then-pasteurized milk: effects of short term and long term ingestion on lactose absorption and mucosal lactase activity in lactase deficient subjects. *American Journal of Clinical Nutrition* 49: 823-827.

Marcoux, S., Brisson, J. & Fabia, J. 1991. Calcium intake from dairy products and supplements and the risks of pre-eclampsia and gestational hypertension. *American Journal of Epidemiology* 133: 1266-1272.

Martini, M.C., Lerebours, E.C., Lin, W-J., Harlander, S.K., Berrada, N.B., Antoine, J.M. & Savaiano, D.A. 1991. Strains and species of lactic acid bacteria in fermented milks (Yogurts): effect on *in vivo* lactose digestion. *American Journal of Clinical Nutrition* 54: 1041-1046.

Medical Research Council. 1991. The Caerphilly and Speedwell Prospective Heart Disease Studies. Progress Report No. 7.

Mettlin, C. & Graham, S. 1979. Dietary risk factors in human bladder cancer. *American Journal of Epidemiology* 110: 255-263.

Micheli, H., Schuchan, C. & Bachmann, C. 1982. Plasma cholesterol in four Swiss cities: relationship with alcohol and milk consumption. In: *Lipoproteins and coronary atherosclerosis* (ed. G. Noseda, Fragiacomo, R. Fumagalli, R. Paoletti). Elsevier, Amsterdam.

Murosaki, S., Yoshikai, Y., Kubo, C., Ishida, A., Matsuzaki, G., Sato, T., Endo, K. & Nomoto, K. 1990. Influence of intake of skim milk from cows immunized with intestinal bacterial antigens on onset of renal disease in (NZB) x NZW)F_1 mice fed *ad libitum* or restricted energy intake. *Journal of Nutrition* 121: 1860-1868.

Papenburg, R., Bounous, G., Fleiszer, D. & Gold, P. 1990. Dietary milk proteins inhibit the development of dimethylhydrazine-induced malignancy. *Tumour Biology* 11: 129-136.

Pariza, M.W. 1991. CLA, a new cancer inhibitor in dairy products. Bulletin of the IDF 257: 29-30.

Petschow, B.W. & Talbott, R.D. 1991. Response of *Bifidobacterium* species to growth promoters in human and cow milk. *Pediatric Research* 29: 208-213.

Prince, R.L., Smith, M., Dick, I.M., Price, R.I., Webb, P.G., Henderson, N.K. & Harris, M.M. 1991. Prevention of post-menopausal osteoporosis. A comparative study of exercise, calcium supplementation and hormone replacement therapy. *New England Journal of Medicine* 325: 1189-1195.

Renner, E., Knie, G., Schatz, H., Stracke, K., Weber, K., Minne, H.W. & Leidig, G. 1991. On the incidence of osteoporosis in relation to the calcium intake with milk and milk products. *International Dairy Journal* 1: 77-82.

Sentipal, J.M., Wardlaw, G.M., Mahan, J. & Matkovic, V. 1991. Influence of calcium intake and growth indexes on vertebral bone mineral density in young females. *American Journal of Clinical Nutrition* 54: 435-438.

Silva, M.F. de A., Jenkins G.N., Burgess, R.C. & Sandham, H.J. 1986. Effects of cheese on experimental caries in human subjects. *Caries Research* 20: 263-269.

Silva, M.F. de A., Burgess, R.C., Sandham H.J. & Jenkins, G.N. 1987. Effects of water-soluble components of cheese on experimental caries in humans. *Journal of Dental Research* 66: 38-41.

Staehelin, H.B., Eichholzer, M. & Gey, K.F. 1992. Nutritional factors correlating with cardiovascular disease: results of the Basel study. *Bibliotheca Nutritia Dieta* 49.

Stocks, P. & Karn, M.N. 1933. A cooperative study of the habits, home life, dietary and family histories of 450 cancer patients and an equal number of control patients. *Annals of Eugenics* 5: 237-280.

van der Meer, R. & Lapre, J.A. 1991. Calcium and colon cancer. International Dairy Federation Bulletin 255: 55-59. International Dairy Federation, Brussels.

van't Veer, P., Dekker, J.M., Lamers, J.W., Kok, F.J., Schouten, E.C., Brants, H.A.M., Sturmans, F. & Hermus, R.J.J. 1989. Consumption of fermented milk products and breast cancer: a case-control study in The Netherlands. *Cancer Research* 49: 4020-4023.

Wargovich, M.J., Lynch, P.M. & Levin, B. 1991. Modulating effects of calcium in animal models of colon carcinogenesis and short term studies in subjects at increased risk for colon cancer. *American Journal of Clinical Nutrition* 54: 202S-205S.

Weaver, C.M. & Heaney, R.P. 1991. Isotopic exchange of ingested calcium between labelled sources. Evidence that ingested calcium does not form a common absorptive pool. *Calcified Tissue International* 49: 244-247.

Dairy Products in Human Health and Nutrition, Serrano Ríos et al. (eds) © 1994 Balkema, Rotterdam, ISBN 90 5410 359 0

Evolution of nutritional impact produced by milk and dairy products intake in Spain

C. Martí-Henneberg, V. Arija, G. Cucó & J. Fernández-Ballart
Research Unit on Human Nutrition and Growth, Faculty of Medicine, University Rovira i Virgili, Reus, Spain

ABSTRACT: Spain is a mediterranean country which maintains the characteristics of a diet which is typical to this area of the world. Traditionally it has been a low consumer of dairy products.

It is the third country in milk production in the European Mediterranean area. The milk intake has gradually increased from 1966 to 1986 but many data confirm that recently this trend is being reversed. All the rest of dairy products are increasing in their frequency of consumption as well as their quantity in the diet.

The contribution of milk and dairy products to lipids intake in the population studied is moderate, except in some groups of age. The intake of whole milk in the third year of life implies 23% of the lipid content of the diet. In the same age, 30% of children eat fresh cheese which contributes 20% to their lipid intake.

1 INTRODUCTION

Although the Mediterranean diet is an ideal model which is set as an example of good eating habits in occidental countries, we still are a long way from defining the basic characteristics of this type of diet (R. Giacco et al.1991). The first difficulty lies in the fact that this definition of diet, is not all that real because it encompasses the diet of many different countries with differing cultures and varied economic status.

Some general characteristics which define this diet are: a greater intake of cereals, fruit and vegetables and a smaller intake of meat, sugars, milk and dairy products than in other European countries. The balance of lipid intake is characterized in these countries by a great intake of oil and a smaller consumption of animal fats compared to the other western countries.

The cooking of pulses in our community is traditionally frequent but is quickly decreasing.

All these characteristics are still valid, but perhaps with the socioeconomic changes which we are going through, are producing rapid changes in our eating habits.

From an epidemiological point of view the mediterranean. diet has been related to a lower incidence of cardiovascular disease, as well as a lower incidence of hypertension, obesity, diabetes, and some types of malignant diseases.

In Spain during the last twenty years we have changed from eating habits based on cereals, pulses, olive oil, potatoes, fruits, vegetables, eggs and a low consumption of meat and milk to eating habits in which cereals and potatoes decrease and meat, milk and dairy products increase. Vegetable protein intake is less and animal protein intake increases (Ministerio de Agricultura Spain 1991).

Nevertheless the Spanish diet at the present moment, can be considered good enough and satisfies the nutritional needs of the population. From the traditional diet, it maintains the ingestion of olive oil, fruit, vegetables and fish which enrich nutrition with essential fatty acids, fibre, vitamins and minerals.

On the contrary it diminishes bread, rice and cereal products which decreases the intake of complex carbohydrates and fibre.

The decrease in the use of pulses diminishes the contribution of good quality proteins without fats. On the contrary, the increase of foods of animal origin produces an excessive amount of saturated fats, which leaves us far from some of the essential characteristics of the mediterranean diet.

We observe an increase in transformed products like meat derivatives, some of which are typical of the country but others, which have been introduced recently Another of the mediterranean characteristics which is diminishing, is the intake of wine.

In our culture there are remnants from ancient habits which testify that the intake of milk and preparation of dairy products was common in the mediterranean countries (G. Ottogalli et al.1991) .

The culinary culture of ancient Greece and Rome has left written witnesses of the preparation of varied cheeses kept in olive oil with aromatic herbs from our mountains.

Nevertheless in our countries there still exist many differences in the origin of milk and the quantity of its production. France (FAO 1986 in ASSOLATE 1987) is the greatest cow's milk (92% of the total) producer. Greece, which is a low milk producer consumes an equivalent of 5% of the milk produced in France. Italy produces 35% compared with French production.

There are few countries in which we have enough facts which enable us to know the evolution of the consumption of dairy products during these last decades. In France (FAO 1985 in ASSOLATE 1987) between 1966 and 1986 the intake of liquid milk, changed from 103 litres per year per person to 79 litres. Whereas the intake of fermented milk passed from 4,2 litres to 13.0 l. Cheese from 12,1 Kg to 21,1 kg and butter goes down from 9. kg to 7,5 kg always by year and person. In Italy, on the contrary, during this same period, an increase in intake of liquid milk took place, from 66.8 litres to 78.5. Fermented milk increased from 0,5 litres to 3,2 litres, cheese from 9,1 kg to 17,3 kg. Butter has increased slightly from 1,6 kg to 2,2 kg.

Using facts from FAO we know that in mediterranean countries the nutritional contribution of dairy products to the diet represents between 6,5% to 10% of the total caloric intake, between 13% and 24% of the protein intake and 9% and

Table 1. Evolution of diary products consumption in Spain

	1987	1990
Whole milk	* 342	299
Skimmed milk	37	44
Fermented milk	23	21
Fresh cheese	5	5
Other Cheeses	12	11
Total	413	374

ml-g/inh/day
* Mean
Source: Ministerio de Agricultura. España, 1991

19% of the lipid intake. The countries where the caloric intake from dairy products is greater. are France, Italy and Malta. This implies that in a country like Malta where the global lipid intake is low, 77,9 gr. per day the lipid intake from dairy is

15,1 gr per day, which represents the greatest proportion in all Mediterranean countries.

In Spain there is a global production of milk of 7.344.000 tons which represents one fifth of the French production. From this total, cow's milk is 92%.

The evolution of dairy product intake in this country has suffered a paradoxic change. We proses data from 1966 to 1986. The FAO obtained data from the market supplies and in this way we know that the intake of liquid milk per person has increased during this period of time from 71.0 litres per year to 108,1 litres, but the data from the Spanish agricultural department which obtains them from the housewives shopping, show us a decrease in dairy product shopping from 1987 to 1990 (table 1) from 413 ml inhabitant day in 1987 to 374 ml in 1990. The data show clearly a decrease of buying whole milk and a rise of the buying of skimmed milk. We did not see any changes in the other dairy products.

If we look again at the results of the FAO investigation, we can see that the consumption of fermented milk in Spain is rising also. From 1,2 l/inh/ year to 6,9 l/inh/ year, and the cheese rise from 2,1 kg /inh/ year to 5,1 kg /inh/ year. On the country, the butter is stabilizing from 0,3 kg /inh/ year to 0,5 kg /inh/ year.

The mean caloric intake per person in Spain was 3303 kcal day by the market supplies method in 1985. The milk and dairy products contributed 269 kcal that is the 8% of the total.The total protein consumption was 88,7 g /inh/d ; dairy contributed to the total amount 14,5 g /inh/d that is 15%. The lipids in the diet are 137,8 g /inh/d and the dairy products 15,6 g /inh/d that is 10,8%.

All these important results, as we say, brought by the study of the market supplies of the housewives shopping are references for other studies that try to know the real intake of the population by ages and sexes.

2 DAIRY INTAKE IN THE MEDITERRANEAN SPANISH AREA

This study took place in Reus, which is city with 89.496 inhabitants, located 5 km from the sea. In 1982 (J. Salas et al. 1985 A) the sample was randomized from the total number of families in the city. The family was the unit of randomization. The sample represented all the districts in the city. 345 families were studied, all of them with a son younger than 10 years. The sample was, them, formed by 1397 people, from 6 m. of age to 65 years.

In 1993 we studied again the same population.

From the total of the families still living in the city, 177 (59% of the total in 1983) accepted to collaborate again . We randomized using the same method of 1983, obtaining another group of 120 families, with a minimum of a son younger than 10

years. Now the sample was composed by 1138 people.

The method used to collect the intake amount of each person in the family was the "24 h. recall", repeated three days a week.

3 RESULTS

Between 1983 (J. Salas et al. 1985 B) and 1993 the dairy intake has been stable, but this result in its globality implies important changes (table 2). The intake of whole milk is less, but skimmed milk is rising and the fermented milk, fresh cheese and other cheese intake are also growing.

Table 3 shows the changes in the milk intake by groups of age and sexes. First we realize that the total number of consumers of milk is rising if we compare with the data from 1982 in the same population. Groups of age of which only 60% were consuming milk in 1982 are disappearing. Only people older than fifty years are still consuming milk less frequently than the other groups in 1992.

Table 2. Evolution of diary products intake in Reus (Spain)

	1983	1993
Whole milk	* 244 (187)	205 (191)
Skimmed milk	18 (64)	47 (110)
Fermented milk	18 (38)	25 (49)
Fresh cheese	2 (11)	5 (15)
Other Cheeses	12 (19)	15 (21)
Total	294 (195)	300 (193)

ml-g/inh/day
* Mean (SD)
Source: Reus (Spain) Study, 1993

Table 3. Evolution of milk intake in Reus (Spain)

Groups				Whole + skimmed milk [1]	
Age (years)	Sex	n		1983	1993
		1983	1993		
0.5-1	M & F	14	24	* 347 (196)	338 (196)
2	M & F	20	21	388 (207)	451 (356)
3-4	M & F	57	30	365 (154)	361 (189)
5-6	M & F	68	41	332 (176)	306 (181)
7-10	M	82	45	356 (141)	339 (164)
	F	81	40	324 (154)	311 (127)
11-15	M	90	74	371 (266)	314 (186)
	F	98	50	275 (160)	281 (147)
16-20	M	46	59	282 (182)	277 (192)
	F	79	63	241 (136)	241 (167)
21-30	M	60	69	200 (165)	251 (194)
	F	91	84	256 (187)	252 (200)
31-50	M	204	170	154 (151)	169 (153)
	F	222	197	242 (155)	229 (167)
51-65	M	48	63	175 (186)	142 (146)
	F	35	62	198 (167)	210 (143)

[1] ml/inh/day
n = number of individuals
* Mean (SD)
M = Males; F = Females
Source: Reus (Spain) study, 1993

Some adults in our population still maintain the old habits of a small intake of milk, typical of the mediterranean area.

But we can observe, on the contrary, that the amount of milk drunk is going down in the majority of the groups.

There are a few exceptions like the third year of life in which the intake of milk has increased and in males from 20-50 years in which the same is true, which reflect this increase in milk taking habits.

The contribution of whole milk in the caloric content of diet (tables 4 and 5) is decreasing from the first year of life to adulthood as would be expected, observing that in the third year it still represents 18% of the total caloric content of the diet.

These figures confirm the data from the FAO 1985 (ASSOLATTE 1987) as our milk consumption places this food in an inferior nutritional range than in other countries.

Our data also confirm that whole milk has an important part in the proteic and lipid intake of the child, as we can see in the third year of life. During puberty 10% of the lipids in the diet come from whole milk. This is also the same proportion found in women over 50 years of age.

The consumers of skimmed or semi skimmed milk increase with age being frequent in women from 16-50 years.

The contrary is observed in the amount of consumers of fermented milk which decreases with age. The intake of yoghurt is frequent during the third, fourth and fifth year of life. The contribution of yoghurt to the total caloric intake (table 6) in the youngest never exceeds 4%. Its part in lipid ingestion is also small.

Between 1983 and 1993 an increase in the ingestion of fermented milk has taken place which is obvious in all groups of age. As we have said the intake of fresh cheese is on the increase in our population. The figures which show the proportion of consumers (table 7) prove that this is a nutrient which is introduced at a later age than fermented milk. The greatest figure of consumers is observed among children 4-5 years old. From this period onwards, the quantities of consumption decrease to proportions which are lower than 20%. The age at which intake is lower is the young adult.

The consumers of highest quantities of, of fresh cheese, are children of 3-4 years, this represents 6-8 % of the total caloric content of the diet, 10,6 % of proteic intake and 11,7 % of lipid intake. At the

Table 4. Energy and macronutrients intake Reus (Spain)

Groups		Intake (units/inh/day)			
Age (years)	Sex	Energy (Kcal)	Proteins (g)	Lipids (g)	CHO (g)
0.5-1	M & F	1114 (305)	52 (16)	39 (19)	134 (33)
2	M & F	1609 (511)	69 (22)	70 (27)	166 (57)
3-4	M & F	1690 (373)	65 (18)	78 (24)	173 (38)
5-6	M & F	1849 (445)	69 (18)	81 (27)	196 (52)
7-10	M	1929 (408)	71 (16)	85 (22)	206 (52)
	F	1853 (434)	68 (18)	79 (23)	202 (51)
11-15	M	2470 (619)	93 (24)	113 (33)	256 (80)
	F	2152 (417)	79 (17)	98 (27)	220 (52)
16-20	M	2390 (632)	88 (22)	110 (32)	244 (77)
	F	1861 (452)	71 (18)	83 (21)	194 (64)
21-30	M	2366 (576)	87 (22)	112 (30)	228 (80)
	F	1855 (546)	68 (21)	86 (23)	185 (76)
31-50	M	2298 (617)	82 (21)	102 (32)	224 (73)
	F	1795 (507)	66 (18)	82 (27)	180 (60)
51-65	M	2039 (540)	74 (20)	89 (25)	207 (82)
	F	1640 (499)	63 (18)	78 (33)	161 (57)

M=Males; F=Femeles

Source: Reus (Spain) study, 1993

Table 5. Contribution of whole milk to nutritional intake in Reus (Spain)

Groups		Contribution to nutritional intake			% Cons
Age (years)	Sex	Energy %	Proteins %	Lipids %	
0.5-1	M & F	18.1 (9.8)	21.4 (12.3)	29.0 (13.9)	74
2	M & F	17.9 (10.9)	23.4 (15.0)	23.1 (15.4)	95
3-4	M & F	13.4 (6.5)	19.6 (9.8)	15.7 (8.4)	100
5-6	M & F	10.5 (6.5)	15.6 (9.5)	13.0 (8.0)	93
7-10	M	12.0 (5.1)	17.7 (7.4)	14.5 (6.3)	91
	F	9.5 (4.7)	14.6 (8.1)	12.0 (6.6)	93
11-15	M	8.7 (4.6)	12.6 (6.6)	10.4 (5.7)	91
	F	8.8 (4.7)	13.1 (6.8)	10.4 (5.7)	88
16-20	M	8.2 (4.4)	12.0 (6.3)	9.6 (5.2)	90
	F	8.8 (5.6)	12.4 (7.6)	10.3 (6.3)	76
21-30	M	7.5 (4.7)	11.2 (7.4)	8.5 (5.5)	87
	F	4.4 (6.0)	11.2 (8.8)	8.3 (6.5)	85
31-50	M	5.0 (3.6)	7.8 (6.0)	6.2 (5.0)	81
	F	7.2 (6.6)	10.8 (9.6)	8.5 (7.7)	78
51-65	M	5.3 (3.8)	8.1 (5.9)	6.8 (5.2)	67
	F	9.2 (5.9)	13.3 (9.1)	10.6 (6.7)	63

% Cons = Percentage of consumers   Source: Reus (Spain) study, 1993
M = Males; F = Females

Table 6. Contribution of fermented milk to nutritional intake in Reus (Spain)

Groups		Contribution to nutritional intake			% Cons
Age (years)	Sex	Energy %	Proteins %	Lipids %	
0.5-1	M & F	5.6 (3.7)	8.7 (6.0)	5.6 (4.6)	61
2	M & F	3.9 (2.2)	6.6 (4.1)	3.1 (2.3)	76
3-4	M & F	3.5 (1.7)	6.9 (3.0)	2.5 (1.8)	77
5-6	M & F	2.5 (1.3)	4.9 (2.4)	1.9 (1.1)	56
7-10	M	2.8 (2.1)	5.4 (3.6)	2.1 (2.0)	56
	F	2.6 (1.9)	5.0 (3.4)	1.9 (1.5)	55
11-15	M	2.2 (1.6)	4.0 (2.5)	1.5 (1.0)	46
	F	1.8 (1.0)	3.7 (2.6)	1.3 (0.8)	28
16-20	M	2.5 (1.6)	4.9 (2.8)	1.5 (1.0)	20
	F	3.4 (1.9)	6.6 (3.8)	2.4 (1.8)	22
21-30	M	2.5 (2.4)	4.9 (3.9)	1.6 (1.6)	30
	F	3.1 (2.3)	6.1 (4.5)	1.7 (1.1)	29
31-50	M	2.2 (2.1)	4.5 (4.3)	1.9 (1.6)	22
	F	3.0 (2.7)	5.6 (4.7)	1.7 (1.7)	25
51-65	M	3.0 (2.5)	6.0 (5.4)	1.4 (1.0)	21
	F	2.6 (1.3)	4.9 (2.3)	1.2 (1.1)	24

% Cons = Percentage of consumers   Source: Reus (Spain) study, 1993
M = Males; F = Females

Table 7. Contribution of fresh cheese to nutritional intake in Reus (Spain)

Groups		Contribution to nutritional intake			% Cons
Age (years)	Sex	Energy %	Proteins %	Lipids %	
0.5-1	M & F	8.8 (2.5)	12.1 (3.0)	16.2 (3.9)	13
2	M & F	10.7 (8.4)	15.1 (12.5)	20.3 (17.1)	29
3-4	M & F	6.8 (4.6)	10.6 (6.7)	11.7 (7.6)	50
5-6	M & F	5.0 (3.3)	7.9 (4.1)	9.7 (6.0)	17
7-10	M	5.9 (3.6)	9.3 (5.1)	11.2 (6.1)	20
	F	3.6 (3.1)	5.7 (4.8)	6.5 (4.8)	18
11-15	M	4.2 (3.1)	7.0 (4.9)	7.2 (4.9)	14
	F	2.3 (2.2)	4.2 (4.0)	3.9 (3.7)	18
16-20	M	4.0 (3.5)	6.2 (4.7)	6.7 (6.1)	12
	F	3.3 (2.6)	5.3 (3.4)	4.9 (3.9)	17
21-30	M	1.8 (1.4)	3.4 (2.7)	2.8 (3.0)	9
	F	2.2 (1.2)	4.2 (2.4)	3.4 (2.6)	7
31-50	M	1.7 (1.5)	3.2 (2.7)	2.7 (2.9)	10
	F	2.3 (2.4)	3.7 (2.5)	3.2 (2.9)	14
51-65	M	1.3 (0.7)	2.1 (1.0)	2.0 (1.1)	10
	F	2.2 (2.1)	3.3 (2.6)	3.4 (3.7)	16

% Cons = Percentage of consumers
M = Males; F = Females

Source: Reus (Spain) study, 1993

Table 8. Contribution of other cheese to nutritional intake in Reus (Spain)

Groups		Contribution to nutritional intake			% Cons
Age	Sex	Energy %	Proteins %	Lipids %	
0.5-1	M & F	4.5 (3.6)	5.1 (3.4)	8.0 (6.4)	19
2	M & F	3.6 (2.8)	5.3 (4.2)	6.3 (4.9)	67
3-4	M & F	2.3 (1.2)	3.6 (1.7)	3.6 (1.9)	43
5-6	M & F	4.1 (2.8)	6.5 (4.2)	6.9 (5.0)	56
7-10	M	3.5 (2.4)	5.0 (3.3)	5.5 (3.9)	49
	F	2.4 (1.8)	3.8 (2.7)	4.2 (2.5)	60
11-15	M	4.8 (3.5)	7.1 (4.8)	7.6 (5.4)	57
	F	4.8 (3.7)	7.1 (4.9)	7.4 (5.1)	70
16-20	M	4.6 (3.5)	7.1 (5.0)	7.8 (5.6)	69
	F	4.4 (3.6)	6.4 (5.2)	7.1 (5.6)	63
21-30	M	4.4 (4.4)	6.7 (3.4)	6.4 (5.9)	65
	F	4.5 (3.9)	6.9 (5.3)	7.1 (6.1)	70
31-50	M	4.3 (2.9)	6.9 (4.4)	7.2 (4.8)	59
	F	4.1 (3.7)	5.9 (4.8)	6.5 (5.6)	58
51-65	M	4.3 (2.8)	6.8 (4.3)	6.9 (4.7)	58
	F	4.3 (2.9)	6.1 (4.3)	6.7 (4.3)	42

% Cons = Percentage of consumers
M = Males; F = Females

Source: Reus (Spain) study, 1993

same age we found that whole milk intake com be a low consumer of fresh cheese although we must state that in some children the intake of fresh cheese is an important lipid contribution to the diet. We should analyse carefully this fact before reaching further conclusions.

Fresh cheese consumption has increased in our country between 1983-1993 and this is clear at all ages. This nutrient was consumed in very small amounts after the beginning of puberty in 1983.

The intake of cheese is clearly present in the diet of a majority of our population since the 3rd year of life.

The consumption of cheese has increased in all mediterranean countries amongst our population although the increase is small, and it is only clearly observed among young males and adults. Cheese is a growing contribution of lipids in adults from our sample (table 8).

4 CONCLUSION

Spain is still a moderate consumer of milk and dairy products. In spite of the fact that during these bast decades the intake has been on the increase. The study of the recent evolution shows us that there is an increase in the number of consumers in all these types of food.

There is a slight decrease in the consumption of whole milk. The rest of dairy products clearly are increasing only during the first years of life the dairy products have an significant place in the lipid contribution to diet.

REFERENCES

Associazione Italiana Lattiero-Casearia (ASSOLATTE). 1987. Relazione del Presidente. Supplemento della Rivista Il Mondo del Latte:157.

Giacco, R. & G. Ricardi 1991. Comparison of Current Eating Habits in Various Mediterranean Countries. In G.A. Spiller (ed.),The Mediterranean diets in healts and disease: 3-9. New York: Van ostrand Reinhold.

Ministerio de Agricultura (Spain) 1991. La alimentación en España.

Ottogalli, G. & G. Testolin 1991. Dairy Products in G.A. Spiller (ed.), The Mediterranean diets in healts and disease: 135-159. New York: Van Nostrand Reinhold.

Salas, J., I. Font, J. Canals, L. Guinovart, C. Sospedra & C. Marti-Henneberg 1985. (I) Consumo global por grupos de alimentos y su relacion con el nivel socioeconómico y de instrucción. 84: 339-343.

Salas, J., I. Font, J. Canals, L. Guinovart, C. Sospedra & C. Marti-Henneberg 1985. (III) Distribución por edad y sexo del consumo de leche, derivados de la leche, grasas visibles vegetales y verduras. 84:470-475.

Dairy Products in Human Health and Nutrition, Serrano Ríos et al. (eds) © 1994 Balkema, Rotterdam, ISBN 90 5410 359 0

Epidemiologic topics in nutrition and health relevant to dairy industry

F.J. Kok
Department of Epidemiology and Public Health, Wageningen Agricultural University, Netherlands

ABSTRACT: Recent epidemiologic findings relevant to dairy industry are discussed. It is concluded that cholesterol-lowering drugs seem to be beneficial only for subgroups who are at very high risk of death from coronary heart disease (CHD). Furthermore, consumption of partially hydrogenated vegetable oils (trans fatty acids) may increase the risk of CHD. Antioxidants, like vitamin E and beta-carotene may be protective against CHD. Finally high intake of calcium and fermented milkproducts may reduce colon cancer risk.

I Lowering cholesterol and mortality

It's well-known that elevated serum cholesterol increases the risk of coronary heart disease (CHD). Adequate diet may lower serum cholesterol to a maximum of about 15-20%, whereas very effective drugs may go to 50%. The last decade there has been a tremendous increase in prescription of cholesterol-lowering drugs, e.g., in Great Britain prescription increased more than sixfold between 1986 and 1992 (1). The question is whether drug and dietary interventions are of help in lowering CHD risk. Recent meta-analysis of drug and non-drug trials indicate that cholesterol-lowering is beneficial in only a small proportion of patients at very high risk of death from CHD. Overall risk of CHD should be the main focus of clinical and dietary guidelines (1). In intervention trials, beneficial effects on CHD are often observed, however, death from other causes such as cancer and accidents, suicide and violence are sometimes increased, resulting in no net effect on total mortality (1,2). On average

the risk of cancer mortality is 50% higher for those receiving treatment, however, extremely low cholesterol is probably a consequence rather than a cause of cancer. The approximately 75% higher risk of death from external causes, as observed in some drug trials is based on low numbers, lacks a biological explanation and may be due to confounding.

II Evolution of the role of fat in coronary heart disease

The development of the scientific knowledge on the role of fat in CHD is illustrated in figure 1. In the dotted squares the types of fat that elevate cholesterol are indicated. From the saturated fats only lauric acid (C12:0), myristic acid (C14:0), and palmitic acid (C16:0) increase cholesterol. Palmitic acid is less effective than lauric and myristic acid. Stearic acid (C18:0) may lower cholesterol and short chain fatty acids are neutral. Depending on the dietary habits dairy products may contribute quite substantially

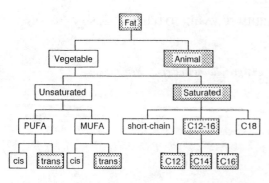

Figure 1. Evolution of the role of fat in coronary heart disease

to saturated fat intake, however, are also rich in short-chain fatty acids and moderately rich in stearic acid. Moreover, dairy products contain reasonable amounts of mono-unsaturated fats, of which it has been shown that they may lower cholesterol.

Unsaturated fatty acids may depending on their configuration increase cholesterol. These so-called trans fatty acids are formed when liquid vegetable oils are partially hydrogenated to form margarine and shortenings. Thus processed vegetable fats may contain between 5 and more than 30% of these trans-isomers. Trans fatty acids are also formed in the rumen of cattle and make up about 5% of dairy and beef fat. Trans isomers constitute about 5-6% of dietary fat consumed in the USA with a wide variation (3). It has been shown recently that high trans fatty acid intake may almost double the risk of CHD. About 60% of the trans fatty acid intake was derived from vegetable fats (margarine, cookies, cake, white bread), and 40% came from animal sources (mainly beef and dairy products). The increased risk of CHD was completely due to trans fatty acids from vegetable sources.

III Antioxidants and coronary heart disease

Relatively new in cardiovascular research is the potentially protective role of antioxidants in the intitiation and pro-

gression of atherosclerosis. It is well-established that elevated levels of LDL-cholesterol are associated with increased risk of CHD. The mechanism of the atherogenic effect of LDL has become more clear in recent years. It has been shown that LDL cholesterol after oxidative modification becomes 3-10 times more atherogenic compared to native LDL. In the LDL particle, the unsaturated fatty acids in the cholesterol esters and phospholipids are an important substrate for oxidation. Fat-soluble antioxidants (e.g. vitamin E, beta-carotene), which are transported in the plasma through LDL, protect the fatty acids from oxidation. Oxidation of unsaturated fatty acids may occur either by exogenous or endogenous free radicals. If the antioxidants are consumed a chain reaction of lipid peroxidation is initiated. There is considerable experimental and clinical evidence for this theory and it is hypothesized that low antioxidant levels may increase CHD risk through LDL oxidation.

Recent epidemiological data suggest a protective role for vitamin E, however, only at extremely high dosis. In two prospective studies based on large US cohorts the incidence of CHD was decreased with about 40% only among those who used daily vitamin E supplements (4,5). Moreover, within the normal intake range of beta-carotene, a high intake was associated with an overall reduced risk of 26%. A more detailed analyses, showed that especially current and ex-smokers benefit from high beta-carotene intake.

In the EURAMIC Study, a multicenter case-control study in 10 centers in Europe and Israel, we studied the protective role of the antioxidants vitamin E and beta-carotene, as measured in adipose tissue, and risk of a first myocardial infarction (6). Adipose tissue levels of antioxidants reflect longterm intake. By comparing levels of cases (n=683) and controls (n=702), and making the necessary adjustments for confounding variables, no relevant difference was observed for vitamin E and strongly reduced levels for beta-carotene revealed, which again were confined to current and ex smokers. The null findings for vitamin E are compatible with the results in the US cohorts, i.e., only supplement users benefit.

The preventive implications from these epidemiologic studies are not yet clear. Sofar the scientific basis to advice the use of vitamin E supplements is to small. The effects are probably comparable to what previously was concluded for cholesterol-lowering drugs, namely only small groups may benefit. If the evidence accumulates that antioxidants may reduce the risk of CHD, than a balanced diet is the first advice, to reach the requirements. If much higher antioxidant intakes than the RDA's are beneficial only, than one could think of enrichment of food products, including dairy products.

IV Dairy products and colon cancer

In the fourth and last part the role dairy products may have in the etiology of colon cancer will be addressed. Figure 2 shows the proposed mechanism of calcium in colon carcinogenesis. The normal sequence in colon carcinogenesis includes: normal turnover of mucosal cells; hyperproliferation of cells; growth to

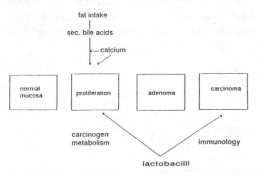

Figure 2 Dairy products and colon cancer: mechanisms for a protective role of calcium and fermented milkproducts

adenomatous polyps; further development to malign tumour. Calcium may be implicated in colon cancer by neutralizing secundary bile acids or directly prevent cells from hyperproliferation.

The general picture from epidemiologic studies suggests a potential beneficial effect for high calcium intake. The most recent study by Stemmerman et al (7) showed a 40% lower risk for those in the highest tertile of the calcium intake distribution. More evidence for a protective role of calcium is coming from intervention studies where the effect on cell proliferation was studied (8,9). By supplementing groups with high familial risk of colon cancer with high daily dosis of calcium (1250 mg on top of the average 700 mg per day) during three months, proliferation was reduced with 60% (8). And the proliferation rate came back to levels that are normal for individuals with low colon cancer risk.

An independent protective effect on colon cancer risk is suggested for fermented milkproducts. The biological mechanism for fermented milkproducts is related to lactobacilli (figure 2). Lactobacilli may inhibit the conversion of procarcinogens to carcinogens in the colon. Furthermore, they may stimulate the immune respons by activating lymphocytes and macrophages and the production of cytokines.

Ecologic findings suggest high incidence of colon cancer in countries like USA, UK and Ireland with low per capita consumption of fermented milkproducts. Low colon cancer incidence and high fermented dairy consume is observed in countries like Sweden, Finland, Denmark and the Netherlands. Case-control studies show similar beneficial results for fermented milkproducts. For example, Young and Wolf (10) observed in a study with 350 colon cancer cases and 600 controls a protective association for fermented milkproducts. For those using 8 versus 1 serving per month the risk was reduced with 35%. Peters et al.(11) observed similar findings for yoghurt. However, no effects of fermented milkproducts on the risk of adenomatous polyps were observed by Kampman et al (12) in two large US prospective studies.

Thus, in contrast to calcium for fermented milkproducts, the benefits in relation to colon cancer are less clear.

Conclusions

Cholesterol-lowering drugs in the prevention of CHD seem to be beneficial only for subgroups who are at initially high risk of developing coronary disease. Trans fatty acids from margarines may increase the risk of CHD. Antioxidants, especially vitamin E and beta-carotene may protect against CHD by protecting LDL cholesterol from oxidation. Finally high intake of calcium and fermented milkproducts may reduce colon cancer risk.

Literature

1. Davey Smith G, Song F, Sheldon TA. Cholesterol lowering and mortality: the importance of considering intitial level of risk. Br Med J 1993;306:1367-73.

2. Muldoon MF, Manuck SB, Matthews KA. Lowering cholesterol concentrations and mortality: a quantitative review of primary prevention trials. Br Med J 1990;301:309-14.

3. Willett WC, Stampfer MJ, Manson JE et al. Intake of trans fatty acids and risk of coronary heart disease among women. Lancet 1993;341:581-5.

4. Stampfer MJ, Hennekens CH, Manson JE et al. Vitamin E consumption and the risk of coronary disease in women. N Engl J Med 1993;328:1444-9.

5. Rimm EB, Stampfer MJ, Ascherio A et al. Vitamin E consumption and the risk of coronary heart disease in men. N Engl J Med 1993;328:1450-6.

6. Kardinaal AFM, Kok FJ, Ringstad J et al. Antioxidants in adipose tissue and risk of myocardial infarction. (submitted)

7. Stemmerman GN, Nomura A, Chyou PH. The influence of dairy and nondairy calcium on subsite large-bowel cancer risk. Dis colon rectum 1990;33:190-4

8. Lipkin M, Newmark H. Effect of added dietary calcium on colonic epithelial-cell proliferation in subjects at high risk for familial colonic cancer. N Engl J Med 1985;313:1 1381-4.

9. Wargowich MJ, Lynch PM, Liven B. Modulating effects of calcium in animal models of colon carcinogenesis and short-term studies in subjects at increased eisk for colon cancer. Am J Clin Nutr 1991;54:202S-5S.

10. Young Th, Wolf DA. Case-control study of proximal and distal colon cancer and diet in Wisconsin. Int J Cancer 1988; 42:167-75.

11. Peters RK, Pike MC, Garabrant D, Mack TM. Diet and colon cancer in Los Angeles County, California. Cancer Causes and Control 1992;3:457-73.

12. Kampman E, Giovannucci EL, Van 't Veer P, et al. Calcium, vitamin D, dairy foods and the occurrence of colorectal adenomas amon men and women in two prospective studies. Am J Epidemiol 1993 (in press).

Dairy Products in Human Health and Nutrition, Serrano Ríos et al. (eds) © 1994 Balkema, Rotterdam, ISBN 90 5410 359 0

Dairy products in the third world: An overview

F. Monckeberg
Institute of Nutrition and Food Technology, University of Chile, Santiago, Chile

ABSTRACT: Malnutrition in underdeveloped countries is prevalent, mainly in pre-school children. At the same time, milk consumption per capita is very low. Cow's milk can be a very important factor in prevention of malnutrition. National milk supplementation program, has been implemented in Chile, with very successfull results. The experience is analized.

Today the population living in Third World countries, represents two thirds of the whole population, and according to the last report from FAO, 1.156 million live in poverty or in precarious conditions. There is a high prevalence of preventible diseases and chronic undernutrition that affects mainly pregnant women and children (Institute on Hunger and Development, 1992). Although ciphers vary from country to country, at present, more than 50% of children under 6 years of age, living in the underdeveloped countries, present undernutrition of different degrees (UNICEF, 1993). This means an increased susceptibility to infections and a significant growth and developmental retardation also affecting their intellectual capacities. The perspectives for the future are not promising, due, among other factors, to the very rapid population growth. It has been calculated that by the year 2015, the world's population will be more than 7.500 millions, and that 85% of this increment will be in the underdeveloped world (PNUD, 1992). Poverty continues to increase: a recent report of the UNDP (1993) points out that between 1970 and 1990 the countries concentrating the richest 20% of the world's population, increased their participation in the international GNP from a 70% to 82%, while those countries in the poorest 20%, had their participation reduced from a 2.3% to a 1.4%. On the other hand, (according to a recent report of the World Bank, 1993), in 40 underdeveloped countries which accumulate a population of 800 millions inhabitants per capita income has fallen during the last decade.

The present diet in underdeveloped countries is insufficient in quantity and quality. Different studies report that approximately 1.500 millions inhabitants receive less calories than required for their normal growth and development and to obtain adequate nutritional conditions. As a consequence, approximately 500 million individuals in their great majority children, present undernutrition. The protein content and the quality of the diet is also insufficient, since cereal grains are the principal source of protein (80%) (World Bank, 1993).

In underdeveloped countries, individuals are undernourished not because they do not have access to adequate amounts of their usual diet, but mainly because they do not have enough income to obtain a qualitatively and quantitatively adequate diet. For this reason, it is very difficult to prevent undernutrition unless, there is an improvement in family income which means that there must be a previous decrease of poverty levels. Food donations might help in hunger situations, but evidently they are not a solution for a chronic sub-alimentation situation which is a characteristic of these countries.

It is true that in poor countries there is also a bad distribution of income, but even if this could be balanced, the total income would not be enough to erradicate undernutrition. While in developed countries, an average of 15% to 22% of the income is used in foods, in underdeveloped countries this percentage increases to ciphers ranging from 60% to 85% according to different regions (Monckeberg, F.,

1990). It must be considered that almost two thirds of the population living in underdeveloped countries has an annual "per capita" income of under US$400 (World Bank, 1992). According to these antecedents, it is difficult, if not impossible, to prevent undernutrition if the conditions of underdevelopment are not improved. In spite of this, there are some examples of a few underdeveloped countries, that during the last decades have been able to improve the nutritional situation of their populations, even in underdevelopment conditions. This is the case of Chile, that during the last three decades has experienced a significant progress in this respect (Monckeberg F., 1990). It is true, that in order to obtain this result, a political decision has been necessary with a very high social investment in the areas of health, nutrition education, housing and environmental sanitation (Schlesinger, L. et al., 1983).

Undernutrition is the result of the adding of different adverse factors inherent to poverty, and for its prevention, the implementation of nutritional programs is not enough.

CHARACTERISTICS OF UNDERNUTRITION

It is a general rule that in poor countries, undernutrition affects mainly the infantile population, during the process of rapid growth; because in this stage of life, nutritional requirements are higher and more specific. It is also a rule that undernutrition affects pregnant and lactating mothers, because they also increase their nutritional needs due to the greater caloric and nutritional expense that signifies pregnancy and breast feeding (Monckeberg F., 1992).

In countries with high proportions of rural areas, undernutrition generally starts after the first year of life, when breast feeding decreases. Because of the migration of masses of impoverished individuals to the cities, the process is reverted and undernutrition starts at earlier ages, which is mainly due to disappearance of breast feeding, to a lack of purchasing power required to substitute this, or to the bad sanitary conditions leading to frequent gastrointestinal and infections disturbances. Early malnutrition constitutes a severe problem, with a high risk of death, a very difficult and expensive treatment; and for those who survive, long lasting physical and intellectual sequelae (Monckeberg, F., 1992).

Unfortunately, during the last decades, the process of rural migration has increased continuously, specially in Latin America and some Asian countries, and this tendency will continue to increase in the near future. For example in Latin America, 72% of the population is urban, and the trend continues to increase. This migration process is also acquiring importance in the greater part of Asian countries. For this reason, early undernutrition (first months of life) is becoming more prevalent.

IMPORTANCE OF MILK

In the case of the infant, there is no doubt that breast feeding is the first alternative, because of its nutritional composition, the presence of immunological factors that prevent infections, and because of psychological aspects, so important in the first periods of life. This is why all efforts should be directed primarily to its preservation.

Unfortunately, success in not always attained, or it is only partial, because of the present tendency to substitute it for bottle feeding. The migration to the cities of impoverished peasants, and their incorporation to this new way of life means an imitation of habits, such as bottle feeding, which appears to symbolize the new life in town, abandoning breast feeding prematurely, since it appears to them as an out moded habit (Monckeberg, F., 1975). On the other hand, maternal undernutrition, that is prevalent at these levels of poverty means that the quantity and duration of breast feeding is very often insufficient. Finally, as a consequence of their incorporation into a new way of life, many mothers are forced to work away from their homes, and this again leads to an early abandonment of breast feeding. Under these conditions there is no other alternative than bottle feeding with cow's milk, which is not always possible because of the cost this signifies. Moreover, the bad environmental sanitary conditions causes contamination and consequently gastrointestinal disturbances.

There is no doubt that cow's milk can be a very important factor in the prevention of undernutrition, because it contains the lowest cost, protein from animal origin, and although it differs to the composition of human milk, it is the best as regards the quantity and quality of nutrients needed during this period of rapid growth, as well as a very high digestibility for the child.

Unfortunately, the present availability of

milk in underdeveloped countries is not enough. Its cost is quite elevated in relation to family incomes. In these countries, the production and elaboration of milk is scarce. Recent reports form FAO, have demonstrated that while in the developed world lives less than the fifth part of the population, there lies four fifths of the total production of milk of the world. In other words, where there lives four fifth of the world's population, only one fifth of the world's milk production is produced (FAO, 1992). The problem is not only in the number of cows, but the efficiency of the cows to produce milk, it is six times less in the underdeveloped world in comparison to the developed world (FAO, 1992). To this we must add that the industrialization of the milk is also very precarious, so the consumption of dairy products is also very low. All this means that the consumption of milk per inhabitant, as an average, is ten or more times lower in the poor world, in relation to the developed world.

It is a fact that milk is not a habit in the feeding of children nor in adults in underdeveloped countries. Maybe this is why there is such a high lactose intolerance, that in some countries reaches 100% of the adult population. This situation should be reverted, in order to improve the nutritional situation of underdeveloped countries, but it needs a strong support from the respective governments. In this aspect, the experience observed in Chile during the last decades, can be extraordinarily useful (Monckeberg, F., 1990).

CHILEAN EXPERIENCE

During the last thirty years, a progressive and continuous improvement in the health and nutrition of infants and preschool children has taken place in Chile. In these results, the free distribution of powdered milk to every child and pregnant and lactating mother has played a very important role.

The situation was quite different prior to the early 1960s. Chile had one of the highest infantile mortality rates in Latin America (120 per thousand live birth). This decreased to 16 per thousand in 1992, one of the lowest in the region. This decline in the infantile death rate resulted from a remarkable decrease in the mortality from respiratory and diarrheal diseases specially in children under one year old. A similar trend has been observed in preschool children mortality, than has declined from 14 per thousand in

1960, to 0.8 per thousand in 1992 (Monckeberg, F., 1992).

At the same time, the percentage of children with malnutrition has also been reduced, from 37% in 1960, to 6.5% in 1992. Second and third degree malnutrition similarly decreased from 5.9 percent to 0.4 percent. Maternal nutrition has also improved if we consider that the percentage of newborns with low birth weight (below 2.5 kg) has diminished from 12 percent to 6.2 percent from 1975 to 1992. All the biomedical indicators show that Chile has reached one of the highest levels in the region, very similar to a well developed country, although during this period the gross national product (GNP) per capita has not changed substantially (Monckeberg, F., 1992).

These enormous changes have been the consequence of the implementation of a health and nutritional policy, in which four main areas have been considered: health, nutrition, environmental sanitation and education. At a first stage, it was necessary to create a health infrastructure that could offer at least, free primary health care to the whole population and especially to the lower socioeconomic groups. In the beginning only a small percentage of the population was covered, but at present it has been extended to the whole country, excluding only those who can afford private medical care. The National Health Service has 35.000 Hospital beds and 1.480 Health Clinics and Health Centers throughout the country. The National Health Service employs 58.000 persons, including 4.400 physicians, 1.365 dentists, 2.090 registered nurses, 1.690 midwives, 768 social workers, 710 nutritionists and 24.600 nurses aides.

Since the beginning, a program of nutritional intervention was implemented through the National Health Service (González, N. et al., 1983). It includes free distribution of powdered milk (25% fat) to every child up to two years of age and weaning foods containing powdered milk (25%), cereals, vitamins and minerals. The program also includes powdered milk distribution to lactating and pregnant mothers. Each child from 0 to 5 months of age receives once a month, in the Health Center, tree kilograms of powdered milk (25% fat). Between 6 to 23 months old receive 2 kilograms of powdered milk (25% fat) and between 2 to 5 years of age receive weaning food, 1,5 kilograms. Pregnant mothers receive 2 kilograms of powdered milk and nursing mothers 3 kilograms of powdered milk once a month. At present the total amount of milk distributed through the Health System reaches 30 millions of powdered milk annually.

As we have said, the food is distributed through the primary Health Centers and this food distribution becomes a motivation for undertaking other health care activities. Milk distribution had been extremely important not only from the nutritional point of view but also as a mechanism to attract the mothers to the Health Centers. To achieve these goals, the products distributed and their packaging display have been of excellent quality. Special care has been taken to avoid the feeling that these programs are designed for poor people. The same products and services compete successfully in the open market.

When food distribution started, the amount of milk dispensed was limited but increased gradually as the National Health Service developed. It was interesting to observe a close relationship between the amount of milk distributed and the number of visits to Primary Health Care facilities. During some periods, milk distribution declined, in parallel the number of visits also declined and when this increased, the number of visits also increased. The linkage between attendance at Health Care Centers and milk distribution means that in the public mind both programs are interrelated and complementary (González, N. et al., 1983)

In short, an efficient Health Care infrastructure and rational nutritional programs have been two basic factors that explain the dramatic decline in malnutrition and infant and preschool mortality in Chile. The implementation of the Health System with its broad coverage has led not only to effective nutritional programs oriented at target groups but also to other interventions such as family planning, health control, immunizations, health and nutritional education and promotion of breast feeding. Then, during the thirty years that the Service has been in operation, coverage has not only been extended but it has been made more effective. At the same time, during this period health personnel has developed a special attitude of service and commitment to the community, gaining their respect. In turn, the population has become aware of their rights and responsibilities in relation to health care. Thus, for example, pre-natal examinations have increased considerably, 98 percent of births now take place in hospitals and an estimated 95% of all children are regularly given immunizations. Regular ckeck'ups of children have become a routine and provide

weight-for-age data for over 90 percent of the preschool children, who are evaluated every three months. In summary, it is a fact that at present, the community has developed a true "culture of health" and has awakened to the need to preserve it through the health service and this is of paramount importance.

MILK DISTRIBUTION VERSUS BREAST FEEDING

One of the main objections against free milk distribution in underdeveloped countries, is the negative effect that it might have upon breast feeding. This is true if milk distribution is not paralleled by an intensive program of breast feeding promotion. In Chile, the decline in breast feeding had started before the initiation of the milk distribution program, and this was the reason for a high prevalence of undernutrition during the first year of life. Studies done in those years, demonstrated that undernutrition already affected more than 40% of children under one year of age. This is why, at present, together with a free distribution of milk a very wide program of promotion of breast feeding in also developed, using both mass media (eg radio, television, magazines) and formal education. In particular a firm stand was taken on this issue in the professional medical community and in schools training professionals related to child health care such as midwives, nurses, health educators. Professionals and auxiliary personnel have received special instructions provided by the National Health Service. Printed materials illustrating the importance of breast feeding and how to promote it, have been prepared and distributed.

As a consequence of all this, at present more than 62% of mothers now breast feed their children during the first ninety days, and malnutrition during the first year of life affects only 4% of infants in the country (Ministerio de Salud, Chile, 1992).

COW MILK VERSUS HUMAN MILK

During the last years many modifications have been introduced to cow milk in order to have a product more similar to human milk. Nevertheless, all of them raise the price of the product, so it becomes unpractical to use it massively in programs in underdeveloped countries were costs are important limiting factors.

In our initial experience, we have used unmodified powdered milk, that the mother dilutes at two thirds, adding carbohydrates to increase caloric density. This same formula has been used for the treatment of children with severe undernutrition under one year old (Monckeberg, F. and Riumallo, J., 1983). The studies of nitrogen balance, as well as the clinical observation demonstrate that this formula is adequate including those children in whom tolerance could be diminished. To increase caloric density vegetable oil can be added.

So, it is possible to make modifications by decreasing the protein content of the formula and by replacing in part, animal fats by vegetable fats. This does not increase the price, and in our case, this modified formula well be used proximately in our National Program.

Another interesting aspect of a National Program of milk distribution and/or weaning foods is the possibility to use it as a vehicle to prevent specific deficiencies of some minerals, such as a iron, or other trace elements, such as fluoride, or vitamin deficiencies. All of these are being studied and it is probable that milk will be enriched with these elements in a near future, which evidently means an additional benefit for children under 6 years old.

MILK SUPPLEMENTARY FEEDING PROGRAM AND DAIRY INFRASTRUCTURE

Another very advantageous aspect observed in the milk Supplementation Program of the National Health Service, has been the development of and industrial infrastructure for the elaboration of milk and dairy products. Before this program was started, in Chile there were no industries that could elaborate milk or produce dairy products. In the first years the milk used was imported, while at present, almost all of it is produced locally. As the state created a very important purchasing power the private sector was encouraged to build milk industries in different regions of the country and now in Chile milk industry is one of the best in Latin America. As a consequence, milk production has increased in the number of cows as well as in efficiency. At present, this is very similar to that of developed countries and in our country there are 16 dairy processing plants. All this has led to an adequate availability of dairy products and a notable growth in the per capita milk consumption. In 1940 this only reached to forty liters per person per year, today it

is more than 120 liters per person per year (Ministerio de Agricultura, 1992).

REFERENCES

Brown L. 1992. The World Bank Development Report. State of the World 1992. New York: W.W. Nowton. 1992.

FAO, 1992. Anuario de Comercio. Roma

González, N., Infante, A., Schlesinger, C. and Monckeberg, F. 1983. Effectiveness of Supplementary Feeding Programs in Chile. In: Underwoord, B. ed. Nutrition Intervention Strategies in National Development. New York: Academic Press, 101.

Informe sobre de Desarrollo Humano 1992. 1993. Programa de las Naciones Unidas para el Desarrollo (PNUD). Washington.

Institute on Hunger and Development: Hunger 1992. 1992. Cohen M. y Hoehn R. editors. 802 Rhode Island Avenue, N.E., Washington D.C. 20018.

Ministerio de Agricultura. 1992. Boletín de Leche, Santiago, Chile.

Monckeberg, F. 1990. Integrating National Food, Nutrition and Health Policy. The Chilean Experience. In: Symposium: Advance in Nutrition. Washington, D.C.: Smithronian Institution.

Monckeberg, F. 1981. The possibilities for Nutrition Intervention in Latin America. Food Technology. September, 115.

Monckeberg, F. 1993. Urbanization, underdevelopment and the child. International Child Health, 3:1.

Monckeberg, F. 1975. Artificial Feeding in Infants: Hight Risk in Unederdevelopment countries. In: Gabor M. editor. At. Risk Factors and the Health and Nutrition of Young children. Cairo University, Cairo.

Monckeberg, F., and Riumallo, J. 1983. Nutrition Recovery Centers: The chilean experience. In: Underwood B. ed. Nutrition Intervention strategies in: National Development. New York: Academic Press, pag. 189

Schlesinger, L., Weinberger, J., Figueroa, G., Secure, M.T., Gongález, N. and Monckeberg, F. 1983. Environmental Sanitation. In: Underwood, R. ed. Nutrition Intervention Strategies in National Development. New York: Academic Press, 241.

The World Bank: Human Resources in Latin
America and the Caribbean. January 1993.
The World Bank. Washington D.C. 20577.
U.S.A.

3 Life styles, vital cycles and dairy products consumption

Dairy Products in Human Health and Nutrition, Serrano Ríos et al. (eds) © 1994 Balkema, Rotterdam, ISBN 90 5410 359 0

Dairy products and physical activity

P.W.R.Lemon
Kent State University, USA

ABSTRACT: For most of the twentieth century nutritionists have believed that exercise does not affect dietary protein requirements. However, this opinion is based primarily on data from studies which used individuals that were sedentary or only moderately active. In contrast, athletes (especially those involved in strength/power exercise) have routinely consumed diets containing 2-4 times the current recommended dietary allowance (RDA) for protein. During the past 20-25 years a great deal of new information has become available from studies utilizing subjects who were actively training. These data suggest that the RDA for protein may need to be as high as 1.7-2.0 g/kg body weight · d⁻¹ (212-250% of the current RDA) for strength athletes and 1.2-1.4 g/kg · d⁻¹ (150-175% of the current RDA) for endurance athletes. Some of these recent data indicate that muscle size gains with strength training may even be enhanced if protein intakes are about 175-200% of the current RDA. However, greater protein intakes do not produce larger gains. Despite these observations, physically active individuals need not take protein supplements because these quantities of protein can be obtained in a normal diet that contains sufficient high quality protein sources. Care must be taken to consume adequate total energy (dietary carbohydrate is very important because it is the major source of exercise fuel) to cover the high expenditures of training because insufficient energy intake will further elevate dietary protein requirements.

1 INTRODUCTION

For most of the twentieth century nutritionists have believed that physical activity does not significantly alter dietary protein requirements (Åstrand & Rodahl, 1977). In contrast, athletes (especially those involved in strength or power training) regularly consume diets that contain two-four times (Grandjean, 1988; Steen, 1991) the recommended dietary allowance for protein (US Food & Nutrition Board, 1989; Food & Agricultural Organization, 1985). The athletic opinion is based primarily on uncontrolled, trial and error self-experimentation and has undoubtedly been influenced by the deceptive testimonial approach often utilized by manufacturers to sell dietary protein supplements. The scientific opinion is based primarily on experiments completed 25-125 years ago (Cathcart, 1925; Lemon, 1991a). Although it is not yet possible to state a precise dietary protein requirement for active individuals, a great deal of new information has become available over the past 20-25 years as a result of the phenomenal growth of exercise science. Most of these data

indicate that regular exercise leads to an increased dietary requirement for protein. Therefore depending on an individual's current protein intake, dietary modifications may optimize performance capacity or even the health of individual athletes. If so, high quality protein foods, such as dairy products could play a significant role in the diets of active individuals. This paper reviews some of the scientific data which have led investigators to modify their view regarding the quantity of dietary protein necessary for active individuals.

2 METHODS TO ASSESS DIETARY PROTEIN REQUIREMENTS

Traditionally, dietary protein requirements have been assessed via nitrogen (protein contains 16% nitrogen) balance studies (assessments of dietary nitrogen intake minus total nitrogen excretion). Dietary requirements are determined as the quantity of a particular nutrient necessary to elicit balance (intake = excretion). The recommended dietary allowance (RDA) for a particular nutrient equals the requirement plus a safety margin (equal to two standard deviations) necessary to prevent a deficiency from occurring in 95% of the population (Food & Agricultural Organization, 1985). The vast majority of studies have utilized sedentary or only moderately active individuals and have estimated the RDA for protein to be 0.8 g/kg body weight · d^{-1} (Food & Agricultural Organization, 1985; US Food & Nutrition Board, 1989). For those involved in a regular, intense exercise program the RDA for protein is less clear and, in fact, considerable controversy currently exists (Butterfield, 1991; Lemon, 1991b). In addition, there are a number of factors which must be considered when the nitrogen balance technique is used, especially when assessing the requirements of exercising individuals. Specific examples which can invalidate experimental observations include: inadequate energy intake (whether the result of low intake or excessive expenditure) (Munro, 1951; Goranzon & Forsum, 1985), insufficient accommodation to experimental dietary changes (Scrimshaw et al, 1972), and difficulties in precisely quantifying all nitrogen intake and excretion (Oddoye & Margen, 1979). Finally, this technique is labor intensive, relatively expensive, and limited in that it does not assess how protein metabolism is regulated. More recently, metabolic (radio/stable labeled) tracers have been utilized extensively to assess protein needs. This technique allows one to investigate the various processes of metabolism, ie, amino acid oxidation, protein synthesis, etc (Young et al, 1989). As such, it provides important information which can be used with nitrogen balance data to more adequately assess dietary protein requirements.

3 EFFECTS OF CHRONIC ENDURANCE EXERCISE ON DIETARY PROTEIN NEEDS

Based on nitrogen balance methodology (Figure 1), it appears that a dietary protein intake of 1.0 g/kg · d^{-1} (125% RDA) is inadequate for previously sedentary individuals during the initial few days of an aerobic exercise program (Gontzea et al, 1974). This apparent increased protein need does not only exist during the initial stages of an endurance exercise training program because several studies have determined the protein requirement to be about 1.2-1.4 g/kg · d^{-1} for individuals who have been training for years (Tarnopolsky et al, 1988; Brouns et al, 1989; Friedman & Lemon, 1989; Meredith et al, 1989).

It is now known that the amino acid alanine is produced in muscle (Figure 2) in an exercise intensity-dependent manner (Felig & Wahren, 1971; Odessey et al, 1974). This observation is especially important relative to dietary protein needs for individuals engaged in regular endurance exercise because it suggests that amino acids from either muscle or liver (the two major sites of body protein) can provide exercise energy (via oxidation of the carbon skeletons of the branched chain amino acids which contribute their NH_2 group to pyruvate forming alanine). This suggestion has been directly confirmed in oxidation studies using acute endurance exercise (Figure 3) and either ingestion or injection of radio/stable labeled branched chain amino acids (White & Brooks, 1982; Lemon et al, 1982; 1985; Babij et al, 1983; Evans et al, 1983). The explanation for this increased amino acid oxidation is likely related to the exercise intensity-

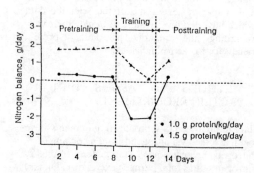

Figure 1. Effect of acute endurance exercise on nitrogen balance while consuming 125 vs 188% of the RDA for protein. (n=30/group). From Gontzea et al (1974).

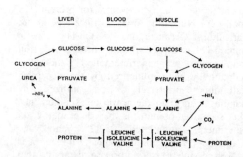

Figure 2. Metabolic pathway showing alanine and urea formation as well as branched chain amino acid oxidation. From Felig & Wahren (1971) and Odessey et al (1974).

142

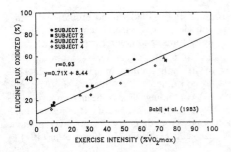

Figure 3. Effect of exercise intensity on oxidation of the amino acid leucine. From Babij et al (1983).

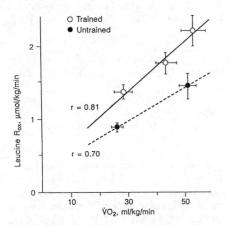

Figure 4. Effect of endurance training on oxidation of the amino acid leucine. (n=16-19/group). From Henderson et al (1985).

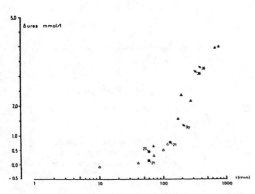

Figure 5. Effect of exercise duration at 60-70% VO₂max on serum urea concentration. Numbers indicate data from different studies. From Haralambie & Berg (1976).

Table 1. Leucine Oxidation During Endurance Exercise (2h at 55% VO₂max) in Humans (Evans et al, 1983).

Treatment	Rate (umol/kg · h⁻¹)	% of Daily Requirement
Rest	14.8±1.3	28±2
Exercise	46.1±9.7*	86±18*

values are means±SE; n=8 subjects/treatment
*significantly (P<0.05) greater than Rest

dependent activation of the limiting enzyme (branched chain ketoacid dehydrogenase) in the branched chain amino acid oxidation pathway (Kasperek & Snider, 1987). The magnitude of this oxidation can be substantial because a 2 h exercise bout (at 55% VO₂max) can represent as high as 86% (Table 1) of the current daily requirement for at least one of the branched chain amino acids (leucine) (Evans et al, 1983). Moreover, it appears that chronic endurance exercise (training) further increases (Figure 4) branched chain amino acid oxidation (Dohm et al, 1977; Henderson et al, 1985), although the underlying mechanism responsible is unclear (Hood & Terjung, 1987). Unless a dramatic reduction in oxidation occurs between exercise bouts, these data indicate that endurance exercise would increase daily leucine needs. This could contribute to an increased dietary protein need; however, the overall significance of exercise amino acid oxidation must await further study because the magnitude of the exercise-induced increased oxidation may vary among different amino acids (Wolfe et al, 1984).

Using data from several laboratories, Haralambie & Berg (1976) observed that the concentration of the major end product of amino acid oxidation (urea) in the blood increased exponentially after about 1 h of continuous exercise at 60-70% VO₂max (Figure 5). They suggested this meant that total amino acid oxidation must be substantial because reduced urea removal from the blood (by the kidney) could not account for the observed increases. Reduced glycogen (major fuel for exercise) availability is probably responsible for the increased amino acid oxidation during this type of prolonged exercise because glycogen stores are known to be significantly depleted after approximately 1 h at this intensity (Hermansen et al, 1967). Moreover, similar exercise when glycogen stores are initially low results in earlier

143

increases in blood urea, as well as dramatic increases in urea excretion via exercise sweat (Lemon & Mullin, 1980) and greater activation of the branched chain ketoacid dehydrogenase (Wagenmakers et al, 1991). Although indirect, these data suggest that total amino acid oxidation is substantial during prolonged exercise.

Several other types of evidence indicate that regular endurance exercise alters protein metabolism such that dietary protein need might be increased. These include: increased urinary excretion of 3-methylhistidine (an amino acid which is quantitatively excreted in the urine following contractile protein degradation) (Dohm et al, 1987), increased skeletal muscle urea content (Lemon & Dolny, 1986), increased muscle ammonia (end product of amino acid metabolism), total and essential amino acids (ones that cannot be produced in the body) without increases in branched chain amino acids (MacLean et al, 1991), and increased urinary urea excretion (Refsum & Stromme, 1974; Dohm et al, 1982, Tarnopolsky et al, 1990). Taken together, all of these data from a variety of experimental approaches suggest that dietary protein needs of individuals who regularly engage in endurance exercise are greater than their more sedentary counterparts. Based on the nitrogen balance data and using conventional linear regression techniques (Food & Agricultural Organization, 1985), it appears that the RDA for protein for individuals who regularly engage in endurance exercise should be about 1.2-1.4 g/kg · d⁻¹ (150-188% RDA) (Lemon, 1991b).

4 EFFECTS OF CHRONIC STRENGTH/ POWER EXERCISE ON DIETARY PROTEIN NEEDS

Theoretically, increased protein intake when combined with the anabolic stimulus of strength training could lead to increased muscle protein synthesis (and therefore bigger and stronger muscles). Unfortunately when attempting to document this effect, most investigators have used nitrogen balance methodology and many have not adequately controlled the various factors that can invalidate the results of these types of studies (see above). As a result, the dietary protein requirement of strength athletes is at least as controversial as those of endurance athletes (Lemon, 1991c). However, recent data from several laboratories provide some experimental support for the suggestion that supplemental dietary protein in combination with strength training may enhance muscle size/strength development.

Frontera et al (1988) found greater gains in thigh muscle area (from computer axial tomography scans) and greater urinary creatinine (an index of total muscle mass) following 12 weeks of strength training in untrained, elderly men who consumed a daily dietary supplement (2,345 kJ) containing 23 g protein compared to controls who did not. However, it is interesting to note that strength gains did not accompany these size gains (Table 2). Fern et al (1991)

Table 2. Effect of Protein Supplementation During 12 Weeks of Strength Training (Frontera et al, 1988).

Group	Thigh Muscle Area (cm²)	Urinary Creatinine (g/d)	1RM[a] (kg)
Control	+6.1±2.4	-0.05±0.07	+19.0±2.9
Supplement	+14.6±1.5*	+0.16±0.05*	+20.2±2.1

values are mean gains±SE; n=5 or 6/treatment
[a]1 repetition maximum strength
*significantly (P<0.02) greater than Control

observed a significantly greater gain in lean body mass (body weight gain =2.8±0.9 vs 1.5±0.6 kg) over four weeks of strength training when subjects (initial training status was not indicated) increased their protein intake from 1.3 to 3.3 g/kg · d⁻¹. Moreover, metabolic tracer data indicated that although the strength training increased protein synthesis on both protein intakes, the increase on the higher protein diet was about 5 fold greater. These data are fascinating because they suggest

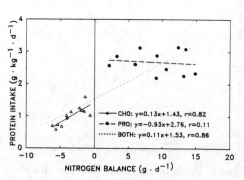

Figure 6. Protein requirements during strength training calculated from protein intake and nitrogen balance. (n=12/group). From Lemon et al (1992).

144

that an intake of protein approximately 4 times the RDA can enhance muscle size gains. However, no strength data were reported and the very large increase in amino acid oxidation (159%) observed in these subjects may indicate that the optimal protein intake was exceeded. Using nitrogen balance methodology (Figure 6), Lemon et al (1992) determined the protein requirement (intake necessary to elicit nitrogen balance) to be 1.5 g/kg · d⁻¹ and the recommended dietary protein allowance (requirement+2 SD) to be 1.7 g/kg · d⁻¹ for novice body builders during the first month of training. Surprisingly, the observed gains in strength (both voluntary and electrically evoked) and size (computer axial tomography scan, needle biopsy) were similar in subjects with a protein intake of 1.35 vs 2.62 g/kg · d⁻¹, despite a negative nitrogen balance on the lower protein intake. Although future work is necessary to fully understand why the strength/size gains were similar, it could be that short term negative nitrogen balance does not adversely affect muscle gains because it is possible to use endogenous nitrogen reserves to make up the deficit. How long this might continue it unclear, but it is likely that gains would be affected at some point. If so, a protein intake in excess of 1.35 g/kg · d⁻¹ should benefit body builders, at least during the first month of training. Combining nitrogen balance and metabolic tracer methodology in the same experiment, Tarnopolsky et al (1992) have shown that the optimal protein intake for individuals engaged in active strength training is between 1.4 and 2.4 g/kg · d⁻¹. Based on nitrogen balance, the RDA for protein was calculated (linear regression methodology) to be 1.76 g/kg · d⁻¹ for strength athletes and 0.89 g/kg · d⁻¹ for sedentary individuals. From the tracer data, they determined that increasing dietary protein intake from 0.86 to 1.4 g/kg · d⁻¹ with the strength athletes resulted in an increased rate of protein synthesis without an increase in amino acid oxidation. For the sedentary individuals, the same dietary protein increase did not increase protein synthesis. These data indicate a beneficial effect of the additional dietary protein for the strength athletes. In addition, when protein intake was increased from 1.4 to 2.4 g/kg · d⁻¹ in the strength athletes no further increase in protein synthesis occurred but an increased amino acid oxidation was observed. These data indicate a condition of protein overload. Taken together, these recent studies with strength exercise suggest that it is possible to enhance muscle size gains if strength training is combined with a dietary protein intake around 1.7-2.0 g/kg

· d⁻¹ (212-250% RDA). For more experienced strength athletes (who have already realized most of their potential), a lower protein intake of about 1.2 g/kg · d⁻¹ may be adequate (Tarnopolsky et al, 1988). The difference is probably explained by the fact that the greatest increases in muscle mass/strength occur early in a strength program. Later, less protein is needed to maintain the mass that has been accumulated. Although strength gains with supplemental dietary protein are less apparent in these studies, these gains are usually proportional to size increases (but are difficult to demonstrate consistently due to other confounding factors, ie, motivation, etc) and, therefore, it is likely they will be documented as future studies over longer time periods are completed.

5 POSSIBLE ADVERSE EFFECTS OF HIGH PROTEIN INTAKE

Although it is commonly believed that excessive protein intakes are hazardous, most of the information available has been extrapolated from studies on patients with compromised kidney function (Brenner et al, 1982). There is no published evidence that the high protein intakes that strength athletes routinely consume lead to kidney disease. Further, studies with rodents fed massive protein intakes (80% of energy intake) for more than 50% of their life span produced minimal problems (Zaragoza et al, 1987). Apparently, the health concern regarding high protein intakes has been overstated, at least in individuals with normal kidney function. At present, there is certainly no reason to believe that protein intakes in the range of those recommended (1.2-2.0 g/kg · d⁻¹) would cause any health concerns.

6 SUMMARY AND CONCLUSIONS

Dietary protein requirements for active individuals have been debated for many years. Current dietary recommendations are based on experiments utilizing subjects who were either sedentary or, at best, moderately active. Recent studies employing nitrogen balance and metabolic tracer methodology indicate that active individuals have higher dietary protein requirements than their sedentary counterparts. Based on the most recent information, it appears that the recommended protein intake for individuals engaged in regular endurance exercise should be about 1.2-1.4 g/kg · d⁻¹ and for strength exercise about 1.2 (experienced strength athletes)-1.7 or 2.0 g/kg · d^{-1} (novice strength athletes). Despite these observations, it is not necessary to consume large quantities of protein supplements to attain these dietary protein intakes. Rather, one should evaluate her/his existing diet to be certain it contains sufficient protein and energy (carbohydrate intake is critical here because protein needs are elevated if energy intake is inadequate) to obtain the desired effect (increased strength/size for strength athletes and maintenance of muscle mass in endurance athletes). If the diet is inadequate, additional protein can be obtained via high quality protein foods (dairy products, meats, vegetables, nuts) and additional carbohydrate from high or moderate glycemic index foods (bread, pasta, cereal, potatoes, chocolate, honey, some fruits, sport drinks).

ACKNOWLEDGEMENTS

The work cited from the author's laboratory has been supported by Weider Health & Fitness, National Institutes of Health, Ross Laboratories, and Kent State University's Office for Graduate Studies & Research.

REFERENCES

Åstrand, P-O. & K. Rodahl 1977. *Textbook of work physiology.* New York:McGraw-Hill.

Babij, P., S.M. Matthews & M.F. Rennie 1983. Changes in blood ammonia, lactate and amino acids in relation to workload during bicycle ergometer exercise in man. *Eur. J. Appl. Physiol.* 50:405-411.

Brenner, B.M., T.W. Meyer & T.H. Hostetter 1982. Protein intake and the progressive nature of kidney disease: the role of hemodynamically mediated glomerular sclerosis in aging, renal ablation, and intrinsic renal disease. *N. Eng. J. Med.* 307:652-657.

Brouns, F., W.H.M. Saris, E. Beckers, H. Adlercreutz, G.J. van der Vusse, H.A. Keizer, H. Kuipers, P. Menheere, A.J. Wangenmakers & F. ten Hoor 1989. Metabolic changes induced by sustained exhaustive cycling and diet manipulation. *Int. J. Sports Med.* 10, Suppl. 1:S49-S62.

Butterfield, G.E. 1991. Amino acids and high protein diets. In: *Perspectives in exercise science and sports medicine, Vol 4, Ergogenics-The enhancement of exercise and sport performance* (edited by M. Williams & D. Lamb). Indianapolis:Benchmark Press.

Cathcart, E.P. 1925. Influence of muscle work on protein metabolism. *Physiol. Rev.* 5:225-243.

Dohm, G.L., A.L. Hecker, W.E. Brown, G.J. Klain, F.R. Puente, E.W. Askew & G.R. Beecher 1977. Adaptation of protein metabolism to endurance training. *Biochem. J.* 164:705-708.

Dohm, G.L., R.T. Williams, G.J. Kasperek, & A.M. van Rij 1982. Increased excretion of urea and N$^\tau$-methylhistidine by rats and humans after a bout of exercise. *J. Appl. Physiol.* 52:27-33.

Dohm, G.L., E.B. Tapscott & G.J. Kasperek 1987. Protein degradation during endurance exercise and recovery. *Med. Sci. Sports Exercise* 19(5,suppl):S166-S171.

Evans, W.J., E.C. Fisher, R.A. Hoerr & V.R. Young 1983. Protein metabolism and endurance exercise. *Phys. Sportsmed.* 11:63-72.

Felig, P. & J. Wahren 1971. Amino acid metabolism in exercising man. *J. Clin. Invest.* 50:2703-2714.

Fern, E.B., R.N. Bielinski & Y. Schutz 1991. Effects of exaggerated amino acid and protein supply in man. *Experientia* 47:168-172.

Food & Agricultural Organization 1985. World Health Organization, United Nations University. *Energy and protein requirements.* Geneva:World Health Organization Technical Report Series 724.

Friedman, J.E. & P.W.R. Lemon 1989. Effect of chronic endurance exercise on the retention of dietary protein. *Int. J. Spt. Med.* 10:118-123.

Frontera, W.R., C.N. Meredith & W.J. Evans 1988. Dietary effects on muscle strength gain and hypertrophy during heavy resistance training in older men. *Can. J. Spt. Sci.* 13(2):13P.

Gontzea, I., P. Sutzescu & S. Dumitrache 1974. The influence of muscular activity on the nitrogen balance and on the need of man for proteins. *Nutr. Rep. Int.* 10:35-43.

Goranzon, H. & E. Forsum 1985. Effect of reduced energy intake versus increased physical activity on the outcome of nitrogen balance experiments in man. *Am. J. Clin. Nutr.* 41:919-928.

Grandjean, A.C. 1988. Current nutritional beliefs and practices in athletes for weight/strength gains. In: *Muscle development: Nutritional alternatives to anabolic steroids* (edited by W.E. Garrett, Jr. & T.R. Malone). Columbus:Ross Laboratories.

Haralambie, G. & A. Berg 1976. Serum urea and amino nitrogen changes with exercise duration. *Eur. J. Appl. Physiol.* 36:39-48.

Henderson, S.A., A.L. Black & G.A. Brooks 1985. Leucine turnover in trained rats during exercise. *Am. J. Physiol.* 249:E137-E144.

Hermansen, L., E. Hultman & B. Saltin 1967. Muscle glycogen during prolonged severe exercise. *Acta Physiol. Scand.* 71:129-139.

Hood, D.A. & R.L. Terjung 1987. Effect of endurance training on leucine in perfused rat skeletal muscle. *Am. J. Physiol.* 253:E648-E656.

Kasperek, G.J. & R.D. Snider 1987. Effect of exercise intensity and starvation on the activation of branched-chain keto acid dehydrogenase by exercise. *Am. J. Physiol.* 252:E33-E37.

Lemon, P.W.R. & J.P. Mullin 1980. Effect of initial muscle glycogen levels on protein catabolism during exercise. *J. Appl. Physiol.* 48:624-629.

Lemon, P.W.R., F.J. Nagle, J.P. Mullin & N.J. Benevenga 1982. In vivo leucine oxidation at rest and during two intensities of exercise. *J. Appl. Physiol.* 53:947-954.

Lemon, P.W.R., N.J. Benevenga, J.P. Mullin & F.J. Nagle 1985. Effect of daily exercise and food intake on leucine oxidation. *Biochem. Med.* 33:67-76.

Lemon, P.W.R. & D.G. Dolny 1986. Role of individual body tissues in urea production. *Can. J. Appl. Spt. Sci.* 11(3):26P.

Lemon, P.W.R. 1991a. Does exercise alter dietary protein requirements? In: *Advances in nutrition and top sport* (edited by F. Brouns). Med Sport Sci., Vol 32. Basel:Karger.

Lemon, P.W.R. 1991b. Effect of exercise on protein requirements. *J. Spt. Sci.* 9:53-70.

Lemon, P.W.R. 1991c. Protein and amino acid needs of the strength athlete. *Int. J. Spt. Nutr.* 1:127-145.

Lemon, P.W.R., M.A. Tarnopolsky, J.D. MacDougall & S.A. Atkinson 1992. Protein requirements and muscle mass/strength changes during intensive training in novice bodybuilders. *J. Appl. Physiol.* 73:767-775.

MacLean, D.A., L.L. Spriet, E. Hultman & T.E. Graham 1991. Plasma and muscle amino acids and ammonia responses during prolonged exercise in humans. *J. Appl. Physiol.* 70:2095-2103.

Meredith, C.N., M.J. Zackin, W.R. Frontera & W.J. Evans 1989. Dietary protein requirements and protein metabolism in endurance-trained men. *J. Appl. Physiol.* 66:2850-2856.

Munro, H.N. 1951. Carbohydrate and fat as factors in protein utilization and metabolism. *Physiol. Rev.* 31:449-488.

Oddoye, E.B. & S. Margen 1979. Nitrogen balance studies in humans: long-term effect of high nitrogen intake on nitrogen accretion. *J. Nutr.* 109:363-377.

Odessey, R., E.A. Khairallah & A.L. Goldberg 1974. Origin and possible significance of alanine production by skeletal muscle. *J. Biol. Chem.* 249:7623-7629.

Refsum, H.E. & S.B. Stromme 1974. Urea and creatinine production and excretion in urine during and following prolonged heavy exercise. *Scand. J. Clin. Lab. Invest.* 33:247-254.

Scrimshaw, N.S., M.A. Hussein, E. Murray, W. M. Rand & V.R. Young 1972. Protein requirements of man: Variations in obligatory and fecal nitrogen losses in young men. *J. Nutr.* 102:1595-1604.

Steen, S.N. 1991. Precontest strategies of a male bodybuilder. *Int. J. Spt. Nutr.* 1:69-78.

Tarnopolosky, L.J., J.D. MacDougall, S.A. Atkinson, M.A. Tarnopolsky & J.R. Sutton 1990. Gender differences in substrate for endurance exercise. *J. Appl. Physiol.* 68:302-308.

Tarnopolsky, M.A., J.D. MacDougall & S.A. Atkinson 1988. Influence of protein intake and training status on nitrogen balance and lean body mass. *J. Appl. Physiol.* 64:187-193.

Tarnopolsky, M.A., S.A. Atkinson, J.D. MacDougall, A. Chesley, S. Phillips & H.P. Schwarcz 1992. Evaluation of protein requirements for trained strength athletes. *J. Appl. Physiol.* 73:1986-1995.

US Food & Nutrition Board 1989. *Recommended dietary allowances*, Vol 10. Washington:National Academy Press.

Wangenmakers, A.J.M., E.J. Beckers, F. Brouns, H. Kuipers, P.B. Soeters, G.J. van der Vusse & W.H.M. Saris 1991. Carbohydrate supplementation, glycogen depletion, and amino acid metabolism during exercise. *Am. J. Physiol.* 260:E883-E890.

White, T.P. & G.A. Brooks 1981. [U-^{14}C] glucose, -alanine, -leucine oxidation in rats at rest and during two intensities of running. *Am. J. Physiol.* 240:E155-E165.

Wolfe, R.R., M.H. wolfe, E.R. Nadel & J.H.F. Shaw 1984. Isotopic determination of amino acid-urea interactions in exercise in humans. *J. Appl Physiol.* 56:221-229.

Young, V.R., D.M. Bier & P.L. Pellet 1989. A theoretical basis for increasing current estimates of the amino acid requirements in adult man with experimental support. *Am. J. Clin. Nutr.* 50:80-92.

Zaragoza, R., J. Renau-Piqueras, M. Portoles, J. Hernandez-Yago, A. Jorda & S. Grisolia 1987. Rats fed prolonged high protein diets show an increase in nitrogen metabolism and liver megamitochondria. *Arch. Biochem. Biophys.* 258:426-435.

Dairy Products in Human Health and Nutrition, Serrano Ríos et al. (eds) © 1994 Balkema, Rotterdam, ISBN 90 5410 359 0

Recent aspects of nutrition with milk and dairy products

C.A. Barth

Institut für Ernährungsforschung, Bergholz-Rehbrücke, Germany

Cow's milk contains the three macronutrients, which are of essential importance to energy metabolism of human beings: protein, carbohydrates and fat. Figure 4.1.-1 shows the energy-content proportion of these three main nutrients.

Further, cow's milk contains a great variety of essential nutrients, which human metabolism has to be provided with by food in order to keep the organism healthy. These essential nutrive substances are: essential amino-acids, minerals, trace elements and vitamins. Figures 4.1.-2 to 4.1.-4. show, that milk in fact contains 22 - i.e. nearly half of the about 40 to 50 - nutrients, which are essential for human metabolism. These 22 nutrive substances sufficiently exceed the R. D. A. In other words: if one would live on milk exclusively, the metabolic demand for 22 out of 40 to 50 essential nutrients would already be met. Although no reasonable nutritionist or physician would advise such a diet, this theoretical experiment demonstrates emphatically that - apart from macronutrients - a great variety of essential nutrive substances are being provided to metabolism by cow's milk.

Beyond these facts that are well-known among nutrition experts and physicians, the following article discusses some important modern aspects of nutrition with milk and dairy products.

4.1.1. Milk Protein

The above mentioned facts about the nutrient density of essential amino-acids have already explained that milk protein is highly suitable to cover the organism's demand for nutrients of children and adults. In fact, several comparisons have shown that milk's protein content with essential amino-acids even exeeds demand. PORTER, for instance, proved this on the basis of former FAO/WHO-

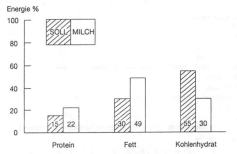

figure 4.1-1 energy portion of macro nutrients in cow's milk (3.5 per cent fat): Soll: recommended; Milch: milk.
Source: Recommandations of the Deutsche Gesellschaft für Ernährung (German Society of Nutrition)

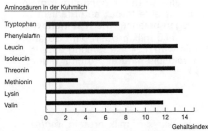

figure 4.1-2 nutrient density of essential amino-acids in cow's milk.
formula to calculate the content index:
content of nutrients / R. D. A. of nutrients
----
energy content / R. D. A. of energy

recommandations about the demand for amino-acids (figure 4.1.1.-1.). These conclusions (see figure 4.1.1.-2.) have been approved by the newly calculated FAO/WHO values of demand. The human nutrition experiments concerning the

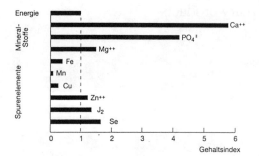

figure 4.1-3 nutrient density of minerals and trace elements in cow's milk

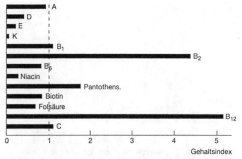

figure 4.1-4 nutrient density of vitamins in cow's milk

evaluation of milk proteins have proved that milk proteins excellently meet the adult's protein demand. Calculating the biological value from the minimum protein dose, which is able to put an organism into a nitrogen balance, the result shows that unskimmed milk protein with 88 and lactalbumin with 124 are ranking among the most valuable natural proteins (figure 4.1.1.-3.)

4.1.1-1

amino-acid values of milk protein (mg/g) and protein values recommended according to proposals by FAO/WHO (2)

	proteins of unskimmed milk	casein	proteins of whey	values recommended by FAO/WHO
isoleucine	61	61	62	40
leucine	100	92	123	70
lysine	83	82	91	55
methionine	27	28	23	35
cystine	09	03	34	35
phenylalamine	49	50	44	60
tyrosine	58	63	30	60
threonine	49	49	52	40
tryptophan	17	17	22	10
valine	69	72	57	50

4.1.1-2

comparison of recommended amino-acid composition of food protein with the composition of protein of eggs, milk and meat

	recommended demand	egg	composition cow's milk	beef
		mg/g protein		
histidine	19	22	27	34
isoleucine	28	54	47	48
leucine	66	86	95	81
lysine	58	70	78	89
methionine + cysteine	25	57	33	40
phenylalamine + tyrosine	63	93	102	80
threonine	34	47	44	46
tryptophane	11	17	14	12
valin	35	66	64	50

figure 4.1.1-3
minimum supply of milk protein to achieve N-balance

	g/kg/day	biological value[a]
unskimmed milk	0,57	88
lactalbumin	0,48	124
casein	0,70	72

[a] according to Jekat and Kofrany (3)

Surely, there is a close connection to the fact, that metabolism can use very effectively milk protein - either being isolated or being a component of milk or dairy products. The reason is that milk protein, on the one side, is not being accompanied by substances that impair absorption, e.g. substances as tannins, trypsin inhibitors or lectins and, on the other side, it does not cause a loss of amino-acids by increased secretion of endogenous proteins (enzymes of pancreas or shedding of intestinal epithelium) (figure 4.1.1.-4).

	casein-diet
N-resorption (percentage of supply)	99,4 + 0,52
endogenous N-secretion (g Protein/24 h)	8,9 + 0,46
(% der Zufuhr)	14

figure 4.1.1.-4 absorption and endogenous secretions during the digestion of casein; Homarginine-technique; Steady state; adult minipig(4)

The bioactive peptides in casein - so-called casomorphines -, described by BRANDL and his collaborators for the first time in 1979, may exercise an influence on the function of the gastro-intestinal tract and possibly on the digestive process, too (5). In the meantime, effects on the whole animal after intake of ß-casomorphins have been described. Scientists were able to find out, that the speed was reduced at which the contents of stomach and intestines pass the body under the influence of ß-casomorphine (6). If there will be a possibility in the future to exploit this effect - described for experimental animals - for the therapy of diarrhia can not be stated yet.

In connection with the phosphorylated sequences of casein - so-called phosphopeptides - high expections had come up. Some of the results from chemical experiments indicated that the phosphopeptides set free in the gastrointestinal tract may be conducive to the intestinal absorption of essential nutrients such as calcium and zinc. So far, no laboratory was able to support these theoretical expectations by experiments (7).

What a valuable supplement milk and milk protein is to the nutrition of adolescent organism is going to be discussed in the following highlights. Tropical physicians again and again reported that foodstuffs available in these countries are relatively poor in nutrients and protein. Especially the huge volume of such a diet based on starch-containing foodstuffs often is filling without meeting the demand for essential amino-acids and nutrients in the way it has become usual in the developed industrialized countries of the northern hemisphere. The following comparison between a typical African and an European diet of a small child should illustrate this. Comparing the weight of a child's ration for one day in Uganda with that in England it becomes obvious that the weight of solid food in Uganda is for times the weight of solid food in Europe. Another problem is the typical higher viscosity of food in tropical countries (e.g. porridge made of foodstuffs, which are rich of starch) (8).

The importance of milk for the nutrition of an infant becomes obvious out of conclusions reached by the American nutritionist Vernon Young, too. Figure 4.1.-5 demonstrates how much the nutritional status of an infant is improving by supplementing her/his pure-vegetable tropical nutrition with 200 ml of milk. It becomes really obvious that, in case of such a supplementation, more than 40 per cent of protein, more than 50 per cent of limiting lysine, more than 30 per cent of calcium and nearly the entire vitamin B 12 are covered by the supplement. There is no better way of showing milk's considerable importance to a child's

nutrition than by such a theoretical experiment. In this connection, it is important to note that lysine, which is limiting in nearly all vegetable food, is being plenty provided by milk protein, and this applies also to calcium and vitamin B 12 - two nutrients of considerable importance to the growth of children. All these thoughts underline the paediatricians'demands for supplying children sufficiently with milk.

Alter der Kinder	kcal	Prozentuale Bedarfsdeckung durch 200 ml Milch			
		protein	lysin	calcium	vitamin B12
6-11,9 months	14	46	59	44	< 100
1-2 years	10	46	66	30	100
2-4 years	9	41	58	30	70
4-6 years	8	37	53	30	70

figure 4.1.1-5 children's demand for protein and other nutrients und the covering of this demand by 200 ml of milk a day (9)

In this connection, one should mention that the less a consumer eats meat the more milk is ging to be the only source of vitamin B 12. For lacto-ovo-vegetarians milk is the only source of vitamin B 12 - a vitamin that is essential for the undisturbed formation of haemoglobin and the formation of red blood cells in general.

The essential amino-acid lysine, which milk protein contains in large quantities, is the reason for the fact that milk and grain - two basic elements of our nutrition - are ideal supplements for an optimum supply with nutrients. On the one hand, lysine, which is a limiting amino acid of cereal protein, is supplemented by milk protein. And on the other hand, a meal mixed of grain and milk guarantees a sufficient supply with carbohydrates because grain is very rich of starch.

There are quite a lot of reports on the different effects of vegetable and animal protein on human fat metabolism. There are unanimous reports that rabbits provided with a semi-synthetic casein-rich diet respond in case of change from casein to soya protein by a low cholesterol level in the blood. This finding strongly worried nutritionists and physicians because the question arose: Should consumers be recommended to do without animal protein and eat more vegetable protein?

A lot of laboratories have been working at this problem and the situation could be clarified:
· A recently published finding by Beynen

and West could classify the former findings about rabbits. Beynen and West reported that - under the condition of a moderate low supply with cholesterol, which is appropriate for this species, - there are no more different effects of casein vs. isolated soy protein if both diets contain exactly the same quantity of cholesterol, whole fat and unsaturated fatty acids (10).
· All attempts to demonstrate the different effects of milk protein and soya protein by **controlled** nutrition experiments with healthy test persons failed. Now and then, a serum cholesterol-reducing effect of vegetable protein was described but only in those experiments where a strictly controlled food intake could not been guaranteed (11).

Thus, there is no reason for advising consumers a reduced consumption of animal protein because of its pretended hypercholesterolemic effect.

Sources and references

(1) FAO/WHO 1990: Protein Quality Evaluation. Report of a Joint FAO/WHO Expert Consultation held in Bethesda, Md., U.S.A., 4-8 December 1989. Food and Agricultural Organization of the United Nations. Rome, 1990

(2) PORTER, J.W.G., 1980 The Role of Milk and Milk Constituents in the Human Diet. In: Factors affecting the yields and contents of milk constituents. Int. Dairy Fed. Document 125, p. 14 ff.

(3) JEKAT, F., KOFRANYI, E., 1970. Zur Bestimmung der biologischen Wertigkeit von Nahrungsprotein, XV Milch und Milchprodukte, Hoppe-Seyler`s Zschr. Physiol. Chem. 351: 47-51

(4) HAGEMEISTER, H., ERBERSDOLBER, H., 1985. Chemical labelling of dietary protein by transformation of lysine to homoargienine: a new technique to follow intestinal digestion and absorption. Proc. Nutr. Soc. 44: 133 A

(5) BRANDL, V., TESCHEMACHER, H., HENSCHEN, Agnes und LOTSPEICH, F., 1979. Novel opiod peptides derived drom casein (ß-casomorphins) I. Isolation from bovine casein peptone. Hoppe-Seylers Zeitschrift Physiologische Chemie 360: 1211-1216

(6) DANIEL, H., HAHN; A.,1990: ß-Casomorphine - opioidaktive Peptide aus der Milch, Ernährungsumschau 37, 3: 95 -101

(7) SCHOLZ-AHRENS, Katharina E., KOPRA, Nina, BARTH, C.A. 1990. Effect of casein phosphopeptides on utilization of calcium in minipigs and vitamin-D-deficient rats. Z. Ernährungswiss. 29: 295-298

(8) WHITEHEAD, R. G.: The protein need of malnourished children in: Proteins and Human Nutrition (Porter, J.W.G. und Rolls, B.A. Hrsg.) Academic press, London 1973, p. 103 ff

(9) YOUNG, V.R., PELLET, P.L. 1988. How to evaluate dietary protein. In: Milk Prteins. Hrsg. Barth, D.A., Schlimme, E., Steinkopff-Verlag, Darmstadt, 7-36

(10) LOVATI, Maria, WEST, C., SIRTONI, C.R., BREYNEN, A.C., 1990, Dietary animal proteins and cholesterol metabolism in rabbits, Brit. J. Nutr. 64: 473-485

(11) Barth, C.A., PFEUFFER, Maria, 1988, Dietary protein and atherogenesis. Klin. Wochenschr. 66: 135-1430

4.1.2 Milk fat

Nearly all recommendations for nutrition in western countries advise to reduce the consumption of fat from about 40 per cent energy at present to 30 or 25 per cent energy in future. The demand for this essential change in nutrition results from recent findings on human metabolism. Namely fat is the only macronutrient which is not removed from metabolism by oxidation when ingested to excess but deposited in fat depots. Undoubtedly a too high total energy intake in the form of dietary fat is the main risk factor as to overweight. Special importance is therefore attributed to fat ingestion causing overweight widespread among the elderly population in western industrialized countries (1).

For this reason, preventing overweight among the population has to be given priority under the aspect of medical prevention. It has to do with the overweight paving the ground for other metabolic imbalances which, on their part, increase the risk of chronic degenerative diseases. Metabolic imbalances of this kind are the increase of blood fats (hypertriglyceridemia, hypercholesterolemia), high blood pressure (essential hypertension), maturity-onset diabetes (type-II diabetes) and hyperuricemia (high risk of gout). What is important about these metabolic imbalances is the fact that they increase the risk of being affected by atherosclerotic blood-vessel changes. In other words: through these metabolic imbalances overweight increases the risk of cardiovascular disease and ischemic heart disease among the population generally. These diseases account for the main cause of death in the Federal Republic of Germany.

In addition, in the last few years findings were obtained on the effect different fats have on the blood fat levels, particularly on serum cholesterol. The latter one is an important risk factor for the occurence of cardiovascular diseases - as numerous epidemiologic studies have shown (2). Of prime importance here is the serum cholesterol fraction being transported in low-density lipoproteins. Not all the saturated fatty acids increase this metabolic parameter, only those with a chain length of carbon atoms of C12 to C16 do. Stearic acid (C18 : O) has proven not to be hypercholesterolemic. Trans-fatty acids increase LDL cholesterol in blood plasma and reduce HDL cholesterol fractions. Oleic acid, a monounsaturated fatty acid, reduces LDL cholesterol and increases HDL cholesterol; a finding that could explain why in Mediterranean populations there is a lower incidence of myocardial infarction than in Northern Europeans. The question whether polyunsaturated fatty acids of the n-6 type are possibly less protective than those of the n-3 type is intensely discussed at the moment and has not been answered yet (3).

As a conclusion it can be stated that priority should be given to a reduced ingestion of all fats when it comes to advising the general population. The underlying cause for this advice is to prevent the widespread overweight which - as mentioned above in detail - paves the ground for other risk factors of cardiovascular diseases.

Sources and references

(1) BARTH, C.A. 1991. Animal products and human health: consequences for agriculture and some new approaches. VI. Internt. Symp. Protein Metabol. and Nutr. Herning, Denmark 9.-14.6.1991, p. 7-22

(2) KANNEL, W.B., CASTELLI, W.P., GORDON, T., 1979. Cholesterol in the prediction of atheroscle-rotic disease. New perspectives bases on the Framingham study. Ann. Intern. Med. 90: 85-91

(3) LEAF, A., WEBER, P.C., 1988. Medical progress. Cardiovascular effects of n-3-fatty acids. New   Engl. J. Med. 318/9: 549-557

4.1.3 Milk sugar

Due to an intestinal ß-galactosidase (lactase) deficiency the cleavage and subsequent absorption of lactose occurs in many - particularly non-European - adults in such a slow way that after ingesting milk larger quantities of indigested lactose get into the colon. It serves the bacterial flora as a fermentable substrate there. Consequences of this process may be gastrointestinal complaints like belching, flatulence, winds, nausea, belly-aches, lower abdominal spasms and diarrhoea. Diminished lactose digestion is generally referred to as lactose malabsorption; the above mentioned symptoms are referred to as lactose intolerance.

From the international point of view lactose malabsorption is rather the rule. More than 70% of the adult world population belong to the lactose malabsorbers (1). Whereas among Northern and Central Europeans and their descendants in North America less than 15% are affected by lactose malabsorption, this value amounts to 40% in Mediterranean countries and to almost 100% among the African black population and in the Far East.

Lactose intolerant adults, however, are generally better capable of tolerating fermented milk products than milk. Interestingly enough, in countries with a widespread lactose intolerance milk is primarily consumed in form of fermented products.

KOLARS and co-workers (2) could show that the biochemical signs of lactose malabsorption, namely an increased exhalation of hydrogen bacterially generated in the colon, were reduced after lactose ingestion in form of yoghurt. The authors could also show that this effect was caused by the catalytic activity of bacterial ß-galactosidase (lactase) in yoghurt. So, in a simple way, it can be concluded that lactase in fermented products substituted the enzyme missing in the intestinal wall.

In the mean time this finding could be repeatedly confirmed (3,4). The supporting effect of microbial lactase on lactase cleavage and resorption could also be directly proven in animal experimentation through the measurement of increased postprandial plasma galactose levels after ingestion of native Kefir in comparison to heated Kefir (5).

The fermented milk product itself has got two more functions. Due to the good buffer effect of milk protein the acid pH-value per definition found in the stomach is buffered to such a degree that microbial ß-galactosidase passes through the stomach without irreversible activity loss. In addition, in comparison to milk ingestion the gastro-intestinal passage of lactose is slowed down after yoghurt ingestion, favouring milk sugar cleavage and absorption even at low lactase activity (5).

Sources and references

(1) GILAT, T. 1979. Lactase deficiency: the world pattern today. Israel J. Med. Sciences 5: 369-373

(2) KOLARS, J.C., LEVITT, M.D., AOUJI, M., SAVAIANO, D.A. 1974. Yogurt - an autodigesting source of lactose. New England J. Med. 310: 1-3

(3) SAVAIANO, D.A., ABOUELANOUAR, A., SMITH, D.E., LEVITT, M.D. 1984. Lactose malabsorption from yogurt, pasteurized yogurt, sweet acidophilus milk, an cultured milk in lactase-deficient individuals. Am. J. Clin. Nutr. 40: 1219-1223

(4) DEWIT, O., POCHART, P., DESJEUX, J.T. 1988. Breath hydrogen concentration and plasma glucose , insulin and free fatty acid levels after lactose, milk, fresh or heated yoghurt ingestion by healthy young adults with or without lactose malabsorption. Nutrition 4: 131-135

(5) de VRESE, M., FLOURIE, B., POCHART, P., CHAASTANG, C. et al. 1990. Effect of heated and native Kefir an lactose absorption in pigs. Br. J. Nutr. 67: 67-75

(6) MARTEAU, P., FLOURIE, B., POCHART, P., CHAASTANG, C. et al. 1990. Effect of microbial lactase activity in yoghurt on the intestinal absorption of lactose: an in vivo study in lactase-deficient humans. Br. J. Nutr. 64: 71-79

4.1.4 Milk calcium

Table 4.1.4 -1 represents the calcium intake recommended by the German Society of Nutrition on the basis of its conclusions 1985 and 1991. As published at the consensus conferences, American nutritionists recommended an even higher intake for women after menopause.

Table 41.4-1 Recommended calcium intake

age	calcium recommended intake mg/day	
	1)	2)
sucklings		
0 to under 4 months	500	500
4 to under 12 months	500	500
children		
2 to under 4 years	600	600
4 to under 7 years	700	700
7 to under 10 years	800	800
10 to under 13 years	1000	900
13 to under 15 years	1000	1000
adolescents and adults		
15 to under 19 years	800-1000	1200
19 to under 25 years	800	1000
25 to under 51 years	800	900
51 to under 65 years	800	800
65 years and more	800	800
pregnants	1200	1200
breast feeders	1200	1300[a]

a   in compensation of losses during pregnancy
1)   German Society of Nutrition "Recommendations for nutrient intake", Umschau Ffm 1985

2)   German Society of Nutrition "Recommendations for nutrient intake", Umschau Ffm 1991

The Dutch nutritionist SCHAAFSMA has made a model calculation where he compared the intake of those nutrients which are important for the health of the bone assuming that no milk products would be contained in Dutch nutrition (table 4.1.4-2). The importance of milk and milk products for the calcium intake is resulting therefrom.

These figures indicate that the calcium demand of more than 800 mg/day could not be met, if milk and milk products were not consumed. In addition it follows that the ratio of calcium to phosphorus is nearly and the ratio of calcium to protein is entirely tripled, when Dutch nutrition comprises the consumption of milk products. This proves to be important because a highest possible ratio of calcium to phosphorus and of calcium to protein in food is a target worth aiming at in order to give stability to the bone skeleton. Moreover, considering that lactose promotes the calcium resorption in the small bowel, a high quotient of lactose to calcium in milk product consumption has to be rated favourably, too.

An analysis of the consumption behaviour among the German population in the mid 80ies resulted in the conclusion that the recommendations given for nutrition are by no means followed by all sections of the population - as far as calcium intake is concerned. In adolescents particularly, the mean calcium intake does not at all reach the set standards. This is also the reason for the unanimous recommendation given by nutritionists and physicians in advocacy of a higher milk consumption among the population.

Table 4.1.4.-2 Model calculation

	model calculation with milk products	without milk products
Ca (g)	0,94	0,23
P (g)1.63	1,63	1,12
protein (g)	88	67
Ca/P	0,58	0,21
Ca/protein	10,7	3,2
lactose/Ca	24,5	0

Consumption data NL (1975)

Source: according to Schaafsma 1983

Consequently, the Ernährungsbericht of 1984 called upon "adults to drink 400 ml of milk, that are 3 cups of milk per day" (1).

The underlying cause is a life-long, regular calcium intake being a condition for the prevention of osteoporosis ocurring at older age. What is understood by osteoporosis is a depletion in osseous substances, particularly in women after menopause, leading to a higher incidence of fractures in the femoral neck, the vertebral column and the forearm. In the second half of a lifetime a steadily progressing decomposition of osseous substances takes place depending on age (Fig. 4.1.4-1). It is the reason why, given

(3) BIRGE. S. et al. 1967. Osteoporosis, intestinal lactase deficiency and low dietary calcium intake. New. Engl. J. Med. 275: 445-448

(4) NEWCOMER, A. et al. 1978. Lactase deficiency: prevalence in osteoporosis. Ann. Intern. Med. 89: 218-220

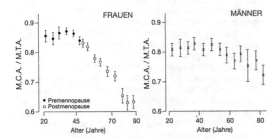

Fig. 4.1.4-1 Bone loss depending on age analyzed radiographically

growing overaging of the population, more and more people suffer from symptoms of senile osteoporosis.

A connection between regular calcium intake with nutrition and spreading of osteoporosis is suggested by the following observations:
- It was repeatedly reported that female patients with senile osteoporosis more frequently than healthy patients of the same age admitted to have abstained from milk all their lives, thus ingesting less calcium (2).
- Such a connection is also indicated by the observation of more lactose intolerant people among patients with osteoporosis than in a control group (3,4).
- It was reported from Yugoslavia that in a comparison of two districts different mineral densities in bones and incidences of femoral neck fractures could be stated in dependence on calcium intake.

Sources and references

(1) Deutsche Gesellschaft für Ernährung, Frankfurt am Main, Ernährungsbericht 1984, p. 36

(2) SANDLER, R. et al. 1985. Postmenopausal bone density and milk consumption in childhood and adolescence. Am. J. Clin. Nutr. 42: 270-274

4.1.5 Summary

The following conclusions can be summarized:
· A sufficient intake of calcium with food - especially during the period of growth - contributes to a sufficient mineralization and to the stability of the bone skeleton.
· If the density of minerals and the bone tissue is higher during the third decade of life - this is a more favourable starting position for the higher age, because the critical point of the density of minerals of $1g/cm^2$ will be reached later.

Therefore, every consumer should keep in mind that a steady intake of calcium by a constant nutrition with milk and dairy products all life long are highly recommendable. In this conection, it should not be forgotten that other important measures to prevent senile osteoporosis are:
to supply women with oestrogens after menopause and to guarantee sufficient physical exercise in women and men.

Sources and references

HAGEMEISTER, H., PRECHT, D., BARTH; C.A., 1988. Zum Transfer von Omega-3-Fettsäuren in das Milchfett bei Kühen. Milchwissenschaft 43 (3): 153-158

HAGEMEISTER, H., PRECHT, D., FRANZEN, Maike, BARTH; C.A. 1991. α-Linolenic acid transfer into milk fat and its elongation by cows. Fat. SCI. Technol. 93/10: 387-391

HAGEMEISTER, H., BARTH, C.A., 1987. Homogenisierung der Milch aus ernährungsphysiologischer Sicht. Schriftenreihe Verbraucherdienst, Hrsg. AID, P. 19-22

BAERTH, C.A., 1982. Milch und Milcherezugung. Hülsenberger gespräche. VTV-Verlag Hamburg, Schriftenreihe der Schaumann Stiftung zur Förderung der Agrarwissenschaften, p. 13, p.3

BARTH, C.A., 1988, Ernährungsphysiologie beurteilt die Käsequalität, schweizerische Milchzeitung, Nr. 13, p.3

SICK, H., BARTH, C.A., 1986. Der Einfluß der molkereitechnischen Bearbeitung von Rohmilch auf den ernährungsphysiologischen Wert der Kosummilch. AID-Verbraucherdienst 31, Heft 4: 75-81

BARTH, C.A., KRUSCH, U., MEOSEL, H., PROKOPEK, D., Schlimme, E., de VRESE, M., 1989 . Möglichkeiten und Grenzen der Reduzierung des Kochsalzgehaltes in Schnittkäse. Kieler Milchwirtschaftliche Forschungsberichte 41: 105-136
PROKOPEK, D., BARTH, C.A., KLOBES, H., KRUSCH, U., MEISEL, H., SCHLIMME, E., de VRESE, M., WOTHA, H.J., 1990. Reduzierung des Kochsalzgehaltes in Edamer Käse bei industrieller Herstellung. Kieler Milchwirtschaftliche Forschungsberichte 41: 565-596

BARTH, C.A., SVHOLZ-AHRENS, Katharina E., KOPRA, Nina, 1988. Bedeutung des Nahrungscalciums für die Prävention der Altersosteoporose. Deutsche Milchwissenschaft 43: 1461-1463

de VRESE, M., BARTH, C.A., 1991. Gesundheitliche Bedeutung von lebenden Keimen in fermentierten Milchprodukten. dmz - Lebensmittelindustrie und Milchwirtschaft 32/33: 988- 991

KERSTING, Mathilde, SCHÖCH, G. 1984. Praktische Ratschläge zu aktuellen Problemen der Ernährung von Klein- und Schulkindern. Sozialpäd. Prax. Klin. 6/5: 254-265

KERTING, Mathilde, SCHÖCH, G., 1985. Milch - ein wichtiges Thema in der pädiatrischen Ernährungsberatung. Sozialpäd. Prax. Klin. 7/6: 180-182

Dairy Products in Human Health and Nutrition, Serrano Ríos et al. (eds) © 1994 Balkema, Rotterdam, ISBN 90 5410 359 0

Milk consumption and level of risk on health and nutrition in grouped countries in the world

F. Mardones-Restat
Instituto de Nutrición y Tecnología de los Alimentos y Facultad de Medicina Campus Oriente, Universidad de Chile, Santiago, Chile

ABSTRACT: The impact of milk consumption on Nutrition and Health level in the vulnerable groups of the Third World is attempted to demostrate by grouping the countries as established by UNICEF in its book: The Situation of Infancy in the World. 1993. The funcional damage is expressed in a quotient, amplified by one thousand, between deaths of children under 5 years and total birth, from now TMM5. Four different level of the damage are related with the amount of milk products available in each group of countries by inhabitants. The association is strong, but also with a set of indicators of the levels of life. Some highlitgths of the policy of health and nutrition in Chile are discussed, in wich the priority in promotion of national milk production and its distribution in social programs, is considered.

1. Looking for an association of the probability of global health risk damage (TMM5) and milk products consumption. The distribution of the population by level of TMM5 and by continent is presented.

The table 1 illustrate the distribution of the population at risk of TMM5 in four level: very high, high, middle and low, by continent and is association with the availability of milk products by inhabitants.

The figure 1 and 2, shows the population distribution by continents and by risk of TMM5.

In the figure 3 is illustrate the different proportion of population and new born by level of damage. In the very high risk group the proportion of new born is twice the proportion of peoples and the contrary happen in the low group of risk.

In the figure 4 the association of milk availability and level of health risk is presented.

2. Indicators of the level of life by the four categories of probability of health damage and milk availability.
In the table 2, a set of indicators of categories of life are presented in association with the four categories of health damage (TMM5 UNICEF), and the milk products availability. Strong associations

Table 1. Population of countries distributed in four categories according: "Probability of functional damage: TMM5." (Columns Z,Y,X y V) by continents (rows F,H,J,L y N).
Levels of Probability of risk (TMM5)

		Very High	High	Middle	Low	World
		Z	Y	X	V	O
A.	TMM5					
	1960	262	231	174	48	177
B.	1991	197	116	26	11	67
C.	Decrease %	33.	50.	85.	77.	62.
D.	Population	502	1672	2226	959	5359
E.	%	9.4	31.2	41.5	17.9	(100.)
F.	Continents:					
F.	Africa	84.6	12.1	2.2	–	617
G.	%	(62.9)	(29.9)	(7.2)		(100.)
H.	Asia	15.4	80.1	80.5	22.0	3403
I.	%	(2.3%)	(39.2)	(52.3)	(6.2)	(100.)
J.	America	–	3.3	15.9	30.8	765
K.	%		(7.8)	(50.6)	(41.6)	(100.)
L.	Europe	–	0.3	1.6	45.0	547
M.	%		(1.0)	(7.4)	(91.6)	(100.)
N.	Oceania	–	–	–	2.2	27
O.	%				(100.)	(100.)

P. Milk products consumption*
lt/inh/year 25. 29. 72. 264. 96.

is observed not only with the static indicator for one year (circa 1991) but also with their trends, mainly in the last three decades.

TMM5

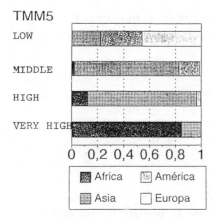

Figure 1. Percentaje of populations distributed by continents according categories of health damage (TMM5)

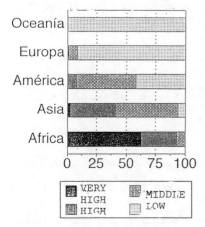

Figure 2. Percentage of population distributed by categories of health damage (TMM5), according continents

3. Patterns of birth rate and level of health risk.

In the demographic and also in the social situation of women indicators presented in the table 2, it can be seen that global fertility of women (number of babies at the term of the fertility period of women) is highly associated with the rate of infant mortality (mainly of the one that consider those below 5 years).

In the figure 3. the different proportion of newborn and total populations bay level of risk conuntry group is presented.

Roughly the newborn are in the proportion of 20 por cent in the very high risk group, 30 % in the high, 40 % in the middle and

Table 2. LEVEL OF LIVE INDICATORS ACCORDING THE CATEGORIES OF RISK: TMM5.

CATEGORIES OF RISK

TMM5: Very high high median low world
Indicators:

Population					
(millions)	502	1672	2226	959	5359
% 1991	9.4	31.2	41.5	17.9	(100.)
Tmm5 1960	283	231	174	48	202
1991	197	116	36	11	91
Decrease %	30.	50.	79.	77.	55.
Milk consuption milk					
l/i/y	25.	29.	72.	264.	96.
GNP: us$/inh.					
1990	355	525	1465	17580	3927
Infant mortality rate					
1960	164	143	114	38	125
1991	114	80	29	9	61
Decrease %	30.	44.	75.	76.	51.
Births					
(millions)	23.6	53.6	50.4	13.4	141
1991 %	17.	38.	36.	9.	(100.)
Life expectation at birth					
1991 (years)	50	59	69	76	65
Adult literate					
1991 %	48	54	7	94	79
Schooling Basic					
1986-90	64	93	120	103	100.
Nutrition					
birth weight					
< 2500 g %	16	27	10	7	17
Breastfeeding at one year old					
%	82	77	41	10	58
Calories consumption,					
80 % of requirment					
	91	105	116	133	113
Health:					
drinking					
water					
total %	43	75	76	-	72*
urb. %	62	83	89	100*	80*
Rur. %	35	71	67	85*	57*
Enviroment					
total %	43	23	67	-	47*
urb. %	66	56	83	-	54*
Rur. %	33	10	48	-	29*
Access to Health Services					
%	52	61	87	-	66*
Inmunization:					
tb	62	86	93	77	84
dpt	47	80	87	89	78
polio	46	80	92	88	80
measles	46	76	89	78	80
Pregnant women:					
tetanus	28	65	54	-	63*

only 10 % in thelow one. By the contrary the populations in the four groups are only 10 % in the very high 30 % in the high, 40% in middle and 20 % in the low one.

160

TMM5: Very high high median low world
indicators:
_____

Demography (1991)
less than
16 years 276   707   738   213   1934
age   %   14.   37.   38.   11. (100.)
Less than
5 years 106   244   243   67   660
age   %   16.   37.   37.   10. (100.)
Annual growth rate:
1965-1980 2.6   2.5   2.1 0.9   2.0
1980-1991 3.0   2.3   1.7 0.7   1.8
Fertility rate
1980   50.   44.   36.   21.   37.
1991   47.   32.   23.   14.   26.
Decrease % 6.   27.   36.   33.   30.
Global fertility rate
1991   6.6   4.2   2.7   1.8   3.4
Urban population
91 %   25   30   41   75   42
Growth of urban population
(% year)
1980-1991 5.3   3.8   3.3   1.0   3.2
Economy
  annual rate of growth
  1965-80 2.4   2.6   4.2   -   3.2
  1980-91 - .8   1.8   1.4   2.5   1.5
Annual inflation
average
1980-90   24   23   94   5   49
Guvernamental expenditure:
% in health 3   3   7   13   6
  education 9   9   11   4   9
  defence   -   15   10   14   13
Services of ext.Debt %
of exportations
  1970   5   15   12   -   12
  1990   15   20   16   10   16
Women situation:
literace % men
           62   62   80   -   71
Schooling women/men
- basic
1986/90   74   80   93   100   81
- medium
1986/90   58   64   87   102   80
Use of contraceptives %
women
15-49 years 6   33   66   72   51
Professional care
of birth % 33   35   87   97   54
Maternal mortality rate
by 100 000
birth   640   440   100   12   311
Rhythm of Progress
Childrem mortality rate
0-5 y. (Tmm5)
1960   263   231   174   48   194
1980   221   165   69   17   126
1991   197   116   36   11   91

TMM5: Very high high median low world
Indicators:
_____

Ch.M.Rate < 5 years
Index 100=
1960
1980   84   71   40   43   65
1991   75   50   21   23   47
Global fertility
rate:1960 6.6   6.1   5.1   3.0   5.5
     1980 6.8   5.1   3.1   1.9   4.4
     1991 6.6   4.2   2.7   1.8   3.4
Global fertility
rate index 100=
    1960
    1980 103   84   61   63   80
    1991 100   69   53   60   62
_____

* estinated figures.

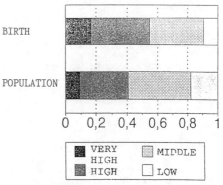

BIRTH

POPULATION

0   0,2 0,4 0,6 0,8   1

| VERY HIGH | MIDDLE |
| HIGH | LOW |

Figure 3. Newborns populations groups of
populations with veri high, high middle and
low level of TMM5.

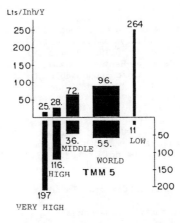

Lts/Inh/Y

Figure 4. Consumption of milk products and
categories of health damages of TMM5.

4. Apparent consumption of milk products and categories of health damages (TMM5).

The table 4 display the association of the consumption of milk and the categories of health damage (TMM5). From this information it is deduce the importance of the milk avalaibility in control the health and nutrition risk, but at the same time that the development of industry require political and economical decisions, that not always recive the adecuate priority in socio- economical Policies.

REFERENCES

UNICEF, 1993. Situation of Infancy in the World. Edit. Unicef. New York.

FAO, 1991. Annuaries on Production, Commerce and Balance of foods   sheets. Edit. FAO. Rome.

Puffer R, Serrano C, 1989 Patterns on birthweight Scientific Publication OPS/OMS № 504. Washington D.C.

Mardones Restat F. Jones G. Diaz M. Dach N. Prediccting Poor Growth in infants. PAHO Bulletin 21 (4), 1987, pp:341-357.

Mardones-Restat F. Jones G, Mardones S F, Diaz M, Lara M.E, Dachs N, Habicht J-P. Growth Failure Prediction in Chile. Int J of Epidemiology 1989;18, Supplement 2, ISNN 0300-5771, pp:S44-S49 England U.K.

Monckeberg F. Mardones-Restat F. & Valiente S
The evolution of malnutrition and mortality in infant and young children over the past 20 years in Chile.In: Hansluska H, López AD, Porapakkham Y, Prasartkul P, Eds . New development in the analysis of mortality and cases of death. Bangkok: Mahdol University. Faculty of Public Health. Institute for Population & Social Research, 1986, pp:295-321.

Rosselot J. & Mardones-Restat F. Antecedentes Históricos de la Seguridad Alimentaria infantil y familiar en Chile. Rev Pediatr (Santiago) 1988; 31:115-131

Rosselot J. & Mardones-Restat F. Salud de la Familia y Paternidad responsable. La experiencia de Chile 1965-1988. Rev Méd de Chile 1990; 118:330-338.

Cruz-Coke E Preventive and Oriented Medicine. 1938. Editorial Nascimento.

Dragoni F, Burnet I. Report on Food and Nutrition in Chile. Rev.Méd de Higiene, Salubridad y Medicina del Trabajo 1937

Foxley A, Raczynsky D. Vulnerables groups at recesives situation. The children and youth case in Chile. Colección Estudios CIEPLAN 13.

González N, Hertrampft E, Mardones S F, Rosso P, Verdugo C. Evaluación preliminar del programa de Fomento de la Lactancia Materna. Rev Ch Pediatr 1983;54(1):36-40.

Howard J, Monckeberg F, Mardones-Restat F, y cols. Eds. Manual for Primary and Secondary malnutrition treatment. Editorial CRECES, 1991.

Infante A, Mardones-Restat F Health and Nutrition Statistics. In: La realidad en cifras. Gómez S, Ed. FLACSO. Stgo. Chile. 1992.

Jones G, Mardones-Restat F   Methodologics consideration in the nutritional and food distribution programs. Cuad Méd Soc 1980;21(4):39-53. Santiago-Chile

Mardones-Restat F Breastfeeding and lenght in a cohort of 1151 born alive in 4 maternal in Santiago of Chile. Rev Chil Pediatr 1990;61(6):233 (Letter of Editor).

Mardones J, Cox R, Eds. Food and feeding in Chile. Editorial Universitaria, 1942. Santiago Chile.

Mardones S F Breastfeeding actual and historical situation in Chile. Rev Méd Chile 1979; 167:750-760.

Mardones-Restat F Materanl and Child Health in the last 30 years. Rev Chil Pediatr 1990;61(6):281-286.

Mardones-Restat F Paternidad Responsable y Salud Familiar: Una opción gubernamental Rev Pediatr (Santiago) 1983;26:116-123.

Mardones-Restat F Birthweight and Infant Mortality rate of adolescents mothers deliveries. Chile, Macro-Region Rev Chil Pediatr, 1989;60(5):305 (Letters of Editor).

Mardones-Restat F Statistical models in the estimation of the scemaries for planning and classification of the population Cuad Méd Soc 1993;XXXIV(1):55-67.

Mardones-Restat F Social Security benefits for mother and children Care in Chile REv Chil Nutr 1984;12:23-27

Mardones-Restat F, Díaz M, Risopatrón F Children at risk according the level of live of the county of residence. Rev Chil Pediatr 1991;62(2):132-141.

Molina S Basis for a program against poverty in a political democratic system. In: Social Development of the 80. UNICEF/ILPES/CEPAL 1980;233-240.

Monckeber F, Riumalló J Centers for undernutrition recovery . In: Extrem Poverty and infancy UNICEF/ILPES/CEPAL 1981.

Monckeberg F, Oxman S, Lacassie I Infants nutritional conditions and level of live at the province of Curicó. Chile. Rev Chil Pediatr 1967;38:491.

Monckeberg F   Trends of undernutrition and of infant mortality rate in the last 20 years in Chile. Cuad Univ Chile 1985;4:165-204.

Raczynsky D, Oyarzo C ¿Why fall infant mortality rate in Chile? Colec Estudios Cieplan № 6.

Rosselot J, Avendaño O, Borgoño JM et al
    Report of the policies for fertility
    regulation at the National Health
    Service in Chile. Rev Méd Chile
    1966;744-750.
Taucher E The influence of family planning
    on infant mortality levels. UN, Dept of
    Int Affairs Population Studies 1985, Nº
    ST/ESA/SER.
Becerra C, Mardones S F, Montesinos N,
    Manual de fomento para la Lactancia
    Materna. UNICEF/MINSAL 1989. Editorial
    UNICEF Santiago. Chile.
Viel B, Campos W La planificación familiar
    en Chile y su efecto en los índices de
    Salud. Bol APROFA 1988;24:7-12.
Vio F, Albala C, Salinas J, Mardones S F,
    Truffello I Tabaquismo y Lactancia
    Materna Rev. Méd Chile 1987;115(7):611-
    615.
Vio F, Salazar G, Infante C Smoking during
    pregnancy and lactation its effects on
    breat-milk volume. Am J Clin Nutr
    1991;54:1011-1016.

Dairy Products in Human Health and Nutrition, Serrano Ríos et al. (eds) © 1994 Balkema, Rotterdam, ISBN 90 5410 359 0

Dairy products in infant nutrition

E.Casado de Frías & C.Maluenda
Hospital Universitario de San Carlos, Madrid, Spain

M.Marco
Hospital Gómez Ulla, Madrid, Spain

Dairy-products have their own characteristics, in the nutrition of infants, which are different from those of the adult person, basically concerning the specific circumstances of this first stage in life.

These differences are basically established in connection with two facts: 1.- the individual for whom they are intended (the infant); 2.- dairy-products themselves.

1.- As regards their relationship whith the infant, dairy products, always an important part in infant nutrition, participate, in the aprropiate proportion with other foods, in the attainment of the main objective of nutrition at these stages of life; to contribute the necessary nutrients to obtain an optimum degree of growth and development.

2.- With respect to the differences deriving from dary-products themselves, we shall only point out that those dairy-products consumed during lactation are exclusive to that stage and certainly different from those which are part of the usual diet of older children and adults.

The most important example of the two above mentioned facts is reflected in the first months of the infant's life. This stage is not only the one in wich the child experiences the highest degree of growth and development but also this growth and development are attained with the only food taken by the child at that time, human milk or infant formula. Tehese peculiarities referred to the infant and diary-products during the first four or six months of its life extend, with some modifications, until the child is one year old. The differences with respect to the previous period are mainly

established in a quantitative manner, decrease in the infant's growth velocity and proportional decrease in the intake of diary-products, when these become no longer the only source of nutrients but instead only part or a diversified feeding system (minimum recommended milk or its derivates intake, 500ml/day, until the child is one year old). From a quantitative point of view, the issue is, if not identical, very similar, high degree of growth and the consumption of special diary-products.

Using these considerations as basis, we will center our exposition in the relationship growth/dairy-products during the first year of life.

In this sense we shall divide the exposition in two parts: in the first we shall tray to summarize the current situation with respect to this subject; in the second, related to the first, we shall set forth some summarized data from several studies carry out at our Departament.

The relationship existing between the milk-fed infant and the type of nutrition it receives, either by breast feeding or by formula feeding, is a currently debated subject of great interest.

In a larger number of publications, different authors describe how formula-fed infants grow taller and gain more weight than breast-fed infants (Boulton 1981). By contrast, in other publications we observe that the development of these parameters follows the same proportion, or is even higher, in breast-fed infants (D'Souza 1979, Sarinen, Taitz 1981).

Nevertheless, a detailed study of the situation enables us to divide publications in tow groups, thouse that were carried out before the seventies and thouse that were carry out after the seventies. Papers wich are chronologically older say formula-fed infants grow faster. Those in the second group, written more recently, question this assertion saying that breast-fed infants grow in the same degree, or more, than formula-fed infants, at least during the first three or four months of their life.

Admitting that the growth pattern of breast-fed infants with respect to formula-fed infants has changed along a period of time, the first thing we have to ask ourselves is what can have happened in connection with this time factor, in each of these cases, separately. In other words, we must ascertain whether the differences in growth we are currently finding, compared with previous years, are causaded by an increase in the growth of breast-fed infants, a decrease in the growth of formula-fed infants, or, finally , by a combination of both circumstances.

Growth in breast-fed infants.-

This subject has been broached by different authors and from different points of view. Some researchers have approached the issue comparing the current infant milk intake (Whitehead 1981), with those referred to in previous (Wallgren 1944). No significant differences have been found in these studies, within a country in particular, or compared with other countries, as long as, logically, the countries concerned have a similar degree of development. Other authors have preferred to base their investigations in the comparison of energy intake of both groups, based in the fact it is directly related with body weight (Chandra 1981). Finally other researchers have approached the subject directly, by comparing body weight in both groups. In this sense we find particulary significant those studies which show the results as the weight increase according to age, in relation to the infant's weight at birth, avoiding thus the mistakes arising from not having an homogeneous population with respect to this last parameter (Stewart 1953, Hooper 1965, Taitz 1981). Those studies that have been carried out in this way show that results are actually very similar,

independently from the period they were carried out.

In short, we can say that when we compare the growth of breast-fed infants in the present day with that of those infants which were also breast-fed during the period under study before the seventies, we perceive that things are very similar. Which brings us to presume, as we had anticipated, that the differences fond between these two periods of time must be related to formula-feeding (Evans 1978, Taitz 1981).

Growth in formula-fed infants.

Once we have established that formula-fed infants are responsible for changing the growth pattern along a period of time, the next step is to look for the reasons implied in this fact. Two facts have been recognised as the most important in this development: changes in the types of infant formula and attitude of the mother towards feeding her infant (Whitehead 1985).

Changes in the type of formula.-

When looking for a substitute for human milk, the objective has been, and still is, always the same: starting with a base of cow's milk the necessary modifications are made to obtain a product which can resemble human milk as much as possible.

Little by little, Nutrition Science and Technology have advanced in such a way that, at each step, the product offered to the infant came nearer human milk itself. Once we have established this, we can distinguish two clearly differentiated periods: before and after the ESPGAN (European Society of Pediatric Gastroenterology and Nutrition) recommendations in the seventies. It was only after the ESPGAN Nutrition Comittee pronounced the aforementioned recommendations, that the infant food industry began to change the composition of the then existing infant milks, for other products which were denominated starting formulas, as they cannot really be called milk. These products have a lower calorie and protein content than the previously existing products, they are more similar to human milk and certainly much better adapted to the needs of the healthy new-born for whom they are intended.

166

These changes were accepted practically unanimously and immediately by the dyetari industry, pediatrists and by the mothers themselves, which means that, in practice, practically all the formula-fed infants from then on have been fed with the new kind of infant formula.

Attitude of the mother

So that these formula may accomplish the purpose for which they have been created, it is essential that they should be adequately reconstituted (proportional mixture of power and water). From this point of view, the parent's attitude, basically the mother's, is of pre-eminent importance. In this sense, the basic change observed has been more adequated food preparation, mainly directed to avoid overdosage. The element directly related to this fact is parents' knowledge of the two main problems arising from overdosage: hypertonic dehydration and obesity, this last problem being also influenced by the current fashion and different concept mothers have these days of their baby's beauty and health.

In fact, if we compare the energy intake of breast-fed and formula-fed infants before the seventies and that of present day infants, we observe that such intake has not varied in breast-fed infants. By contrast, and as was to be expected, it has decreased in formula-fed infants (Beal 1970, Vobecky 1980, Young 1980).

Other factors

There are other factors related to the growth and development of the unweaned infant but, contrary to those mentioned above, the relatinship of these factors is not directly established, i.e., through the characteristics of milk itself, but indirectly, in relation with other circumstances existing around the type of feeding (breast or formula). Whithin this group of factors let us mention two of the most important ones, namely the mother's social and cultural status and the infant's introduction to weaning foods.

The relationship between growth and social class, based in genetic and environmental factors, is a well-known fact (Rona 1981). In this sense, if we study the percentage of mothers who begin to breast-feed their babies and how long they continue doing so, in relation with their social status, we will observe that mothers with the highest social and financial status (the most privileged ones) are those that breast-feed their babies more frequently and for a longer period of time. By conytrast, these in lower status levels are those that less frequently begin to breast-feed their babies and when they do begin, give up much.

Concerning the other factor involved, the infant's introduction to weaning foods, the results can be modified for a series of different reasons, namely:

1.- Weaning foods are included, although the fact is not admitted, in the feeding of infants described as being exclusively formula-fed.
2.- The introduction of weaning foods is done sooner in formula-fed babies than in breast-fed babies.
3.- These days, weaning foods are introduced at a later period than they used to be some years ago.
4.- In practice it has been observed that weaning foods play a different role according to the type of lactancy: as a complement in formula-feeding and as a substitute for breast-feeding.

In short we can say that there are several explanations for the differences found along a period of time in relation with the growth of formula-fed infants. Some of these differences arise from the product itself and others are related to indirect elements.

At present the question at issue is focused in the evaluation of breast-fed and formula-fed infant's growth, but in a different situation, characterized by the following circumstances:
1.- Most formula-fed babies are fed with the new infants formulas, low in solutes and much more similar to human milk.
2.- There is a new attitude and better knowledge on the part of mothers of the different aspects pertaining both to breast-feeding and to formula-feeding.
3.- Bearing in mind those factors indirectly related to the type of feeding and which have not been examined in previous studies.

In our Department we were interested in the study of these problems and we started a series of surveys which, though modest, we think have born interesting results, and we have therefore selected them as part of this paper (Marcos 1989, Casado de Frías 1991).

Our objective was to evaluate the growth both of breast-fed and formula-fed infants during their first year of life, trying to eliminate as much as possible, the interaction of other factors such as the abovementioned indirect factors, i.e., not deriving from nutrition itself.

For this purpose we proceeded to make a pre-selection of the population in order it should fulfill two characteristics: social homogenity (armed forces) and being closely controlled by their respective pediatrician. Selection criteria chosen whith respect to the infant were: healthy full-term new-born infants, with adequate weight for their gestation time, born of a sigle birth and with no pathological obstetric records.

The study took place between July 1986 and January 1988. It started whith 441 infants (226 boys, 215 girls) and was finished with 200 (105 boys, 95 girls). All the babies that arrived to the end of the study were examined every month for whole year. A sociological study was made for each infant at the beginning of the study and at each monthly revision, and we also proceeded at each of these revision to: a) provide counselling services on nutrition folowing ESPGAN recommendation, 2) carry out a dietetic survey, 3) collection of anthropometric data (weight, length, ponderal growth and longitudinal growth).

Infants were divided in four groups, according to the type of food they received: exclusively breast-fed (BF), exclusively formula-fed (FF), breast-fed whith weaning foods (BFWF) and formula-fed whith weaning foods (FFWF).

Results.

1.- Growth in the first quarter.-

Ponderal growth in the first three months in gr/day according to the type of feeding was not different in infants in the BF group (28.1 gr/d) and the FF group (28.6 gr/d). Growth in length in mm/d was higher for the FF group (1.1317 mm/d) than for infants in the BF group (1.067 mm/d), at a significance level of $p<0.01$. There were no significant differences between average weight for the BF group (5.965 gr) and the FF group (6.034 gr) at the end of three months. By contrast, the average length was significantly higher ($p<0.01$) in the FF group (60.47 cm) than in the BF group (59.95 cm).

2.- Growth in the second quarter.-

Average ponderal growth, in gr/day, according to the type of feeding presented differences related to the food received by the infant. Thus, ponderal growth in the FF (21.5 gr/day) or FFWF (21.1 gr/d) groups was higher than those in the BF (17.8 gr/d) or BFWF (17.7 gr/d) groups with a significance level of $p<0.01$. Average longitudinal growth, in mm/day, was lower for the BF group (0.65 mm/d) than for the rest of groups: FF (0.76 mm/d), BFWT (0.72 mm/d), FFWF (0.75 mm/d) with a significance level of $p<0.01$. Infant's weight at the end of the six month period, according to the type of feeding, did not present statistically significant differences, althoug average weight of the FF group infants (7.963 gr) and FFWF group infants (7.828 gr) was higher than that of the BF group (7.599 gr) or the BFWF group (7.622 gr). Average length at the end of sixth months, according to the type of feeding showed a significant difference whith $p<0.01$ in favour of the FFWF group (67.06 cm) with respect to the BF group (65.74 cm). In the comparative study of this parameter whith the rest of groups under study no statistically significant differences were found.

3.- Growth in the third quarter.-

Ponderal growth, in gr/day, during the third quarter reflects a higher gain in the FFWF group (13.8 gr/d) than in the BFWF group (12.8 gr/d) with a significance level of $p<0.01$. Concerning average longitudinal growth, in mm/day, it shows that the FFWF group with (0.519 mm/d) grew more than the BFWF group (0.497 mm/d), with a significance level of $p< 0.01$. The infant's weigth survey at nine months, depending on the type of feeding, reflects a higher degree of weigth in the FFWF group (9.049 gr) than in the BFWF group (8.801 gr), with a statistical significance of p<0.01.

Concernig their length, it was greater in the FFWF group (71.3 cm) than in the BFWF group (70.7 cm), with a statistical significance of p<0.01.

4.- Growth in the fourth quarter.-

No significant differences were observed with respect to ponderal growth, BFWF (10.97 gr/d) and FFWF (10.98 gr/d), or longitudinal growth, BFWF (0.4320 mm/d) and FFWF (0.4471 mm/d), between both groups. Infant's weigth at twelve months of age was higher for the FFWF group (10.015 gr) than for the BFWF group (9.898 gr) although the difference was not significant. What we did find significant was the difference in length at twelve months of age (p<0.01), in favour of the FFWF group (75.4 cm) against the (74.6 cm) in the BFWF group.

Our results, as most of the results to be found in the literature, show once more the existing differences in growth in the first year of life in breast-fed and formula-fed infants.

The differences shown in our survey affect, although not in a simultaneous way, all the parameters we have studied, namely: weight, height, growth velocity and longitudinal growth velocity.

These differences, if any, were always in favour of formiula-fed infants.

Concerning the study of ponderal parameters, significant differences were only found in the second and third quarters. By contrast differences in the study of longitudinal growth on one part and length, were found in the first three quarters and along the first year of life, respectively.

Upon observation of the results in an evolutive form along a period of time, we can say as follows: During the first quarter, formula-fed infants presented a higher longitudinal growth than breast-fed infants, although, there were no differences in ponderal growth. During the second quarter, the

differences found in the first quarter in favour of formula-fed infants were increased by a smaller ponderal gain (gr/day) in breast-fed infants. During the third quarter, at which stage both groups were receiving weanig foods, we found differences in favour of formula-fed infants in all the parameters under study. Along the fourth quarter, differences between both groups decreased, so that both longitudinal and ponderal growth remain the same. There are no significant diffrences between the average weigth of infants in both groups. And the difference between the average lengths attained by the end of the fourth quarter is 0.8 cm lower than that found at the end of the sixth month (1.3 cm). It seems as if infants in the breast-fed group had a slower rate of growth at the beginning but later they tend to catch up the formula-fed group.

We can ourselves whether the differences than have been foud the breast-fed group and the formula-fed group during the first three quarters, which desappear at the end of the fourth quarter, can be indicative or merely represent a more physiological pattern of the growth. This would advocate in favour of recommendation from different authors concerning the need of the availavility of individual growth curves for breast-fed infants, so that these facts can be adequately interpreted as normal and, consequentely, not to suppress, but, on the contrary, to encourage prolonged breast-feeding (for more than three months) (Dewey 1991, Guo 1991, Dewey 1992).

Although, because of the special characteristics of our survey, tye results obtained cannot be considered representative of thouse pertaining to a control population sample, we can asseverate that conclusion obtained in nom pre-selectioned population surveys can also be applied to our survey. On the other hand we allege that our results point out the still existing differences of breast-fed and formula.fed infants and that these differences seem to be related to factors directly involved in the composition of these, at least in certain population like the one we have studied.

REFERENCES

Beal, V.A. 1970. Nutritional intake. In: McCammon, R.W. ed Human growth and development. Spring-field Illinois. 63-100.

Boulton, J. 1981. Nutrition in childhood and its relationships to early somatic growth, body fat, blood pressure and physical fitness. Acta Paediatr Scand (suppl) 284: 1-85.

Casado de Frias, E. Maluenda, C. Marco, M. 1991. Weaning in European and Latin American Countries. Karger 27: 1-14.

Chandra, R.K. 1981. Breast-feeding, growth and morbidity. Nutr Res 1: 25-32.

Dewey, K.G. Heinig, M.J. Nommsen, L.A. Lonnerdal, B. 1991. Adequacy of energy intake among breast-fed infants in the DARLING study: relationships to growth velocity, morbidity and activity levels. J Pediatr 119: 538-47.

Dewey, K.G. Heinig, M.J. Nommsen, L.A. Peerson, J.M. Lonnerdal, B. 1992. Growth of breast-fed and formula-fed infants from 0 to 18 months: the 2DARLING study. pediatrics 89: 1035-41.

D'Souza, S.W. Black, P. 1979. A study of infant growth in relation to the type of feeding. Early Hum Dev 3/3: 245-55.

Evans, T.J. 1978. Growth and milk intake of normal infants. Arch Dis Child 53: 749-51.

Fryer, B.A. Lamkin, G.H. Vivian, V.A. Eppright, E.S. Fox, H.M. 1971. Diets of pre-school children in the North Central Region.J Am Diet Assoc 59: 228-32.

Guo, S. Roche, A. Fomon, S,J. Nelson, S.E. Chandra, W.C. Rogers, R.R. Bonmgartner, R.N. Ziegler, E. Siervogel, R.M. 1991. Reference data on gains in weigth and length during the first two years of life. J Pediatr 119: 355-62.

Hooper, P.D. 1965. Infant feeding and its relationship to weigth gain and illness. The Practitioner 194: 391-5.

Marco, M. 1989. Lactancia crecimiento y morbilidad del lactante. Tesis doctoral. Facultad de Medicina Universidad Complutense. Madrid.

Rona, R.J. 1981. Genetic and environmental factors in the control of growth in childhood. Br Med Bull 37: 265-72.

Sarinen, U.M. Siimes, M.A. 1979. Role of prolonged breast-feeding in infant growth. Acta Paediatr Scand 68: 245-250.

Stewart, A. Westrop, C. 1953. Breat feeding in the Oxford child health survey. Comparison or bottle and breast fed babies. Br Med J i: 305-8.

Taitz, L.S. Lukmanji, Z. 1981. Alterations in feeding patterns and rates of weight gain in South Yorkshire infants 1971-1977. Hum Biol 53: 313-20.

Vobecky, J.S. Vobecky, J. Demers, P.P. Shapcott, D. Blanchard, R. Black, R. 1980. Food and nutrient intake of infants in the first fifteen months. Nutr Rep Int 22: 571-80.

Wallgren, A. 1944. Breast milk consumption of healthy full-term infants. Acta Paediatr Scand 32: 778-90.

Whitehead, R.G. and Paul, A.A. 1981. Infant growth and human milk requirements: a fresh approach. Lancet ii: 161-3.

Whitehead, R. G. Paul, A.A. 1985. Human lactation, infant feeding,and grouwth: secular trends.Raven Press. New York.

Whichelow, M.J. and King, B.E. 1979. Breast-feeding and smoking. Arch Dis Child 54: 240-1.

Yeung, D.L. Hall, J. Leung, M. 1980. Adequacy of energy intake of infants. J Can Diet Assoc 41: 48-52.

Dairy Products in Human Health and Nutrition, Serrano Ríos et al. (eds) © 1994 Balkema, Rotterdam, ISBN 90 5410 359 0

Dairy products and adolescent nutrition

M. Giovannini, A. Rottoli & C. Agostoni
5th Department of Pediatrics, University of Milan, Italy

ABSTRACT: Adolescence is an intense anabolic period. For this reason, the requirements of all nutrients are increased, with particular emphasys for dietary calcium. A balanced intake of the three macronutrients (protein, fats and carbohydrates) is recommended for the prevention of the chronic-degenerative disorders of adulthood. The distribution of the caloric intake also deserves particular attention for a possible role in the homeostatic regulations. Adolescents very often show disorders of the alimentary behavior predisposing them to both obesity and anorexia. A proper dietary intervention in this age should promove the regular consumption of breakfast, a balanced intake of animal and vegetal foods and the increase of calcium supply to maximize the bone density. Dairy products and vegetables (mainly enriched cereals) constitute the dietary basis for a correct diet in adolescents, taking into consideration both the structural needs and the preventive purposes.

1 INTRODUCTION

Anabolic activity is intense during puberty since besides the appreciable increases in anthropometric indices (weight and height), marked changes are also being wrought in body composition: there is an increase in the lean mass, changes in amount and distribution of fatty tissue, and development of internal organs and systems. These events of puberty are the main factors dictating the adolescent's nutritional requirements. Adolescence is the only period of extrauterine life when the rate of growth rises so fast, so nutrition is obviously fundamental. Requirements are closely correlated to the rapid increase in body mass, so that the body's needs, particularly for minerals and micronutrients, are always maximal, rising continuously.
Males gain more weight, faster than females, and their bone growth continues for longer. They deposit more lean mass, while females deposit more fatty mass (Gong, 1988). As lean mass has higher metabolic activity than adipose tissue, the sex-related differences in body composition in this stage of life give rise to nutritional requirements.
On account of the wide differences in the age at which puberty starts, chronological age is not always a good indicator as regards nutritional requirements. Individuals of the same chronological age may differ in their physiological ages. However, national and international recommendations on nutrient requirements obey the need for clear indications ofthe amounts and types of foods needed to fulfil the requirements of maximal growth at any given time. They are therefore the only point of reference, until more precise "markers" become available to indicate when each individual needs increases in specific nutrients.

2 NUTRITION IN ADOLESCENCE

Current nutritional recommendations for adolescents are generally based on estimates of the intake required to assure adequate growth and good health, extrapolated from animal studies or interpolated from studies

in children and adults. There are
still very few direct studies of
adolescents.
Attention has recently focussed on
certain selected topics related to
adolescent nutrition:
1.a study of adolescents' eating
habits and new food fads, to check
whether they lead to any sort of
"malnutrition";
2.prevention of adult
chronic-degenerative pathologies by a
primarily dietary approach to obesity
and by observing national and
international dietary guidelines;
3. a definition of the ideal calcium
intake to ensure maximum bone density
and prevent osteoporosis.
These three points are joined by a
single thread: the need tokeep a
balance of nutrients during a period
when personal choices and preferences
gain priority over eating habits
acquired in the family;
adolescents nowadays often have a
degree of financial independence that
can even if only marginally influence
the quality of their diet. Milk and
dairy products play a vital role, as
we shall see, in reaching this
balance.

2.1 Adolescence: eating habits and
    consumption

We still know little about the
composition of the adolescent'sdiet
and his food preferences. The
picture drawn from studies to date
is complicated by the wide day-
to-day variability in nutrient
intake, and by the different
anthropometric and nutritional
standards employed. Finally,
adolescents are by nature fad-prone,
so their eating habits, like
everything else, tend to shift fast.
Observations in English-speaking
countries in the early Seventies
confirmed the "fast food" habit among
adolescents,in place of traditional
meals (Richardson, 1972). This led
on the one hand to a tendency to skip
meals at normal times (Bender, 1972)
and on the other to take about 25% of
the calorie intake as between-meals
snacks (Thomas, 1973). This was
confirmed in the U.S.A. in a study
which reported the distribution of
macronutrients (Salz, 1983): about
15% of the calorie intake was
protein, 40-50% fats (with saturated
fats amounting to 15-16% of this),
and 45-50% carbohydrates, more than
half of which were simple sugars.

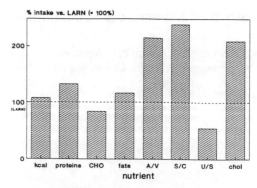

Figure 1. Nutrient intake in a
sample of adolescents in Milan
(Giovannini, 1986).
Comparison with the Italian
Recommended Dietary Allowances
(LARN, 1988)

CHO= Carbohydrates
A/V= Animal/Vegetal protein ratio
S/C= Simple/Complex Carbohydrate
ratio
U/S= Unsaturated/Saturated Fat ratic
Chol= Cholesterol

We found similar figures in a sample
of 335 students aged 12-15 years in
Milan (Giovannini, 1986). Their
energy intake was adequate but their
macronutrient intake was imbalanced,
like in Salz's study, besides which
they consumed a considerable
proportion of animal protein and
dietary cholesterol (Figure 1).
International and national
organisations recommend that
adolescents' diets should contain
less than 10% of protein,25-30 % of
fats (not more than 10% saturated)
and theremaining 60-65%
carbohydrates, less than 25% of
which should be simple sugars.
Dietary cholesterol intake should
not exceed 100 mg/1000 calories.
In the last few years, however, new
observations have been reported from
the U.S.A. on what is considered to
be a "massmedia"-influenced
phenomenon: adolescents,
particularly girls, are increasingly
insecure and dissatisfied with
theirbody image, and frequent resort
to "do-it-yourself" diets to achieve
what they consider an ideal body
status. About two thirds of girls
would like to lose weight, even
though their weight is normal or
even low (Moore, 1988). This is
more frequent in older adolescents,
but has been encountered as early as

eight years old (Maloney, 1992).
The obsession with low-fat,
low-cholesterol diets may, however,
lead to growth deficits resulting
from a lack of essential and
semi-essential nutrients.   This has
been nosologically classified as
"nutritional dwarfing"
(Lifshitz,1987).   This fear of the
possible consequences of high blood
cholesterol not only leads youngsters
to follow low-calorie diets but
sometimes results in their intake of
micronutrients (particularly iron and
zinc) being well below the RDA
(Lifshitz, 1987).   Clinically
detectable "malnutrition" can thus
arise even in the "advanced"
countries, and is most frequent in
adolescence when it may even come
very close to overt anorexia nervosa
(Maloney, 1992).
A questionnaire survey (Moore, 1988)
found that the level of knowledge of
nutritional questions did not seem to
affect teenagers' tendencies and
eating habits.   A fear of one's
image not being up to other people's
expectations seems thus to be
deep-rooted in their social
subconscious. The problem of obesity
certainly exists, but must be
approached in relation to its type
and the measures needed to combat it.

2.2 Prevention of obesity: breakfast

Overweight in adults is associated
with an increased risk of
cardiovascular diseases, gallstones,
diabetes mellitus, atherosclerosis,
gout, arthritis and certain tumours
(Lew,1979).   The possible relations
between overweight in adolescence and
morbidity later in life are less
clear.
A recent study by Must (1992) found
however that overweight during
adolescence (13-18 years) could
predict a series of negative effects
regardless of adult weight, 55 years
later.   The risk of cardiovascular
disease and atherosclerosis was
higher for men and women who had been
overweight as adolescents (body mass
index-BMI-more than the 75th
percentile at two measurements).
The risk of colorectal tumor and gout
was higher for obese males, and
arthritis was a higher risk for
females.
These conclusions agree with earlier
studies which though only few   had
already shown a relation between
overweight during adolescence and
adult health, although for shorter

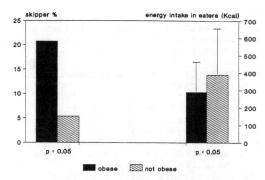

Figure 2. Daily breakfast habits in
obese and not-obese subjects ranging
7yrs-14yrs (Giovannini, 1988)

times and older subjects (Hoffmans,
1988).
There is more to obesity than
merely   disorderly eating. Genetic
and environmental factors such as
baseline energy expenditure and
under stress, inadequate or
inappropriate physical activity,
neuro-hormonal regulation set at
"permissive" levels for energy
sparing and accumulation, besides
eating the wrong types and amounts
of foods, can all contribute to
producing a certain physical
constitution, differing for each
obese person.
However, the first investigational
approach is to check eating
habits.   In a comparative study of
53 overweight and 56 non-obese
children aged between 7 and 14 years
(Figure 2;Giovannini, 1988) both
groups presented the same sort of
macronutrient intake imbalances as
outlined earlier, and were sedentary
for a large number of hours each
day.   The obese subjects, however,
tended to skip breakfast, or ate
only a small proportion of their
calories at that meal.
This finding might be indicative of
some "derangement" in the central
biorhythms regulating the sense of
hunger and satiety through hormonal
interactions (diminished peripheral
insulin sensitivity), metabolism
(high blood levels of neutral
aminoacids) and neurotransmitters
(reduced serotonin synthesis: Bray,
1987; Caballero, 1987).
This tendency to skip breakfast or
to eat the wrong things from a
nutritional viewpoint is widespread
among children, and becomes more
frequent with age (Michaud, 1990;
Cornelius,1991).   In some people

this habit might therefore play a part in producing obesity through a predisposition to early loss of the homeostatic balance mechanisms mentioned. This would not just be an effect or a marker, therefore, but a partial cause.

Eating breakfast has proved an effective means of reducing fat intake and minimizing compulsive snacking, suggesting it could have a useful role in weight reduction programmes (Schlundt,1992). It can also help limit energy intake at subsequent meals (de Graaf, 1992). Serum total cholesterol levels were higher in a population of students who did not eat breakfast (Resnicow,1991).

The association of obesity with eating no breakfast seems thus to identify a metabolic type with a less favourable metabolic "outcome" (Cornelius, 1991), particularly when this is expressed during adolescence. To reestablish the chronorhythm for nutrient intake it thus appears essential to distribute calorie consumption over the whole day, so as to help maintain physiological sensitivity to insulin. Dividing calorie intake over the day seems to result in a better general metabolic balance: better blood glucose control, and lower blood triglycerides and cholesterol (Jenkins, 1989).

2.3 Calcium and bone growth

In the first year of life it is straight forward enough to establish the optimal calcium intake on the basis of what mother's milk would provide, and from metabolic balance studies and the mineral content of bone. In adolescents, however, there is no "standard" against which to establish calcium requirements, so that opinions vary widely on real needs. Daily calcium intake in adolescence can and does vary widely without causing any evident clinical signs of deficit or excess.

Greer (1992) reported that calcium requirements, resulting from net retention, are significantly greater in infancy andadolescence than in any other stage of life. Age is in fact the most important determinant of calcium deposition in bone, age and ethnic origin having less effect. The skeleton contains about 99% of body calcium, and this supports three important events:

1. Skeletal growth length, volume and weight.
2. Skeletal maturation and modelling.
3. Continual redistribution and repair of bone tissue.

The first two are typical of children. Growth is fastest in adolescence, when about 45% of the total body calcium of an adult is deposited (Committee on Nutrition, 1978). Daily calcium deposition reaches 400 mg in males and 240 mg in females (Forbes, 1981).

Figure 3 illustrates the rise in body calcium during adolescence, for both sexes, measured by three different methods (Forbes, 1982; Garn, 1969; Garn, 1970).

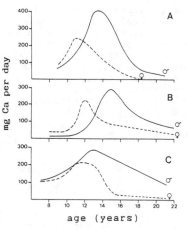

Figure 3. Body calcium increase during adolescence
A) Calculated on the basis of the body mass assuming 21.9 g calcium/kg (Forbes, 1972); B) Calculated on the basis of photodensitometry of the radius and ulna (Garn, 1969);
C) Calculated on the basis of the thickness and length ofthe metacarpal cortex (Garn, 1970)

All these methods show daily calcium rising more steeply and lastingly in males, although the peak is somewhat later than in females. In any event the final accumulation differs for the two sexes in relation to body weight, but once growth is complete it amounts to about 20 g of calcium per centimetre of height (Forbes, 1981).

All this underlines the importance of an adequate dietary intake of calcium in adolescence, and in fact the RDA, like the Italian Recommended Dietary Allowances (LARN), suggest an increase of 50% over the previous age group, rising from 800 to 1200 mg/day.

Although the extent of the positive calcium balance needed to ensure bone growth can be calculated, we still do not understand the genetic potential for its maximum (peak) growth. A recent report (Matkovic, 1992) suggests that calcium intakes below the peak retention capacity are associated with less calcium retention in the body, while exceeding this threshold ensures greater retention.

This does not involve any immediate risk of disease since calcium is an ubiquitous element and there is only one isolated case report of pathology linked to dietary deficits (Pettifor, 1981). However, scant calcium intake during the mineralization phase typical of adolescence could raise the risk of osteoporosis and fractures later in life (Matkovic, 1990).

A recent three-year longitudinal study (Johnston, 1992) compared bone density in two groups of preadolescents and adolescents, one given a supplement of 1 g/day of calcium. Bone mineralometry showed a significantly higher bone density in the supplemented group, but only in the prepuberal age. Another study (Matkovic, 1990), using the same investigational method, found a definite increase in bone density in adolescent females given a calcium supplement. It thus appears that the positive calcium balance, hence also its skeletal accumulation, tends to rise up to a calcium intake about double the current RDA (Anonymous, Nutrition Review, 1992), so that these recommendations could in fact be usefully revised for prepuberal and puberal children, especially considering the medical and social costs of osteoporosis (Norris, 1992). It has also been reported (Sandler, 1985) in post-menopausal women that their bone density was directly correlated with their intake of milk and dairy products at various ages. Adding to the probable inadequacy of the RDA the fact that some studies (Chan, 1991) found that about 85% of adolescents fail to reach the recommended intake anyway, and that intake is adequate (Chan, 1992) only in 15% of girls over 11 years old and 53% of boys, it is clearly essential to ensure adequate dietary sources of calcium, so as to prevent the calcium-lack disorders typical of the elderly particularly females. Chan (1992) listed several main causes of limited consumption of dairy products hence the reduced calcium intake. These included taste, a history of food allergy to milk proteins and diets with low calorie content or low animal fat content. There are of course always some patients with lactose intolerance, which seems to become more frequent with age. Lactose appears to facilitate intestinal calcium absorption, though this is still controversial.

Kocian (1973) gave whole or lactose-free milk to normal subjects and patients with a lactase deficit, and reported that total calcium absorption from whole milk was significantly greater in the normal subjects, but reduced in the lactase-deficient subjects. The two groups presented no differences when lactose-free milk was given. It thus appears that the reduced calcium absorption in lactase-deficient subjects depends either on a low intraluminal calcium concentration or on accelerated intestinal transit, both induced by the osmotic effect of non-absorbed lactose.

These findings were confirmed by studies in which purified substrates (calcium and lactose) were administered in place of milk to low-lactase subjects and normal controls (Cochet, 1983). There are, however, reports (Smith, 1985; Recker, 1988) that absorption of calcium from milk, yoghurt and other dairy products was the same in normal subjects and lactase-deficient patients, so that the higher incidence of osteoporosis in the latter can be attributed to the fact that they purposely avoided milk and dairy products, so as not to induce the symptoms of lactose intolerance.

It therefore appears advisable to recommend a higher intake of calcium-rich foods, but also to supplement certain foods with calcium so as to permit an adequate intake for everyone.

In the U.S.A. between 55-75% of daily calcium intake comes from dairy products (Allen, 1982; Block, 1985) such as milk, cheese and yoghurt. Other dietary sources are leafy vegetables, cereals and the "soft" bony tissues of fish and poultry. If, as we have seen, only a small percentage of "normal" adolescents achieve the recommended daily intake, in certain specific situations such as low-calorie diets, lactose and milk protein intolerance, and "mental" anorexia the risk of lowering the calcium reserves is even greater, with the likelihood of symptoms in adulthood or old age. Lactose intolerance is probably the most frequent of these situations; patients with this disorder are more likely to suffer osteoporosis than the normal population (Newcomer, 1978). These patients can nevertheless absorb calcium well from lactose-free dairy products such as yoghurt and seasoned cheeses, which are therefore an excellent alternative food (Smith, 1985).

3. MILK AND DAIRY PRODUCTS IN THE ADOLESCENT DIET: CREATING A NEW BALANCE FOR HEALTH.

These considerations indicate the main areas where something needs to be done about adolescent nutrition and about much of the Western pediatric population:
   1.Train adolescents to react independently of changing fads, by habituating them young from early infancy to take their meals following a physiological time pattern, with breakfast accounting for 20-25% of the daily calorie intake.
   2.Avoid excessive intake of animal-origin foods, while bearing in mind that iron and calcium must be taken inadequate amounts, in the correct ratio.
   3.Ensure sufficient consumption of nutrients such as fibre, vitamins and minerals that "fast foods" and somehome-prepared convenience foods too often do not cover for various reasons (composition, cooking method, storage time). Calcium is the micronutrient that seems to require most urgent revision of the intake recommendations, since the right amounts can have outstanding beneficial effects on mediumand long-term health.
It is thus clear that milk and dairy products must necessarily be the main source of animal protein on account of their high calcium content; iron is supplied by vegetables, supplemented as necessary, and these also provide complex carbohydrates and fibre.
It is advisable to eat breakfast as a habit for setting the alimentary chronorhythm, since this helps prevent both anorexia and obesity. Its ideal composition based on what we have already noted is milk or yoghurt with cereals enriched in vitamins and minerals. Whole milk and yoghurt contribute to the intake of nutrients needed by the rapidly growing adolescent, such as liposoluble vitamins and essential fatty acids.
Numerous findings are now available on the functions of polyunsaturated fats in pregnancy and early childhood, but we know little about the requirements in adolescence, with its rapid growth and maturation. Milk contains both linoleic and linolenic acid (not a large amount but the ratio is virtually one-to-one), so this food helps balance the overall intake of these molecules which might otherwise be shifted in favour of linoleic acid.
Dairy products should be served as a normal part of the main meals, not just an after thought but an actual dish, so as to raise calcium intake to the maximum levels required. Cheese dishes can be alternated during the week with meat or eggs, fish and legumes, so as to ensure iron intake, long-chain polyunsaturated fatty acids, complex carbohydrates and soluble fibre. Cheese should be eaten with green vegetables, so as to create a balance similar to the milk and cereals in the morning (or as a mid-morning snack).
Children who have stopped taking milk because of presumed intolerance should be told how to eat dairy products so as not to induce symptoms, i.e. by distributing their milk intake over the day, or by selecting products in which the lactose is predigested, or whose composition ensures its "auto-digestion", such as yoghurt.

4 CONCLUSIONS

Milk and dairy products offer a virtually complete macro and micronutrient content for the adolescent diet, apart from iron and fibre. Taken together with vegetable foods with a good iron and vitamin content they help complete

the nutritional spectrum, and this
is an ideal dietary combination for
this age group, considering their
needs and the corrections needed to
compensate current eating trends.
In the light of these remarks, the
dairy products industry might be
interested in the suggestion, already
being implemented in some countries,
that it supply products with
appropriate calcium supplementation,
with modifications to the fat
content as needed from the
quantitative and qualitative
viewpoints raising the ratio of
polyunsaturated to saturated fats.
This would meet requirements for
growth and for disease prevention.
Even earlier in life, though, a child
must get used to eating milk and
dairy products, particularly at
breakfast, and should not drop this
habit of infancy. This will be a
helpful step toward nutritional
education in a stage of life when
eating fads and self-imposed diets
easily oust certain weakly rooted
traditions.

REFERENCES

Allen, L.H., 1982.Calcium
bioavailability and absorption: a
review. Am. J. Clin. Nutr. 35:
783-808

Anonymous 1992.Maximizing peak bone
mass: calcium supplementation
increases bone mineral density in
children.Nutr. Rev. 50: 335- 337.

Bender, A.E., Magee, P. and Nash, AH
1972.Survey of school meals.
Br. Med. J. 2: 383-391.

Block, G., Dresser ,C.M., Hartman,
A.M., et al. 1985.Nutrient
sourcesin the American diet:
quantitative data from the NHANES
II survey. I. Vitamins and
minerals. Am. J. Epidemiol.
122:13-26

Bray, C.A. 1987.Obesity. A disease of
nutrient or energy balance ?
Nutr. Rev. 45: 33-42.

Caballero, B. 1987.Insulin resistance
and amino acid metabolism in
obesity.In: Wurtman R.J., Wurtman
J.J. (eds) "Human Obesity", Ann. N.
Y. Acad. Sci. 499: 84-92.

Chan, G.M. 1991. Dietary calcium and
bone mineral status of children and
adolescents.Am. J. Clin. Nutr. 145:
631-4.

Chan, G.M. 1992. Calcium and bone
mineral deficiency from dieting
children and adolescents.
(Abstract) J. Am. Coll. Nutr. 11:
627.

Cochet, B. and Jung, A. 1983.Effects
of lattose on intestinal calcium
absorption in normal and
lactose-deficient subjects.
Gastroenterol. 84:935-40

Cornelius, L.J. 1991. Health habits
of school-age children. J. Health
Care Poor Underserved; 2:374-395.

Committee on Nutrition 1978. Calcium
requirements in infancy and
childhood. Pediatrics 62:826-33

de Graaf, C., Hulshof, T.,
Weststrate, J.A. and Jas, P. 1992.
Short-term effects of different
amounts of protein, fats and
carbohydrates on satiety. Am. J.
Clin. Nutr. 55: 33-38.

Forbes, G.B. 1982. Growth of the
lean body mass in man. Growth
36:325

Forbes, G.B., 1981. Nutritional
requirements in adolescence. In
Suskind R.M. (Ed.) "Textbook of
Pediatric Nutrition", New York,
Raven Press: 243-268.

Garn, S.M. and Wagner, B. 1969. The
adolescence growth of the skeletal
mass and its implications to
mineral requirements. In "
Adolescent nutrition and
growth",Raven Press New
York:128-149.

Garn, S.M. 1970. The earlier gain
and later loss of cortical bone in
nutrition perspective.
Springfield III Ed., Thomas
Publisher : 165-189.

Giovannini, M., Galluzzo, C.,
Scaglioni, S. et al. 1986.
Indagine nutrizionale nel Comune
di Milano: dati antropometrici,
intake calorici e abitudini
alimentari in età scolare. Riv.
Ital. Pediatr. 12: 533-540.

Giovannini, M., Scaglioni, S.,
Ortisi, M.T. et al.1988. Indagine
nutrizionale sulla popolazione
scolastica di Milano. Rilievi
anamnestici, biochimici e clinici
su due gruppi di bambini: obesi
vs. obesi. Riv. Ital. Pediatr. 14:
365-371.

Gong, E.J., and Heald, F.P. 1988.
Diet, nutrition and adolescence.
In: Modern nutrition in health and
disease (7th Ed.); ME Shils, VR
Young Eds, Lea & Febiger,
Philadelphia: 969981.

Greer, R. 1992. Pediatric calcium
needs and metabolism beyond
infancy. In Tsong R.C., Mimouni F.
eds."Calcium nutriture for mothers
and children". Carnation nutrition
Education Series Vol.3
Glendale/Raven Press, New York:
89-102.

Hoffmans, M.D., Kromhout, D., and de Lezenne Coulander, C. 1988. The impact of body mass index of 78,618 18-year old Dutch men on 32-year mortality from all causes. J. Clin. Epidemiol. 41: 749-756.

Jenkins, D.J.A., Wolever, T.M.S., Jenkins ,A.L. et al. 1989. Nibbling versus gorging: metabolic advantages of increased meal frequency. N. Engl. J. Med. 321: 929-934.

Johnston, C.C., Miller, J.Z., Slemenda, C.W. et al. 1992. Calcium supplementation and increases in bone mineral density in children. N. Engl. J. Med. 327: 82-7

Kocian, J., Skale, I., and Bakos K. 1973. Calcium absorption from milk and lactose-free milk in healthy subjects and patients with lactose intolerance. Digestion 9:311-24.

LARN. Recommended Dietary Allowances for the Italian Population. Revised 1986-87. Istituto Nazionale della Nutrizione, Roma, 1987.

Lew, E.A. and Garfinkel, L. 1979. Variation in mortality by weight among 750.000, men and women. J. Chronic. Dis. 32: 563- 576.

Lifshitz, F., Moses, N., Cervantes , G. and Ginsberg, L. 1987. Nutritional dwarfing in adolescence. Sem. Adolescent. Med. 3: 255-256.

Lifshitz, F. and Moses, N. 1987. Growth failure: a complication of hypercholesterolemia treatment. J. Am. Coll. Nutr.6: 450 (Abstract).

Maloney, M., Morrison, J., Turns, M., et al. 1992. The prevalence of dieting behavior and atypical eating attitudes in children. J. Am. Coll. Nutr. 11: 626 (Abstract 98)

Matkovic, V., Fontana, D., Tominac, C. et al. 1990. Factors that influence peak bone mass formation: a study of calcium balance and the inheritance of bone mass in adolescent females. Am. J. Clin. Nutr. 1990; 52:878-88

Matkovic, V. 1991. Calcium metabolism and calcium requirements during skeletal modeling consolidation of bone mass. Am. J. Clin. Nutr. 54 (Suppl 1): 2455-2605

Matkovic, V. 1992. Calcium intake and peak bone mass. N. Engl. J. Med. 327: 119-120

Michaud, C., Musse, N., Nicolas, J.P. et al. 1990. Nutrient intakes and food consumption in the adolescent's schoolday breakfast in Lorraine (France). Nutr. Res. 10: 1195-1203.

Moore, D.C. 1988. Body image and eating behavior in adolescent girls. Am. J. Dis. Child. 142: 1114-1118.

Must, A., Jacques, P.F., Dallal, G.E., et al. 1992. Long term morbidity and mortality of overweight adolescents. N. Engl. J. Med. 327: 1350-5.

Newcomer, A.D., Hodgson, S.F., Mc Gill, D.B., et al. 1978. Lactase deficiency: prevalence in osteoporosis. Ann. Intern. Med. 89:218-20

Norris, R.J. 1992. Medical costs in osteoporosis. Bone 13:511-6

Pettifor, J.M., Ross, F.P., Travers, R., et al. 1981. Dietary calcium deficiency: a syndrome associated with bone deformities and elevated serum 1,25-dihydroxyvitamin D concentrations. Metab. Bone Dis. Relat. Res. 2:301-5

Recker, R.R., Bammi, A., Barger-Inx, M.J. et al. 1988. Calcium absorbability from milk products, an imitation milk, and calcium carbonate. Am. J. Clin. Nutr. 47:93-5

Resnicow, K. 1991. The relationship between breakfast habits and plasma cholesterol levels in schoolchildren. J. Sch. Health 61: 81-85.

Richardson, D.P. and Lawson, M. 1972. Nutritional value of mid- day meals in senior school children. Br. Med. J. 4: 697-702.

Salz, K.M., Israel, T. and Ernst, N. 1983. Selected nutrient intakes of free-living white children aged 6-19 years: the lipid research clinics (LRC) program prevalence study. Pediatr. Res. 17: 124-331.

Sandler, R.B., Slemenda, C.W., La Porte, R.E., et al. 1985. Postmenopausal bone density and milk consumption in childhood and adolescence. Am. J. Clin. Nutr. 42:270-4

Schlundt, D.G., Hill, J.O., Sbrocco, T., et al.1992. The role of breakfast in the treatment of obesity: a randomized clinical trial. Am. J. Clin. Nutr. 55: 645-651.

Smith, T.M., Kohlars, J.C., Savoiano, D.A. et al. 1985. Absorption of calcium from milk and yogurt. Am. J. Clin. Nutr. 42: 1197-200

Thomas, J.A., and Call, D.L. 1973. Eating between meals: a nutrition problem among teenagers. Nutr. Rev. 31: 137-141.

Dairy Products in Human Health and Nutrition, Serrano Ríos et al. (eds) © 1994 Balkema, Rotterdam, ISBN 90 5410 359 0

Peptide hormones and growth factors in bovine milk

O. Koldovský
Department of Pediatrics and The Steele Memorial Children's Research Center, University of Arizona, College of Medicine, Tucson, Ariz., USA

ABSTRACT: Bovine milk, as milk of other species, contains various peptide hormones and growth factors. Their concentration is changed during the duration of lactation and by hormonal treatment of the lactating cow. Pasteurization has, in many cases, no effect, whereas heating decreases considerably their concentration in dairy milk. In infant formula they are either absent or present, only in low concentrations, as compared to dairy milk or human breast milk. The potential significance of peptide hormones and growth factors present in dairy milk and milk products is discussed.

1. PRESENCE IN BOVINE MILK

It is well established that the milk of various mammals contain hormones and growth factors (GF). In this review, we will discuss in detail only bovine milk; the interested reader may find information about other aspects and especially comparison with human milk in recent reviews (Koldovský & Thornburg 1987, Koldovský 1989a, 1989b, 1993, Koldovský et al. 1993).

Table I lists hormone growth factors detected in bovine milk. Most of the data were obtained from cows after the birth of their offspring; some studies report data on dairy milk.

2. FACTORS AFFECTING THEIR CONCENTRATIONS IN BOVINE MILK

In Table II, I have compiled data about factors that affect their concentrations in milk. With the exception of somatostatin, the other five peptides studied were found to be more concentrated in colostrum than in the milk. Changes during lactation were reported only for GRP and PHrP.

Treatment of lactating cows with recombinant bovine growth hormone (bGH), called also bovine somatropin (bST), did not increase the bGH concentration in the milk of treated cows (Groenewegen et al. 1990, Torkelson et al. 1987) but caused an increase in insulin-

TABLE I. Hormonally active peptides in bovine milk.

HYPOTHALAMO–HYPOPHYSEAL HORMONES

Bovine Growth Hormone	Groenewegen et al. 1990, Juskevich & Guyer 1990, Torkelson et al. 1987
GnRH	Baram et al. 1977
Prolactin	Akers & Kaplan 1989, Erb et al. 1977, Malven 1977, Malven et al. 1987a, McMurtry et al. 1975
TRH	Baram et al. 1977

GASTROINTESTINAL REGULATORY PEPTIDES

GRP	Jahnke & Lazarus 1984, Takeyama et al. 1989, Takeyama et al. 1990
Somatostatin	Takeyama et al. 1990
VIP	Takeyama et al. 1990

PARATHYROID HORMONE RELATED PEPTIDE

Budayr et al. 1989, Goff et al. 1991, Ratcliffe et al. 1990, Thurston et al. 1990, Erb et al. 1977, Law et al. 1991, Stewart et al. 1991

GROWTH FACTORS

EGF & related GF	Carpenter 1980, Klagsbrun & Neumann 1979, Shing & Klagsbrun 1984, Tapper et al. 1979, Yagi et al. 1986
IGF-I	Campbell & Baumrucker 1989, Juskevich & Guyer 1990, Malven et al. 1987b, Nagashima et al. 1990, Prosser et al. 1989, Schams & Einspanier 1991
IGF-II	Juskevich & Guyer 1990, Malven et al. 1987b
Insulin	Malven et al. 1987b, Nowak 1989, Slebodzinski et al. 1986
TGFß	Cox & Burk 1991, Stoeck et al. 1989a, Stoeck et al. 1989b, Tokuyama & Tokuyama 1989

TABLE II. Changes in concentrations of hormonally active peptides in bovine milk.

FACTORS	EFFECTS
Higher in colostrum	GRP: Takeyama et al. 1990 IGF-1: Malven et al. 1987b Insulin: Malven et al. 1987b Prolactin: Erb et al. 1977, Malven 1977 VIP: Takeyama et al. 1990
Similar in colostrum and milk	Somatostatin: Takeyama et al. 1990
Decrease during duration of lactation	GRP: Takeyama et al. 1990
Increase during duration of lactation	Parathyroid hormone related peptide: Goff et al. 1991
Effect of breed and and cow treatment	bGH: same levels in bGH and non-bGH treated controls, Groenewegen et al. 1990, Torkelson et al. 1987. IGF-1: increased in milk of lactating non-pregnant cows treated s.c. with bGH, Prosser et al. 1989. Parathyroid hormone related peptide: Jersey cows exhibit 20% higher values than Friesian, Goff et al. 1991. Prolactin: increased in milk of cows kept at low or high extreme temperatures, McMurtry et al. 1975.
Pasteurization and heating	bGH: heat treatment reduces the values to 10%, Juskevich & Guyer 1990. EGF+undefined growth factors: pasteurization reduces values by 50%, Yagi et al. 1986. IGF-1: pasteurization does not destroy, but heating does, Juskevich & Guyer 1990. Parathyroid hormone related peptide: present in similar concentrations in commercial whole, low - and no-fat milk; about 20 x lower in buttermilk and chocolate milk, Budayr et al. 1989. No effect of pasteurization, Ratcliffe et al. 1990.
Infant formulae	EGF: absent: Carpenter 1980, Tapper et al. 1979, Yagi et al. 1986, our own unpublished data. IGF-1: low to absent: Nagashima et al. 1990, Juskevich & Guyer 1990. Insulin: very low: Read et al. 1985. Parathyroid hormone related peptide: about 10% as in bovine milk; one formula had higher values (33%); in soya-based formula was not detectable, Budayr, et al. 1989.

like growth factor-1 (IGF-1) levels in their milk. The problems of eventual health hazards from the presence of bGH and IGF-1 in milk from cows treated with recombinant bGH were discussed at the NIH Technology Assesment Conference "Bovine Somatotropin" in December 7, 1990. Abstracts of presentations at this meetings were published by the Office of Medical Application of Research of the National Institues of Health, Bethesda, Maryland, USA. It is known that bGH has no effects in humans and its chances to "survive" in the gastrointestinal tract of human adults are minimal. A reported increase of IGF-1 in the milk of bGH treated dairy cows was also considered negligible. The conference thus concluded that bGH treatment of dairy cows does not possess an endocrine risk for the human population, but recommended further studies to explore possible effects of orally-consumed IGF-1 on the gastrointestinal tract. Several papers and comments concerning the problem of treating cows with bGH were published in scientific journals (Anderson 1990; Anonymous 1991; Cherfas 1990; Epstein 1990, 1991a, 1991b; Erickson 1990; Gibbons 1990a, 1990b Juskevich & Guyer 1990, 1991; Kronfeld 1991; Reotutar 1990; Shulman 1989; Sun 1989; Weldon 1991).

Interestingly, pasteurization does not affect concentration of EGF and related peptides, IGF-1 and PHrP (as assayed by radioreceptor assay, which is not specific for EGF and actually authentic EGF [Carpenter& Baumrucker 1989, Klagsbrun & Neumann 1979, Shing & Klagsbrun 1984, Tapper et al. 1979, Yagi et al. 1986] might not be present in bovine milk at all). Heating (boiling) on the other hand reduces considerable bGH and IGF-1 milk levels.

From a pediatric nutritional point of view, it is interesting that several peptides, present in human breast milk (Koldovský 1989b, Koldovský et al. 1993) are low or absent in infant formulae.

3. FUNCTIONAL SIGNIFICANCE OF MILK-BORNE HORMONES FOR THE HUMAN

This question relating to the nutrition of newborn infants has been actively explored in recent years using laboratory animals. Available data allow us only to speculate about the effect of bovine milk-borne hormones and growth factors on adult human subjects. From the preceeding review, it is clear that we have only little data about the presence of these peptides in pasteurized milk. Furthermore, most of the data were obtained by radioimmunoassays. It is well established, that the immunological reactivity of peptides does not prove their biological activity; other characterizations, including biossays, are needed.

Be as it may, "survival" (i.e., resistance to proteolytic degradation) in the stomach is necessary if ingested peptide is to function within the gastrointestinal tract. As a first approach to this question in the human neonate, Britton, et al. (1989) have shown that degradation of ^{125}I-human recombinant EGF by the gastric juices of preterm infants *in vitro* is negligible. Similar findings were obtained with gastric juices of suckling and weanling rats (Britton, et al. 1988). Studies with gastric contents demonstrated only a small decrease in EGF "survival" with maturation. Studies with intestinal luminal content indicate developmental changes. In suckling rats the degradation was low,

however, it increased in weanling rats (Britton, et al. 1988). Similar preliminary studies performed in our laboratory with gastric juices of adult subjects indicate a developmental increase of EGF degradation, but there is still considerable "survival" of EGF. Studies performed *in vivo* have shown that orogastrically administered ^{125}I-EGF to suckling rats was degraded very little in the stomach and small intestinal lumen (Thornburg et al. 1984, Thornburg et al. 1987). Similar results were seen in suckling mice (Popliker et al. 1987) and lambs (Read et al. 1987). In mature rats the degradation was increased, but still some ^{125}I-EGF remained intact and was absorbed (Thornburg et al. 1987).

It is noteworthy that intraluminally administered EGF affects several functions in maturing or mature rats. In weaned rats, EGF given enterally reduced mucosal permeability to HCl (Tepperman & Soper 1989). The addition of EGF to the jejunal perfusate in adult rats increased within 20 minutes absorption of H_2O, Na^+, Cl, and glucose (Opleta-Madsen et al. 1991). Contraversy exists about the trophic effect of EGF administered for a longer period.

Goodlad et al. (1987) found no effect after intraluminal administration, but Ulshen et al. (1986) reported a trophic effect of intraileally administered EGF on the rat gastroduodenal mucosa.

4. CONCLUSIONS

It is clear that we know many facts about this problem, but many more studies must to be performed to conclude whether hormones and growth factors in bovine milk have any effect on the gastrointestinal tract (or even beyond) of the adult human consumer. If effects are found, they might have both positive and negative effects.

REFERENCES

Akers, R.M. & R.M. Kaplan. 1989. Role of milk secretion in transport of prolactin from blood into milk. *Horm. Metabol. Res.* 21:362-365.

Anderson, G.C, 1990. Health worries over use of milk hormone. *Nature* 345:280.

Anonymous. 1991. Safety of bovine growth hormone. *Science* 251:256-257.

Baram, T, Y. Koch, E. Hazum, & M. Fridkin. 1977. Gonadotropin-releasing hormone in milk. *Science* 198: 300-302.

Britton, J.R., C. George-Nascimento & O. Koldovský. 1988. Luminal hydrolysis of recombinant human epidermal growth factor in the rat gastrointestinal tract: Segmental and developmental differences. *Life Sci.* 43:1339-1347.

Britton, J.R., C. George-Nascimento, J.N. Udall & O. Koldovský. 1989. Minimal hydrolysis of epidermal growth factor by gastric fluid of preterm infants. *Gut* 30:327-332.

Budayr, A.A., B.P. Halloran, J.C. King, D. Diep, R.A. Nissenson & G.J. Strewler. 1989. High levels of a parathyroid hormone-like protein in milk. Proc. Natl. Acad. Sci. 86:7183-7185.

Campbell, P.G. & C.R. Baumrucker. 1989. Insulin-like growth factor-I and its association with binding proteins in bovine milk. *J. Endocrinol.* 120:21-29.

Carpenter, G. 1980. Epidermal growth factors as a major growth promoting agent in human milk. *Science* 210:198-199.

Cherfas, J. 1990. Europe: Bovine growth hormone in a political maze. *Science* 249:852-853.

Cox, D.A. & R.R. Burk. 1991. Isolation and characterisation of milk growth factor, in transforming-growth-factor-β2-related polypeptide, from bovine milk. *Eur. J. Biochem.* 197:353-358.

Epstein, S.S. 1990, Potential public health hazards of biosynthetic milk hormones. *Int. J. Health Serv.* 20:73-84

Epstein, S.S. 1991a. Potential public health hazards of biosynthetic milk hormones. *Int. J. Health Serv.* 21:372:373.

Epstein, S.S. 1991b. A reply to Virginia Weldon. *Intl. J. Health Serv.* 21:563-564.

Erb, R.E., B.P. Chew, H.F. Keller & P.V. Malven. 1977. Effect of hormonal treatments prior to lactation on hormones in blood plasma, milk, and urine during early lactation. *J. Dairy Sci.* 60:557-565.

Erickson, D. 1990. Trojan Cow. An embattled hormone raises social questions [news]. *Sci. Am.* 263:26.

Gibbons, A. 1990a. FDA publishes bovine growth hormone data. *Science* 249: 852-853.

Gibbons, A. 1990b. NIH panel: bovine hormone gets the nod. *Science* 250:1506.

Goff, J.P., T.A. Reinhardt, S. Lee & B.W. Hollis. 1991. Parathyroid hormone-related peptide content of bovine milk and calf blood assessed by radioimmunoassay and bioassay. *Endocrinology* 129:2815-2819.

Goodlad, R.A., T.J.G. Wilson, W. Lenton, H. Gregory, K.G. McCullagh & N.A. Wright. 1987. Intravenous but not intragastric urogastrone-EGF is tropic to the intestine of parenterally fed rats. *Gut* 28:573-582.

Groenewegen, P.P., B.W. McBride, J.H. Burton & T.H. Elsasser. 1990. Bioactivity of milk from bST-treated cows. *J. Nutr.* 120:514-520.

Jahnke, G.D & L H. Lazarus. 1984. A bombesin immunoreactive peptide in milk. *Proc Natl. Acad. Sci. USA* 81:578-582.

Juskevich, J.C. & C.G. Guyer. 1990. Bovine growth hormone: human food safety evaluation. *Science* 249: 875-884.

Juskevich, J.C. & C.G. Guyer. 1991. Response to Kronfeld. *Science* 251:256-257.

Klagsbrun, M. & J. Neumann. 1979. The serum-free growth of BALB/c3T3 cells in medium supplemented with bovine colostrum. *J. Supramol. Struct.* 1:349-359.

Koldovský, O. 1989a. Hormones in milk: their possible physiological significance for the neonate. *Textbook of Gastroenterology and Nutrition in Infancy,* 2nd Edition. Raven Press Ltd, New York.

Koldovský, O. 1989b. Critical review: Search for role of milk-borne biologically active peptides for the suckling. *J. Nutr.* 19:1543-1551.

Koldovský, O. 1993. Do hormones in milk affect the functions of the neonatal intestine? Presented at the American Society of Zoologist Meeting, December 1992, Vancouver BC. *Amer. Zool., in press.*

Koldovský, O. & W. Thornburg. 1987. Hormones in milk: A review. *J. Pediatr. Gastro. Nutr.* 6:172-196.

Koldovský, O., W. Kong, R.K. Rao & P. Schaudies. 1993. Milk-borne peptide growth factors. *Immunophysiology of the Gut,* Vol. 11 of the Bristol-Myers Squibb/Mead Johnson Nutrition Symposia, in press.

Kronfeld, D. 1991. Safety of bovine growth hormone. *Science* 251:256.

Law, F.M. , P.J. Moate, D.D. Leaver, H. Diefenbach-Jagger, V. Grill , P.W. Ho & T.J. Martin. 1991. Parathyroid hormone-related protein in milk and its correlation with bovine milk calcium. *J. Endocrinol.* 1281:21-6.

Malven, P.V. 1977. Prolactin and other protein hormones in milk. *J. Animal Sci.* 46:609-616.

Malven, P.V., H. H. Head & R.J. Collier. 1987a. Secretion and mammary gland uptake of prolactin in dairy cows during lactogenesis. *J. Dairy Sci.* 70:2241-2253.

Malven, P.V., H.H. Head, R.J. Collier & F.C. Buonomo. 1987b. Periparturient changes in secretion and mammary uptake of insulin and in concentrations of insulin and insulin-like growth factors in milk of dairy cows. *J. Dairy Sci.* 70:2254-2265.

McMurtry, I.F., P.V. Malven, C.W. Arave, R.E. Erb & R.B. Harrington. 1975. Environmental and lactational variables affecting prolactin concentrations in bovine milk. *J. Dairy Sci.* 58:181-189.

Nagashima, K., K. Itoh & T. Kuroume. 1990. Levels of insulin-like growth factor in full and preterm human milk in comparison to levels in cow's milk and in milk formulas. *Biol. Neonate* 58:343-346.

Nowak, J. 1989. Changes of insulin concentration in colostrum and milk of women, cows and sows. *Acta Physiologica Polonica* 40:349-355.

Opleta-Madsen, K., J. Hardin & D.G. Gall. 1991. Epidermal growth factor upregulates intestinal electrolyte and nutrient transport. *Am. J. Physiol.* 260: G807-G814.

Popliker, M., A. Shatz, A. Avivi, A. Ullrich, J. Schlessinger & C.G. Webb. 1987. Onset of endogenous synthesis of epidermal growth factor in neonatal mice. *Dev. Biol.* 119:38-44.

Prosser, C.G., I.R. Fleet & A.N. Corps. 1989. Increased secretion of insulin-like growth factor I into milk of cows treated with recombinantly derived bovine growth hormone. *J. Dairy Res.* 56:17-26.

Ratcliffe, W.A., E. Green, J. Emly, S. Norsbury, M. Lindsay, D.A. Heath & J.G. Ratcliffe, 1990. Identification and partial characterization of parathyroid hormone-related protein in human and bovine milk. *J. Endocrinol.* 127:167-178.

Read, L.C., G.L. Francis, J.C. Wallace & F.J. Ballard. 1985. Growth factor concentrations and growth-promoting activity in human milk following premature birth. *J. Dev. Physiol.* 7:135-145.

Read, L.C., S.M. Gale & C. George-Nacimento. 1987. Intestinal absorption of epidermal growth factor in newborn lambs. *Human Lactation 3: The Effects of Human Milk on the Recipient Infant.* Plenum Press, New York.

Reotutar, R. 1990. Bovine growth hormone raises national concern. *J. Am. Vet. Med. Assoc.* 196:1018.

Schams, D. & R. Einspanier. 1991. Growth hormone, IGF-I and insulin in mammary gland secretion before and after parturition and possibility of their transfer into the calf. *Endocr. Regul.* 25:139-43.

Shing, Y.W. & M. Klagsbrun. 1984. Human and bovine milk contain different sets of growth factors. *Endocrinology* 115:273-282.

Shulman. S. 1989. U.S. opposition to milk hormone. *Nature* 340:667.

Slebodzinski, A.B., J. Nowak, H. Gawecka, & A. Sechman. 1986. Thyroid hormones and insulin in milk: A comparative study. *Endocrin. Exper.* 20:247-255.

Stewart, A.F., T.L. Wu, K.L. Insogna, L.M. Milstone & W.J. Burtis. 1991. Immunoaffinity purification of parathyroid hormone-related protein from bovine milk and human keratinocyte-conditioned medium. *J. Bone Miner. Res.* 6:305- 310.

Stoeck, M., C. Ruegg, S. Miescher, S. Carrel, D. Cox V. Von Fliedner & S. Alkan. 1989a. Comparison of the immunosuppressive properties of milk growth factor and transforming growth factors b1 and b2. *J. Immunol.* 143:3258-3265.

Stoeck, M., H. Sommermeyer, S. Miescher, D. Cox, S. Alkan & M. Szamel. 1989b. Transforming growth factors b1 and b2 as well as milk growth factor decrease anti-CD3-induced proliferation of human lymphocytes without inhibiting the anti-CD3-mediated increase of $[Ca^{2+}]^i$ and the activation of protein kinase C. *FEBS Lett.* 249:289-292.

Sun, M. 1989. Market sours on milk hormone. *Science* 246:876-877.

Takeyama, M., K. Kondo, Y, Hayashi & H. Yajima. 1989. Enzyme immunoassay of gastrin releasing peptide (GRP)-like immunoreactivity in milk. *Int. J. Pept. Protein Res.* 34:70-74.

Takeyama, M., N. Yanaga, K. Yarimizu, J. Ono, R. Takaki, N. Fujii & H. Yajima, 1990. Enzyme immunoassay of somatostatin (SS)-like immunoreactive substance in bovine milk. *Chem. Pharm. Bull.* 38:456-459.

Tapper, D., M. Klagsbrun & J. Neumann. 1979. The identification and clinical implications of human breast milk mitogen. *J. Pediatr. Surg.* 14:803-808.

Tepperman, B.L. & B. D. Soper. 1989. Effect of epidermal growth factor on the ontogenic response of gastric mucosa to H+. *Am. J. Physiol.* 257:G851-G859.

Thornburg, W., L. Matrisian, B. Magun, O. Koldovský. 1984. Gastrointestinal absorption of epidermal growth factor in suckling rats. *Am. J. Physiol.* 246:G80-G85.

Thornburg, W., R.K. Rao, L.M. Matrisian, B.E. Magun & O. Koldovský. 1987. Effect of maturation on gastrointestinal absorption of epidermal growth factor in rats. *Am. J. Physiol.* 253:G68-G71.

Thurston, A.W., J.A. Cole, L.S. Hillman, J.H. Imo, P.K. Thorne, W.J. Krause, J.R. Jones, S.L. Eber & L.R. Forte. 1990. Purification and properties of parathyroid hormone-related peptide isolated from milk. *Endocrinology* 126:1183-1190.

Tokuyama, H. & Y. Tokuyama. 1989. Bovine colostric transforming growth factor-b-like peptide that induces growth inhibition and changes in morphology of human osteogenic sarcoma cells (MG-63). *Cell Biol. Internat. Repts.* 13:251-258.

Torkelson, A.R., K.A. Dwyer, G.J. Rogan & R.L. Ryan. 1987. Radioimmunoassay of somatotropin in milk from cows administered recombinant bovine somatotropin. *Proc. Dairy Sci. Meeting,* University of Missouri.

Ulshen, M.H., L.E. Lyn-Cook & R.H. Raasch. 1986. Effects of intraluminal epidermal growth factors on mucosal proliferation in the small intestine of adult rats. *Gastroenterology* 91:1134-1140.

Weldon, V.V. 1991. A response to Samuel Epstein's article on synthetic bovine growth hormone. *Int. J. Health Serv.* 21:561-562.

Yagi, H., S. Suzuki, T. Noji, K. Nagashima & T. Kuroume. 1986. Epidermal growth factor in cow's milk and milk formulas. *Acta Pediatr. Scand.* 75:233-235.

Dairy Products in Human Health and Nutrition, Serrano Ríos et al. (eds) © 1994 Balkema, Rotterdam, ISBN 90 5410 359 0

Metabolic interactions during pregnancy in preparation for lactation

E. Herrera, P. Ramos, P. López-Luna & M. A. Lasunción
Departamento de Investigación, Hospital Ramón y Cajal, and Departamento de Bioquímica y Biología Molecular, Universidad de Alcalá de Henares, Madrid, Spain

1 INTRODUCTION

Gestation is a physiological condition in which the fetus develops at the cost of nutrients crossing the placenta. Among these nutrients, glucose is quantitatively the most important, followed by amino acids (Herrera et al. 1985; Lasunción et al. 1987), and the continuous dependence of the fetus on these compounds is well known. This causes the tendencies in the mother to develop both hypoglycemia and hypoaminoacidemia.

In order to support this continuous extraction of nutrients by the fetus, the mother has to adapt her own metabolism. One of the parameters most affected in the mother is her lipidic metabolism, in spite of the fact that with the exception of ketone bodies and free fatty acids, the placenta is practically impermeable to lipids (Herrera et al. 1990; Herrera et al. 1992a).

Altough it has been long known that the mother accumulates a great proportion of fat depots and develops hyperlipidemia during gestation (Hytten, Leitch, 1971; Beaton et al. 1954), the functional role of such adaptations has not been known until more recently. Now we know, that besides being an alternative source of energy and of gluconeogenetic substrates (Herrera et al. 1992c), these lipids play an essential role in the preparation for lactation. This is the reason why we will analyze here the accumulation of fat depots in the mother during gestation and its physiological consequences, with special emphasis on its role in mammary gland preparation for lactation.

2 MATERNAL BODY FAT ACCUMULATION AND DEVELOPMENT OF HYPERLIPIDEMIA

During gestation, the increase in maternal body weight corresponds not only to the growth of the fetal-placental unit, but to her own structures. The latter is mainly the result of an increase in fat depots, which has been demonstrated both in humans (Hytten,

Leitch, 1971) and in the rat (Herrera et al. 1988; López-Luna et al. 1986; Beaton et al. 1954). This change occurs during the first two thirds of gestation (Herrera et al. 1988; Beaton et al. 1954) and has a relationship with the maternal hyperphagia since it disappears with condition of food restriction (Lederman, Rosso, 1980; Moore, Brassel, 1984; Fain, Scow, 1966).

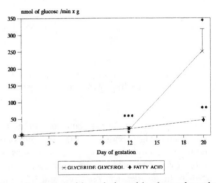

Figure 1.- Fatty acids and glyceride glycerol synthesis by periuterine adipose tissue *in situ* during gestation in the rat. Methodological details have been previously described (Palacín et al., 1991). Values are means ± SEM. Statistical comparisons versus virgin rats (0 days of gestation) are shown by astherisks.

Maternal increase in fat depots is also a consequence of the metabolic changes occurring during the first two thirds of gestation. On the one hand, as shown in figure 1, the synthesis of both fatty acids and glyceride glycerol from glucose in the periuterine fat pad from rats studied *in situ* increases progressively up the 20th day of gestation (Palacín et al. 1991) indicating that triglyceride synthesis is enhanced. On the other hand, we have previously shown that the activity of lipoprotein lipase (LPL) in lumbar fat pads is increased at day 12 of gestation in the rat as compared to virgin controls (Herrera et al. 1992b).

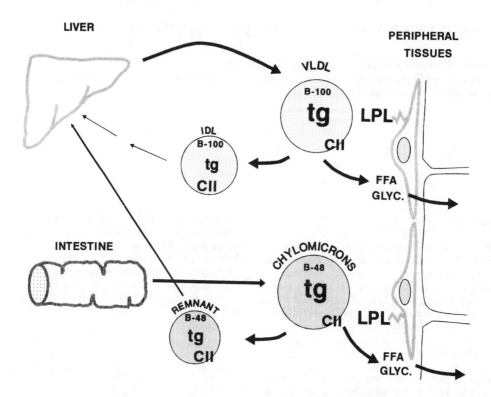

Figure 2.- Role of lipoprotein lipase (LPL) present in the capillary endothelium on the metabolism of triglyceride-rich lipoproteins and the hydrolysis and tissue uptake of circulating triglycerides.

This enzyme is present in the capillary endothelium and hydrolyses the triglycerides that circulate in blood associated to either chylomicrons or very low density lipoproteins (VLDL), which are converted into lipoproteins of higher density, remnants and IDL and LDL respectivelly (figure 2). In this way, LPL facilitates the uptake by the tissue of the hydrolytic products, FFA and glycerol, for their reesterification and storage (Lasunción, Herrera, 1983). The increased activity of LPL found at mid gestation in pregnant rats therefore must also contribute to their fat depots accumulation.

The tendency to accumulate fat in the mother ceases during the last trimester of gestation (Herrera et al. 1988; Hytten, Leitch, 1971; Beaton et al. 1954; López-Luna et al. 1986). This is due to the fact that maternal lipid metabolism switches to a catabolic condition, as shown by an increase in adipose tissue lipolytic activity (Knopp et al. 1970; Chaves, Herrera, 1978) and a reduction in adipose tissue uptake of circulating triglycerides (Herrera et al. 1987) secondary to a decrease in LPL activity (Herrera et al. 1988; Otway, Robinson, 1968; Hamosh et al. 1970;

Ramírez et al. 1983). Besides, during late gestation the augmented lipogenetic activity in maternal adipose tissue decreases rapidly (Palacín et al. 1991), and all these changes cause a net accelerated breakdown of the fat depots.

The lipolytic products, free fatty acids (FFA) and glycerol increase in maternal plasma during late gestation (Herrera et al. 1987). The liver is the main receptor organ for these products, where they can be reesterified to be reexported to the circulation in the form of VLDL-triglycerides (Carmaniu, Herrera, 1979). Increased adipose tissue lipolytic activity during late gestation therefore would cause an enhancement in maternal liver VLDL production, which has been directly demonstrated in experimental models (Wasfi et al. 1980; Kalkhoff et al. 1972). This condition is also accompanied by an enhancement in intestinal absorption of dietary lipids (Argilés, Herrera, 1989), all of which causing an exaggerated increase in the level of triglycerides in maternal plasma (Knopp et al. 1975; Herrera et al. 1988; Otway, Robinson, 1968; Stemberg et al. 1956; Knopp et al. 1978; Russ et al. 1954; Konttinen et al. 1964; Scow et al. 1964;

Herrera et al. 1969; Argilés, Herrera, 1981).

2.1 Role of the accumulation of body fat during the first half of gestation on maternal hypertriglyceridemia during late gestation

In order to determine how maternal hypertriglyceridemia during late gestation is influenced by the accumulation of fat depots during earlier stages, we studied pregnant rats made diabetics by treatment with streptozotocin (*D*) and receiving a substitution dose of insulin for different periods. Streptozotocin (45 mg/Kg) was given intravenously prior to mating, at which time they were divided into 3 groups: 1) *D-Controls*, which received a daily subcutaneous replacement insulin therapy (1.5 IU/100 g body weight); 2) *D12-20* that received the same treatment from day 0 until day 11th of gestation, and were kept diabetic between days 12 and 20: or 3) *D* that did not receive any treatment throughout pregnancy. All the animals were studied at day 20 of gestation, at which time it was found (Herrera et al. 1990) that the lumbar fat pad weight was much lower in *D* than in *D12-20* rats, whose value was similar to that of *D-Controls*, indicating that diabetes during the first part of gestation, but not during the second, impairs maternal capacity to maintain lipidic maternal stores.

In this same experiment it was found (Herrera et al. 1990) that plasma triglycerides were augmented in *D* and *D12-20* animals as compared to the *D-Controls*, but values in the *D12-20* rats were even higher than in *D*. Since lipidic stores were exhausted in the *D* animals the efficient lipolytic activity required to sustain the endogenous triglycerides overproduction was not possible. We therefore think that this is the reason for *D* rats developing a milder hyperlipidemia than those diabetic animals receiving insulin therapy during the first half of gestation (*D12-20*), where fat depots were built up to the same level as in the *D-Controls*, and therefore were able to sustain a greatly augmented lipolytic activity.

A similar experiment to that for the diabetic rats was carried out by us with thyroidectomized animals. Rats were mated and thyroidectomized on the same day. Some animals were kept without treatment and killed on day 12 or 21 of gestation, whereas others were subsequently treated with L-thyroxine (1.8 ug/100 body weight) for either the first 12 days and then not treated from that time until day 21 or else not treated for the first 12 days and then treated from days 12-21. It was found that (Bonet, Herrera, 1991; Bonet, Herrera, 1988) on day 12 of gestation, maternal net body weight (free of the conceptus), which is an index

of the mass of maternal structures, was much smaller in the rats not receiving thyroxine treatment than in those receiving the treatment, and this difference was maintained until the 21st gestational day, even though untreated rats during the first half of gestation received the thyroxyne treatment during the second half, and were euthyroid at the time of sacrifice. All those thyroidectomized rats where the anabolic changes were impaired during the first half of gestation showed a lower hypertriglyceridemia during late gestation, independently of receiving the thyroxine treatment during the second half of gestation (Bonet, Herrera, 1991).

It may be concluded then, that maternal fat store accumulation during the first half of gestation has a pivotal importance on the development of maternal hypertriglyceridemia during late gestation.

3 CONSEQUENCES OF MATERNAL HYPERLIPIDEMIA

These adaptations in maternal lipidic metabolism have important consequences for the mother and her offspring. Both the accumulation of fat depots and the enhaced lipolytic activity in adipose tissue increase glycerol levels in maternal circulation (Chaves, Herrera, 1980). Since the placental transfer of glycerol is much smaller than other hydrosoluble compounds such as glucose or amino acids (Herrera et al. 1992a), the mother uses this metabolite for other pathways. We have shown previously that the conversion of glycerol into glucose in the pregnant rat is even greater than that of the more classical gluconeogenic substrates such as alanine or pyruvate (Herrera et al. 1991; Zorzano, Herrera, 1986; Zorzano et al. 1986). We may therefore conclude, that maternal glycerol actively contributes to the synthesis of glucose that is needed for both placental transfer and maternal tissues. Through this way we see how, in an indirect manner, the fetus benefits from maternal hyperlipidemia, which in fact is greatest during the phase of maximal fetal growth.

Maternal hyperlipidemia may also constitute a "floating" energetic store for both the mother and the fetus, to be used under conditions of a shortage of other nutrients, as in starvation. This reasoning justifies the great ketogenesis that is seen in the late pregnant mother during fasting (Herrera et al. 1969; Scow et al. 1958; Girard et al. 1977). The synthesis of ketone bodies is carried out by the liver from those free fatty acids that are taken up by this organ from both those released to plasma through the lipolytic activity in adipose tissue and those being released

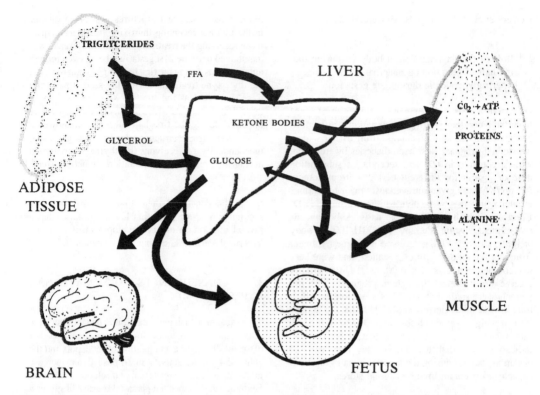

Figure 3.- Role of lipolytic activity in adipose tissue as an important source of substrates for ketogenesis and gluconeogenesis in the fasting condition during late pregnancy, and its consequent availability of metabolites for the fetus.

at the liver capillaries by the action of lipoprotein lipase over circulating triglycerides. We have previously shown that these two processes are greately enhanced in the fasted pregnant rat (Knopp et al. 1970; Chaves, Herrera, 1978; Herrera et al. 1988). The enhanced arrival of ketone bodies to maternal tissues and their use as alternative fuels allows to save other more limited and essential substrates for the fetus, such as amino acids and glucose.

The fetus also receives maternal ketone bodies through the placenta, and their use seems to play an important metabolic role under conditions of maternal nutritional deprivation. Figure 3 summarizes the maternal response to starvation. We see then the important role that maternal fat depots accumulated during early gestation has as main source of substrates for ketogenesis and gluconeogenesis during late gestation, under conditions of food deprivation. In this way, the availability of essential substrates for the fetus is guaranteed.

Despite that maternal hypertriglyceridemia is one of the most striking features of maternal metabolism during late gestation, the transfer of triglycerides through the placenta is practically negligible (Herrera et al. 1992a)). The fetus therefore does not directly benefit from maternal hypertriglyceridemia. As indicated above, the metabolism of circulating triglycerides requires their previous hydrolysis by the LPL action, and with few exceptions, the activity of this enzyme does not change or even decreases in most maternal tissues (Herrera et al. 1988). Within these exceptions is the mammary gland. As shown in figure 4, whereas LPL activity is very similar in 20 pregnant rats and virgin controls in the heart, lung and liver, it is decreased in lumbar fat pads in the former group but it is enhanced in the mammary gland. The functionality of such a change plays an important role in the maternal preparation for lactation, and we therefore should dedicate attention to this specific aspect.

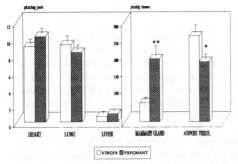

Figure 4.- Lipoprotein lipase activity in different tissues from 20 day pregnant rats and virgin controls. The enzyme activity was measured in acetone-ether extracts, as previously described (Ramírez et al., 1983). Means ± SEM. Statistical comparison versus virgin is shown by astherisks (*).

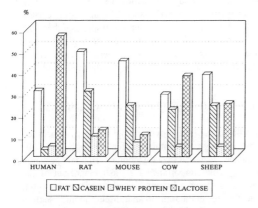

Figure 5.- Percentual distribution of solid components in the milk of different species (adapted from Mepha,. 1976).

4 LIPIDS IN THE MILK AND THEIR SOURCE

As shown in figure 5, in most species lipids are the main solid components of the milk, and even in humans they are so after lactose (Mepham, 1976). Besides, in the suckling infant, maternal lipids constitute up to 50% of the total nutrient calories (Martínez, Dodds, 1983), and they are the vehicle for liposoluble vitamins and essential fatty acids (Ali et al. 1986; Kohn, 1992).

The major components of milk lipids are triglycerides which in human's milk represent up to 98% of the total lipids, whereas phospholipids are just 1% and cholesterol and cholesterol esters around 0.5%

(Lammi-Keefe, Jensen, 1984). All this indicates the importance of lipids in the milk and the preponderant role of triglycerides on it.

Milk triglycerides may come from either those synthesized in the mammary gland or those being taken from circulation, which are derived from the diet or from other tissues. From studies in the rat, it is known that the activity of lipogenic enzymes are very low in the mammary gland during gestation and is not induced up to 48 h after parturition (Martyn, Hansen, 1981; Grigor et al. 1982). In spite of low lipogenic activity, as shown in figure 6, the mass of mammary glands and their lipidic content progressively increases from mid gestation and is almost ten times higher prior to parturition (day 21 of gestation in the rat) than in virgin controls. Besides, it is known that the newborns initiate the suckling process before the lipogenic activity of mammary glands becomes fully enhanced (Martyn, Hansen, 1981). This indicates that during the perinatal phase the circulating triglyceride-rich lipoproteins, chylomicrons and VLDLs, constitute the major source for mammary glands triglycerides. This conclusion has been experimentaly supported both in women (Hachey et al. 1987) and in the rat (Ramírez et al. 1983; Argilés, Herrera, 1989).

5 ROLE OF MATERNAL HYPERTRIGLYCERIDEMIA DURING LATE GESTATION ON MILK LIPIDS

Once the importance of circulating triglycerides has as a source of milk lipids around parturition is recognized, we will analyze the role that maternal hypertriglyceridemia has on this, and how they are driven to the mammary gland.

Maternal hypertriglyceridemia disappears around parturition both in women (Miller, 1990; Kallio et al. 1992) and in the rat (Ramírez et al. 1983). This change occurs with minor changes in adipose tissue LPL activity, but it is coincident with an intense and rapid increment in mammary gland LPL activity (Ramírez et al. 1983). Besides, as shown in figure 7, such an increase in mammary gland LPL activity is coincident with an intense increase in the uptake by the same tissue of ^{14}C-lipids 4 hours after an oral load of ^{14}C-tripalmitin to 20 day pregnant rats as compared with virgin rats used as controls. These findings indicate that the induction of LPL activity in the mammary gland during late gestation allows this tissue to increase its capacity to take up circulating triglycerides for milk production.

Since it is known that prolactin is an important

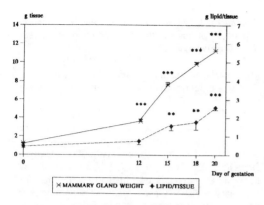

Figure 6.- Fresh weight and lipidic content of mammary glands during gestation in the rat. Experimental protocol was as previously described (López-Luna et al., 1986). Statistical comparison versus virgin rats (0 days of gestation) is shown by astherisks (*).

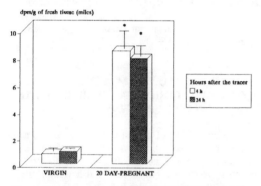

Figure 7.- Appearance of labelled lipids in mammary gland of 20 day pregnant rats and virgin controls at 4 and 24 h after oral administration of ^{14}C-tripalmitate. Experimental details were previously described (Argilés and Herrera, 1989). Means ± SEM. Statistical comparison versus virgin is shown by astherisks (*).

hormonal factor inducing LPL expression in mammary glands around parturition (Spooner et al. 1977), we inhibited the peak of prolactin in the late pregnant rat by giving progesterone treatment and studied its consequences on both mammary gland LPL activity and circulating triglycerides (Ramírez et al. 1983). It was found that progesterone treatment completely inhibits the increase of LPL activity in mammary gland of late pregnant rats and blocks the reversion of maternal hypertriglyceridemia normally occurring in

the rat just prior to parturition. These findings, therefore, indicate that besides its role in driving circulating triglycerides to the mammary gland for their uptake, the induction of LPL activity in this tissue plays a key role in the disappearance of maternal hypertriglyceridemia around parturition, a fact that has been well documented both in women (Knopp et al. 1992; Kallio et al. 1992) and in the rat (Ramírez et al. 1983).

Figure 8 summarizes most of these changes occurring in the pregnant mother around parturition: the intense lipolytic activity in adipose tissue facilitates the release of substrates, FFA and glycerol, to the circulation, that are mainly taken up by the liver, where they are reesterified for triglyceride synthesis and reexported into circulation associated to VLDL. These lipoproteins are pooled with those synthesized in the intestine from lipids mainly derived from the diet, chylomicrons, causing an exaggerated increase in the overall total body production of "triglyceride-rich lipoproteins". The decrease in LPL activity in certain maternal tissues, mainly adipose tissue, together with the induction of LPL in the mammary gland drives these lipoproteins to this tissue, where the triglycerides contribute very actively to the synthesis of milk.

6 SUMMARY AND FINAL CONCLUSIONS

On the basis of the above findings it may be concluded that although placental transfer of lipids is small, sustained maternal hyperlipidemia during late gestation is of pivotal importance for the metabolism of the mother and her offspring. Besides aporting essential metabolites to the fetus in an indirect manner, such as glucose synthesized in maternal liver from glycerol released from adipose tissue, the active lipidic metabolism in the mother allows the availability of high amounts of circulating triglyceride-rich lipoproteins for milk synthesis in preparation for lactation. The induction of LPL activity in the mammary gland is important for this function, and warrants the availability of essential fatty acids from the diet to be present in the milk, as well as contributes to the disappearance of maternal hyperlipidemia around parturition. Besides, maternal hyperlipidemia constitutes a floating energetic store to be used under conditions of food deprivation to ensure the availability of alternative substrates for maternal tissues, such a ketone bodies, and to save essential metabolites for the fetus. Maternal hyperlipidemia is the result of numerous and dynamic metabolic adaptations that have to be controlled very finely. Any deviation from this control may alter maternal lipoprotein profile and even be responsible for an alteration in the milk composition, as it has been

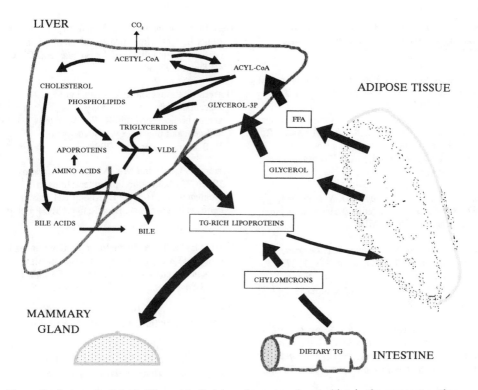

LIVER

CO₂

ACETYL-CoA

ACYL-CoA

ADIPOSE TISSUE

CHOLESTEROL

PHOSPHOLIPIDS

GLYCEROL-3P

FFA

TRIGLYCERIDES

APOPROTEINS

VLDL

AMINO ACIDS

GLYCEROL

BILE ACIDS

BILE

TG-RICH LIPOPROTEINS

CHYLOMICRONS

MAMMARY
GLAND

DIETARY TG

INTESTINE

Figure 8.- Summary of the lipidic metabolic interactions around parturition in the pregnant mother.

already reported in dyslipidemic mothers (Myher et al. 1984; Steiner et al. 1985).

7 ACKNOWLEDGEMENT

The work was supported by Grant 92/0407 from the Fondo de Investigaciones Sanitarias de la Seguridad Social. The authors thank Ms. Shirley McGrath for her editorial help.

8 REFERENCES

Ali J, Kader HA, Hassan K, Arshat H, 1986. Changes in human milk vitamin E and total lipids during the first twelve days of lactation. Am J Clin Nutr 43:925-930

Argilés J, Herrera E, 1981. Lipids and lipoproteins in maternal and fetus plasma in the rat. Biol Neonate 39:37-44

Argilés J, Herrera E, 1989. Appearance of circulating and tissue 14C-lipids after oral 14C-tripalmitate administration in the late pregnant rat. Metabolism 38:104-108

Beaton GH, Beare J, Ryv MH, McHewry EW, 1954. Protein metabolism in the pregnant rat. J Nutr 54:291-313

Bonet B, Herrera E, 1988. Different response to maternal hypothyroidism during the first and second half of gestation in the rat. Endocrinology 122:450-455

Bonet B, Herrera E, 1991. Maternal hypothyroidism during the first half of gestation compromises normal catabolic adaptations of late gestation in the rat. Endocrinology 129:210-216

Carmaniu S, Herrera E, 1979. Conversion of (U-14C)-glycerol, (2-3H)-glyecrol and (1-14C)-palmitate into circulating lipoproteins in the rat. Rev Esp Fisiol 35:461-466

Chaves JM, Herrera E, 1978. In vitro glycerol metabolism in adipose tissue from fasted pregnant rats. Biochem Biophys Res Commun 85:1299-1306

Chaves JM, Herrera E, 1980. In vivo glycerol metabolism in the pregnant rat. Biol Neonate 37:172-179

Fain JM, Scow RO, 1966. Fatty acid synthesis in vivo in maternal and fetal tissues in the rat. Am J Physiol 210:19-25

Girard J, Ferre P, Gilbert M, Kervran A, Assan R, Marliss E, 1977. Fetal metabolic response to maternal fasting in the rat. Am J Physiol 232:E456-E463

Grigor MR, Geursen A, Sneyd MJ, Warren SM, 1982. Regulation of lipogenic capacity in lactating rats. Biochem J 208:611-618

Hachey DL, Thomas MR, Emken EA, Garza C, Brown Booth L, Adlof RO, Klein PD, 1987. Human lactation: maternal transfer of dietary triglycerides labeled with stable isotopes. J Lipid Res 28:1185-1192

Hamosh M, Clary TR, Chernick SS, Scow RO, 1970. Lipoprotein lipase activity of adipose and mammary tissue and plasma triglyceride in pregnant and lactating rats. Biochim Biophys Acta 210:473-482

Herrera E, Knopp RH, Freinkel N, 1969. Carbohydrate metabolism in pregnancy VI. Plasma fuels, insulin, liver composition, gluconeogenesis and nitrogen metabolism during gestation in the fed and fasted rat. J Clin Invest 48:2260-2272

Herrera E, Palacín M, Martín A, Lasunción MA, 1985. Relationship between maternal and fetal fuels and placental glucose transfer in rats with maternal diabetes of varying severity. Diabetes 34(Suppl.2):42-46

Herrera E, Gómez Coronado D, Lasunción MA, 1987. Lipid metabolism in pregnancy. Biol Neonate 51:70-77

Herrera E, Lasunción MA, Gómez Coronado D, Aranda P, Lopez Luna P, Maier I, 1988. Role of lipoprotein lipase activity on lipoprotein metabolism and the fate of circulating triglycerides in pregnancy. Am J Obstet Gynecol 158:1575-1583

Herrera E, Lasunción MA, Gómez-Coronado D, Martín A, Bonet B, 1990. Lipid metabolic interactions in the mother during pregnancy and their fetal repercussions. In: Cuezva JM, Pascual Leone AM, Patel MS (eds.), Endocrine and biochemical development of the fetus and neonate. New York: Plenum Press, pp. 277-282

Herrera E, Lasunción MA, Palacín M, Zorzano A, Bonet B, 1991. Intermediary metabolism in pregnancy. First theme of the Freinkel era. Diabetes 40 Suppl 2:83-88

Herrera E, Lasunción MA, Asunción M, 1992a. Placental transport of free fatty acids, glycerol and ketone bodies. In: Polin R, Fox WW (eds.), Fetal and neonatal physiology. Philadelphia: W.B.Saunders, pp. 291-298

Herrera E, Lasunción MA, Martín A, Zorzano A, 1992b. Carbohydrate-lipid interactions in pregnancy. In: Herrera E, Knopp RH (eds.), Perinatal biochemistry. Boca Raton: CRC Press, pp. 1-18

Herrera E, Martín A, Montelongo A, Domínguez M, Lasunción MA, 1992c. Serum lipid profile in diabetic pregnancy. Avanc Diabet 5 (Supl. 1):73-84

Hytten FE, Leitch I, 1971. The physiology of human pregnancy, Oxford: Blackwell Scientific

Kalkhoff RK, Bhatia SK, Matute ML, 1972. Influence of pregnancy and sex steroids on hepatic triglyceride biosynthesis. Diabetes 21(Suppl.1):365-369

Kallio MJT, Siimes MA, Perheentupa J, Salmenperä L, Miettinen TA, 1992. Serum cholesterol and lipoprotein concentrations in mothers during and after prolonged exclusive lactation. Metabolism 41:1327-1330

Knopp RH, Herrera E, Freinkel N, 1970. Carbohydrate metabolism in pregnancy.VIII. Metabolism of adipose tissue isolated from fed and fasted pregnant rats during late gestation. J Clin Invest 49:1438-1446

Knopp RH, Boroush MA, O'Sullivan JB, 1975. Lipid metabolism in pregnancy. II. Postheparin lipolytic activity and hypertriglyceridemia in the pregnant rat. Metabolism 24:481-493

Knopp RH, Montes A, Warth MR, 1978. Carbohydrate and lipid metabolism. In: Committee on Nutrition of the Mother and Preschool Child (ed.), Laboratory indices of nutritional status in pregnancy. Washington: National Academy of Sciences, pp. 35-88

Knopp RH, Bonet B, Lasunción MA, Montelongo A, Herrera E, 1992. Lipoprotein metabolism in pregnancy. In: Herrera E, Knopp RH (eds.), Perinatal biochemistry. Boca Raton: CRC Press, pp. 19-51

Kohn G, 1992. Human milk and fatty acids: quantitative aspects. In: Ghisolfi J, Putet G (eds.), Essential fatty acids and infant nutrition. Paris: John Libbey Eurotext, pp. 79-88

Konttinen AT, Pyorala T, Carpen E, 1964. Serum lipid pattern in normal pregnancy and preeclampsia. J Obstet Gynaecol Br Commonw 71:453-458

Lammi-Keefe CJ, Jensen RG, 1984. Lipids in human milk: A review. 2: Composition and fat-soluble vitamins. J Pediatr Gastroenterol Nutr 3:172-198

Lasunción MA, Herrera E, 1983. Changes with starvation in the rat of the lipoprotein lipase activity and hydrolysis of triacylglycerols from triacylglycerol-rich lipoproteins in adipose tissue preparations. Biochem J 210:639-643

Lasunción MA, Lorenzo J, Palacín M, Herrera E, 1987. Maternal factors modulating nutrient transfer to the fetus. Biol Neonate 51:86-93

Lederman SA, Rosso P, 1980. Effects of food restriction on maternal weight and body composition in pregnant and non-pregnant rats. Growth 44:77-88

López-Luna P, Muñoz T, Herrera E, 1986. Body fat in pregnant rats at mid and late gestation. Life Sci 39:1389-1393

Martínez GA, Dodds DA, 1983. Milk feeding patterns in the United States during the first 12 months of life. Pediatrics 71:166-170

Martyn P, Hansen A, 1981. Initiation of lipogenic enzyme activities in rat mammary glands. Biochem J 198:187-192

Mepham B, 1976. The secretion of milk, London: Edward Arnold Pub. Ld.

Miller VT,, 1990. Dyslipoproteinemia in women. In: La Rosa JC (ed.), Endocrinology and Metabolism. Clinics of North America. Lipid Disorders. Philadelphia: W.B. Saunders co., pp. 381-398

Moore BJ, Brassel JA, 1984. One cycle of reproduction consisting of pregnancy, lactation, and recovery: effects on carcass composition in ad libitum-fed and food-restriced rats. J Nutr 114:1548-1559

Myher JJ, Kuksis A, Steiner G, 1984. Milk fat structure of a patient with type 1 hyperlipidemia. Lipids 19:673-682

Otway S, Robinson DS, 1968. The significance of changes in tissue clearing-factor lipase activity in relation to the lipaemia of pregnancy. Biochem J 106:677-682

Palacín M, Lasunción MA, Asunción M, Herrera E, 1991. Circulating metabolite utilization by periuterine adipose tissue in situ in the pregnant rat. Metabolism 40:534-539

Ramírez I, Llobera M, Herrera E, 1983. Circulating triacylglycerols, lipoproteins, and tissue lipoprotein lipase activities in rat mothers and offspring during the perinatal period: effect of postmaturity. Metabolism 32:333-341

Russ M, Eder HA, Barr DP, 1954. Protein-lipid relationships in human plasma.III. In pregnancy and the newborn. J Clin Invest 33:1662-1669

Scow RO, Chernick SS, Smith BB, 1958. Ketosis in the rat fetus. Proc Soc Exp Biol Med 98:833-835

Scow RO, Chernick SS, Brinley MS, 1964. Hyperlipemia and ketosis in the pregnant rat. Am J Physiol 206:796-804

Spooner PM, Garrison MM, Scow RO, 1977. Regulation of mammary and adipose tissue lipoprotein lipase and blood triacylglycerol in rats during late pregnancy. Effect of prostaglandins. J Clin Invest 60:702-708

Steiner G, Myher JJ, Kuksis A, 1985. Milk and plasma lipid composition in a lactating patient with type I hyperlipoproteinemia. Am J Clin Nutr 41:121-128

Stemberg L, Dagenais-Perusse P, Dreyfuss M, 1956. Serum proteins in parturient mother and newborn: an electrophoretic study. Can Med Assoc J 74:49-61

Wasfi I, Weinstein I, Heimberg M, 1980. Hepatic metabolism of [1-14C]oleate in pregnancy. Biochim Biophys Acta 619:471-481

Zorzano A, Lasunción MA, Herrera E, 1986. Role of the availability of substrates on hepatic and renal gluconeogenesis in the fasted late pregnant rat. Metabolism 35:297-303

Zorzano A, Herrera E, 1986. Comparative utilization of glycerol and alanine as liver gluconeogenic substrates in the fed late pregnant rat. Int J Biochem 18:583-587

Dairy Products in Human Health and Nutrition, Serrano Ríos et al. (eds) © 1994 Balkema, Rotterdam, ISBN 90 5410 359 0

Dairy products during perinatal stage: Relevance of their calcium and long chain polyunsatured fatty acids content

M. Moya
Hospital Universitario de San Juan, Universidad de Alicante, Spain

ABSTRACT: The importance of milk and dairy products are analyzed in the pregnant women and thereafter in the preterm and term infants. Adequate transfer to the fetus will require non only a normality of placental transfer mechanisms but a reasonable maternal nutritional status allowing such transport. The present approach will be limited to the calcium and long chain polyunsatured fatty acids. Taking as a model breast milk cuantitative studies are presented concerning to the content of calcium, free calcium and different fatty acids in two used formulas. The different absorption rates were measured through metabolic balance studies.

Nutrition in the newborn is milk based. Breast milk or formula feedings normally ensure the maintenance of the living body, the normal growth rate and the repair costs in case of disease, at least for the first few months of life. At this age the genetic potential is probably of less importance towards growth. Less well known are the procedures governing the intrauterine growth, probably due to the fact that the invasive study techniques can be harmful by themselves and because it is difficult to know to what extent, small deviations in maternal nutrition can affect the fetus, and particularly when they will normally be only assessed by somatometry related to gestational age. With this in mind it is necessary to know how each increase of weight for height category in the young mother during the second part of pregnancy will increase the mean birthweight (1).

If breast feeding were universally used for term infants during the first 6 months of life, much of the present concern about infant nutrition would not exist. This utopia hardly corresponds with our present situation. Between 1984 and 1989, the rate of initiation of breast-feeding in the US, declined 13% and 24% at 6 month postpartum. This happened despite the claims of health care providers, that breast feeding is the preferred way of nursing in the first semester (2). Once the mother is out of the little but still coercive atmosphere of the maternity wards, it is totally abandoned, at least in our means (3), because the desire of returning to work, or because of an active nursing attitude by the father now contemplated by the law or by other well known circumstances, such as cosmetic or being totally tied to the babies 24 hours a day.

Maternal spontaneous supplementation constitutes more of a marker than the cause of breast-feeding problems. On the other hand it is difficult to define the clear advantages of breast feeding (protection against infection, maternal bonding ...), that create a certain scepticism in unconvinced nursing mothers. In a developed society the advantages of breast-feeding if ever they can be felt by the mother, will have a social counterpart (work facilities ..). All this causes stabilization or even an increase in formula feeding from the beginning.

The alternative of low costly cow milk is not acceptable for the newborn infant because it is well known that the excess of protein or sodium or the lacking of vitamin D, or ω3 long chain fatty acids. Therefore new formulas for the first and second semester have been produced not only for securing a comparable growth and development pattern to that obtained with breast milk but for covering special situations such as prematurity or definite clinical conditions that can be the inborn errors of metabolism. Precisely the possibility of modifiying or introducing some nutrients has opened a vast field for making almost every hypothesis and sometimes with a too rapid application, without taking into account important side effects (4).

Because the broad nutritional extent presented by dairy products, a limitation has been made to two aspects in this presentation: calcium and LCPs fatty acids.

CALCIUM MATERNO PLACENTAL ASPECTS

The main source for dietary calcium in the pregnant woman are dairy products (5). Relevant changes in maternal calcium metabolism occur during pregnancy, which eventually lead to a positive calcium balance. Despite a reversible pattern of bone resorption found in early pregnancy, the bone structure and bone mineral content normally remain unchanged at the end of gestation (6, 7). If that happens it is because two mechanisms become activated, one is the rise of 1,25 dihydroxyvitamin D (1,25D) in maternal plasma, improving the intestinal calcium absortion (8) and the other is related to the action of calcitonin protecting the maternal skeleton (9). Routine obstetrical care should include some nutritional questioning particularly with regard to certain supplements and not merely the assessment of the optimal weight gain. The influence of prenatal nutrition on the genesis of neonatal osteopenia is not well known. But if the placental transfer of Ca and Pi decreases, whether by intrinsic impairment (pre-eclampsia) or by a reduction of them in the maternal side, osteopenia appears to be more common (10).

TABLE I. Minerals and fatty acids content in the formulas used in the two periods of balance. Values after 33 samples analyzed.

mg/dL	F + LCPs	F	p
Total Ca	72.3(9.1)	57.0(7.3)	‹0.001
Free Ca	24.5(16.0)	8.5(4.9)	‹0.001
Mg	6.3(0.8)	6.9(0.9)	NS
Pi	37.3(3.4)	38.5(3.2)	NS
Total Fat	3700(500)	3600(200)	NS
C12	175(53)	126(33)	‹0.001
C14	142(31)	103(70)	‹0.005
C16	789(188)	1333(156)	‹0.001
C18	143(31)	138(15)	NS
C18:1	1143(287)	1092(134)	NS
C18:2	484(100)	391(32)	‹0.001
C18:3	56(20)	36(9)	‹0.001
C20:5	6.8(4.1)	-----	
C22:6	4.3(3.5)	-----	

m (SD)

TABLE II. Balance of total fat and individual saturated fatty acids in eleven babies.

(mg/Kg/day)	C12	C14	C16	C18	TOTAL FAT
INTAKE					
F + LCPs	362(112)	292(62)	1630(392)	295(63)	7791(1534)
F	251(71)	197(65)	2650(460)	277(60)	7282(1746)
FECAL EXCR.					
F + LCPs	0.9(1.1)	10.0(4.7)	189(41)	52(14)	1200(569)
F	0.5(0.8)	8.3(4.3)	339(136)	54(25)	1691(711)
NET. RET.					
F + LCPs	361(111)	282(61)	1440(384)	243(61)	6591(1683)
F	251(71)	189(105)	2311(396)	223(48)	5591(1729)
% ABSORPTION					
F + LCPs	99.7(0.3)	96.5(1.7)	88.0(3.2)	81.9(5.2)	84.0(7.9)
F	99.8(0.3)	95.4(2.5)	87.4(4.3)	80.8(7.1)	76.4(8.9)

m(SD)   • $p<0.01$ •• $p<0.001$

After a normal pregnancy term the fetus contains 30 g of calcium (11) due to a progressive accumulation ranging from 110 mg/kg/d in the 24th week up to 150 mg/kg/d in the 36th week of gestation. This is a result of the positive calcium balance of the mother (12) followed by effective placental transfer, requiring furthermore an adequate activity of calcium regulating hormones (1,25D and PTHrP maternal, placental and fetal).

The calcium crossing mechanism has certain similarities with that occurring in the gut. There are two pathways, one transtrophoblastic, comparable to that of the absorption carried out by the enterocyte and the other is similar to the intestinal paracellular way (13). The resultant materno-fetal flux (J net) out of the substraction of unidirectional fluxes materno-fetal and feto-maternal is not known in humans, but in the rhesus monkey that figure is approximately 70 mg/kg of fetal body weight/day (14). The transcellular mechanisms comportes: i) influx of ionized calcium through the microvillous trophoblastic membrane (maternal side); ii) Cytosolic transport; iii) Efflux of calcium ions through the basolateral trophoblastic membrane (fetal side). In favouring this mechanism, one should consider the stability of cytosolic calcium concentration (range: 10^{-8} M), the presence of CaBP acting as intracytosolic calcium transporter and the presence of cytosolic receptors for 1,25D (15). In the pregnant rat there is a reduced placental transfer of calcium to fetuses suffering from IUGR (16), the mechanism by which it is done is not known but probably it is not restricted to the flow limitation at the maternal side of the placenta (17).

Despite the enormous maternal calcium deposits (1000 g) in relation to the amount transferred to the fetus, "disnutrition" or previous closer pregnancies can affect the appropiate calcium transfer to the fetus although the transfer mechanism were working adequately.

CALCIUM NEONATAL HOMEOSTASIS

Late neonatal hypocalcemia and probably the early one are historical events since new formulas and shorter fasting lapses after birth have been generalized particularly when considering preterm babies. In this population a real problem is still the undermineralization of the bone, known as Osteopenia. Despite the confusing name of prematurity rickets, in this condition the role of vitamin D is less important than the fact of not meeting the preterm requirements of calcium and phosphate. The possibility of developing osteopenia increases as the gestation shortens, because the amounts transferred by the placenta can hardly be supplied by the oral route in terms of volume and Ca and Pi content of the formula feed. This was particularly evident when the survivors weighing less than 1.0 kg were fed with breast milk (18), with such low levels of calcium and phosphate. The study of Ca and Pi in urine and the levels of plasma 1,25D and ALP in laboratory tests are the most important way of detecting this condition. The surveillance and supplements should continue until the infants weigh more than 2.0 kg.

Supplements. From the times when carential rickets was a major problem, a well-absorbed calcium salt has been sought. The formation of insoluble precipitates fears and the initial rules (19) were responsible for formulas with minimums for calcium of 40 mg/dL. Fortunately most of starting formulas contain 70-80 mg/dL, but even such amounts would be absolutely inefficient for preterm babies. Then extemporaneous supplements to the formulas were used, proving to be very effcient. Calcium lactate supplementation (800 mg/kg/d) raised the calcium content in the formulas immediately before feeding from 73 mg/d to 170 mg/dL, which implied net retention of calcium of 42 mg/kg/d and 100 mg/kg/d respectively without clinical problems (20). Ten years later (21), the recommendation for calcium intake ranges from between 70-140 mg/100 kcal, for preterm babies' formulas. Most of them contain nearly 100 mg/dL, in the powder form. The liquid formulas contain less than 80 mg/dL, which will probably need from supplements specially when administered to babies born with weights of 1 kg or less.

Phosphate is better absorbed than calcium and with the normal content of 60 mg/dL in the present formulas, previous hypocalcemia and hypercalciuria have disappeared.

Some specific aspects for full term babies can be considered. The compliance for different ingested amounts of calcium and phosphate or Ca/Pi ratios is greater than the in the preterm. Probably this is due to the more mature compensatory mechanisms operated through the calcium regulating hormones which could prevent at least short term consequences, provided higher amounts than that of breast milk (Ca 30 mg/dL; Pi 15 mg/dL) are supplied by the formula used. Specifically, the low content of Pi in breast milk is enough for term babies because it is coherent with calcium supply (2/1) and covers the minimum required for growing not only the skeleton but other tissues. The excess of Pi will implicate some negative consequences such as raising the serum phosphate level because of the limited neonatal GFR, then increasing the risk of tetany, and furthermore because of the high renal phosphate (and net acid) excretion. On the other hand, a high intake of calcium and phosphate can be a metabolic acidosis risk factor (22). The low Pi content in human milk after six months can prevent the normal mineral accretion despite an adequate repletional vitamin D status (23). The present guidelines for the follow-up formulas (24) support minimum figures of 60 mg/dL for calcium and 40 mg/dL for Pi. These amounts or perhaps the higher ones usually found in formulas are recommended for the second semester, allow a daily calcium intake of 500-600 mg. To meet this, 0.5-0.6 L/d of follow-up formula is necessary because the calcium content of the beikost is very low (5): enriched cereals could contain 100 mg/100 g (and greater amounts for Pi) or 125 mL of cooked spinach, 88 mg. Fresh cow's milk contains 120 mg/100 g of calcium and 95 mg/100 g of Pi, therefore it would not be appropriate at this age, neither would be breast milk. In term infants fed on a cow milk based formula there is a progressive decrease in the bone mineral content/bone width until the 6 first months of life reaching a trough of 160 mg/cm^2 then a constant rise occurs up to 220 mg/cm^2, the amount similar to that found at birth (25). Similar babies fed breast milk supplementd with vitamin D (400 IU/d) will have a parallel "submineralized" (!) BMC/BW pattern (26). But not everything depend on the quality of the diet. Other factors as such summer-born babies, low maternal repletional vitamin D status and maybe race and gender (27) could have a significant long term influence on bone mineralization and perhaps growth (28), the growth after one year, is not related to bone calcium content.

NUTRITIONAL IMPORTANCE OF LONG CHAIN POLYUNSATURATED FATTY ACIDS (LCPs).

The most important nutritional aspect of the LCPs is their "essentiality" character as Burr and Burr adscribed to them in the 30's. That means that the superior organisms are unable to synthesize de novo neither the linoleic acid (LA, C18:2ω6) nor the α-linolenic acid (LNA, C18:3ω3), therefore the diet should contain them. Furthermore a deficiency clinical picture (growth retardation, increased epidermal water loss, scaly dermitis) was described when a rigid exclusion is done through the diet (29), although this is almost impossible to see in clinical practice even in past times when exclusively cow milk based formula were used for nursing the newborn.

The biochemical reasons for their essentiality lay in the inability of the animal kingdom, in introducing double bonds in the fatty acid segment going from omega (ω) methyl end and the subsequent C8. Only plants and particularly unicellular seaweed, contain 12-desaturase and 15-desaturase enzymes (counted from α carboxylic end) permiting the synthesis of polyunsaturated fatty acids from oleic acid (C18:1ω9). In the animal kingdom the farthest possibility of creating a double bond reachs only C9 (9-desaturase).

Elongation and further desaturation. Exogenous LA once reachs the liver will give origin to the ω-6 acids family. By sequential steps of action of the 6-desaturase, elongase, 5-desaturase, the arachidonic acid (AA C20:4ω6) is synthesized. In the case of αLNA, the same sequence will lead to eicosapentaenoic acid (EPA, 20:5ω3) and from that and after another elongation step and 4-desaturase action, docosahexaenoic acid (DHA, C22:5ω3) will be produced. The activity of this enzymatic chain can be affected by a series of factors including the animal species, (humans have lower activity than rats), fasting status or fat intake and particularly the age of the subjects, being lower in the perinatal period when compared with other ages. That gives reason to the consideration of LCPs and particularly the AA, EPA and DHA as "conditionally essential" for the preterm which will be unable to synthesize them in an adequate manner. Their presence in breast milk could support this character.

The nutritional importance of C20s and C22s can be viewed on two aspects. The energetic one probably is of less importance in face that in human milk their content represents, only 1.5% of the total fatty acid. Cow milk has only AA and in a lesser proportion (30).

Nonenergetic importance can be based on the following points: i) when the diet of the preterm contains only the precursors, LA and αLNA, then the concentration of AA and DHA diminishes in phospholipids (31) found in plasma and in the cell membranes (erythrocytes, epithelial cells, neuronal cells, or even adipocytes). ii) Recently (32, 33) it has been reported an improvement in the pattern of the electroretinogram and in the visual-evoked potentials acuity in very low birthweight infants fed with supplemented marine oil formulas. iii) The development of the deficiency picture in patients with a biliariy atresia and with an exclusive fat supply of MCT (34). iv) The fact that LA and AA, are the origin of the eicosanoids. It is well known that ω3 LCPs in the diet supress the convertion of ω6 LA to AA, then modulating the biosynthesis of eicosanoids. It appeared as a new strategy for preventing or ameliorate certain chronic diseases (35). But probably that needs a wider studies, in view to the formation of leukotriene B_5 and docosanoids from dietary EPA and DHA, and to the fact of no adverse effects on the inmmune system when taking fish oil supplements. v) Trans isomers in human pregnancy could have a potential negative effect on early perinatal growth through the mechanism of imparing michrosome desaturation and elongation of LA and αLNA (36). After this rapid considerations on the nutritional importance of LCPs, one could reckon that herbivores can obtain αLNA from the chloroplast lipids they ingest overland; longer ω3 acids are synthesized by algae, fish eating fitoplancton become rich in such products. These constitute an intermediate step in the alimentary chain for furnishing LCPs to the man but not to the newborn babies particularly when they are not breast fed.

LCPs ABSORPTIVE STUDIES.

It is well known that fat is easily absorbed not only by the term infant but even by the preterm (37). Perhaps it is not so well known the absorption rate of individual LCPs and how their progressive length and desaturation can affect it. Another question to be raised is if the different fats can affect the level of the free (soluble and ionized) calcium in the formula. This fraction will be more readibly absorbed than calcium complexes which need from the digestion procedures to solubilize and ionize in part, the calcium and therefore making it absorbable (13).

Balance studies

Formulas. A starting formula has been used under two presentations: a) powder to be reconstructed (13%) and b) liquid ready for use. There are no major differences between them apart from the lipid content (Table I). Powder formula (F+LCPs) contains the following essential fatty acids (% wt/wt of total fatty acids): AA, 0.02; EPA, 0.23 and DHA, 0.24. Palmitic acid (C16:0) were more abundant (40.1%) in liquid formula (F) than in F+LCPs (26.2%). Babies: Eleven preterm babies (GA 35.6 ± 1.9 wk and birthweight of 1.8 ± 0.1 kg) without clinical problems were balanced for two periods of three days, each with one formula. Between both periods a lapse of 6-8 days was established to adapt to the new formula. The baby study followed the usual procedure of the Unit of Nutrition Growth and Metabolism attached to the Department, with the last introduced modifications (4). Fatty acids were extracted from formulas and faeces and through a gas-chromatography procedure identified and quantified. Total calcium and free calcium were quantified from the same samples (plus urine) by means of atomic absorption and calcium selective electrode.

Table II shows the values (mg/kg/day) of intake, fecal excretion, net retention and % of absorption for lauric (C12:0), miristic (C14:0); palmitic (C16:0) and stearic (C18:0) acids. In the last column, total fat balance is shown. A fairly constant finding is the very good absorption of every individual fatty acid. Significant differences in net retention are coherent with the same significant differences in the intake, therefore when considering the percentage absorbed there are not important differences in either formula. The differences in total fat balance can be explained by the presence in F+LCPs of polyenoic acids and a lower content of palmitic acid (we do not know its proportion sterified in position 2 of the triglyceride).

TABLE III. Individual LCPs balance in eleven babies.

(mg/Kg/day)	C18:1	C18:2	C18:3	C20:5	C22:6
INTAKE					
F·+ LCPs	2359(578)	998(206)	116(43)	14.9(9.8)	9.5(7.7)
F	2172(387)	780(142)	75(29)	-	-
FECAL EXCR.					
F + LCPs	169(106)	41(33)	8(9)	1.0(2.7)	1.9(3.4)
F	185(146)	35(36)	9(7)	-	-
NET. RET.					
F + LCPs	2190(572)	957(204)	108(41)	13.9(8.4)	7.6(6.1)
F	1987(442)	745(145)	65(28)	-	-
% ABSORPTION					
F + LCPs	92.7(4.1)	95.9(3.0)	92.2(6.8)	96.3(9.5)	83.6(22.1)
F	91.1(7.4)	95.5(4.5)	87.0(10.2)	-	-

m(SD) • p<0.01

In table III data from LCPs are shown. Oleic acid represents an important quota of the total fat intake. If the amount is added to that of palmitic acid, both acids can represent 70% of the daily total fat ingested (approximately 5 g/kg/d). In these formulas the LA content can guarantee a daily amount of about 1 g per kilo of body weight. When considering longer and more desaturated fatty acids, their contribution is considerably lower, 114 mg/kg/d for LNA, 13 for EPA and 8 for DHA. The percentage of absorption is high, thus permiting substantious retentions for oleic and linoleic acids. In the case of EPA and DHA the net retention shows a wider variation (13±9 and 5±4 mg/kg/d) but still with a reasonable percentage of absorption. It is worth noticing that intake figures obtained in the study are in full agreement with the theoretical content given by the manufacturer. Other data from that balance studies deserve some comment. The daily number and weight of stools, apart from giving information about the digestive tolerance of the formula, constitutes a very good mechanism for estimating the balance accuracy. In the present study the fecal evacuation was during the period on F+LCPs formula 8.3±2.3 g/kg/d and during the period on conventional formula (F), 10.3±4.3 g/kg/d. These figures are in agreement with our own previous experience as were the number of stools per day.

The second aspect dealt with in the present study is to evaluate the total calcium content in both formulas assessed after ashing at 600°C, and the soluble and ionized calcium in the bottle before feeding. Calcium measured figures showed a greater content in F+LCPs, probably due to the higher concentration when reconstucting it, the higher concentration of Mg and Pi will point it out. But the most relevant fact is the considerably reduction of free calcium in the liquid formula. Whether it is due to the absence of LCPs or another characteristic of this ready for use liquid formula, it could represent a pitfall for the initial phase of calcium absorption. It should be remmembered that after the normal digestive procedure most of the complexed calcium fraction will be solubilized and ionized in vivo. The concomitant calcium balances will contribute to lighten if this measurement of free calcium in vitro has clinical relevance.

LCPs absorption in respect to the quantity and quality offered. The recommended supply of 500-700 mg/kg/d (38-40) refers to the addition of ω6+ω3, and keeping a ratio of ω6/ω3 of 5-15/1. The ω6 and ω3 longer than C18 should not represent respectively more than 2% and 1% wt of the total fatty acids. There is some controversy over those figures due to the different degree of lipolysis and further absorption. Some reports (39, 41) would point out a good absorption whereas another (42) shows lower figures. In part it is due to the fact of the wide range of the post-absorptive studies, most of them related to the LCPs presence in the composition of different phospholipids, or on the other hand functional studies on visual and cortex function. The percentage of absorption is well known (43) for certain fatty acids such as C16:0; C18:0 or C18:2. But if this data would be required for LCPs of the ω3 family, there will be considerably less information, probably due to the fact that the amount ingested (about 10 mg/kg/d in the present study) is greatly absorbed. Therefore the amount to be recovered in faeces comports some technical difficulties. Taking into account a previous study (37) and analyzing the percentage of absorption, the following trend is noted: saturated fatty acids showed a lesser absorption as the chain lengthened. This pattern is not shared by LCPs, in which longer chains (and greater desaturation) does not imply the same impairment in absorption seen in the saturated ones. Nevertheless further studies are needed to give more strength to those preliminary results.

It is necessary to consider the fact that the pool of LCPs is a dynamic one and it is not a mere reflex of the intake. The endogenous synthesis is a reality but hardly measurable. According to the data of Carlson et al (44, 45), the biosynthesis of LCPs does not necessarily follow the corporal uses: the AA and DHA content in erythrocyte membrane phospholipids are lesser in the premature infant than in term despite both had similar formulas for comparable period. Furthermore the wide range of AA and DHA content in plasma and erythocyte phospholipids in babies on the same diet, should draw atention to the problem of absorption of individual LCPs.

In conclusion: According to this data, LCPs supplement in formula for the newborn is probably justified due to this good intestinal absorption by the preterm baby. These supplements should be balanced, because of the impossibility of receding to the family ω6 compounds from marine oil.

REFERENCES

1. Hickey C.A., Cliner S.P., Goldenberg R.L., Blankson M.L. Maternal weight status and term birthweoght in first and second adolescent prenacies. J. Adolesc Health, 1992; 13: 561-569.
2. Cronnenwett L, Stukee T, Kearney M et al. Single daily bottle use in the early weeks postpartum and breast-feedings outcome. Pediatrics 1992; 90: 760-66.
3. Diaz N.M., Doménech E., Diaz J.M., Galvain, Barroso A. Influencia de las prácticas hospitalarias y otros factores en la duración de la lactancia materna. Rev Esp Ped 1989; 46: 21-8.
4. Moya M., Cortés E., Ballesterl. Short-term Polycose substitution for Lactose Reduces Calcium Absorption in Healthy Term Babies. J Pediatr Gastroenterol Nutr 1992; 14:57-61.
5. Dairy Bureau of Canada. Nutrient value of Dairy foods. Toronto Ont. Revised 1982.
6. Purdie D.W., Aaron J.E., Selby P.L., Bone hystology and mineral homeostasis in human pregnancy. Br J Obstet Gynecol 1988; 95: 849-54.
7. Christiansen C., Rodbro P., Heinild B., Unchanged total body calcium in normal human pregnancy. Acta Obstet Gynecol Scand 1976; 55: 141-3.
8. Kumar R., Cohen W.R., Silva P., Epstein. Elevated 1,25 dihydroxyvitamin D plasma levels in normal human pregnancy and lactation. J Clin Invest 1976; 63: 342-4.
9. Stevenson J.C., Hylliard C.J., McIntyre I., Cooper H., Whiteheard M.I. A physiological role for calcitonin protection of the maternal skeleton. Lancet 1979; ii: 769-70.
10. Bosley A.R.J., Verrier-Jones E.R., Campbell M.J. Actiological factors in rickets of prematurity. Arch Dis Child 1980; 55: 683-6.
11. Shaw J.C.L. Evidencia de la mineralización esquelética defectuosa en los niños de bajo peso: la absorción de calcio y grasa. Pediatrics (Ed. Española) 1976; 1: 9-18.
12. Gertner J.M., Coustan D.R., Kliger A.S., Mallete L.E., Ravin N., Broadug A.E. Pregnancy as state of physiologyc absorptive hypercalciuria. Am J Med 1986; 81: 451-56.
13. Moya M. Intestinal absorption and excretion of calcium and phosphorus in infancy. Annales Nestlé 1987; 45:7-17.
14. Ramberg C.F., Delivoria-Papadopoulos M., Crandall E.D., Kornfield D.S. Kinetic analysis of calcium transport across the placenta. J Appl Physiol 1973; 35: 662-68.
15. Sweiry J.H., Page K.R., Dacke C.G., Abramovich D.R., Yudelivich D.L. Evidence of saturable uptake mechanism at the maternal and fetal sides of the prefused human placenta by rapid paired tracer dilution: studies with calcium and choline. J Dev Physiol 1986; 8: 435-45.
16. Pike J.W., Gooze L.L., Haussler M.R. Biochemical evidence for 1,25 dihydroxyvitamin D receptor macro molecules in parathyroid, pancreatic, pituitary and placental tissues. Life Sci 1980; 26: 407-14.
17. Mughal M.Z., Ross R., Tsang R.C. Clearence of calcium across in situ perfused placentas of intrauterine growth-retarded rat fetuses. Ped Res 1989; 25: 420-22.
18. Rowe J.C., Wood D.H., Rowe D.W., Raisz L.G. Nutritional hypophosphatemic rickets in a premature infant fed breast milk. N Eng J Med 1979; 300: 293-6.
19. ESPGAN. Committee on Nutrition. Guidelines on infant nutrition. Recommendations for the composition of an adapted formula. Acta Ped Scan 1977; sup 262.
20. Moya M, Doménech E. Role of calcium-Phosphate ratio of milk formulae on calcium balance in low birthweight infants during the first three days of life. Ped Res 1982; 16: 675-681.
21. ESPGAN. Committee on Nutrition. Committee report Nutrition and feeding of preterm infants. Acta Ped Scand 1987; supp 336.
22. Manz F. Why is the phosphorus content of human milk exceptionally low?. Monatsschr Kinderheilkd. 1992; 140: Sup 1 S35-39.
23. De Vizia B., Mansi A. Calcium and phosphorus metabolism in full-term infants. Montatsschr Kinderheilkd 1992; 140 Sup 1: S8-12.
24. ESPGAN Committee on Nutrition. Comment on the composition of cow's milk based follow-up formulas. Acta Ped Scand 1990; 79: 250-54.
25. Steichen J.J., Tsang R.C. Bone mineralization and growth in term infants fed soy-based or cow milk-based formula. J Pediatr 1987; 687-92.
26. Greer F.R., Seary S.E., Levin R.S., Steichen J.J., Steichen-Asch P., Tsang R.C. Bone mineral content and serum 25-hydroxyvitamin D concentrations in breast fe infants with and without supplemental vitamin D: 1 year follow-up. J Pediatr 1982 100: 919-92.
27. Namgung R., Mimouni F., Campaigne B.N., Ho M.L., Tsang R.C. Low bone mineral content in summer-born compared with winter-born infants. J Pediatr Gastroenterol Nutr 1992; 15: 285-88.
28. Steichen J.J., Koo W.N.K. Mineral nutrition and bone mineralization in full term infants. Monatsschr Kinderheilkd 1992; 140 supp 1: S 21-7.9.
29. Hansen AE; Stewart RA; Hugues G and Soderhjelm L. The relation of linoleic acid to infant feeding. A review. Acta Pediatrica 1962, sup. 51, 137-44.
30. Kohn G. Human milk and fatty acids: quantitative aspects. In Essential fatty acids and infant nutrition. Ed by J. Ghisolfi and G. Putet. John Libbey Eurotext. Paris 1992, pag. 79-86.
31. Rhodes PG; Reddy NS; Drowning G et al. Effects of different levels of intravenous α-linolenic acid and supplemental breast milk on red blood cell docosohexaenoic acid in very low birthweight infant. J Pediatric Gastroenterol Nutr 1991; 13:67-71.
32. Uauy R; Birch E; Birch D; Peirano P. Visual and brain function measurements in studies of n-3 fatty acid requirements of infants. J Pediatr 1992; 120: S168-80.
33. Connor WE; Neuringer M; Reisbick S. Essential fatty acids; The importance of n-3 fatty acids in retina and brain. Nutr Rev 1992; 50: 21-29.
34. Pettei MS; Daftary S; Levine JJ. Essential fatty acid deficiency associated with the use of a medium chain triglyceride infant formula in pediatric hepatobiliary disease. Am J Clin Nutr 1991; 53: 1217-21.

35. Boudreau MD; Chanmugam PS; Hart SB et al. α-Linolenic Acid and Prostaglandin Synthesis Nutrition 1992; 8:211-12.
36. Koletzko B. Trans fatty acids may impair biosynthesis of long-chain polyunsaturates and growth in man. Acta Paediatr 1992; 81:302-6.
37. Moya M.; Cortés E; Juste M; Vera A. Absorción de ácidos grasos en recién nacidos pretérmino alimentados con una fórmula conteniendo aceite de pescado. Actualidad Nutricional, 1992 Sup 6:11-15.
38. ESPGAN Committee on Nutrition. Comment on the content and composition of lipids in infant formulas. Acta Ped Scand 1991; 80: 887-896.
39. Clandinin MT and Chappell JE. Long-chain polyenoic essential fatty acids human milk: Are they of benefit to the newborn. In Composition and Physiological Properties of Human Milk. Ed by J. Schaub Elsevier 1955; 213-22.
40. Koletzko B. Minimal, optimal, maximal essential fatty acid requirements during infancy: term infants. In Essential Fatty Acids and Infant Nutrition. Ed. by J. Ghisolfi and G. Putet, John Libbey Eurotext. Paris 1992:147-56
41. Nordoy A; Barstadl L; Connor WE and Hather L. Absorption of n-3 eicopapentaenoic and docosahexaenoic acids as ethyl esters and tryglycerides by humans. Am J Clin Nutr 1991; 53: 1185-90.
42. Verkade HS; Horing EB; Muskiet FAJ et al. Fat absorption in neonates: comparison of long-chain fatty acid and triglyceride composition of formulas, faeces and blood. Am J Clin Nutr 1991; 53:643-51.
43. Clandinin MT; Chappel JE and Van Aerde JEE. Requirements of newborn infant for long chain polyunsaturated fatty acids. Acta Ped Scand 1989, sup 351:63-71.
44. Carlson SE; Cooke RJ, Rhodes PG et al. Effect of vegetable and marine oils in preterm infant formulas on blood arachidonic and docosahexaenoic acid. J Pediat 1992; 120: S159-67.
45. Carlson SE; Cooke RS; Rhodes PG et al. Long-term feeding of formulas high in linolenic and marine oil to very low birthweigh infants: phospholipid fatty acid. Ped Res 1991; 30:404-12.

205

Dairy Products in Human Health and Nutrition, Serrano Ríos et al. (eds) © 1994 Balkema, Rotterdam, ISBN 90 5410 359 0

Dairy products and the elderly

G. Schaafsma
Department of Human Nutrition, TNO Nutrition and Food Research, Zeist, Netherlands

ABSTRACT: As a consequence of decreased physical activity and reduced energy requirements attention should be paid to the nutrient density of the diet of elderly people. Milk consumption contributes to the nutrient density of the diet. Due to its calcium content milk helps to prevent osteoporosis. Moreover, the complex mineral composition of milk may play a role in the prevention of hypertension and colon cancer. Because of their taste, keepability and digestibility, fermented milks, e.g. yogurts, are very popular in the elderly. The nutritional significance of other health aspects of these products is discussed.

1 INTRODUCTION

In many developed countries the population is getting older as a consequence of birth control measurements, improved medical care and prolonged life expectancy. The aging process is associated with an increased incidence of chronic diseases, like cardiovascular disease, cancer, diabetes, hypertension and osteoporosis. These diseases require major medical care which is associated with high costs. Therefore it is important to prevent rather than to treat them. Prevention means a healthy life style, including regular physical activity, no smoking and good nutrition. Regarding the latter, the characteristic of the nutritional needs of the elderly is that energy needs are reduced whereas essential nutrient requirements are not. This implicates that the nutrient density of the diet for the elderly should be higher than that of young adults. In this regard dairy products can play a substantial role. In this paper the nutrient density of milk will be discussed, especially from the view of the specific needs of the elderly. Secondly the nutritional significance of milk with respect to the prevention of chronic diseases will be reviewed. Thirdly a brief discussion will be devoted to health aspects of fermented milk.

2 THE NUTRIENT DENSITY OF MILK

A simple and useful evaluation of the nutritional significance of essential nutrients in milk is obtained by using the concept of nutrient density. This is an index of nutritional quality. For each nutrient the density in a specific food is computed by deviding its concentration in the food per unit of energy by its RDA per energy unit. Usually the nutrient density is expressed as a percentage. A density for a given nutrient of 100% or more indicates that the food, if consumed in sufficient quantities, contributes substantially to the intake of the particular nutrient.

Tables 1 and 2 show the nutrient density of milk, using data on the nutrient composition of milk as given by Renner et al (1989) and the Recommended Daily Allowances for adults as given by the USA Food and Nutrition Board (1989). It can be concluded from tables 1 and 2 that milk has a well balanced nutrient composition and the power to contribute substantially to meeting nutritional needs of the consumer. Nutrients with a high density in milk are: protein, vitamins B2 and B12, calcium, potassium, phosphorus, magnesium and the trace elements zinc, iodine, molybdenum and chromium.

Table 1. Density of essential nutrients in milk: protein and vitamins.

Nutrient density (%)

Protein	233
Vitamin A	164
Vitamin D	44
Vitamin E	44
Vitamin K	193
Vitamin C	110
Vitamin B1	121
Vitamin B2	455
Vitamin B6	175
Vitamin B12	880
Folic acid	110
Patothenic acid	385
Biotin	440
Niacin	19*

* Tryptophane in milk not taken into account.

Table 2. Density of essential nutrients in milk: minerals and trace elements.

Nutrient density (%)

Na	85
K	186
Cl	124
Ca	655
P	514
Mg	149
Fe	9
Cu	15
Zn	121
Mu	6
I	216
Se	80
Mo	318
F	36
Cr	147

2.1 Protein

The high biological value of milk proteins is well recognized. It is generally assumed that the protein content of western diets is in excess of requirements and therefore needs little attention. Moreover, excess dietary protein has been considered as a risk factor for osteoporosis,

Table 3. Calcium metabolism (mg/d) during low and high protein intake in 30 elderly people

	Low-protein	High Protein	P
Intake	860 ± 23	966 ± 24	< 0.001
Faeces	911 ± 56	865 ± 67	NS
Urine	133 ± 11	164 ± 14	< 0.01
Balance	-184 ± 58	-62 ± 64	NS

because of its hypercalciuric action (Yuen et al, 1984). On the other hand there is no direct evidence in man that high protein intake causes bone loss. A recent study in elderly people (Schaafsma et al, 1992) confirmed the hypercalciuric action of protein but this was not associated with a concomitant negative effect on calcium balance. On the contrary, calcium balance tended to be less negative, particularly in elderly women, when protein intake was raised from 13 to 23 en%. Actually, the optimal intake of dietary protein by elderly people is not known. It is possible that dietary protein has an anabolic action by stimulating the synthesis of the insulin like growth factor 1 (IGF1) in the liver (Bonjour, 1992). This might help to prevent the loss of lean tissue which occurs during the aging process.

It should further be stressed that elderly people are more frequently ill because of infections than young adults. This implicates more episodes of recovery which are associated with regain of lost muscle mass and increased protein requirements. This has not been accounted for in RDAs. Other aspects of dietary protein which are not directly related to the nitrogen equilibrium have attracted only little attention. These aspects include effects of specific peptides on the immune system and effects of proteins on gastro intestinal functions (stomach emptying rate, feelings of satiety, intestinal motility and absorption processes). In this regard milk proteins may have beneficial characteristics that are as yet insufficiently recognized.

2.2 Vitamins

Milk is an excellent source of vitamins B2 and B12. Vitamine B2 in milk occurs mainly in the free form, the remainder being present as FAD and FMN. Without dairy products the intake of vitamin B2 would be far from the RDAs. In the Netherlands the contribution of milk and milk products to the intake of vitamin B2 is at least 40%. Vitamin B12 activity in milk is almost entirely cobalamine and occurs bound to the whey protein. For vegetarians milk is the dominating source of this vitamin. There is no evidence that elderly people in western countries experience deficiencies of these vitamins which are attributable to a low intake.

2.3 Calcium and phosphorus

Milk contributes substantially to the intake of these nutrients. No less than 75% of the calcium in the western diets originates from milk. An adequate intake of calcium by elderly people is required to reduce the age related loss of bone tissue which may lead to the development of osteoporosis. The ratio between calcium and phosphorus in milk (1.2 on a weight basis) is higher than that in most other foods. This is considered favourable since low calcium to phosphorus ratios may stimulate parathyroid hormone secretion and accellerate bone loss. There is no direct evidence in man that phosphopeptides formed during the digestion of milk casein enhance calcium absorption. Phophorus deficiency in the human is rare, since phosphorus is distributed widely in foods. Passive calcium absorption is known to be enhanced by lactose in milk. The nutritional significance of this for elderly people is uncertain.

2.4 Magnesium and potassium

The contribution of milk to the intake of these nutrients has been estimated at about 20% (Renner et al, 1989). In elderly people who are treated with diuretics increased urinary losses of potassium occur. Like fruits and vegetables milk is a good source of potassium. The ratio of sodium to potassium in milk is low as compared to that in total diets. Therefore and because of its calcium and magnesium, milk may help to prevent hypertension, which has a high prevalence in elderly people. It is possible that magnesium requirements of elderly people are higher than those of young adults, because of reduced capacity to maintain adequate intracellular magnesium concentrations at low intakes.

2.5 Trace elements

An adequate intake of zinc by elderly people is important for tissue repair (wound healing) and the immune system. The contribution of dairy products to the intake of zinc is about 25% (Renner et al, 1989). The iodine content of milk depends on the iodine concentration of the soil and the use of iodophores as udder disinfactants. Iodine is essential for the synthesis of thyroid hormones. The contribution of dairy products to the iodine intake may be as high as 36% in the UK and is about 13% in the Netherlands. Chromium and molybdenum in milk and dairy products have been reported to make up 21 and 36% of the total intake of these elements respectively (Renner et al, 1989). Molybdenum deficiency in man is unknown, whereas chromium deficiency causes decreased glucose tolerance and increased serum lipid levels. The nutritional significance of milk in data this regard is difficult to assess since quantitative data on human requirements of chromium and molybdenum are uncertain.

3 PREVENTION OF CHRONIC DISEASES

Adequate consumption of milk will most probably lower the risk for the development of three diseases which have a high prevalence in elderly people: these are osteoporosis, hypertension and colon cancer.

3.1 Osteoporosis

It is now widely recognized that adequate intake of calcium during growth is required for the attainment of the peak bone mass at adult age. Since the rate of bone loss in later life is not dependent on the initial bone mass, attainment of peak bone mass is very important for osteoporosis prevention. At older age adequate calcium intake may slow down the rate of bone loss. In practise it is not possible to meet the RDA without consumption of dairy products, unless calcium pills are used. Calcium pills, however, are lacking the nutritional value of milk. When calcium intake is too low, calcium will be released from the skeleton in order to maintain the extracellular calcium concentration. On a long term basis this will cause osteoporosis.

3.2 Hypertension

Many health authorities point to the importance of salt restriction for the prevention of hypertension which is a significant risk factor for cardiovascular disease and stroke. The contribution of milk to the intake of sodium is modest. Moreover the sodium to potassium ratio in milk (0.31) is low as compared to that in the total diet (about 1.8). This makes sense, because a low ratio between these elements may be more important than sodium restriction alone. A low calcium intake could be another factor contributing to hypertension. Epidemiological studies have suggested the existence of an inverse relation between dietary calcium and blood pressure. Clinical trials provided however conflicting results. It is possible that the inverse relation-ship between dietary calcium and blood pressure is caused by the total complex of minerals in milk (e.g. potassium, magnesium and calcium), rather than by calcium alone. Van Beresteijn et al (1990) have investigated this possibility in a double blind placebo-controlled trial with young normotensive female students. As a placebo an imitation milk which contained essentially the same macronutrients as normal milk, but not the milk minerals was used. It was found that even in these normotensive healthy females supplementation with milk (1 l per day) as compared to placebo significantly decreased systolic blood pressure while the students were on a low calcium diet. From the present knowledge it can be concluded that milk consumption helps to prevent hypertension.

3.3 Colon cancer

Evidence exists that colon cancer development is related to nutritional factors, including low intake of dietary fiber, high consumption of meat and fat and low calcium intake. However, as yet no final statements can be done. In a recent prospective study by our institute no significant relationship appeared between colon cancer incidence and either fat or meat intake (Van den Brandt & Bausch-Goldbohm, 1993). Experimental studies in rats and humans have demonstrated that calcium or calcium phosphate salts can bind cytotoxic bile acids and fatty acids in the colon (Lapré, 1992). This leads to less irritation of the epithelial cells, to decreased proliferation and most probably to a decreased risk of colon cancer. In this regard milk may exert a beneficial effect.

4 HEALTH ASPECTS OF FERMENTED MILK

The popularity of fermented dairy products is increasing, as appears from consumption statistics of the International Dairy Federation. Excellent taste, prolonged keepability and health aspects contribute to this popularity. The health aspects include: improved digestibility, immune stimulating effects and beneficial effects on the intestinal flora. There is no doubt that yogurt is tolerated better than milk by lactase deficient people. Since the prevalence of symptoms of lactose intolerance increases with age, even in Caucasians, yogurt is very popular by many elderly people. Possible beneficial effects of lactobacilli and fermented milk on the immune system and the gastro intestinal function, including the metabolic activity of the gut flora, are currently being investigated all over the world. A critical evaluation of the available scientific evidence leads to the conclusion that not all research has been done properly and that interpretation of the results of many studies is hindered by the huge number of different strains of lactobacilli used and by poor experimental designs (IDF, 1992). Moreover, results obtained in experimental animals may not be extrapolated directly to the human. Nevertheless, beneficial effects have clearly been demonstrated and it should be considered as a challenge to the dairy industry to develop further this important area.

5 CONCLUSIONS

- Because of their nutrient density dairy pro-

ducts fitt excellent in the diet of the elderly.
- Milk consumption is essential for the prevention of osteoporosis and probably also for that of hypertension and colon cancer.
- Fermented milk can exert beneficial effects on the immune system and the intestine, but the nutritional significance has not yet been completely established.

6 REFERENCES

- Bonjour, J-P. 1992. Action of IGF-1 on bone. Proceeding of the First Workshop on Protein Intake and Bone Health, Paris.
- Food and Nutrition Board 1989. Recommended Dietary Allowances. Washington: National Academic Press.
- International Dairy Federation 1991. Cultured Dairy Products in Human Nutrition. Bulletin of the International Dairy Federation, no. 255.
- Lapré, J. 1992. Dietary calcium as a possible anti-promotor of colon carcinogenesis. Thesis, Wageningen, Agricultural University.
- Renner, E., G. Schaafsma & K.J. Scott 1989. Micronutrients in milk. In: E. Renner (ed). Micronutrients in milk and milk-based food products. London and New York: Elsevier Applied Science, pp 1-70.
- Schaafsma, G. 1992. Protein intake and calcium metabolism in elderly subjects. Proceedings of the First International Workshop on Protein Intake and Bone Health, Paris.
- Van Beresteijn, E.C.H., M. van Schaik & G. Schaafsma 1990. Milk: does it affect blood pressure? A controlled intervention study. J. Int. Med. 228:477-482.
- Van den Brandt, P. & S. Bausch-Goldbohm 1993. A prospective cohort study on diet and cancer in the Netherlands. Thesis, Maastricht, State University Limburg.
- Yuen, D.E. et al 1984. Effect of dietary protein on calcium metabolism in man. Nutr. Abstr. Rev. 54:447-459.

4 Dairy products and metabolic impact

dairy products and meat processing chapter 4

Dairy Products in Human Health and Nutrition, Serrano Ríos et al. (eds) © 1994 Balkema, Rotterdam, ISBN 90 5410 359 0

Milk and scientific knowledge of nutrition

F.Grande Covián
Departamento de Bioquimica Molecular y Celular, University of Zaragoza, Spain

There is little I can add to what has been said here about the role of milk in human feeding and nutrition. Therefore, and in order to avoid repetitions, I think it would be useful to take advantage of this opportunity to deal with something which I believe has not been considered in detail, namely the role performed by the study and knowledge of milk and its properties in the enhancement of the scientific knowledge of nutrition.

DIFFERENCES IN COMPOSITION BETWEEN MILKS FROM DIFFERENT SPECIES

Milk is undoubtedly the only single foodstuff specifically intended for feeding the new-born from the different mammal species during the first stage of their lives. It is therefore surprising that such remarkable differences should exist in the composition, in terms of nutrients, of milk produced by the females of different mammal species. One could say, from a teleological point of view, that the considerable differences in composition between different milks show us that the nutritional needs of the new-born from the different species are also different, in contrast with the relative consistency of nutritional needs of adults of the different mammal species.

Gustav von Bunge was apparently the first person to realize this important fact and to give a lot of his time and attention to this question.

In his Treatise on Physiology (II vol. p. 121, 1901) we are able to read: "The composition of milk from the different mammal species is considerably different. As far as I know, nobody has tried to explain these differences before. Preliminarly, at least, I find a possible teleological explanation in the different speeds of growth experimented by the suckling young. A priori, it is possible to think that milk from those animals with the highest growth rate would be the richest in those nutritional matters which preferably serve for building up tissues, namely, proteins and inorganic salts. This relationship attracted my attention when I published the analysis of milk in 1979."

Mammals include over 3500 species (Morowitz) which show remarkable differences in size and growth speed. The smallest mammal, the shrew (Suncus etruscus) can weigh as little as 1.6 grams whilst the blue whale (Balaenoptera musculus) can weigh 135 Tm. The whale is therefore almost 100 million times larger than the shrew.

There are also remarkable differences between their growing speed. It can take the human new-born baby between 120 and 140 days to double its weight at birth while it takes sheep only about 35 days and rats or rabbits some four to six days.

But also, the time needed to reach the characteristic adult size varies also from one species to another. The rat needs about ten months, while the human being needs almost 20 years.

The size of the cells which constitute the different organs and tissues of mammals is practically the same whatever the size of the animal. The cells which constitute an elephant's liver, for example, are no bigger than those constituting the liver of a rat. Red blood cells in mammals are practically all of the same size, whatever the size of the adult animal to which they belong.

One would be inclined to think that the increase in body size which takes place during the growing stage is only due to the increase in the number of cells which make up the body. But this is not so, because the increase in body size is accompanied by changes in the proportion in which different organs and tissues contribute to the total weight. The brain of a 70 kg man weighs approximately 1.4 kgs, i. e. around 2 per cent of his body weight; but the brain of a 3.5 kg new-born baby weighs between 380 and 390 grams, which is approximately 11 per cent of its total weight.

Factors determining body size and growing speed

The size of the different animal species is determined by two types of factors, genetic and nutritional. It is not very difficult to understand the genetic factor if we consider that each animal species has a characteristic size which remains constant, within certain limits, from one generation to another. In the case of mammals, the mother's size is a basic factor to determine the size of the new-born. More than 50 years ago, Walton and Hammond crossed large Shire draft-horses with very small Shetland mare ponies (and Shire mares with Shetland male ponies). The size of the colts at birth was proportional to that of their mothers, but as they became older, the paternal influence started becoming noticeable. The resultant adult horses from each of these crossings did not show outstanding differences in size between each other.

Nor is it difficult to understand the importance of the nutritional factor. Pediatricians know very well that undernourished children show signs of backwardness in growth, and stock breeders know it just as well. It is a well known fact that an insufficient contribution of energy or of essential nutrients causes retardment or stops growth in experimentation animals. In fact, the use of growing animals as a way to evaluate the nutritional value of a diet has been one of the most used procedures in experimental nutritional studies.

One of the methods that is universally used for evaluating the nutritional condition of human populations is measuring growth speed. But it is important to remember that retardment in growth is a non-specific manifestation of inadequate nutrition, consequent to an insufficient contribution of energy or of one of the essential nutrients.

According to Moulton, it is generally accepted that the maximum size that can be attained by a given animal species is determined by genetic factors. But that such size should be ever reached, or, better still, the realization of the genetic potential, depends on the food received during the growing stage. It will not be necessary to say, on the other hand, that to be plentifully fed, with the best kind of food, during the growing period can hardly make the animal surpass the maximum size determined by genetic factors.

Critical stages in growth

The effects, on growth, of a period of malnutrition depend not only on the intensity and length of such a period. They also depend on the moment in the animal's life in which such malnutrition period occurs. The lines (in percentiles) of the growth curves normally used these days describe the growth of normal children. Along the different stages of its growth, a normal child will follow one of the curves. But if this child suffers a period of inadequate nutrition, he will stop growing, or slow down. His or her measurements will shift towards curves smaller than the "standard" curve they used to follow. When the child is once again adequately fed, he or she will gain weight quickly and return to his or her former curve. If the child's appetite does not decrease after having reached the "standard" curve, he or she might surpass it, but it does not often happen that by simply consuming a large amount of food the child will surpass the size which corresponds to him or her. This phenomenon is described as "compensating growth" and it reflects the capacity of the body to compensate the lack in growth caused by a period of inadequate nutrition.

Chronically undernourished children present a different situation. It is a well-known fact that children in chronically undernourished (hyponutrition) populations present lower weight and size figures than those observed in normally well-fed children of the same race. We carried out two different surveys in Madrid just after the Spanish Civil War which showed important differences between school-children belonging to population groups from different social levels. The weight and size figures as well as the bone development radiographic studies showed remarkable backwardness in somatic growth in the groups of children belonging to the less-favoured groups of population.

But the effects of an inadequate nutrition on physical development not only depend on the intensity and length of the hyponutrition period. It also depends, as has already been said, on the moment in which the food restriction period takes place. This fact is clearly proved by comparing different mammal species. The guinea-pig and the pig behave in a similar way to the human species while the rat behaves differently.

MacCance and Widdowson use an ingenious method to produce hyponutrition in the rat during the lactancy period which has become widely popular. Two litters of new-born rats are distributed in such a way that one of the mother-rats will suckle, for example, only four baby rats, while the other will suckle fourteen baby-rats. Three weeks later, after the lactancy period is over, all the little rats are fed "ad libitum". After 80-100 days of "ad libitum" feeding, the rats from the first group weigh approximately 500 grs while those in the second group only weigh 300 grs. Therefore, rats subject to food restrictions in the lactancy period do not show compensating growth later on.

MacCance and Widdowson have introduced the concept of "Critical periods in growth" to describe this phenomenon described by Dobbing as "vulnerable periods".

In contrast, rats who were suckled in small groups and who were fed "ad libitum" after weaning, lost weight when they were subjected to food restrictions for a short period of time, but gained it again when they were fed once again without restrictions, therefore showing "compensating growth."

Something similar happens with proteic restriction as we were able to prove with Doctor Galdeano some years ago (Grande 1989). Rats subject to proteic restrictions after weaning stop growing and the slowdown in their growing speed is proportional to the proteic content limitation in their diet. But these rats show compensating growth when re-fed with a protein-rich diet.

Considering these facts we can now approach the problem of the relationship between the composition of milk and growth speed in the different mammal species. But we should not forget, what Brody (1945, p. 805) wrote: "The situation is too complex for a simple generalization, although there is no doubt that growth speed, composition and physiological age of the new-born are important facts determining the evolutive trends of milk." And he adds (p. 807) "While the composition (of milk) tends to vary with the maturing speed of the new-born, other facts confuse this relationship."

Protein content in milk and growth speed of the new-born

Bunge used 9 mammal species (horse, goat, pig, rabbit, cat, man, sheep, dog and cow) in his original study, having observed an inverse relationship between the necessary time for doubling the weight at birth and protein concentration in milk. But although Bunge believes that the relationship keeps a remarkable regularity, it is not difficult to observe that the figures for men and rabbits show a marked deviation. The linear correlation coefficient we have calculated is of only r -0.675 which means that the protein content variance explains less than 50 per cent of the variances for the necessary time for doubling the weight at birth. We must also bear in mind that in the case of man, Bunge's figures overestimate the protein content in human milk as well as the necessary time for doubling the weight at birth.

In view of this, Dr. Galdeano and myself studied this relationship with more recent

218

data from 15 different species (horse, goat, pig, guinea-pig, rabbit, cat, man, acaca mulatta, sheep, dog, rat, mouse and cow). In the case of the guinea-pig and the rabbit, the data from the literature were completed with other analysis carried out at our Laboratory using a total of 32 data pairs. After trying different mathematical models we arrived at the conclusion that there is an inverse relationship between the decimal logarithm of the protein concentration in milk and the decimal logarithm of the number of days necessary for doubling the weight at birth. The linear correlation coefficient for the 32 pairs of facts was of r   - 0.929.

The regression equation derived from such data was:

$$y = 2.2822 - 1.3972 \; x$$

in which y represents the decimal logarithm of the number of necessary days for doubling the weight at birth, and x represents the decimal logarithm of the protein concentration in milk (g/dl).

If we represent the growth speed by the reciprocate of the number of days necessary for doubling the weight at birth, and we express this equation in an exponential way, we find that growth speed is proportional to protein concentration at power 1.4. But this does not mean, evidently, that growth speed in all species is proportional at such power of protein concentration in milk because the data obtained from different species really represent protein concentration and characteristic growth speed interaction in each of the species analized. What seems most probable is that the milk produced by each species has the most adequate

protein concentration for its own young to reach their respective genetically determined growth speed.

On the other hand, it is important to remember that proteins are not the milk component presenting the highest degree of variability. The data we have show that the minimum concentration is to be found in human milk, which is in the order of 1 g per decilitre. The figures 1.2 to 1.4 g which are found in the literature are due to the fact that they were obtained by means of the Kjeldahl method which also includes non-proteic nitrogen, and human milk has a higher non-proteic nitrogen content than that from other species, as has been proved by the surveys published by Swedish authors (Hambreus). In our laboratory, the research carried out by Villacampa has proved that protein concentration in human milk, measured by the biuret reaction, is no higher than 1 g per dl. At the other end of the spectrum, the highest concentration according to the data we have is found in doe rabbit milk with almost 14 g per dl. The protein concentration rank is undoubtedly much more restricted than the fat concentration rank as we shall now see.

Fat content in milk

The milk from polar carnivores and sea-mammals presents the highest degree of fat concentration, much higher than the protein concentration figures we have just seen. The grey seal's (Halychoerus grypus) milk, for example, has a fat concentration in the order of 52 g per dl and the white bear's (Thalarctos maritimus) milk has a 33 g. per dl fat concentration. In the cetaceans we find that porpoise's (Phocoena phocoena) milk has a 47 g /dl. fat content, dolphin's (Tursiops truncatus) milk 33 g /dl. and blue whale's milk 42 g /dl.

Within the group of earth mammals, the lowest fat concentrations are found in perisodactiles's milk. Mare's (Equus caballus) milk has under 2 g /dl and donkey's (Equus asinus) milk is in the order of 1.4 g /dl. The most surprising case is the rhinoceros (Diceros bicornis), where the female produces a type of milk with practically no fat content.

Therefore we can say that the mammary gland is unable to produce milk with a proteic content over 14 g /dl. while it is able to produce milk with a 52 g /dl. fat content.

Composition of the fatty acids in milk

The different kinds of milks produced by the females of the different mammal species not only differ in their fat content. They also differ in the fatty acid composition of the fat and the effect of the mother's diet on such composition. In certain species, one of them the human species, the fatty acid composition in milk fat is influenced by the amount and type of fat in the mother's diet (Alling et al 1973, Insull et al 1959, Mallies 1979, Potter & Nestel 1976, Villa-campa 1981). This does not happen in other species, particularly in ruminants.

Using data from the literature and from analysis carried out in our laboratory and collected in our previous publication

(Grande & Galdeano 1980) and bearing in mind the limitations of the information within our reach, it is possible to detect some differences I would like to point out now. Generally speaking, the two most abundant fatty acids are Palmitic acid (C16:0) and Oleic acid (C18:1, n-9). They make up, in fact, between 50 and 60 per cent of all the fatty acids. Fats in goats', sheeps' and cows' milk are specially known for being very rich in saturated short chain fatty acids (C4.0 -C10:0) which constitute 22.5 per cent of all fatty acids in goats' milk, 16 per cent in sheeps' milk and 8 per cent in cows' milk.

Rabbit milk is specially known for its high fatty acid content with 8 and 10 carbon atoms (Caprilic and Capric) which amount to 52 per cent of its total fatty acids content. Fat in human milk contains only 1 per cent capric acid (C10:0) according to Villa-campa's data, and pig's milk 0.9 per cent caprilic acid (C8:0).

Fats in rodents' milk (guinea-pig, rat, mouse) contain respectively 0.1, 11 and 5.5 per cent saturated fatty acids C8:0, C10:0 and C12:0.

The importance of knowing the fatty acid composition of fat in the different types of milk is because we need to know their essential fatty acid (EFA) content. We should not forget that nutritional needs of the suckling infant have been often calculated based on the composition and quantity of milk consumed by infants whose development is considered normal (Fomon1974, Grande 1980).

Some years ago, Crawford and

his co-workers (1972, 1981) pointed out the similarity existing between the content of certain long chain n-3 polyunsaturated fatty acids (PUFA) in milk and in the brain. This fact has led them to think that these fatty acids, belonging to the alpha-linoleic family (C18.3, n-3), might be essential for the development of the brain. It is a well-known fact that such fatty acids are less efficient than linoleic acid for treating the signs of experimental deficiency of essential fatty acids in rats. For this reason, the FAO Experts Committee to which I belonged (1977) proposed a recommended figure for linoleic acid but not for those acids from the alpha-linoleic family. Nevertheless, in the FAO publication (1977, p. 19) we can read: "Because of the possible essential role of this family of fatty acids in specialized tissues, alpha-linoleic acid (C18:3 n-3) should be considered an essential part of the diet. But it is necesary to clarify the role of this family of fatty acids (n-3) in the human diet."

The presence of long chain n-3 polyunsaturated fatty acids in human milk such as Eicosapentaenoic (C20:5 n-3) and Docosahexaenoic (C22:6 n-3) has been repeatedly confirmed (Villacampa, 1981) and their role as essential fatty acids is today generally admitted. The estimated proportion of n-6 polyunsaturated fatty acids (linoleic) and n-3 polyunsaturated fatty acids that should be present in the diet, ranges from 4-1 and 10-1 (Neuringer et al. 1989, Dupont, 1990).

In the recent Conference on essential fatty acids and Eycosanoids which took place in Australia (1992) there were several papers on this topic. The authors of these papers (Connor et al, Bourre et al and Bjerva et al) agree in pointing out the need of having an adequate supply of n-3 long chain polyunsaturated fatty acids to guarantee a normal development of the brain and the retina, both in men and animals. The presence of these fatty acids in human milk and the higher linoleic acid content in this type of milk therefore justify the opinion of Crawford et al concerning the superiority of human milk against cows' milk to supply essential fatty acids (EFA).

It seems evident that the development of the brain requires the presence of fat in the milk consumed by the suckled new-born. I remember some years ago, discussing with Doctor Crawford my surprise at the absence of fat in rhinoceros' milk. He said : "Don't be surprised, the rhinoceros has a very small brain". More recently, at the meeting held in Vitoria in February 1993, Dr. Crawford showed photographs of the new-born rhinoceros and its tiny brain.

But the amount of fat in milk is not, evidently, the only determinant of the size of the brain. Cows' milk and human milk both have approximately the same amount of fat. But a two year old calf can weigh 200 kgs while its brain weighs no more than 350 grs. A child of the same age might weigh around 15 kgs but its brain will weigh 1 kg or more. The child's brain is therefore about 3 times bigger than the calf's, in absolute terms, and some 40 times larger if it is expressed as a percentage of the respective body weight.

The proof of the presence of n-3 long-chain polyunsaturated fatty acids in milk has been the starting point which has led to establish the essential role of such fatty acids and their importance for the development of the brain and the retina in man and experimental animals.

These studies have also led to explain the reason of the dolphin's brain remarkable size. A 155 kg dolphin's brain will weigh approximately 1.6 kg, which is about 1 per cent of its body weight. It is the only one of the large mammals with a brain approximately the size of the human brain.

The research carried out by Crawford et al, compiled in the recently published book by Crawford and Marsh (1989) shows that there is approximately a 1:1 relationship between n-3 and n-6 polyunsaturated fatty acids in the brain. The dolphin, as Crawford and Marsh point out, has a considerable advantage over earth mammals because it feeds on food which is rich in n-3 polyunsaturated fatty acids, particularly docosahexaenoic acid.

It has been said (Crawford and Sinclair, 1972) that the brain of carnivorous mammals is larger than that of herbivorous mammals because the food eaten by the former is richer in essential n-3 fatty acids than the food eaten by the latter. In fact, large carnivorous mammals have a relatively small brain in comparison with their body weight. Their somatic growth exceeds the growth of their brain.

The traditional idea is that man's brain has passed from the 450 grams weighed by the chimpanzee's brain to the actual 1400 gramms weighed by

the brain of man these days. Recent surveys show, as I have pointed out, that there is a 1:1 proportion of n-3 and n-6 polyunsaturated fatty acids in brain lipids. The analysis of dolphin's tissues shows that in this animal the proportion of n-3 and n-6 polyunsaturated fatty acids is 1:1, both in the muscles and in the brain, while in fish the relationship is 1:40.

Crawford and Marsh conclude from these studies that dolphins behave as mammals, which they are, and not as fish. But they have an advantage over earth mammals in being able to enjoy a plentiful supply of n-3 polyunsaturated fatty acids, mainly docosahexaenoic acid (C22:6, n-3). They believe therefore that in the course of Evolution, earth mammals have increased their body size because they had available supplies of n-3 essential fatty acids, but not of n-6 essential fatty acids, necessary for the development of their brain. Consequently, they believe that primitive forms of human life which developed along the shores of the sea were able to enjoy a plentiful supply of both kinds of essential fatty acids, necessary to ensure their somatic and their cerebral development.

I am no authority to try to analize in detail this interesting Evolution Theory which tries to explain the difference between the development of the human brain and that of his primate forbears. What has been said should be enough to be able to understand that the study of milk fats has helped to establish the essential role of n-3 polyunsaturated fatty acids and an evolutive theory which tries to explain the cerebral development in our species.

MILK AND THE DISCOVERY OF VITAMINS

The experiments carried out by Lunin (1880) in Bunge's Laboratory in Dorpat (Estonia) are often quoted as the first experiments where the results led to think of the existence of those essential nutrients we now call "Vitamins". But these experiments are not often correctly described in the literature and very few papers consider Bunge's participation in the setup and interpretation of the experiments.

In the excellent revision of the historical development of the discovery of vitamins, published by the British Medical Research Council (1932, p. 12) it is acknowledged that Lunin's conclusion "A natural food, like milk, must therefore contain, apart from its known components, small quantities of unknown substances, essential for life." is the first indication of the existence of the essential nutrients we now call "Vitamins". But the analysis of Lunin's experiments is incomplete and the reader, in the end, does not know the reasons which motivated them.

Henriette Chick's description (1975) is also incomplete and full of incorrections.

Lunin's work was originally published as a Doctoral Thesis at the University of Dorpat (1880) and in the Hoppe Seylers Zeitschrift in 1881.

Background for Lunin's experiment

Considering the differences in composition of the abovementioned types of milk, with respect to their mineral content, Bunge concluded it is impossible to determine the mineral needs of adult mammals by studying the composition of milk ashes. This is what Bunge wrote in his Treatise on Physiological Chemistry (1894): "This is how we arrived at the experiment. We would be able to keep an adult animal alive by feeding it exclusively on organic foodstuffs, determine how long it is able to survive and the kind of disorders it shows. This basic metabolical experiment has only been made once by Forster, Voit's assistant at the Munich Laboratory in 1873."

The study Bunge proposes to Lunin as the theme for his Doctoral Thesis seeks an interpretation of the results obtained by the German researcher. Let us not forget that Lunin's Thesis had the following title: "Über die Bedeutung der anorganischen Salze für die Ernährung des Thieres" (Grande, 1992).

Lunin's experiment and its results.

Bunge believes that Forster's results are due to the absence of bases in the diet, necessary for neutralizing the sulphuric acid formed in the body by the oxidation of sulphur in proteins. Bunge points out that proteins contain around 1 per cent sulphur and that 80 per cent of this sulphur contained in proteins appears in the urine in the form of sulphate. But Lunin's experiments show that the neutralization of sulphuric acid doubles the length of survival time in mice, but does not stop them from dying.

Consequently, a second experiment is carried out. This time a mixture of all the inorganic components in milk, in the same proportion as they exist in milk in relation with its organic components, is added to the mineral-free diet.

The mice fed on this diet only survive between 20 and 31 days, that is to say, no more than those fed on the ash-free diet with addition of sodium carbonate. Another 3 mice were fed only with fresh cows' milk and, except one who died 47 days later, apparently from intestinal obstruction, the other two lived quite normally for two and a half months, increasing in body size. This result justifies Lunin's above-mentioned conclusion.

On the other hand, Bunge writes in his Treatise on Physiological Chemistry and in his Treatise on Physiology: "This is something to be seriously considered. Animals, fed exclusively on milk, are able to live, but if we put together all the components of milk, which according to our current knowledge are necessary for the upkeep of the body, animals will also quickly die."

After considering several possible explanations, Bunge makes a fundamental question: "Can it be that, as well as fats and carbohydrates, milk also contains some other organic substances which are also essential for life?" and he adds: "It would be worthwhile to continue with this research."

I do not know the reasons why Bunge did not continue with this research. The fact is that Bunge was the first person to consider that those substances, essential for nutrition, present in milk, could be of an organic nature,

that is carbon compounds, as in fact are the 13 essential vitamins for man that we know today.

It will not be neccessary to add that 25 years after Lunin's experiments, Pekelharing proved that mice fed on an artificial diet were able to live and to develop normally if a small amount of fresh milk was added to their diet. This amount would be, by itself, insufficient to keep the mice alive. In 1912, Hopkins, without knowing Pekelharing's findings, obtained the same results with rats.

Therefore, milk appears closely associated with the discovery of vitamins and with their classification in two groups: liposoluble and hydrosoluble.

LACTOSE INTOLERANCE

Lactose, or milk sugar, like all other disaccharides, is not absorbed by the intestine. To be absorbed, it has to be split up in the two monosaccharides which constitute it, glucose and galactose. Intestine cells in new-born mammals contain lactase which splits lactose, thus enabling its absorption.

Lactase defficiency is a very infrequent congenital metabolic error which hampers lactose absorption (Holzel et al, 1962). It is also known that there are a number of intestinal diseases, such as gluten enteropathy and certain infections which are accompanied by Lactase defficiency (Dahlqvist, 1984) and that the consumption of milk can cause diarrhoea and other digestive alterations in those patients.

But we now also know that most "normal" adult human beings, maybe 90 per cent of the total adult population, suffer Lactase defficiency and are therefore intolerant to Lactase in milk. Lactase defficiency of the human adult was first acknowledged in 1963 (Dahlqvist et al.).

The series of observations carried out at the end of the II World War, when the U.S.A. literally flooded the world with powdered milk, with the aim of improving the nutritional condition of the most needy groups of population, contributed to the discovery of this important fact. It was possible to observe then that adults from many of these groups were intolerant to milk in a higher or lower degree (Anderson et al., 1973).

In contrast with congenital Lactase defficiency, adult Lactase defficiency is not total.

The research carried out by Scandinavian authors has proved that in fact, adult people from those population groups intolerant to Lactose are able to tolerate 5 g of this disaccharide but not 10 g. The fact is that, as has already been said, most human adults show a limited tolerance to Lactose. Most adults from coloured races (blacks, yellow-coloured, American indians, Eskimos, etc.) are intolerant to Lactose. One exception are the members of some African tribes basically dedicated to cattle-herding, who include milk in their usual diet.

Individuals belonging to the white race generally tolerate Lactose, although there are some differences. In Europe, for example, more than 90 per cent of the adult Danish and Swedish populations tolerate Lactose perfectly well, but the rate of adults intolerant to this disaccharid increases when travelling from North to South in Europe. An excellent summary of the geographical distribution of Lactose tolerance can be found in Fickler and Leitzmann's work (1980). It has been proved that the continuous administration of Lactose to those individuals who show intolerance to this disaccharid does not increase the activity of Lactase in the intestine (Rosenszweig 1974).

It is currently believed that the reduction of Lactose activity in the intestine once the lactancy stage is over is a "normal" phenomenom which affects all mammal species, including human ·adults intolerant to Lactose. In human adults intolerant to Lactose the decrease of Lactase activity in the intestine seems to start showing at 5 years of age.

The question is how to explain the process which has allowed to preserve intestinal Lactase activity along the adults' life.

It is assumed that some primitive human groups, basically dedicated to cattle-herding in Africa, underwent some 10000 years ago a mutation which enabled the preservation of Lactase.

Dairy Products in Human Health and Nutrition, Serrano Ríos et al. (eds) © 1994 Balkema, Rotterdam, ISBN 90 5410 359 0

Milk and dairy products as dietary supplements

A.Gil
*Department of Research and Development of PULEVA & Department of Biochemistry and Molecular Biology,
University of Granada, Spain*

ABSTRACT: Milk and milk ingredients are being used as the basis of many products designed for nutrition of infants, children and adults. Infant formulas and special diets utilized for the dietary treatment of children suffering a sort of diseases form part of a selection of supplements in which milk and milk byproducts are the main components. In addition to those products enteral clinical nutrition diets and dietary supplements for the adults are increasingly being used to maintain the nutritional status of patients and populations. Milk ingredients also form part of those supplements. In this paper we review the nutritional significance of milk components and consider the criteria of formulation and choice for those products.

1 INTRODUCTION

Dietary supplements are increasingly being used both in infancy and adulthood as a consequence of the diversity of nutritional requirements that have the humans during their life. Dietary supplements serve as nutritionally structured foods aiding to fully sastisfy the requirements of specific groups of populations which may present nutritional deficiencies because of an unadequate intake or malabsorption of nutrients derived from the presence of a particular disease, a convalescence period, increased nutritional needs related to a period of rapid growth and a high metabolic rate generated by the existence of a pathology (Gil, 1992a).

Milk formulas for normal and low-birth weigth infants are currently used in a number of countries to fed, exclusively or as supplementary food mixtures, to newborns unable to be fed on human milk because of mother disease and in many cases because of social reasons. Moreover, baby foods form part of the diet in infancy and childhood in most occidental countries; these products are frecuently based on milk ingredients. Furthermore, special diets for the treatment and nutritional repletion of infants affected of congenital inborn errors metabolism and many adquired diseases such as gastroenterological pathologies which in turn lead to malnutrition are based in milk ingredients. The use of manufactured dairy products in infancy and childhood to adolescence is very extended worldwide. In general, each country has developed specific products and a number of them have elaborated recommendations for their utilization (ESPGAN, 1972; ESPGAN, 1981; Codex Alimentarius Commission, 1988; Commission of the European Communities 1986).

Protein energy malnutrition (PEM) is not only a phenomenon linked to an unadequate dietary nutrients intake but to the presence of disease which is able to generate it. PEM is highly prevalent in all hospitals trough the world with independence of the degree of development of the country, the incidence being dependent of the particular disease and the pharmacological and nutritional routine within the hospital. In a great number of patients the supply of conventional foods is not enough to maintain a good nutritional status because of the existence of anorexia, swallowing difficulties, and food restriction. Those patients must be nourished using special diets that are normally administered by enteral via usually trough fine nasoenteral tubes. Patients recovering from surgical operations are also fed with enteral clinical nutrition formulas allowing a better an rapid outcome. Most of the formulas currently being used in developed countries have dairy ingredients to assure a high nutritional value of the final products. On the other hand, in many diseases the use of a dietary supplement together with the comsumption of conventional foods can contribute to avoid malnutrition or to provide specific nutrients that otherwise are not normally supplied; that is the case for special diets used to maintain the nutritional status in elderly people and patients afeccted of chronic diseases, namely gastroenterological pathologies such as liver cirrhosis an inflammatory bowel diseases in which the food intake is usually restricted.

Fermented milks and lactic milk drinks have been used for centuries as healthy foods. The rapid progress in bacteriology, biochemistry and physiology during the last decades have increased the possibilities of making positive use of the beneficial effects of fermented milks particularly as agents to maintain the intestinal ecology in subjects suffering intestinal abnormalities (Gil, 1992b).

This paper reviews the potential uses of milk and dairy ingredients in infant formulas and baby foods as well as in dietetic supplements to be administered in different metabolic situations both in infancy and adult life. We will consider the nutritional significance and value of milk ingredients and the reasons they should have part of supplementary foods. In addition, we will focus on the nutritional and technological basis of design of infant milk formulas, enteral clinical nutrition products, and milk supplements for use in human nutrition.

2 NUTRITIONAL AND PHYSIOLOGICAL VALUE OF MILK COMPONENTS

Milk is a complex biological fluid secreted by mammals for the nourishment of their young. Through the centuries, evolution has produced a stable fluid which is a concentrated source of protein, carbohydrate and lipid with an unusual stability becoming a valuable foodstuff. Furthermore, milk is an important source of vitamins and minerals since the infant growth must be supported during a relatively long period exclusively from that food.

The nitrogen content of the milk is inversely correlated to the growth speed of the newborn. Cow's milk contains about 3-3.5 g/l of nitrogenous substances and human milk only about 1-1.2g/l. Caseins account for 80% of total proteins in cow's milk whereas human milk only has 30% of their proteins as caseins. Conversely, whey soluble proteins represent about 20% in cow's milk and 70% in human milk. Casein is a heterogeneous protein mixture formed by several proteins of relatively low molecular weight (19,000-23,000 daltons); alpha, beta, and kappa caseins being the most important components of the micellae estructure. α-casein, the major component is calcium sesnsitive, contains about 1% phosphorus and does not contain carbohydrates. α-casein is soluble in low amounts of calcium and contains 0.5% of phosphorus. κ-casein is poor in phosphorus (0.2%), contains a number of sialic acid residues and does not precipitate in the presence of calcium. The whey proteins are formed by lactalbumin, ß-lactoglobulin, serum albumin, proteose-peptones and other minor proteins including lactoferrin, lysozyme, and a number of enzymes. The specific profile of whey proteins is species specific; human milk does not contain ß-lactoglobulin but has high amounts of lactoferrin and lysozyme and the levels of immunoglobulins, specially those of Ig A, are also elevated as compared to ruminant milks which dominant immunoglobulin is Ig G (Gil, 1992b; Sánchez-Pozo, 1986a; Gil, 1989).

The quality of a protein for a human being may be defined by the smallest amount of this protein in a balanced diet, which maintains continuous health. At the same time one has to take into account that different requirements exist for different age groups, during pregnancy and lactation, and may exist also in the case of malnutrition, chronic diseases, postoperative periods and for sportmen. The quality of a protein for human nutrition depends primarily on the content of each of the indispensable amino acids. Non-essential amino acids under some circumstances may also contribute to the quality of a protein. The scoring patterns of the essential amino acids for cow's milk in comparison to other sources and for pre-school children, school children and adults have been reported (FIL/IDF, 1988; FIL/IDF, 1990).

Milk proteins are rich in essential amino acids specially branched chain amino acids and lysine. Whey proteins have a high content of sulfur amino acids particularly cysteine whereas caseins are rich in methionine. Milk proteins present a relative high content of serine and threonine (Hagemeister, 1990). Moreover, the content of some indispensable amino acids such as glutamic acid and glutamine is high; these amino acids are important for the maintenance and development of some tissues like the intestine and the skeletal muscle (Faus, 1984). The nutritional requirements of branched chain amino acids seem to be altered in hard exercise and in chronic liver disease (Young; Holm, 1986). The rate of leucine oxidation is significantly enhanced during exercise and due to the high clearance of branched chain amino acids in liver disease their plasma levels are low. These observations support the importance of the content of branched chain amino acids for the nutritive value of proteins. Milk and whey proteins are excellent and their biological value is reached only by egg and meat. On the other hand, casomorphines are formed following proteolitic degradation of milk proteins during the digestive processes; these peptides modulate the motility of intestinal tract and influence the release of insulin and glucagon playing an important role in food intake regulation (Brantl, 1981; Levin, 1986; Schusdziarra, 1983). Milk proteins also influence the bioavailability of mineral elements namely Ca, Zn, Mn and Fe; this is because of the high number of serine phosphate residues in caseins which bind divalent metal ions (Lönnerdal 1984). Caseins increase the absorption of calcium and phosphorus (Mykkänen, 1980) whereas bioavailability of zinc is apparently decreased by the consumption of bovine milk. However, human milk fed infants exhibit a better absorption of Zn than those fed milk formulas based on cow's milk (Sandström, 1983).

Curd formation from milk in the stomach contributes to a delayed emptying and causes better predigestion of the proteins facilitating the digestive capacity of the intestine. Furthermore, the milk proteins stabilize the intestinal microflora which is particularly important for the health of the infant (FIL/IDF, 1990).

Milk proteins are also implicated in the maintenance of the immune system. Not only immunoglobulins present in high amounts in colostrum but also a number of proteins namely, lysozyme, lactoferrin, lactoperoxidase, and xanthine oxidase play a role in the defense mechanisms of the humans particularly during infancy (Reiter, 1985). In addition to proteins there has been described the presence of a number of enzymes and hormones in milk (Koldovsky, 1987). Some of these substances infuence the growth of the young infant although their physiological role have not been fully established. Moreover, milk from diverse mammals contains non protein nitrogen compounds; human milk has more than two hundred non protein substances for which urea accounts for about 50%, creatine, creatinine, free amino acids and nucleotides are also present in relatively high amounts (Gil, 1985).

The content of taurine in human milk is high and could have a role in fat absorption and in the visual function, specially in premature infants (Gaull, 1977). Taurine dietary supplementation results in a better fat absorption in patients with cystic fibrosis since it leads to an increase in the ratio of taurine to glycine conjugated biliary acids (Darling, 1985; Thompson, 1987).

Infants fed formulas have lower levels of carnitine in plasma than those fed human milk what suggests a better availability of that nutrient in the latter (Warshaw, 1987). Carnitine plays an important role in the mitochondrial fatty acid oxidation and it has been demonstrated that the supplementation of carnitine to the diet in low birth weight infants decreases the free fatty acid to ß-hidroxybutirate ratio (Schmidt-Somerfield, 1981).

Human milk also contains poliamines which may have a role in the intestine development during early life (Sanguansermrri, 1974).

Milk has a species specific pattern of acid-free soluble nucleotides. Human milk has at least 13 nucleotides, cytidine, adenosine, and uridine derivatives being the more abundant. On the contrary, cow's milk has low levels of cytidine and adenosine derivatives and orotate is present in relatively high amounts in ruminant milk but it is absent in human milk (Kobata, 1962; Gil, 1981; Janas, 1982; Deutsch, 1960; Gil, 1982) Dietary nucleotides, particularly inosine facilitates the absorption of iron (Mazur, 1958); moreover, infant formulas supplemented with nucleotides in similar concentrations to those found in human milk result into higher levels of intestinal bifidobacteria and lower levels of enterobacteria (Gil, 1984). Dietary nucleotides have also a role in the lipoprotein metabolism during infancy contributing to increase the levels of HDL through a rise in the biosynthesis of apoprotein A-I (Sánchez-Pozo, 1986b). In addition, nucleotides influence the metabolism of polyunsaturated fatty acids during the immediate postnatal period; nucleotides apparently modulate the activity of fatty acid desaturases either in the intestine or in the small intestine or both increasing the levels of long chain fatty acids of the n-6 and n-3 series in plasma lipid fractions and in erythrocyte membranes (Uauy, 1985; Gil, 1986; DeLucchi, 1987a; Gil, 1988). Furthermore, dietary nucleotides have a role in the maintenance of the inmune system in humans and experimental animals (Kulkarni, 1986;Carver, 1990; Van Buren, 1983) and participate in the development and regeneration processes of the intestine (Uauy, 1988; Núñez, 1990).

The cow's milk fat content is about 3.5%, thus representing 49% of its total energy. Daily milk consumption of milk and dairy products is different according to countries; however, it oscillates between about 10 and 40 g which represent 12-25% of the total fat consumption of the population. In Spain the energy derived from dairy products accounts only for 10% of the total and the fat consumption 13% of the total fat energy (Gil, 1992b).

Milk fat is mainly formed by triglycerides which represent 98% of the total mass. Fat membrane also contains minor amounts of phospholipids and sterols. In addition, there are liposoluble vitamins and carotenoids. Milk fat contains more than 200 different fatty acids, many of them being only in trace amounts. Saturated, unsaturated, as well as branched chain and hydroxy fatty acids are present. The contents of short and medium chain fatty acids are relatively high in ruminants' milks and in human milk. Likewise, the contents of stearic, and palmitic acids are high in all milk types. Oleic acid is the most quantitatively important fatty acid (Webb, 1974).

Short and medium chain fatty acids are easily absorbed by the intestine since they pass directly into the enterocyte and are vehicled to the liver though the porta vein whithout intervention of the pancreatic lipase. These fatty acids represent a direct energy supply for the human being in a period of life in which there exist a deficiency in pancreatic lipase.

The content of essential fatty acids is relatively low in ruminants'milks. However, the concentration of these fatty acids in human milk and in mammals whose development at birth is relatively small, is high. Moreover, long chain fatty acids, specially arachidonic and docosahexaenoic acids are present in milk of a diversity of mammals the content of these fatty acids being negatively correlated with the degree of development of the species. The supply of long chain polyunsaturated fatty acids may be of importance for the preterm infant since the enzymatic systems which participate in the biosynthesis of long chain fatty acids are inmature even at birth (DeLucchi, 1987b).

Milk fat is easily absorbed by infants and children and its digestibility is very high in adolescent and adults. Reasons for a good digestibility of milk fat are found in the degree of dispersability of fat globules and in their fatty acid composition. In addition, the melting point of most of the fatty acid constituents of the milk fat is lower than the body temperature thus contributing to their absorption. A significant part of the milk fat is not fully hydrolysed in the intestine and it is absorbed directly by enterocytes though a pinocytosis process which is enhanced in homogenized milk (Renner, 1983).

Milk fat contains 30-50 mg of phospholipids per deciliter. The nutritional importance of phospholipids in milk is related to their influence in absorption and digestion. Furthermore, phospholipids are important as lipotropic agents contributing to the lipid transport from liver and intestine to the peripheric tissues. Phospholipids can be synthetized by the human body; however, a direct supply to the diet ameliorates the absorption of lipids and have a role in the reduction of plasma triglycerides (Gil, 1992b).

Cholesterol is the major component in the sterol fraction of milk. However, the cholesterol content of ruminants' milks is low in comparison with other animal foods. The average content of cholesterol in milk is 13 mg/dl, corresponding to a concentration of 3 mg/g of fat (Renner, 1983). The colesterol content in dairy products represents 0.25 to 0.40% of total lipids; thus, the consumption of cholesterol

trough dairy products is heavily depending on their percentage of fat.

Milk and dairy products only contribute to 10% of the total carbohydrate energy intake in adults and 13-20% in children (Gil, 1992b). Lactose is the main carbohydrate present in milk of diverse mammals. This compound serves as a source of energy for the neonate and to supply galactose for the development of the nervous central system. Moreover, lactose is partly utilized in the large bowel by bifidobacteria and other intestinal bacteria making organic acids which protect the newborn against diseases caused by enteric organisms (Gil, 1984). Cow's milk contains about 4.8% lactose and human milk about 7%. The latter has in addition to lactose more than fifty oligosaccharides; they are formed by tri- to octosaccharides mainly composed of N-acetylglucosamine and N-acetylneuraminic acid. The structure of these compounds are currently well known; they account for 12-14 g/l in colostrum decreasing their concentration with advancing lactation to approximately 0.7 g/l (Gil, 1989). Oligosaccharides are also present in caseins and in gangliosides but their structure is different to that of soluble oligosaccharides.

Intestinal bifidobacteria are stimulated by the presence of lactose and free oligosaccharides containing syalic acid, fucose, and N-acetylglucosamine. On the other hand, oligosaccharides in human milk exhibit structures which are analogous to that of epithelial receptors thus contributing to reduce the incidence of infectious diseases and inflammation blocking the binding of bacteria to the surface of enterocytes (Anderson, 1985). Gangliosides represent about 1-2% of the total fat in bovine milk. Ninety per cent of them are located in the fat globule membrane GM_3 and GD_3 being the most important (Keenan, 1974). GD_3 is the main ganglioside in human colostrum. GM_1 is also present in minor amounts exhibiting inhibitory properties against enterotoxins from *V. cholerae* and *E. coli* (Laegreid, 1987). GM_3 is the most abundant ganglioside in mature human milk.

Lactose intolerance is well documented specially among black people. However, inborn lactose malabsorption is a less frequent phenomenon. Using fermented dairy products is a valid alternative to the consumption of dairy products in lactose intolerants. Dietary intake of fermented milk products with active lactase due to the presence of microorganisms leads to a better digestion and absorption of lactose (Renner, 1991). This compound in turn promotes the absorption of some mineral elements namely calcium and magnesium. Cultured dairy products contribute to low the intestinal pH limiting the adhesion of pathogens and producing anti-bacterial substances and they seem to exhibit anti tumoural properties (Gorbach, 1988; Friend, 1984). Microorganisms in fermented products may also contribute to the enhancement of the immune system of the host favouring T cell proliferation (de Simone, 1986). We have previously suggested that nucleic acids and nucleotides produced during fermentation may have a role in the stimulation of the intestinal immune response (Gil, 1992b).

Milk contains variable amounts of minerals and vitamins according to the requirements of the species. Cow's milk has a content of minerals of about 7.3 g/l whereas human milk accounts for only 2.4 g/l. In addition to calcium, magnesium, phosphorus, sodium, potassium, and chlorine a number of trace elements are present. The importance of calcium and phosphorus in dairy products has been extensively documented since they contribute to the growth and maintenance of the bone structure. Milk is a good source of vitamins specially vitamin A and vitamins B_2, B_1, B_6, B_{12}, and panthotenic acid. Dairy products supply a significant part of the total daily requirements of vitamins in developed countries. Children diet may be deficient in vitamin A and in some vitamins of the group B and this is an argument to regularly supply milk and dairy products in the school.

3 MILK AND MILK BYPRODUCTS AS SOURCES FOR DIETARY SUPPLEMENTS

3.1 Formulas for infancy and childhood

Infant formulas are products designed for feeding infants from birth to 1-3 years of life. These products sustitute partially or totally human milk satisfying the nutritional requirements of the normal infants. There are two main types of infant formulas; the first is intended for use in infants from birth to 4-6 months of age and the second one is designed as a follow-up formula until the first to third year of life. The composition of an adapted milk formula should be as similar as possible to human milk covering the nutritional requirements of the infant and should be adapted to the tolerance of specific nutrients during early life. Practically, infant formulas are based on cow's milk and certain milk byproducts together with additions of vegetable oils and other types of fats and carbohydrates, minerals, and vitamins.

Adapted milk formulas have a protein content of about 1.8-2.8 g/100 kcal and follow-up milk formulas 3.0-5.5 g/100 kcal (ESPGAN, 1977;

ESPGAN, 1981). The specific profile of amino acids in human milk is achieved by adding to cow's milk isolated and demineralised whey proteins. Human milk has a ratio of whey proteins to casein of 70:30 whereas cow's milk has a ratio of 82:18 and casein has a high content of aromatic amino acids and a relative low content of cysteine (Sánchez-Pozo, 1986a). The addition of whey proteins to cow's milk results into a similar human milk methionine to cysteine ratio permitting to low the phenylalanine and tyrosine content of cow's milk.

Dietary intakes of 2.25 g/kg/day with a whey protein to casein ratio of 60:40 result in similar amino acid plasma profiles than those obtained in human milk fed infants (ESPGAN, 1977). On the contrary, infants fed predominant casein formulas present high concentrations of aromatic amino acids as well as methionine and excrete relative high levels of amino acids in urine.

The fat composition in infant formulas should be adjusted in such a way that allows an absorptive value of 85% (ESPGAN, 1977; ESPGAN, 1981). In practical terms the fatty acid composition of fat should be as much as similar to that found in human milk. There is no prove that mixtures of vegetable oils are better than mixtures of vegetable and animal oils and fats. Mixing cow's milk fat with a rich monounsaturated fatty acid oil and a rich essential fatty acid oil i.e. olive oil and soy oil permits an adequate adaptation of the fatty acid profile of the formula maintaining a high digestibility and a good palatability.

Lactose should be the main carbohydrate in infant formulas specially during the early postnatal period. Glucose polymers may be added when osmolarity restriction is needed. Starch and small amounts of sucrose can be added only in follow-up infant formulas. Finally, vitamins and minerals contents are adjusted taking into account the human milk concentrations of those substances as well as their bioavailability.

In western countries milk forms part of cereals. This is justified when the product is able to be recombined in water and the mixture contains at least 3 g/100 kcal of dairy proteins (ESPGAN, 1981). Lower levels of milk leads to a low intake of protein and calcium. Using hygienized cow's milk to make cereals at home is a good practice to cover the nutritional requirements during infancy and childhood.

Low birth weigth infants (LBWI) have special nutritional requirements due to their immaturity. A daily intake of 130 kcal should satisfy the energy requirements of LBWI making possible a similar growth rate to that achieved in utero. The maximum volume intake should be 200 ml/kg what may be obtained using an infant formula with an energy density of 65 kcal which is the minimum recommended (Commission of the European Communities, 1986).

Formulas for LBWI are also based in cow's milk. The protein content is usually higher than 2.25 g/100 kcal but it should not exceed 3.1 g/100 kcal. The ratio between whey proteins and casein must be adjusted to provide a similar pattern of amino acids to that of human milk. Concerning the supplementation of non-protein nitrogen substances, taurine has been shown to influence the development of the visual and auditive functions in very LBWI. The addition of nucleotides to infant formulas for LBWI results in the stimulation of the immune response; infants fed with these formulas have higher concentrations of Ig A and Ig M than those fed with a nucleotide free standard formula (Gil, 1993). Nucleotides also affect the development of the gut in early life; we have recently observed that dietary nucleotides contribute to decrease the intestinal permeability and to accelerate the gut closure in preterm neonates.

The ESPGAN has recommended that infant formulas for LBWI must contain 3.6-7.0 g/100 kcal (Commission of the European Communities, 1986). Fat mixtures of animal fat, including milk fat, and vegetable oils are being used with succes to fed LBWI. Those formulas usually include medium-chain triglycerides which are well absorbed by the neonates although levels higher than 40% of the total fatty acids are not recommended. Linoleic acid content should oscillate between 4.5 and 20% of the total energy of the formula and linolenic acid should represent a minimum of 55 mg/100 kcal (Commission of the European Communities, 1986).

Infant formulas for preterm newborns must contain lactose in a certain proportion since it is not clear the total requirements of galactose for the development of the central nervous system can be satisfied by the *de novo* synthesis from glucose. Moreover, lactose is implicated in the establishment of a Gram positive microflora and enhance the absorption of calcium, magnesium and other divalents cations which are important for growth and development. In addition to lactose, formulas may contain other carbohydrates namely, corn syrup solids, glucose polymers, and sucrose; the incorporation of starch is not recommended.

The mineral content of formulas for LBWI must be higher than those for normal infants. Calcium and phosphorus concentrations must be increased to permit an adequate bone development; 70 mg of calcium and 50 mg of phosphorus per 100 kcal are envisaged as the minimum figures. The maximum dietary intake of calcium is considered to be 140 mg/100 kcal with an optimum Ca/P ratio of 2.2. Recommendations for intakes of mineral and vitamins has been documented by several nutrition committees (Commission of the European Communities, 1986; American Academy of Pediatrics, 1977).

During the last three decades special diets for the nutritional replection of children affected of many diseases have been designed and marketed in developed countries. A series of those formulas are devised for the dietary treatment of inborn errors of metabolism. Most of these formulas are based in protein milk hydrolysates which undergo different processes to eliminate or low the concentration of specific amino acids involved in the pathogenesis of the disease. Another series of special diets are intended for the dietary treatment of gastroenterological diseases which are frequent in infancy. Primary and secondary lactose intolerance as well as galactosemie are treated with formulas which lack that carbohydrate. Furthermore, protein intolerances in atopic children and in infants suffering other diseases associated to malnutrition and malabsorption can be treated with a sort of products based in protein hydrolysates with reduced antigenicity. Those hydrolysates are usually derived from casein and whey proteins permitting the maintenance of an adequate biological value and an amino acid profile similar to that of human milk.

Modular formulas are now being increasingly used in the nutritional replection of hospitalized children; burn, trauma, septic, and major surgery patients as well as cardiovascular and renal patients are enterally fed using polimeric diets similar to those used in adults or specific diets formulated considering the special requirements of children and adolescents or modular diets which are formulated in the hospital according to the particular needs of the patient. Milk and milk components are frequently utilized as the basis for the formulation of those diets.

3.2 Enteral diets and supplements in adult life

Protein-energy malnutrition has a negative impact on the structure and functionality of many organs and tissues. The intestine is particularly affected by malnutrition both at the morphological and functional levels; there is a reduction in the absorption surface due to the decrease in the number of villous and the alteration in the structure of microvilli and a drop in the digestive juices secretion. The liver activity is also affected and the secretion of plasma proteins is severely decreased. Moreover, the immune system response is impaired and the malnourished patient is susceptible to suffer many infectious diseases (Gil, 1992a).

Artificial nutrition and particularly enteral nutrition is now being used as a support for many patients both at home and in hospitals. Malnourished patients due to anorexia, therapeutic nutritional deficit, chronic disease, and malabsorption syndromes and stressed patients with multiple fractures, sepsis, burns, and surgered patients are candidates to be nourished using enteral nutrition. This type of nutrition present many advantages on parenteral nutrition, namely less metabolic, mechanical, hepatic, and sepsis complications, and prevents the intestinal hypoplasia favouring the tolerance of oral foods. Even in intestinal pathologies enteral nutrition may be used with a high succes.

Once it has been decided to provide nutritional support via the enteral route the best formulation to meet the nutritional requirements of the individual patient must be selected. A large number of enteral diets are now commercially available; those diets cause less infection problems than those home brew. The succes of enteral nutrition is based on two aspects: type of diet and administration method. The first enteral diets were based on mixtures of amino acids provided they will be fully absorbed; carbohydrates sources were mainly glucose and sucrose and different mixtures of fats and oils were used. Those products had an intense osmolarity and provoked diarrhea. The increase knowledge in physiology, biochemistry, and pathophysiology has derived into the formulation of new diets with low osmolarity and adjusted to the special requirements of particular diseases.

Most of the enteral diets currently used have a source of nitrogen based on full protein; those are named polymeric diets. Proteins must be of a high nutritional value; concentrated whey proteins and casein and caseinates are widely used. These substances should be almost free of lactose specially when the diet is intended for use in gastroenterological patients in which lactase activity may be severely affected. Using concentrate whey proteins results into products with a relatively low methionine to cysteine ratio which is advisable in septic patients and in chronic liver diseases where the liver cistathionase activity is usually compromised. Moreover, the biological value of whey proteins is higher than that of casein and the palatability of products increase.

Predigested chemically defined diets are designed for use in patients with severely impaired gastrointestinal function. The source of nitrogen for these diets is usually a protein hydrolysate manufactured from milk proteins. The peptide distribution should be studied to provide low molecular compounds (<3000 daltons) to avoid absorption of active antigenic peptides and subsequent allergenic reactions; tri- and dipeptides must represent a high percentage of the mixture since those compounds are readily absorbed by the enterocyte elliminating the competition in amino acid absorption that occurs when amino acid mixtures are exclusively used. Finally, the concentration of free amino acids should be lower than 30% of the total nitrogen to preserve the final osmolarity of the formula.

Lipids are important components of the diet since they serve as high energy substrates and because they supply essential fatty acids and liposoluble vitamins. The importance of preventing essential fatty acid deficiency needs emphasizing, particularly as it may occur when gut function is impaired and long chain triglycerides (LCT) are poorly assimilated. Medium chain triglycerides (MCT) are a good source of energy and they are widely utilized in clinical nutrition. They are absorbed in the absence of pancreatic lipase and their hydrolysis is rapid whithout giving to changes in the pancreatic secretion; moreover, they are oxydized in the mitochondria avoiding the carnitine shuttle. Short chain fatty acids (SCFA) are also rapidly absorbed and represent a direct source of energy for the colon. MCT and SCFT are components of milk fat; thus it can be efficiently used when mixed with other types of fat, namely high monounsaturated oils like olive oil, high oleic sunflower oil, and canola oil, and essential fatty acid rich oils such as corn, sunflower, and soy oils. Milk fat contributes to give a pleasant flavour to formulas for enteral nutrition and their use in percentages oscillating 20-40% must be encouraged. An optimum ratio between saturated, monounsaturated, and polyunsaturated fatty acids can be obtained mixing milk fat, and vegetable oils to provide a good taste and flavour which is important for the acceptance of the diet in conscious patients.

Glucose polymers are by far the most used carbohydrates in enteral clinical nutrition. However, it has not been demonstrated that small amounts of lactose may cause disturbs in patients having a good intestinal functionality. Mixing maltodextrines with small amounts of lactose can result in a better absorption of minerals and in a more physiological intestinal microflora.

There are a number of situations in which feeding with conventional foods is not enough to maintain the nutritional status of particular patients or populations. Elderly people, for example, do not normally intake sufficient vitamins and minerals since they restrict the consumption of a variety of foods and women after the menopause do not currently satisfy their needs in calcium and phosphorus to maintain an adequate bone mineral density. In those and other situations namely, anorexia, swallowing difficulties, chronic diseases, etc, the usual diet may be completed with dietary supplements. These products can be enriched in particular nutrients such as minerals, vitamins, essential fatty acids, amino acids, thus depending of the nutritional status of the patient and the basic pathology. In other situations due to the presence of the disease the supplement can be lower in one or more nutrients. That is the case for patients suffering chronic encephalopathy and renal chronic insufficiency to which protein restriction may be necessary.

Dietary supplements can be formulated using a variety of ingredients. However, milk and dairy byproducts are extensively used particularly concerning the source of nitrogen. Products designed to avoid malnutrition in risk populations like elderly people and menopausic women are also frequently based in milk products.

4 REFERENCES

American Academy of Pediatrics: 1977. Committee on Nutrition. Nutritional needs of low birth weight infants. *Pediatrics*; 60: 519-30.

Anderson B, Porras O, Hanson LA, Svanborg-Eden C, Leffler H. 1985. Nonantibody containing fractions of breast milk inhibit epithelial attachment of Streptococcus pneumoniae and Haemophilus influenzae. *Lancet I* 643.

Brantl V, Teschemacher H, Blasig J, Henschen A, Lottspeich F. 1981. Opioid activities of beta-caso-morphins. *Life Sci* 28: 1903-1909.

Bulletin of the International Dairy Federation. 1988. Milk products and health, nº 222.

Bulletin of the International Dairy Federation. 1990. Role of milk protein in human nutrition, nº 253.

Carver JD, Cox WI, Barness LA. 1990. Dietary nucleotide effects upon murine natural killer cell activity and macrophage activation. *JPEN* 14: 18-22.

Codex Alimentarius Commission. 1988. Codex standards for foods for special dietary uses including foods for infants and children and related code of hygienic practice. *Codex Alimentarius*, vol IX, Suppl 3. Rome: FAO/WHO

Commission of the European Communities. 1986. Modified proposal for a council directive on the approximation of the laws of the member states relating to infant formulae and follow-up milks. *COM*: 564.

Darling PB, Lepage G, Leroy C, Masson P, Roy CC. 1985. Effect of taurine supplements on fat absorption in cystic fibrosis. *Pediatr Res* 19: 578-582.

de Simone C, Bianchi SB, Negri R, Ferrazzi M, Baldinelli L, Vesely R. 1986. The adjuvant effect of yogurt on production of gamma-interferon by Con A-stimulated human peripheral blood lymphocytes. *Nutr Rep Int* 33: 419-433

DeLucchi C, Pita ML, Faus MJ, Molin JA, Uauy R, Gil A. 1987a. Effects of dietary nucleotides on the fatty acid composition of erythrocyte membrane lipids in term infants. *J Ped Gastr and Nutr* 6: 568-574.

DeLucchi C, Pita ML, Faus MJ, Periago JL, Gil A. 1987b. Changes in the fatty acid composition of plasma and red blood cell membrane during the first hours of life in human neonates. *Early Human Development* 15; 85-93.

Deutsch A, Mattsson S. 1960. Acid-soluble nucleotides in cow's milk and colostrum. Milk and dairy research *Report No. 63*, Alnarp, Sweden.

ESPGAN Committee on Nutrition. 1981. *Guidelines on infant nutrition. II.* Recommendations for the composition of follow-up formula and Beikost. Acta Paediatr Scand; 70: Suppl 287.

ESPGAN Committee on Nutrition. 1977. *Guidelines on infant nutrition. I.* Recommendations for the composition of an adapted formula. Acta Paediatr Scand; 66: Suppl 262.

Faus O, López-Morales J, Faus MJ, Periago JL, Bueno A, Gil A, Martínez-Valverde A. 1984. Contenido de aminoácidos libres en leche humana española. *An Esp Pediatr* 6: 557-563.

Friend BA, Shahani KM. 1984. Antitumour properties of lactobacilli and dairy products fermented by lactobacilli. *J Food Protect* 47: 717-723.

Gaull GE, Sturman JA. Räihä NCR, Heinonen K. 1977. Milk protein quantity and quality in low-birth-weight infants. III. Effects on sulfur amino acids in plasma and urine. *J Pediat* 90: 348-355.

Gil A, Sánchez-Medina F. 1981. Acid-soluble nucleotides of cow's, goat's and sheep's milk at different states of lactation. *J Dairy Res* 48: 35-44.

Gil A, Sánchez-Medina F. 1982. Acid-soluble nucleotides of human milk at different stages of lactation. *J Dairy Res* 49: 301.

Gil A. 1984. *Nucleótidos en la leche humana fundamento para su empleo en leches infantiles.*

Granada: Europea de Dietéticos y Alimentación, S.A. EDDA.

Gil A. 1985. Nucleótidos de la leche humana y otras especies. En: *"Avances en Nutrición de la Infancia"*. Ed. Gráficas del Sur, Granada, p. 103-112.

Gil A. Pita ML, Martínez A, Molina JA, Sánchez-Medina F. 1986. Effect of dietary nucleotides on the plasma fatty acids in at term neonates. *Hum Nutr Clin Nutr* 40c: 185-195.

Gil A, Lozano E, De-Lucchi C, Maldonado J, Molina JA, Pita M. 1988. Changes in the fatty acids profiles of plasma lipid fractions induced by dietary nucleotides in infants born at term. *Eur J Cl Nutr* 42: 473-481.

Gil A. 1989. Factores de crecimiento y desarrollo de la leche humana. En: *Avances en nutrición de la infancia*. Vol 3, Gil A (ed)., Grafsur, Granada.

Gil A, Gassull MA. 1992a. *Nutrición Enteral: Cuándo y cómo debe utilizarse*. Barcelona.

Gil A. 1992b. La leche y los productos lácteos en la nutrición humana. *Revista Española de Lechería*, Julio/Agosto: 19-30.

Gil A, Jiménez J, Navarro J, Núñez MC. 1993. *Nucleótidos y Nutrición*. Doyma, Barcelona.

Gorbach SL, Vapaatalo H, Saminen S. 1988. Studies of *Lactobacillus* GG in humans. In Symp Intes Microecol. Alghero.

Hagemeister H, Sick H, Barth CA. 1990. Nitrogen balance in the human and effects of milk constituents. *Bulletin of the International Dairy Federation* nº 253.

Holm E, Leweling H, Staedt U, Striebel JP, Tschepe A, Uhl W. 1986. Protein und Aminosauren-stof-twechsel bei Leberinsuffizienz. Infusions therapeutische und diatetische Folgermgen. Verh. Dt. Ges. *Innere Med* 685-737.

Janas LM, Picciano MF. 1982. The nucleotide profile of human milk. *Ped Res* 16: 659-662.

Keenan TW. 1974. Composition and synthesis of gangliosides in mammary gland and milk of the bovine. *Biochim Biophys Acta* 337: 255-270.

Kobata A, Ziro S, Kida M. 1962. The acid-soluble nucleotides of milk. I. Quantitative and qualitative differences of nucleotide constituents in human and cow's milk. *J Biochem Tokyo* 51: 277-287.

Koldovsky O, Thornburg W. 1987. Hormones in milk. *J Ped Gastroenterol Nutr* 6: 172-196.

Kulkarni A, Fanslow WC, Drath DB, Rudolph FB, Van Buren CT. 1986. Influence of dietary nucleotide restriction on bacterial sepsis and phagocytic cell function in mice. *Arch Surg* 121: 169-172.

Laegreid A, Otnaess ABK. 1987. Trace amounts of ganglioside GM_1 in human milk inhibit enterotoxins from *Vibrio cholerae* and *Escherichia coli*. *Life Sci* 40: 55-62.

Levin AS, Morley JE, Gosnella BA, Billington CJ, Krahn DD. 1986. Neuropeptides as regulator of consummatory behaviors (Critical review). *J Nutr* 116: 2067-2077.

Lönnerdal B, Cedesblad A, Davidson L, Sandstrom B. 1984. The effect of individual components of soy formula and cow's milk formula on zinc bioavailability. *Am J Clin Nutr* 40: 1064-1070.

Mazur A, Green S, Saha A, Carleton A. 1958. Mechanism of release of ferritin iron in vivo by xanthine oxidase. *J Clin Invest* 37: 1809-1817.

Mykkänen HM, Wasserman RH. 1980. Enhanced absorption of calcium by casein phosphopeptides in rachitic and normal chicks. *J Nutr* 110: 2411-2148.

Núñez MC, Ayudarte MV, Morales D, Suárez MD, Gil A. 1990. Effect of dietary nucleotides on intestinal repair in rats with experimental chronic diarrhea. *JPEN* 598-604.

Reiter B. 1985. The biological significance of the non immunoglobulin protective proteins in milk: Lysozyme, lactoferrin, lactoperoxidase. In: Fox, PF (Ed). Developments in Dairy Chemistry, Vol 3, *Appl. Sci. Publ.* London, New York, 281-335.

Renner E. 1983. Milk and dairy products in human nutrition. N-GmbH, Volkswirtschaftlicher Verlag, München.

Renner E. 1991. Cultured dairy products in human nutrition. *Bulletin IDF* nº 255.

Sánchez-Pozo A, López J, Pita ML, Izquierdo A, Guerrero E, Sánchez-Medina F, Martínez-Valverde A, Gil A. 1986a. Changes in the protein fractions of human milk during lactation. *Ann Nutr Metab* 30: 15-20.

Sánchez-Pozo A, Pita ML, Martínez A, Molina JA, Sánchez-Medina F, Gil A. 1986b. Effects of dietary nucleotides upon lipoprotein pattern of newborn infants. *Nutr Res* 6:763-771.

Sandström B, Cederblad A, Lonnerdal B. 1983. Zinc absorption from human milk, cow's milk and infant formulas. *Am J Dis Child* 137: 726-729.

Sanguansermrri J, György P, Zilliken F. 1974. Polyamines in human and cow's milk. *Am J Clin Nutr* 27: 859-865.

Schmidt-Somerfield E, Penn D, Wolf H. 1981. The influence of maternal fat metabolism on fetal carnitine levels. *Early Human Develop* 5: 233-238.

Schuszdziarra V, Schick R, De La Fuente A, Holland A, Brantl V, Pfeiffer EF. 1983. Effect of ß-casomorphines on somatostatin release in dogs. *Endocrinol* 112: 1948-1951.

Thompson GN, Robb TA, Davidson GP. 1987. Taurine supplementation, fat absorption, and growth in cystic fibrosis. *J Pediatr* 111: 501-6.

Uauy R, Gil A. 1985. Fatty acid metabolism in the neonate. Effect of age, diet and nucleotides. *Proceedings III International Symposium on Infant Nutrition and Gastrointestinal Disease.* Brussels Belgium. pp 65-75.

Uauy R, Stringel G. 1988. Effect of dietary nucleotides on growth and maturation of the developing gut in the rat. *J Pediatr Res* 23: 494A.

Van Buren CT, Kulkarni AD, Schandle VB, Rudolph FB. 1983. The influence of dietary nucleotides on cell-mediated immunity. *Transplantation* 36; 3: 350-352.

Warshaw JB, Uauy R. 1987. Metabolsimo de los ácidos grasos durante el desarrollo. En: *Avances en Nutrición de la Infancia.* A Gil, ed. Jarpyo Eds, Madrid. p. 7-18.

Webb BH, Johnson AH, Alford JA. 1974. *Fundamentals of dairy chemistry*, 2nd Ed. Westport Connecticut. The AVI Publishing Company, Inc.

Young VR. Protein and amino acid metabolism in relation to physical exercise. En: Winnick, M (ed). *Nutrition and Exercise*. John Wiley and Sons, New York.

Dairy Products in Human Health and Nutrition, Serrano Ríos et al. (eds) © 1994 Balkema, Rotterdam, ISBN 90 5410 359 0

Artificial nutrition: Historical evolution

H. Joyeux
Institut Curie, Paris, France

Artificial nutrition has a fascinating historical evolution, showing that all the scientific progresses took their origin in manhood courage.

Yet in the Vth Century b.c., Hippocrates was writing in his "Antiqua Medicine": "Therefore, I firmly trust that every physician has to study human nature and wounder carefully if he really wants to fulfil his obligations, what relations exist between man and his food, his drinks, all his way of life, and what sort of influence each thing has on each one".

For a very long time, man has been trying to feed himself artificially when it was not possible by the natural routes. He has tried the digestive tube and when it was not working, tried the vascular system. Here is the story of men and artificial nutrition.

According to HERODOTE, in ancient Egypt, "emetics and enema were used three times a month to preserve health.

1210 IBN al NAFIS born in Damas. Physician and philosph.- The first to develope the small circulation of blood theory (pulmonary circulation), openly contradicting with the accepted ideas of GALIEN and IBN SINA (AVICEN). In his prescriptions: "He never prescibed a medicine as long as he was able to prescribe an alimentary diet, just as he was never prescribing a composed medicine as long as he was able to content himself of a simple drug".

1492 Transfusion to Pope INNOCENT VIII.- "Pope INNOCENT VIII's strengthes were quickly decliving, he was for some time in such a somnolence, that sometimes he seemed to be dead. All the means to awaken his exhausted life had been used. A jewish physician proposed to obtain the expected result with transfusion, by the mean of young people blood. Then, was exchanged the old pontif blood with the blood of a young man. Threee times the experience was renewed in exchange for the life of three young men. Probably there was air in the blood of those. But no effect was obtained, the Pope died on April 25th, 1492".

1495 "Blood is a "special sap", with the loose of blood escapes life too... Marsilio FICINO recommends to an old man to drink the blood of a young man...". "Blood, food of life..." "And why our old men, who are dismissed of all help, would they not suck a young girl's milk? and the blood of a young boy, who would accept it, who would be healthy, gay, quiet, and having a much good blood and

237

by chance abundant?... "Let them suck it then from the vein of the left arm... Up to one or two ounces...".

1542 Jean FERNEL.- Birth of "physiology": "La nature de l'homme sain, de toutes ses fonctions".

1598 CAPIVACCEUS.- Introduces artificially nutrients into the esophagus.

1601 At this time lemons and oranges are supplied regularly on the ships of the English East India Company...

1604 Magnus PEGEL.- First descriptions of arterio-arterial blood transfusions..

1615 Andréas LIVABIUS.- Further descriptions of arterio-arterial blood transfusions..

1616 William HARVEY (18th April).- Discovery of the blood circulation... set forth in his work "Exercitatio anatomica", 1628.

1617 FABRICIUS and AQUAPENDENTE.- use a silver tube passing through the rhinopharynx to feed a tetanus patient.

1650 Francis POTTER.- In England: "First animal transfusion experiment ... without result".

1651 Dom Robert des GABETS.- This benedictine monk works on "blood communication", and fully describes the method and instrumentation", the latter being extremely easy has two small silver tubes connected to a leather pounch, that fills up on the arrival of the blood and empties under pressure...

1655 Sir Christopher WREN (astronomer and architect of the London Saint Paul Cathedral).- "Injection intraveineuse de vin, de bière et de morphine au chien". This operation was then called infusion.

1657 Doctor Robert BOYLE.- "Première transfusion de chien à chien".

1658 Doctor Robert BOYLE (friend of Sir Christopher WREN).- "Inyection intraveineuse d'une solution d'opium au chien".

1662 Richard LOWER in Oxford.- "Description de la mèthode de perfusion...". "Transfusion de sang de mouton à mouton".

1664 Caspar SCOTUS.- "Injection intraveineuse de vin au chien".

1665 Johann Sigmund ELSHOLTZ.- "Clysmatica Nova", a book published in Holland. Description of the perfusion technique from the arm to the leg ....

1667 Jean-Baptiste DENIS.- Doctor of Louis XIV and Paul EMMEREZ - his surgeon. "Première transfusion de sang d'un agneau à l'homme: de la carotide d'un agneau à la veine du bras d'un homme"... The first transfusion did not show any complications... They carried out this type of transfusion several times, (especially on mental patients), but the death of a transfusion patients led to the prohibition of this method in France.

"Carrying out a transfusion", says DENIS, "merely stands for imitating the example of nature which, in order to feed the fetus in the mother's womb, is a steady transfusion of the umbilical vein. Having a transfusion done simply means feeding in a shorter way than usual, i.e. receiving ready made blood in the veins instead of food that only becomes blood after several changes. This shortened way of feeding is preferable to the other method, since oral food-intake goes to several parts which are often badly placed and therefore may develop different bad qualities before reaching the veins.

In Germany Matthaus GOOTTFRIED-PURMANN, would transfuse lamb blood to man. Increasing criticism based on medical and religious grounds, led to the prohibition of this practice all over Europe at the end of the 17th Century.

1667 Fr. REDI.- Injecting air into the blood causes death...

1668 Edmond KING and Thomas COXE.- Vein-to-vein transfusion from calf to sheep...

1670 Dictionary of Arréts de Brillon (MDCCXVII), Article "Chirurgien": "Défense à tous médicins et chirurgiens d'exercer la transfusion du sang, à peine de punition corporelle". Arrét du Parlament de Paris (Prohibition for all doctor and surgeons to carry out blood transfusions on pain of corporal punishment - Decree of the Paris Parliament) on 10th January, 1970. Journal des Audiences, tome III, Livre X, chap. XV.

1679 William COURTEN in Montpellier.- "Injection intraveineuse d'huile d'olive chaude au chien".

1692 KETELAER.- Uses the term "SPRUE" for the first time.

1749 Birth of Nicolas APPERT, creator of the preservation of food based on the heat technique.

1775 Oxford Dictionary.- Definition of denutrition.

1780 Antoine-Laurent LAVOISIER.- Differenciates base, acid, salt, oxide....

1790 John HUNTER.- Successfully feeds a man suffering from muscular palsy from deglutition with a tube connected to a vesica.

1796 Antoine-Auguste PARMENTIER.- "L'oxygène a une influence sur la couleur du sang".

1801 J.J.C. LEGALLOIS.- Thesis for the doctorate: "Le sang est il indentique dans tous les vaisseaux qu'il parcourt".

1810 Philip SYNG PHYSICK (Philadelphia) uses the first orogastric tube to save a "Poisened patient".

1818 James BLUNDELL.- English surgeon.- Takes up for the doctorate: "Recherches sur la force du coeur aortique"... Creation of the hemodynamometer.

1825 Jean-Louis POISEUILLE.- Doctoral Thesis: "Recherches sur la force du coeur aortique"... Creation of a Hemodynamometer.

1828 W. PPROUT.- "Equilibre des saccharides, des graisses et des albumines dans l'alimentation humaine..." Essay published in Philadelphia in 1834.

1830 Doctor LATTA in Scotland.- "Perfusion de solutiom salée dans Philadelphia in 1834".

1839 François MAGENDIE.-"Lectures on the blood", published in Philadelphia.

1839 MULDER.- Invents the term "PROTEINS".

239

1839 J.B. BOUSSINGAULT.- French chemist and agronomist carries out the calculation of "nitrogen balance".

1841 James Prescott JOULE.- Draws up the laws namend after him on the release of heat produced by electric power in a conductor... he uses this "Joule effect" when measuring heat pertaining to the mass.

1842 LIEBIG.- Shows the calorific value of the different food values ... the cause of each vital phenomenon lies in the energy supplied by food.

1843 Claude BERNARD.- "Infusion de soluté de glucose". Lectures at the Collège de France: "La physiologie expérimentale appliquée à la médecine". Thesis for the Medicine: "Du suc gastrique et de son role dans la nutrition".

1851 J.F. REEVE.- Describes, in Lancet, an enteral nutrition apparatus to feed those who refuse to eat.

1854 Claude BERNARD.- "Notes of M. Bernard's lectures on the blood", published in Philadelphia. He also injects hen's egg albumin.

1855 François MAGENDIE.- Carries out research work on the effects that diets of different compositions have on dogs.

1857 C.E. BROWN-SEQUARD.- Shows the evidence of surviving red cells transfused to the receptor ...

1860 Joseph LISTER.- Surgery professor in Glasgow states the importance of asepsis.

1863 Fr. GOLITZ.- Recommends intravenous fluid supply in the case of abdominal haemorrhage....

1865 Claude BERNARD.- Concept of the "milieu intérieur" deriving from the concept of "secrétion interne". The blood is the distributor of food reserves and the necessary energetics to the constancy of cell activities...

1867 KUSSMAUL.- Uses a flexible orogastric tube to decompress the stomach.

1869 MENZEL and PERCO.- Are the first to systematically experiment the possiblity of parenteral hypercalorific supply. They inject different oil types kinds, by the subcutaneous route, to a dog and state a complete absorption in 4 to 48 hours.. They tried it on man but the painful reaction made them give up.

1873 Edward M. HODDER in Toronto.- Milk perfusion in cholera... After a 400 ml infusion to a patient declared moribund by a doctor without any hope left a real improvement took place and the patient regained life....

1873 L. LANDOIS.- Dog serum causes red cell hemolysis in rabbits...

1878 Claude BERNARD.- Lectures on the phenomenon of animals and plants coexisting: There is only one way of life, a one and only physiology for all living beings....

1879 H. KRONECKER and J. SANDERS.- Salted serum perfusion can save the life in case of haemorrhage....

1880 Louis PASTEUR creates the microbiology.

1880 Samuel GEE.- Shows interest of the diet without gluten (one pint of oysters every day) in the cealiac sprue.

1880 HAYEM.- "Etude expérimentale précise de la transfusion..".

1884 Kazimierz FUNK, polish biochemist.- Invents the word "VITAMINE", eager to design a nitrogen substance (amine) wich is essential for life.. Now, many vitamines are not amines or even nitrogen substances and the avitaminoses are not necessarily fatal ....

1885 S. RINGER.- "Naissance des solutions de Ringer... "(Birth of Ringer solutions).

1890 A. BIEDL and R. KRAUS in Germany.- "Perfusion de glycise....".

1891 Rudolph MATAS (New Orleans).- "Perfusion de glucose...".

1895 W. LEUBE in Germany.- "Injection sous-cutanée d'huile camphrée comme source de caloríes...".

1895 W.A. MORRISON.- Reports in Boston Med. Journal a directly intragastric nutrition of 28 dyphteric palsy cases.

1896 Christian EIJKMAN (Novel price of Medicine in 1929).- "Le Bébéri est dü à la Consommation de riz décortique". (Béribéri is due to the consumption of husked rice).

1898 Georges CRILE, surgeon in Cleveland.- "Mise au point des sutures vasculaires et d'une canule pour transfusion".

1900 Karl LANDSTEINER from Vienna.- Discovers the human blood groups.

1902 Otto LOEWI produces for the first time, a protein and free peptides from cattle pancreas that keep dogs at nitrogen balance.

1904 E. ABDERHALDEN and P.RONA.- "Découverte de l'hydrolyse des protéines..". They fed dogs with casein hydrolysat, starch, lard and bone power hydrolysat for two months and a half... It is the first concept of a complete synthetic diet.

1904 FRIEDRICH from Leipzig Supplies a peptone solution by subcutaneous route as well as a lipid-salt and glucose mixture. He is the first research worker proposing the complete parenteral nutrition.

1906 E. ABDERHALDEN and A. SCHITTENHELM in Germany.- "Nutrition artificielle par voie rectale".

1910 M. EINHORN.- Invents the duodenal nutrition.

1912 Gabriel BERTRAND, French chemist and biologist.- Defines the role and term of trace elements.

1913 V. HENRIQUES and A.C. ANDERSEN.- "Perfusion d'hydrolysats de caséine chez la chrèvre"...".

1914 Johann THIESS.- "Réinfusion de sang dilué, à partir de la cavité abdominale...".

1914 HUSTIN from Brussels.- "La tranfusion ne présente de difficultés parce que le sang est coagulable..., il découvre la transfusion citratée". (The transfusion does not any difficulty as blood is clottable...). He discovers the citrated transfusion.

1915 J.R. MURLIN and J.A. RICHE.- "Lipides sériques et production d'énergie..".

1915 WOODYATT and COLL.- Prove that intravenous glucose infusion can supply 6000 calories per day. They also show that 0,10 g glycose infusion per hour and kilogramme does not determine glycosuria.

1915 Lewis d'AGOTE.- "Organizes in Buenos Aires, the first blood dibation of 2000 voluntaries blood donors.

1917 Emmanuel HEDON in Montpellier claims the absolute innocousness of citrated transfusion diffused by E. JEANBRAU during the war.

1918 A.F.R. ANDRESEN.- Publishes in Ann. Surg. The Enteral Nutrition immedeiately after a gastro-enterostomy he starts on operating table.

1920 T. NOMURA and S. YAMAKAWA.- "Perfusion d'une huile de Castor Yanol" given up in Japan and USA in 1930.

1921 Franz OEHLECKER.- Veno-venous transfusion apparatus.... Compatibility test before transfusion.

1923 Dr. Florence SEIBERT in Philadelphia.- "Découverte des substances pyrogènes". (Discovery of pyrogenic substances).

1928 P. SAXL and F. DONATH in Viena.- "Perfusion d'huile (olekiniol) aux animaux et à l'homme...".

1931 W.C. ROSE.- "les acides aminés essentiels..".

1932 D.P. CUTHBERTSON.- "Catabolisme protéique post-traumatique...".

1933 C.M. JONES and F.B. EATON in Boston.- "Oedème de malnutrition post-opèratoirs.."(Post-operative malnutrition edema..).

1936 Robert ELMAN (Saint Louis).- "Perfusion d'hydrolysat de protéines chez le chien..". (Protein hydrolysat perfusion to dogs).

1936 First blood bank in Rome.

1936 B. FANTUS.- Blood bank in Chicago.

1936 John ELLIOT.- First plasma perfusion.

1939 W.O. ABBOTT and A.J. RAWSON invent a double lumen enteral nutrition tube.

1940 SHOHL and BLACKFAN prove the possibility to use a synthetic amino-acid solution wich is biologically comparable with the solutions prepared by enzymatic methods. (12 Dextrogyrus amino-acids and 13 Levegyrus amino-acids).

1940 Karl LADSTEINER, Alexander SALOMON and A.S. WIENER.- Discover the rhesus factor.

1942 J.E. RHOADS.- "Influence de l´hypoprotéinémie sur la formation du cal après fracture osseuse". (Influence of hypoproteinemia on callus formation after bone fracture).

1942 J.L. GAMBLE.- "Anatomy and pattology of the fluid compartment...".

1943 P.A. PANIKOV from Russia.- Describes a feeding method for abdomen injured patients hit during the war.

1944 Edwin E. COHN.- "Séparation des fractions de plasma..."

1944 A. WRETLIND in Stockholm makes the first amino-acids solution, will tolerated by men.

1944 P.R. CANNON, R.W. WISSLER (Chicago).- "Relations entre déficit protéique et infection ...".

1947 R. ELMAN.- "Parenteral alimentation in surgery", 1 vol. (New York).

1949 F. D. MOORE.- "Adaptation of supportive treatment to needs of surgical patient". (J.A. MA 1949, 141, 646).

1949 H. C. MENG (Nashville).- "Study of complete parenteral alimentation in dogs".

1950 R. AUBANIAC (Algeria).- "L'injection intraveineuse sous-claviculaire..". (Subclavicular intravenous injection).

1950 A. KESO, J. BROZAK and Al. (Mineapolis).- Publish "The biology of human starvation". Minnesota.

1954 M.D. PAREIRA and R. ELMAN.- Report on enteral Nutrition Exclusive supplied by tube to 240 patients.

1955 E. WENNING in Germany.- Perfuses honey by venous route.

1958 Fernando PAULINO in Brazil.- Alimentaçao Parenteral en Cirurgia.

1960 A. WRETLIND in Stockholm creates Intralipid, soja oil emulsified by the phosphatides of the egg yolk, being the only lípid emulsion unanimously accepted all over the world.

1960 R.B. COUCH and WINITZ report on the first experiments with "Elemental diet" and the firt long term study has been supported by NASA in order to study the possibilites of alimentary application on cosmonauts.

1960 O. SCHUBERTH in Stockholm reports on the first case of making the guts rest, (patient, 22, suffering from Crohn's disease) by total parenteral alimentation during 5 months.

1964 M. N. MUNRO AND J.B. ALLISON (Glasgow) publish "Mammlian protein metabolism", in IV volumes.

1966 S.J. DUDRICK (Philadelphia).- "Total intravenous feeding and growth in puppies.." Creates the deep intravenous hyperalimentation proving, by means of experiment on dogs, that a long term parenteral hyperalimentation may completely replace feeding.

1969 J.E. RHOADS uses the first time the term "an artificial gastro intestinal tract", retaken by B.H. SCRIBNER under the denominatio of Artificial Gut".

1969 R.V. STEPHENS and H.T. RANDALL.- Assess in "Nature" the interest of elementary diets for cosmonauts.

1972 Cl. SOLASSOL and H. JOJEUX (Montpellier).- Create the concept of venous food mixtures: "All in one" for the long term parenteral nutrition at the hospital or at home.

1973 C. RICOUR (Paris).- Develop the long term parenteral alimentation in a child.

1974 B.R. BISTRIAN.- Evalues alimentary needs of patients in hospitals.

1984 R.J. MERRITT (Los Angeles).- Publishes "Partial peritoneal alimentation in an infant".

1988 H. SAMI and H. JOYEUX.- Publish in Nutrition (vol. 4,269) the modular and steril system, "All in one" in enteral alimentation for ambulatory and home nutrition.

Artificial Nutrition is a steady
evolution. It has become a full
science with all its clinical and
experimental aspects, its
journals, congresses of leading
societies in Europe, USA and
Japan. It follows tha old
Hippocrates' precept "be your food
your medicine".

Dairy Products in Human Health and Nutrition, Serrano Ríos et al. (eds) © 1994 Balkema, Rotterdam, ISBN 90 5410 359 0

Protein sources in enteral nutrition

K.J. Reilly & J.L. Rombeau
Department of Surgery, Hospital of the University of Pennsylvania, Philadelphia, Pa., USA

ABSTRACT: Dietary protein is critical to cellular function. Three enteral forms of protein exist: intact proteins, partially hydrolyzed proteins or crystalline amino acids. Glutamine is an important metabolic fuel for the small intestine, and may have a role as adjuvant treatment in a variety of clinical scenarios. Presented is an overview of options for enteral protein provision and a discussion of possible therapeutic indications for specialized protein diets.

INTRODUCTION

Dietary protein is necessary for normal body function, including muscle contraction, cardiovascular function, immune response, synthesis of hepatic proteins, healing, growth and recovery from illness or injury. Proteins are required for manufacture of vital cell components, such as enzymes and structural proteins, hormones, cytokines, neuromodulating substances and other cell messengers. Protein-calorie malnutrition is associated with alterations in gastrointestinal (GI) tract function, including thinning of mucous membranes, decreased secretory IgA and changes in gut flora, each of which has been implicated in gastrointestinal dysfunction (Schmucker et al., 1986; Van Der Meer, 1988).

Amino acids, the building blocks of proteins, may be divided into two categories: nonessential amino acids (NEAA) and essential amino acids (EAA). Nonessential amino acids are those that the body is able to synthesize de novo. Essential amino acids are those that the body is unable to synthesize, which are consumed during metabolism and only partially recovered for reincorporation during protein synthesis (Stein et al., 1990). Dietary protein should provide protein sources of biologic value, i.e., those that contain higher concentrations of EAA. In the hospitalized patient whose metabolic capabilities may be somewhat compromised, the goal is to provide only what is needed, so as not to overburden the patient's metabolic capacity. The body maintains amino acid levels within very close limits and excess amino acids may be toxic.

PROTEIN DIGESTION AND ABSORPTION

The protein load presented to the GI tract consists usually of whole proteins derived from animal sources, i.e., egg, milk, meat and fish, endogenous proteins (i.e., GI secretions) and desquamated cells from the small intestine. The time required to complete in vitro digestion of protein to free amino acids by the successive actions of pepsin, trypsin and chymotrypsin is on the order of days, and therefore most protein is absorbed in the peptide form (Adibi, 1971; Silk, 1981; Matthews and Adibi, 1976). Normally only 3-5% of ingested nitrogen escapes absorption and is excreted in the stool. (Zaloga, 1993) Digestion of dietary protein administered orally or intragastrically occurs in three phases.

The first phase is the gut lumen phase where acid proteases and pepsin in the stomach initiate protein digestion, yielding a mix of small peptides and a few amino acids. This step has a limited role in normal individuals, but in patients with pancreatic insufficiency, peptic digestion has been shown to enhance intestinal protein absorption (Zaloga, 1993). Under normal conditions, gastric emptying is the rate limiting step in the absorption of ingested protein, not the rate of hydrolysis (Borgstrom, et al., 1957). In conditions where control of gastric emptying is lost, feeding tubes must therefore be placed postpylorically. The gut lumen phase continues in the small intestinal lumen by the specific action of pancreatic enzymes trypsin, chymotrypsin, aminopeptidases and carboxypeptidases.

The second phase of protein digestion is the brush

border phase, where small peptides are further broken down by enterocyte brush border hydrolases to free amino acids, dipeptides, tripeptides and oligopeptides. These brush border enzymes are enterokinases, endopeptidases and aminopeptidases and act primarily on tetrapeptides and larger peptides. Many are substrate-inducible and their activity decreases when nutrients are absent (as in starvation or TPN administration). The final phase of digestion is the cytoplasmic phase whereby peptides absorbed intact by small intestinal cells are hydrolyzed to constituent amino acids by the action of cytoplasmic peptidases. These normal processes may be limited in pancreatic insufficiency or with loss of membrane-associated enzymes following infection, gut atrophy or mucosal damage.

Absorption of dietary peptides and amino acids occurs primarily in the proximal small intestine and is rapid under normal conditions (Silk et al., 1979). Four carrier systems based on structure for transport of free amino acids exist: 1) monoamino, monocarboxylic (neutral amino acids); 2) glycine, proline, hydroxyproline; 3) dibasic amino acids and cysteine; 4) dicarboxylic (acidic) amino acids. Absorption of free amino acids is by active transport and requires the presence of sodium (Matthews, 1991; Matthews and Payne, 1980; Wellner and Meister, 1981). Absorption of dipeptides, tripeptides and oligopeptides occurs by different specific carrier systems which are sodium-independent and stimulated by a proton gradient (Wapnir, 1990). It is unclear whether there is one adaptable peptide transport system, or whether multiple carriers exist (Matthews and Burston, 1984; Rubino et al., 1971).

PROTEIN QUALITY

There are numerous sources of protein used in enteral formulas, and therefore knowledge of protein quality is vital. Protein quality depends on the amino acid profile of the specific protein. The Food and Agriculture Organization/ World Health Organization (FAO/WHO) provide estimates of the optimal proportions of amino acids to ease design of individualized patient formulas. To optimize healing in the injured, seriously ill or undernourished patients, EAA should be $\geq 40\%$ of total amino acid intake. (MacBurney et al., 1990).

To mathematically evaluate the nutritional value of a given protein source, two formulas are used. First the chemical score (CS) compares the amino acid composition of a protein source with a standard amino acid pattern as defined by FAO/WHO (Joint FAO/WHO Report, 1973).

$$CS = \frac{EAA \text{ (product)}/Total \text{ } AA \text{ (product)}}{EAA \text{ (egg)}/ Total \text{ } AA \text{ (egg)}} \times 100$$

Secondly, the biologic value (BV) is a measure of the percentage of nitrogen provided which is returned for growth and maintenance. The BV is expressed as nitrogen retained divided by dietary nitrogen absorbed (Mitchell, 1924)

$$BV = \frac{Dietary \text{ } N - (urinary \text{ } N + fecal \text{ } N)}{Dietary \text{ } N - fecal \text{ } N}$$

The lower the BV, the higher the content of NEAA and the greater protein volume that is required to achieve positive nitrogen balance. The chemical score is a fixed number, while the biologic value may vary with the physiologic state of the patient.

Individual patients may have amino acid imbalances, specific sensitivities or toxicities (MacBurney et al., 1990). Patients with hepatic failure preferentially use branched chain amino acids (BCAA), and therefore special formulas are made with a high ratio of BCAA to aromatic amino acids (AAA) to minimize toxicities and optimize BCAA utilization. In renal failure, protein provision is kept at a minimum to control uremia, and therefore protein given should contain a high ratio of EAA to NEAA.

PROTEIN SOURCES IN FORMULAS

Three forms of dietary protein may be found in enteral formulas: intact protein; partially hydrolyzed proteins (oligo-, tri- and dipeptides); or crystalline amino acids. Intact proteins and protein hydrolysates require further digestion in the small intestine to smaller peptides and free amino acids prior to absorption. Knowledge of the source and form of protein is important, particularly in patients with defects in protein digestion (i.e., pancreatic insufficiency) or absorption (i.e., celiac sprue, short bowel syndrome).

Intact Protein

Intact proteins in enteral formulas are in their complete and original forms as found in whole foods. In general, they are derived from pureed beef, egg white solids, lactalbumin, whey or sodium or calcium casein. (Krey and Murray, 1990). They require complete digestion to smaller peptides and free amino acids before absorption. They do not add appreciably to the osmolality of the formula, but do depend on normal host pancreatic exocrine and brush border enzyme function for complete assimilation, and are therefore of variable digestibility and caloric contribution.

Hydrolyzed Protein

Hydrolyzed proteins are enzymatically or chemically hydrolyzed small peptides derived from the same intact protein sources described above. Tripeptides, dipeptides and free amino acids are absorbed directly; larger peptides need further hydrolysis prior to absorption. Protein hydrolysates often require the addition of free essential amino acids to enhance protein quality (MacBurney, et al., 1990). Most commonly added are methionine, tyrosine and tryptophan. In addition, as protein molecules become smaller, they contribute more to the osmotic load, increasing the incidence of associated diarrhea.

Crystalline Amino Acids

Crystalline amino acids do not require digestion, and are absorbed directly by active transport. Because of their small size, they significantly increase the osmotic load of the formula. These solutions are expensive, and are best reserved for use in specific disease states such as hepatic insufficiency or renal failure.

Also important in choosing a protein source is a knowledge of the characteristics of the various formulas, for example, intact protein formula in general is more palatable than the alternatives, which is important in the patient who is fed orally. Crystalline amino acids may have a bad odor and taste, and in general are used only in tube feedings. There is evidence that when similar amino acid profiles were provided in each of the three forms described, there was no difference found in nitrogen balance in patients with normal GI tracts or with burns (Moriarty et al., 1985; Trocki et al., 1986).

ELEMENTAL DIETS

Elemental diets provide nitrogen in the form of either synthetic amino acids or protein hydrolysates. Elemental diets are advocated by many in a variety of clinical situations where intestinal mucosal integrity may be compromised, where there is decreased effective surface area for absorption, as well as in disorders of amino acid transport, such as Hartnup's disease, cystinuria or exocrine pancreatic insufficiency (Adibi, 1971). Of note, the use of free amino acids in elemental diets was suggested at a time when it was thought that proteins were absorbed only as free amino acids, which we now know to be incorrect (Ziegler et al., 1993).

Amino acids require sodium and ATP for absorption, add significantly to the osmolar load and are expensive. These disadvantages of amino acid use led to the development of protein hydrolysates in elemental diets, which reflects a better understanding of protein digestion and peptide absorption. Although mucosal di- and tripeptide carriers are saturable, their overall capacity for absorption is significantly greater than those for amino acids (Silk, 1981; Ganapathy and Leibach, 1982). Therefore, an enteral diet with protein hydrolysates provides both di- and tri-peptides as well as free amino acids, targeting both absorption systems, as well as reducing the body's role in protein degradation. It has in fact been shown by one group that protein is better absorbed from a mixture of amino acids and small peptides than from the amino acid or whole protein form (Matthews and Adibi, 1976). Therefore, elemental diets of protein hydrolysates alone or combined with a limited quantity of free amino acids have a theoretical advantage over intact protein solutions.

COMPARISON OF PROTEIN SOURCES IN DISEASE

We know that the quantity of dietary protein given to an individual influences overall nitrogen utilization, and, thereby, growth and repair. However, clinical proof of the ideal form of protein is lacking. It should be considered that the individual's nutritional status can alter the absorption response of the GI tract. Specifically, nutritional status can affect the expression of amino acid and dipeptide transport systems on cell membranes as well as alter the activity of brush border hydrolases (Wapnir, 1990). Patients with critical illness following shock, trauma and sepsis may also have altered brush border integrity from sepsis, diminished mucous secretion and gut atrophy from starvation or TPN (Zaloga, 1993). Next presented are studies comparing various forms of protein administration in animal and human models.

In patients with normal gastrointestinal function, a study comparing intact protein, protein hydrolysates and equivalent amino acid mixtures showed no differences in overall nitrogen absorption or utilization. All amino acid patterns were carefully matched. The conclusion drawn was that the normal human small intestine has adequate capacity for efficient absorption and use of whole dietary protein (Silk et al., 1979).

In animal studies, normal and malnourished rats grew faster when fed isocaloric isonitrogenous formulas containing peptides versus intact protein or amino acids. Growth in this study was lowest in those receiving amino acid-based diets (Zaloga et al., 1991; Poullain et al., 1989). In rats following abdominal surgery, growth was highest with an intact protein diet and lowest with an amino-acid-based diet. Of note, rats with pancreatic insufficiency have significantly greater growth with peptide-based diets (Imondi and Stradley, 1974).

Ziegler et al. (1993) studied 12 ICU patients after abdominal surgery requiring one or more stomas. Each was given TPN for 24-48 hours, then continuous enteral nutrition with two diets: a protein hydrolysate (Reabilan) obtained by enzymatic hydrolysis of the native proteins contained in the dietary protein diet (2/3 casein and 1/3 lactoserum). Identical quantities of carbohydrate and lipid were provided.

Patients receiving enteral support with a small peptide-based diet versus a whole protein diet had more effective restoration of normal plasma amino acid levels and nutritional status. Nitrogen balance was identical in both groups, but urinary nitrogen losses tended to decrease with protein hydrolysates. Therefore, the efficiency of protein hydrolysates in postoperative catabolic stress appears to be related to its improvement in nitrogen metabolism.

A recent prospective, randomized study by Wayne-Meredith et al. (1990) comparing whole protein versus peptide-based diets in trauma patients indicated that the peptide-based diet resulted in greater increases in visceral protein levels and decreased diarrhea than did the whole protein diet. Stool nitrogen was similar between the two groups, therefore improved weight gain and nitrogen retention were not the result of better intestinal absorption, but rather of improved nitrogen utilization in the stressed state.

Other support for the administration of protein breakdown products is in patients with Crohn's Disease who show a better nitrogen balance on a peptide diet compared with solid or amino acid-based diets (Smith et al., 1982). In addition, in postoperative cancer patients, improved nitrogen retention has been shown with peptide-based diets (Meguid et al., 1984).

Overall, most evidence indicates a superiority of protein utilization when given in the form of peptides versus whole protein or single amino acids in a variety of disease and injury states. The improved anabolic response to protein hydrolysates may result from greater release by the intestine of trophic hormones (i.e., glucagon) to peptide feedings (Wayne-Meredith et al., 1990). Rerat et al. (1988) demonstrated greater glucagon responses in animals fed peptides versus amino acids. It is also possible that peptide feeds elevate IGF-1 levels, improve intestinal blood flow or are more protective to

intestinal integrity (Zaloga et al., 1991; Poullain, et al., 1989; Monchi et al., 1991).

GLUTAMINE

Glutamine is the most abundant free amino acid in plasma and in body tissues (Scriver & Rosenberg, 1973; Bergstrom et al., 1974). It is a neutral amino acid classically categorized as nonessential, however, it may be conditionally essential during stress or starvation (Chipponi et al, 1982;). More specifically, nearly all tissues possess the prerequisite enzyme necessary to synthesize glutamine from glutamate (glutamine synthetase), yet many organs require large amounts of glutamine from the circulation to maintain cellular metabolism. While skeletal muscle possesses the highest levels of glutamine, it is the intestine that is the major site of glutamine consumption (Bergstrom et al., 1974; O'Dwyer et al., 1990).

Glutamine has a critical role in intestinal metabolism, growth and function. Glutamine is now recognized as a respiratory fuel for the cells of the intestinal mucosa (Roediger, 1982; Windmueller and Spaeth, 1974, 1978) as well as for many other rapidly growing cells, such as stimulated lymphocytes (Ardawi and Newsholme, 1983), cultured cells (Reitzer et al., 1979) and malignant cells (Kovacevic and Morris, 1972). Glutamine also functions as 1) a provider of nitrogen for biosynthetic pathways; 2) a precursor for nucleic acids and nucleotides; 3) a constituent of proteins (Krebs, 1980); 4) a substrate for renal ammoniagenesis (Pitts, 1964; Smith et al., 1985); 5) a potential substrate for hepatic gluconeogenesis (Ross et al., 1967); 6) a possible regulator of muscle protein degradation and 7) the precursor of the two most potent neurotransmitters in the CNS, glutamate, a neuroexcitatory substance, and gamma amino butyric acid (GABA), a neuroinhibitory metabolite (Kovacevic and McGivan, 1983).

Utilization of glutamine by the intestinal mucosa as a respiratory fuel was suggested in 1965 when Neptune reported glutamine conversion to carbon dioxide in an ileal preparation, in preference to glucose (Neptune, 1965; Windmueller and Spaeth, 1974; Smith et al., 1988). Windmueller proceeded to show that an isolated perfused rat intestine will extract up to 33% of plasma glutamine with each pass (Windmueller and Spaeth, 1974). Glutamine is used as a respiratory fuel in its conversion to carbon dioxide, and produces a byproduct, ammonia. Unlike other tissues to which ammonia might be toxic, the gut is well suited for its disposal, as ammonia readily diffuses into the portal system and is extracted by the liver prior to reaching the systemic circulation (O'Dwyer et al., 1990).

The rapid uptake and metabolism of glutamine by the intestine is accelerated in catabolic illness. In dogs, glutamine uptake has been shown to increase by greater than 50% after simple laparotomy (Souba et al., 1985a). There is increased glutamine production and release by skeletal muscle, as well as greater use by the intestine. However, the compensation for increased gut metabolism is not full, and in stress states, plasma glutamine concentrations decrease in approximate proportion to the severity of disease or injury (Miller et al., 1983; Schlienger and Imler, 1980; Roth et al., 1982). A similar response is seen following glucocorticoid administration, suggesting a common mechanism through the pituitary-adrenal axis (Souba et al., 1985b).

As mentioned earlier, glutamine may become an essential amino acid for the intestine and other tissues in catabolic illness, and ill patients are at risk for glutamine deficiency. Currently, glutamine is absent from parenteral solutions and present in only minimal amounts in enteral formulas, as it is considered nonessential. One reason for eliminating glutamine from these solutions is its relative instability in aqueous solution, where it spontaneously degrades to pyroglutamic acid and ammonia (O'Dwyer, 1990).

Glutamine solutions given to healthy volunteers have no adverse effects. Increased plasma levels of glutamate, however, do elicit neurologic symptoms in some individuals (i.e., Chinese restaurant syndrome). There is no evidence of these effects with clinical glutamine administration (Darmain et al., 1986).

The importance of glutamine in nutrition support was highlighted by Hwang et al.(1986) who administered parenteral nutrition lacking glutamine to rats and found mucosal atrophy similar to that seen during TPN administration. When glutamine was added to the same enteral formula in place of other nonessential amino acids, increased cellularity of the jejunum, ileum and colon was observed. When varied concentrations of glutamine were given, a correlation was found between the amount of glutamine intake (but not the absolute nitrogen intake) and the intestinal DNA content.

Glutamine administration has also been studied in models of intestinal injury. In a model of 5-fluorouracil toxicity on rat small intestine, O'Dwyer et al. (1987) observed increased mucosal cellularity, improved nitrogen balance and decreased mortality in animals receiving glutamine-supplemented parenteral diets, versus those given standard nutrient formulas. In addition, Fox et al. (Fox et al., 1987, 1988) observed increased mucosal weight, protein and DNA content in rats with methotrexate-induced enterocolitis who were given enteral glutamine. This group also demonstrated decreased endotoxin translocation from the gut lumen in the same model, suggesting a role for glutamine in intestinal barrier function and immune function.

The provision of oral glutamine to rats after abdominal radiation therapy has been shown to improve gut mucosal morphometrics and barrier function, as well as decreasing morbidity and mortality (Souba et al., 1990). It is hypothesized that the increased mucosal mass improved intestinal function to explain the increased body weight, improved nitrogen balance and decreased overall mortality.

It has been demonstrated that glutamine's role in modulating immune function may depend on the route of administration, with enteral administration faring better. When rats were fed a glutamine-enriched oral diet, mortality from methotrexate was 10% versus 90% in animals given identical solutions parenterally (Alverdy, 1990).

The improvement in mucosal cellularity with enteral glutamine administration observed by O'Dwyer, Fox and others suggests a role in patients following injury to the intestinal mucosa. Specifically, enteral glutamine may be important as a therapeutic adjuvant for the recovery and maintenance of the intestinal mucosa in inflammation, as in inflammatory bowel disease, or following chemotherapy administration. Interestingly, Jacobs et al. (1988) found that the effect of glutamine and epidermal growth factor on small bowel and colonic mucosa were additive. A possible role for glutamine in stress include its preferred use as a respiratory fuel. Dudrick et al. (1992) discovered an increase in mucosal brush border glutamine uptake soon after endotoxemia as well as a decreased consumption of glutamine across the basolateral membrane. They hypothesized that this increased uptake and cellular glutamine concentration may support protein synthesis in sepsis and provides a biochemical rationale for early institution of enteral nutrition in critical illness. Glutamine may also act as a precursor of substances which facilitate cellular reproduction, or as mediator of secretion or action of growth factors or enterotrophic hormones. More information on the mechanism of glutamine's beneficial effects will help us determine possible therapeutic applications in humans.

THERAPEUTIC IMPLICATIONS

It is clear that protein form as well as composition can affect absorption, gut integrity, hormonal and metabolic responses and organ function. Accumulating evidence suggest the ability to generate peptides in the gut lumen has metabolic advantages. Amino acid based diets lack this capacity and are generally associated with poorer metabolic and organ responses. Patients with decreased capacity to process intact protein to peptides may benefit from peptide-based enteral diets. This would include a variety of clinical situations in which gut mucosal integrity may be compromised, as in Crohn's Disease, radiation enteritis or acute mesenteric ischemia; where there is decreased effective surface area for absorption, as in short bowel syndrome or celiac sprue; where there is impaired absorption, as in pancreatic insufficiency; or in stressed, catabolic or septic states.

Table 1: Potential uses of protein hydrolysates in disease

Impaired mucosal integrity
    Radiation enteritis
    Crohn's Disease
    Mesenteric ischemia
Decreased surface area for absorption
    Short bowel syndrome
    Celiac sprue
Impaired absorptive function
    Pancreatic insufficiency
    Post-pancreatectomy
Stressed states
    Postoperative/ICU
    Burns
    Trauma
    Systemic sepsis

One important and common example of the potential application of peptide-based enteral diets is in patients with short bowel syndrome.

SHORT BOWEL SYNDROME

Short bowel syndrome occurs after removal of 70-80% of the small bowel, leading to a massive loss of absorptive capacity of the gut, and resulting in severe diarrhea and malnutrition. Other organ dysfunction occurs, including gastric hypersecretion and decreased secretion of enterohormones such as cholecystokinin and secretin, resulting in decreased gallbladder contraction and pancreatic secretion.

TPN has traditionally been used as the sole form of postoperative nutritional support in these patients despite evidence that in animals (Levine et al., 1974) and humans (Guedon et al., 1986) TPN given alone impairs intestinal growth and function. In fact, intestinal mucosal atrophy is seen in humans after just 3 weeks of TPN (Guedon et al., 1986). The strongest promoter of intestinal growth and function is the presence of food in the intestinal lumen (Johnson, 1987). The effects of enteral contents are both direct and indirect. Food in the intestinal lumen directly augments mucosal cell turnover (Creamer et al., 1961). Furthermore, direct substrate-induced stimulation of the brush border enzymes (peptidases, disaccharidases, lipase) occurs with provision of the appropriate nutrients (McCarthy et al., 1980). Indirect mucosal stimulation by luminal contents occurs via release of enterotrophic hormones, as well as augmentation of blood flow and stimulation of the autonomic nervous system (Rombeau et al., 1993).

The overall protein needs in patients with short bowel syndrome are similar to other surgical patients and depend on the degree of surgical stress and muscle catabolism present. The composition of protein, however, is particularly important in the diet of patients with short bowel syndrome. In a recent study with SBS it was noted that there was lower fecal nitrogen excretion by patients on a diet containing small peptides compared with a control diet containing whole proteins (Cosnes et al., 1990). Elemental diets have been shown to improve adaptation in the remaining gut by increasing intestinal length and stimulating villous hypertrophy (Votik et al., 1973; Votik and Crispin, 1975). However, recent data suggests that polymeric diets are not only advantageous because of the increased stimulation of the mucosa, but are also less expensive (McIntyre, 1985). Although limited studies have been performed in humans, sufficient animal evidence exists to suggest the utility of protein hydrolysates as a complete nitrogen source during intestinal adaptation to short bowel syndrome.

Many therapeutic possibilities for glutamine in enteral formulas exist. The observation that mucosal atrophy can be modified with glutamine suggests an important use in short bowel syndrome. Smith et al. (1988) studied the administration of glutamine-supplemented chow to rats following 60% resection of the midportion of the small bowel. Marked hyperplasia of the remaining small bowel was found in animals receiving glutamine, suggesting stimulation of an adaptive response to short bowel syndrome.

REFERENCES

Adibi, S.A. 1971. Intestinal transport of dipeptides in man. Relative importance of hydrolysis and intact absorption. *J. Clin. Invest.*, 20:2266-2275.

Alverdy, J.C. 1990. Effect of glutamine supplemented diets on immunology of the gut. *JPEN* 14:109S-113S.

Ardawi, M.S.M and Newsholme, E.A. 1983. Glutamine metabolism in lymphocytes of the rat. *Biochem J.* 212:835-42.

Bergstrom, J., Furst, P., Noree, L.O, et al. 1974. Intracellular free amino acid concentration in human muscle tissue. *J. Appl. Physiol.* 36:693-697.

Borgstrom, B., Dahlquist, A., Lundh, G., and Sjovall, J. 1957. Studies of intestinal digestion and absorption in the human. *J. Clin. Invest.*, 36L:1521-1536.

Bounous, G. 1993. Elemental diets in the prophylaxis and therapy for intestinal lesions, In: Buonos, G. (Ed.) *Use of elemental diets in clinical situations*. Boca Raton: CRC Press.

Chipponi, J.X., Bleier, J.C., Santi, M.T., and Rudman, D. 1982. Deficiencies of essential and conditionally essential nutrients. *Am. J. Clin. Nut.* 35:1112-1116.

Cosnes J., Evard, D., Beaugerie, L., et al. 1990. Prospective randomized trial comparing small peptides vs whole proteins in patients with a high jejunostomy. *Clin Nutr.*, 9 Suppl., 111-5.

Creamer, B., Shorter, R.G., and Barnforth, J. 1961. The turnover and shedding of epithelial cells. *Gut* 2:110-18.

Darmain, D., Matthews, D.E., and Bier, D.M. 1986. Glutamine and glutamate kinetics in humans. *Am. J. Physiol.* 251:E117-E126.

Dudrick, P.S., Salloum, R.M., Copeland, E.M. and Souba, W.W. 1992. The early response of the jejunal brush border glutamine transporter to endotoxemia. *J.Surg. Res.* 52:372-377.

Fox, A.D., Kripke, S.A., Berman, J.M., et al. 1987. Reduction of the severity of enterocolitis by glutamine-supplemented enteral diets. *Surg. Forum* 38:43-44.

Fox, A.D., Kripke, S.A., DePaula, J.A., et al. 1988. The effect of a glutamine-supplemented enteral diet on methotrexate-induced enterocolitis. *JPEN* 12:325-331.

Ganapathy, V. and Leibach, F.H. 1982. Peptide transport in intestinal and renal brush border membrane vesicles. *Life Sci.* 30:2137-46.

Guedon, C., Schmitz, J., Lerebours, E., et al. 1986. Decreased brush border hydrolase activities without gross morphologic changes in human intestinal mucosa after prolonged total parenteral nutrition of adults. *Gastroenterology* 90:373-8.

Hwang, T.L., O'Dwyer, S.T., Smith, R.J. and Wilmore, D.W. 1986. Preservation of small bowel mucosa using glutamine enriched parenteral nutrition. *Surg. Forum* 37:56-58.

Imondi, A.R., and Stradley, R.P. 1974. Utilization of enzymatically hydrolyzed soybean protein and crystalline amino acid diets by rats with exocrine pancreatic insufficiency.*J. Clin Invest.* 104:793-6.

Jacobs, D.O., Evans, D.A., Medly, K., et al. 1988. Combined effects of glutamine and epidermal growth factor on the rat intestine. *Surgery* 104:358-364.

Johnson, L.R. 1987. Regulation of gastrointestinal growth, In: Johnson, L.R. (ed.) *Physiology of the gastrointestinal tract*, Vol. 1, 2nd ed. New York: Raven Press.

Joint FAO/WHO Expert Committee Report: Energy and protein requirements. 1973. WHO Technical Report Series, No. 522. Geneva.

Kovacevic, Z. and McGivan, J.D. 1983. Mitochondrial metabolism of glutamine and glutamate, and its physiological significance. *Physiol. Rev.* 63:547-605.

Kovacevic, Z. and Morris, H.P. 1972. The role of glutamine in the oxidative metabolism of malignant cells. *Cancer Res.* 32:326-333.

Krebs, H.A. 1980. Glutamine metabolism in the animal body. In: Mora, J. and Palacios, R. (eds.) *Glutamine: Metabolism, enzymology and regulation*. New York: Academic Press.

Krey, S.H. and Murray, R.L. 1990. Modular and transitional feedings. In: Rombeau J.R. and Caldwell, M.D. (Eds.) *Clinical nutrition: Enteral and tube feeding*. Philadelphia: W.B. Saunders Co.

Levine, G.M., Deren, J.J., Steiger, E., et al. 1974. Role of oral intake in maintenance of gut mass and disaccharidase activity *Gastroenterology* 67:975-82.

MacBurney, M.M., Russell, C., and See Young, L. 1990. Formulas. In: Rombeau, J.R. and Caldwell, M.D. (Eds.) *Clinical nutrition: Enteral and tube feeding*. Philadelphia: W.B. Saunders Co.

McCarthy, D.M., Nicholson, J.A., and Kim, V.S. 1980. Intestinal enzyme adaptation to normal diets of different composition. *Am J. Physiol.* 239:G445-51.

McIntyre, P.B. 1985. The short bowel. *Br. J. Surg.* 72:S92-3.

Matthews, D.M. 1991. Absorption of amino acids, In: Matthews, D.M. (ed.) *Protein absorption*. Chichester UK: Wiley Liss.

Matthews, D.M. and Adibi, S.A. 1976. Peptide absorption. *Gastroenterology* 71:151-161.

Matthews, D.M. and Burston, D. 1984. Uptake of a series of neutral dipeptides including: L-alanyl-L-alanine, glycylglycine and glycylsarcosine by hamster jejunum in vitro. *Clin. Sci.* 67:541-49.

Matthews, D.M. and Payne, J.W. 1980. Transmembrane transport of small peptides. *Curr. Top. Membr. Transp.* 14:331-425.

Meguid, M.M., Landel, A.M., Terz, J.J., and Akrabawi, S.S. 1984. Effect of elemental diet on albumin and urea synthesis: Comparison with partially hydrolyzed protein diet. *J. Surg. Res.* 37:16-24.

Miller, B.M., Ceresosimo, E., McRea, J., et al. 1983. Inter-organ relationships of alanine and glutamine during fasting in the conscious dog. *J. Surg. Res.* 35:310-318.

Mitchell, H.H. 1924. A method of determining the biological value of protein. *J. Biol. Chem.* 58:873-903.

Monchi, M., Vaugelade, P., Vaissade, P., and Rerat, A. 1991. Net protein utilization after duodenal infusion of small peptides or free amino acids, *JPEN*, 15:29S.

Moriarty, K.J., Hegarty, J.E., Fairclough, P.D., et al. 1985: Relative nutritional value of whole protein, hydrolyzed protein, and free amino acids in man. *Gut* 26:694-99.

Neptune, E.M. 1965. Respiration and oxidation of various substrates by ileum *in vitro*. *Am. J. Physiol.* 209:329-332.

O'Dwyer, S.T., Scott, T., Smith, R.J., and Wilmore, D.W. 1987. 5-Fluorouracil toxicity on small intestinal mucosa but not white blood cells is decreased by glutamine. *Clin. Res.* 35:369A.

O'Dwyer, S.T., et al. 1990. New fuels for the gut. In: Rombeau, J.R., Caldwell, M.D. (eds.) *Clinical nutrition: Enteral and tube feeding.* Philadelphia: W.B. Saunders Co.

Pitts, R.F. 1964. Renal production and excretion of ammonia. *Am. J. Med.* 36:720-42.

Poullain, M.D., Cezard, J.P., Roger, L., and Mendy, F. 1989. Effect of whey proteins, their oligopeptide hydrolysates and free amino mixtures on growth and nitrogen retention in starved rats. *JPEN* 13:382-6.

Reitzer, C.J., Wice, B.W., and Kennell, D. 1979. Evidence that glutamine, not sugar, is the major energy source for cultured HeLa cells. *J. Biol. Chem.* 254:2669-76.

Rerat, A., Nunes, C.S., Mendy, F.G., et al. 1988. Amino acid absorption and production of pancreatic hormones in non-anesthetized pigs after duodenal infusions of a milk enzymic hydrolysate or of free amino acids. *Br. J. Nutr.* 60:121-136.

Roediger, W.E.W. 1982. Utilization of nutrients by isolated epithelial cells of the rat colon. *Gastroenterology* 83:424-429.

Rombeau, J.R., Strear, C.M., and Nance, M.L. 1993. Elemental diets and short-bowel syndrome: Scientific rationale and clinical utility. In: Bounous, G. (ed.) *Uses of elemental diets in clinical situations.* Boca Raton: CRC Press.

Ross, B.D., Hems, R., and Krebs, H.A. 1967. The rate of gluconeogenesis from various precursors in the perfused rat liver. *Biochem J.* 102:942-51.

Roth, E., Furnovics, J., Muhlbacher, F., et al. 1982. Metabolic disorders in severe abdominal sepsis: glutamine deficiency in skeletal muscle. *Clin. Nutr.* 1:25-41.

Rubino, A., Field, M., and Schwachman, H. 1971. Intestinal transport of amino acid residues of dipeptides. I. Influx of the glycine residue of glycyl-L-proline across mucosal border. *J. Biol. Chem.*, 246:3542-48.

Schlienger, J.L. and Imler, M. 1980. Variations in blood ammonia and glutamine levels after hepatectomy and/or abdominal evisceration in the rat. *Hepato-Gastroenterology* 27:441-447.

Schmucker, D.L. and Daniels, C.K. 1986. Aging, gastrointestinal infections and mucosal immunity. *J. Am. Geriatr. Soc.* 34:377-384.

Scriver, C.R. and Rosenberg, L.E. 1973. *Amino acid metabolism and its disorders.* Philadelphia: W.B. Saunders Co.

Silk, D.B.A. 1981. Peptide transport. *Clin. Sci.* 60:607-615.

Silk, D.B.A., Chung, Y.C., Berger, K.L., et al. 1979. Comparison of oral feeding of peptide and amino acid meals to normal human subjects. *Gut*, 20:291-99.

Smith, J.L., Arteaga, E., and Heymsfield, S.B. 1982. Increased ureagenesis and impaired nitrogen use during infusion of a synthetic amino acid formula. *N. Engl. J. Med.* 306:1013-18.

Smith, J.L., Artega, C., and Heymsfield, S. 1985. Regulation of protein degradation in differentiated skeletal muscle cells in monolayer culture. In: Khairallah, E., Bond, J., and Bird, J.C. (eds.) *Intracellular protein catabolism.* New York: Liss.

Smith, R.J., O'Dwyer, S., Wang, X-D., and Wilmore, D.W. 1988. Glutamine nutrition and the gastrointestinal tract. In: *The gastrointestinal response to injury, starvation and enteral nutrition. Report of the 8th Ross conference in medical research.* Columbus, Ohio: Ross Laboratories.

Souba, W.W., Klimberg, V.S., and Copeland, E.M. 1990. Glutamine nutrition in the management of radiation enteritis. *JPEN* 14(4):106S-7S.

Souba,W.W., Smith, R.J., and Wilmore, D.W. 1985a. Glutamine metabolism by the intestinal tract. *JPEN* 9:608-17.

Souba W.W., Smith, R.J., and Wilmore, D.W. 1985b. Effects of glucocorticoids on glutamine metabolism in visceral organs. *Metabolism* 34:450-456.

Stein, T.P., Lazarus, D.D., and Chatzidakis, C. 1990. Human macronutrient requirements. In: Rombeau, J.R. and Caldwell, M.D. (eds) *Clinical nutrition: Enteral and tube feeding,* 2nd ed.:54-72. Philadelphia: W.B. Saunders Co.

Trocki, O., Mochizuki, H., Dominioni, L., and Alexander, J.W. 1986. Intact protein versus free amino acids in the nutritional support of thermally injured animals. *JPEN* 10:139-45.

Van Der Meer, J.W.M. 1988. Defects in host-defense mechanisms. In: Rubin R.H. and Yang, L.S. (eds.) *Clinical approach to infection in the compromised host*. 2nd Ed. New York: Plenum Medical Book Company.

Votik, A.J., Eschave, V., Brown, R.A., et al. 1973. Use of elemental diet during the adaptive stage of short gut syndrome. *Gastroenterology* 65:419-26.

Votik, A.J. and Crispin, J.S. 1975. The ability of an elemental diet to support nutrition and adaptation in the short gut syndrome. *Ann. Surg.* 181:220-225.

Wapnir, R.A. 1990. *Protein nutrition and mineral absorption*. Boca Raton: CRC Press.

Wayne-Meredith, J., Ditesheim, J.A., and Zaloga, G.P. 1990. Visceral protein levels in trauma patients are greater with peptide diet than with intact protein diet. *J. Trauma* 30:825-8.

Wellner D. and Meister, A. 1981. A survey of in-born errors of amino acid metabolism and transport in man. *Annu. Rev. Biochem.*, 50:911-68.

Windemueller, H.G. and Spaeth, A.E. 1974. Uptake and metabolism of plasma glutamine by the small intestine. *J. Biol. Chem.* 249:5070-79.

Windmueller, H.G. and Spaeth, A.E. 1978. Identification of ketone bodies and glutamine as the major respiratory fuels *in vivo* for postoperative rat small intestine. *J. Biol. Chem.* 10:69-76.

Zaloga, G.P. 1993. Studies comparing intact protein, peptide and amino acid formulas In:Bounous, G. (ed.) *Uses of elemental diets in clinical situations*:201-217. Boca Raton: CRC Press.

Ziegler, F., Ollivier, J.M., Cynober, L., et al. 1993. Small peptides vs whole proteins in continuous enteral support of abdominal surgery patients In: Bounous, G. (Ed.) *Uses of elemental diets in clinical situations*. Boca Raton: CRC Press.

Dairy Products in Human Health and Nutrition, Serrano Ríos et al. (eds) © 1994 Balkema, Rotterdam, ISBN 90 5410 359 0

Fatty acids, *cis* and *trans*: A metabolic enigma – Role in disease causation

G.J. Brisson
Université Laval, Que., Canada

ABSTRACT: Dietary intake of *trans* fatty acids (tFA), in some countries, may range from 1.6 to 38.7 g/day. *Trans* fatty acids are potent inhibitors of delta-6 and delta-5 desaturases involved in the biosynthesis of precursors of prostaglandins; they exacerbate essential fatty acid deficiency. Dietary tFA may affect membrane-associated enzyme systems. Data suggest placental transfer of tFA in humans; furthermore, the concentration in human milk is directly related to the amount in the diet. Dietary tFA in the diet of pregnant and nursing women should probably be reduced to a minimum. Milk formula, on fat basis, should not contain more than 6 % tFA. Under conditions of normal dietary habits, tFA are not important factors regarding blood cholesterol levels, and may not be a risk factor for atherosclerosis. Cancerogenecity of tFA, or lack of it, when applied to humans, needs further investigation.

1 INTRODUCTION

Dietary fats are made of esters of glycerol and fatty acids. Three molecules of fatty acids are reacted with each molecule of glycerol; the resulting compounds are called triglycerides or triacylglycerols. The physical, chemical and biological properties of dietary fats are determined by the nature of the different fatty acids making up their constituent triacylglycerols.

Fatty acids are chains of carbon atoms saturated or not with hydrogen atoms. If all carbon atoms, except for the carboxyl group, are saturated with hydrogen, they are called saturated fatty acids; if two hydrogen atoms are lacking on two adjacent carbons, the resulting fatty acid shows a double bond and is said to be unsaturated. A double bond in a fatty acid carbon chain permits two possible geometrical arrangements around the point of unsaturation; this phenomenon is called geometrical isomerism; two types of isomers, *cis* and *trans*, are recognized (Brisson, 1981). In one case, the carbon atoms about the point of unsaturation may be said to adopt a linear configuration to give the *trans* geometrical isomer. In the other case, the carbon atoms takes a curved configuration to give the *cis* isomer.

Fatty acids in natural vegetable oils are mostly unsaturated and are all of the *cis* configuration type; *trans* isomers appear when vegetable oils are partially hydrogenated for the purpose of making margarines and shortenings. Some *trans* fatty acids are also found in milk fat and meat because unsaturated fatty acids, taken as constituents of feedstuffs, are partially hydrogenated by rumen microorganisms.

In margarines and shortenings the main *trans* fatty acid has a chain length of 18 carbons and the double bond is between carbon 9 and 10 from the methyl group; it is called elaidic acid and will be given the symbol tC18:1n9. In milk fat and butter the main *trans* fatty acid has also a chain length of 18 carbons but the double bond is between carbon 7 and 8; it is called *trans* vaccenic acid and may be given the symbol tC18:1n7.

The position of the double bond on the carbon chain, as well as the type of geometrical configuration about the double bond, may change considerably the physical properties of fat. For example, elaidic acid (tC18:1n9) has a melting point considerably higher than its *cis* isomer, oleic acid (cC18:1n9). This property is desirable to harden vegetable oils in margarine and shortenings. Early data showing an important consumption of *trans* fatty acids in the form of partially hydrogenated vegetable fats and oils raised concern about possible effects on health.

Early research data were confusing, some raising concern about health, some (mostly from the vegetable oil industry) attempting be to reassuring. "The enigma of the *trans* fatty acids" was presented and documented in an earlier work published in 1981 (Brisson, 1981)

The purpose of the present paper is to reexamine, in the light of recent research, the possible effects of dietary *trans* fatty acids on human health.

2 *Trans* FATTY ACIDS IN FOOD ITEMS

Margarines and shortenings are by far the most important sources of *trans* fatty acids in contemporary human diets. Expressed as percent of total fatty acids, total *trans* fatty acids in margarines vary from 0 % to 52 % (Enig *et al.*, 1983; Enig, Budowski and Blondheim, 1984; Kochhar and Matsui, 1984; Booyens and Katzeff, 1985; Croon, 1987; Coll and Gutierrez, 1989; Ratnayake, Hollywood and O'Grady, 1991). The content varies from country to country and from type to type of margarines. In general, soft margarines contain less total *trans* fatty acids than hard or tub margarines. The content of shortenings is more uniform but may vary from 9 to 35 % (Enig *et al.*, 1983). A great number of food items contain *trans* fatty acids because they contain partially hydrogenated vegetable oils (Enig *et al.*, 1990).

Because as in ruminant animals, the micro flora in the rumen has the property to partially hydrogenate polyunsaturated fatty acids naturally occurring in feedstuffs, dairy fat and red meat also contain small amounts of *trans* fatty acids. In butter, for example, total *trans* fatty acids vary from >1 to about 4 % of total fatty acids (Brisson, 1981; Enig *et al.*, 1983; Lund and Jensen, 1983; Croon, 1987; Brisson, 1992). Both in partially hydrogenated fat and dairy fat, the dominating *trans* fatty acids are C18 monoenes; elaidic acid (*trans*-C18:1n9) dominates in partially hydrogenated fat, and vaccenic acid (*trans*-C18:1n7), in dairy fat. It is important to note the difference between partially hydrogenated vegetable oils and butter fat, with regards to the dominating *trans* isomer.

Trans C18 dienes also appear in partially hydrogenated vegetable oils. For example, Canadian margarines may contain up to 7.6 % *trans*-C18 dienes (Ratnayake, Hollywood and O'Grady, 1991). But, dairy fat, for all practical purposes, contains no *trans*-dienes (Lund and Jensen, 1983).

On a total fatty acid basis, *trans* fatty acids in a particular food item, labeled to contain partially hydrogenated vegetable oils, may vary from 0 % to 52 %. There is no labeling regulation permitting to know the exact *trans* fatty acid content of any food item. This certainly contributes to the enigma of *trans* fatty acids.

3 DIETARY INTAKE OF *TRANS* FATTY ACIDS

Trans fatty acids have been shown to accumulate in all organs and lipid fractions of practically all tissues in the body of both animals and humans (Bonaga *et al.*, 1980; Moore, Alfin and Aftergood, 1980b; Brisson, 1981; Adlof and Emken, 1986). In human tissues, they are exclusively of dietary origin. Furthermore, as shown in animal adipose tissues, their concentration is directly proportional to intake (Enig *et al.*, 1990). It is of importance, therefore, to estimate the possible daily intake of *trans* fatty acids in the general population in order to rationalize properly the possible impact on human health of these molecules, which are considered by some as being "unnatural".

The intake of *trans* fatty acids varies from country to country, depending on food habits and the *trans* fatty acid content of local food items based on partially hydrogenated vegetable oils. Based on available information in 1981, a maximum consumption by the Canadian population was estimated at about 17 g/day with an average of 9 g/day (Brisson, 1981). A recent survey made in U.S.A. showed, for this country, a range of 1.6 to 38.7 g/day; but calculations based on adipose tissues concentration suggested a range of 11 to 28 g/day (Enig *et al.*, 1990). For purposes of comparison, estimates were 17 g/day per person in Holland (Brussaard, 1986), and 7 g per person daily with a maximum of 17 g/day in UK (Nutritional Consultative Panel, 1988).

To obtain an accurate estimate of the consumption of *trans* fatty acids within a given population, the procedure described by Enig *et al.* (1990) should be applied. It is likely then that the maximum daily consumption of *trans* fatty acids would be found higher than that already estimated in most countries.

4 ESSENTIAL FATTY ACIDS

Trans fatty acids accumulate not only in the triacylglycerol fraction of practically all tissues in the body, but also in the phospholipids of all tissues. For example, heart phospholipids may accumulate important amounts of *trans* acids, which is associated with a decrease in essential fatty acids (Hill, Johnson and Holman, 1979). Liver phospholipids may also accumulate appreciable quantities of *trans* fatty acids.

Evidence have been presented that elaidic acid and other members of the *trans*-C18:1 family, as well as members of the *trans*-C18:2 family, found in hydrogenated vegetable oils, are potent inhibitors of delta-6 and delta-5 desaturases. These enzymes are involved in the conversion of the essential fatty acid linoleic acid to arachidonic acid; arachidonic acid is a precursor of prostaglandins (Mahfouz, 1981; Rosenthal and Whitehurst, 1983; Rosenthal and Doloresco, 1984). Linoelaidate (ttC18:2) is even a more potent inhibitor of delta-6 desaturase than members of the *trans*-C18:1 (Rosenthal and Whitehurst, 1983). Furthermore this effect is much more pronounced in a state of essential fatty acid deficiency (De Schrijver and Privett, 1982).

The effect of *trans* fatty acids on enzyme systems involved in the elongation and desaturation of linoleic acid is well documented. *Trans* monoenes and more so *trans* dienes exacerbate essential fatty acid deficiency.

5 PROSTAGLANDINS

Trans-dienes have been shown to be strong inhibitors of the delta-6-desaturase enzyme. The activity of this enzyme system is considered rate limiting in the conversion of linoleic acid to arachidonic acid with possible consequences on the biosynthesis of eicosanoids or prostanoids. Effectively, dietary C18:2tt decreases serum prostaglandin and thromboxane levels in rats (Hwang and Kinsella 1979; Bruckner, Goswami and Kinsella, 1984). It is known also that these metabolites are involved in gastrointestinal, cardiovascular, pulmonary, and renal regulatory functions. Furthermore, some dietary *trans* isomers of linoleic acid may be converted into *trans*-arachidonic acid with possible consequences on the properties of prostaglandins and thromboxanes. This has been and continues to be of concerns with regards to human health (Kinsella *et al.*, 1981).

Intakes of C18:2tt at levels as high as 6.3 % of energy, in rats, had measurable effects of the levels of some prostanoids in various organs, but did not alter platelet aggregation to various agonists (Bruckner, Goswami and Kinsella, 1984). Later studies where two strains of rats were used, confirm that *trans* fatty acids from partially hydrogenated corn oil could affect the biosynthesis of prostanoids (Chiang *et al.*, 1991). But the significance of the effects varied with strains of rats used. In one strain of stroke-prone spontaneously hypertensive rats, dietary *trans* fatty acids altered the ratio PGF2/PGF2a, lowered systolic blood pressure and platelet aggregability. The authors suggested that *trans* fatty acids might prevent thrombotic disorders in these rats. This apparent beneficial effect, however, was not observed in Wistar-Kyoto rats. If such differences in response to dietary *trans* fatty acids are noted between two strains of rats, the question may be raised as to what extent observations made in rats may be extrapolated to humans. Nevertheless, it appears that the influence of *trans* fatty acids on the biosynthesis of eicosanoids may be due to their effect on the enzyme system involved in the biosynthesis of arachidonic acid a precursor of these metabolites, rather than to a direct effect on the eicosanoid-synthesizing enzymes themselves (Zevenbergen and Haddeman, 1989). For that reason, an adequate dietary intake of essential fatty acids may mask the effect of *trans* fatty acids on the biosynthesis of eicosanoids, at least in the rat.

The enigma concerning the possible effects of dietary *trans* fatty acids on the biosynthesis of prostanoids in humans with possible consequences on health remains unsolved.

6 MEMBRANE FUNCTIONS

It is well known that dietary *trans* fatty acids are incorporated in membrane phospholipids. Results on the effects of dietary *trans* fatty acids on membrane fluidity and functions, however, are controversial (Entressangles, 1986). In some cases, membrane fluidity is lowered by feeding *trans* fatty acids (Alam, Banerji and Alam, 1985; Ren *et al.*, 1988; Remmers, Nordby and Medzihradsky, 1990), but in some other, membrane fluidity was not affected (Mahfouz, Smith and Kummerow, 1984).

Some of the early experiments were carried out under experimental conditions where essential fatty acids may have been deficient. But, under conditions where essential fatty acids were supplied in adequate amount, the ATP biosynthesis by liver mitochrondria in rats was still depressed if dietary C18:2tt reached a level of approximately 2.5 % of dietary energy (De Schrijver and Privett, 1984). Growth and efficiency of energy utilization were also depressed. Other work showed that feeding 20 % partially hydrogenated soybean oil (48 % *trans* monoenes) to rats, decreased (Na+ + K+)-ATPase and adenylate cyclase activity in cardiac membranes (Alam, Ren and Alam, 1989). Adding 2 % corn oil to the diet only partially restored the activity of the enzyme system. It may be noted that, in this work, *trans* fatty acids supplied about 18 % of dietary energy, which is more than twice the levels in average human diets.

More work is needed using plasma membranes from different organs and different enzymes systems in several animal species, under varied experimental conditions, before the enigma regarding the role of *trans* fatty acids on membrane functions and possible resulting effects on human health is clarified. Nevertheless, at the present time, there are strong indications that dietary *trans* fatty acids, under certain conditions, may affect membrane-associated enzyme systems with still unknown consequences on human health.

7 NEONATES AND HUMAN MILK

There is an almost one to one correlation between *trans* fatty acids in maternal and cord plasma lipids (Koletzko and Muller, 1990). This would suggest a placental transfer of *trans* fatty acids in humans, and raise the question of their safety in the diet of pregnant women. Furthermore, human milk fat has been reported to contain from 2 % to 18 % *trans* fatty acids (Beare-Rogers and Nera, 1976; Aitchison *et al.*, 1977; Picciano and Perkins, 1977; Hundrieser, Clark and Brown, 1983; Koletzko, Mrotzek and Bremer, 1987). *Trans* dienes, consumed as partially hydrogenated vegetable oils, are also found in measurable quantity in human milk varying from 0.21 % to 0.74 % (Koletzko, Mrotzek and Bremer, 1988). Effectively, the concentration of elaidic acid in human milk is directly related to the amount of this acid in the diet of the previous day (Craig-Schmidt *et al.*, 1984).

Since *trans* monoenes and particularly *trans* dienes are known to decrease the activity of enzyme systems involved in the biosynthesis of arachidonic acid, a precursor of prostaglandins, and exacerbate essential fatty acid deficiency, neonates, under certain conditions, may be at risk with respect to the possible effects on health of dietary partially hydrogenated fat. Effectively, because of rapid growth and limited body stores, infants are more vulnerable to the effects of factors that interfere with essential fatty acid metabolism. Also, brain development, particularly of myelination, in neonates, requires an adequate supply of physiologically active long-chain fatty acids (Crawford, Hassam and Stevens, 1981). For these reasons, intake levels of *trans*-fatty acids in pregnant and nursing women should probably be reduced to a minimum.

Milk formula for neonates may contain some *trans* fatty acids if partially hydrogenated vegetable oils are used in their formulation. Recommendations have been that *trans* fatty acids in milk formula should not exceed 6 % of total fatty acids (Carroll, 1989). Such recom-mendations were based partly on a level of *trans* fatty acids normally found in breast milk, and partly on data showing that the inclusion of *trans* fatty acids in the maternal diet had no apparent effects on the prostaglandin content of either human or rat milk (Craig-Schmidt *et al.*, 1984; Wickwire *et al.*, 1987). Addi-tional work, however, is needed to completely clarify the role of both *trans* monoenes and *trans* dienes in the development and well being of neonates.

Until new and more persuasive data become available, it would appear that levels of *trans* fatty acids in the diet of pregnant and nursing women should be reduced to a minimum, and that milk formula should not contain, on a fat basis, more than 6 % *trans* fatty acids.

8 BLOOD CHOLESTEROL

Serum lecithin:cholesterol acyl transferase (LCAT) is an enzyme involved in the transfer of fatty acids from the beta position of phosphatidylcholines to free cholesterol to yield cholesterol esters, thus preventing the accumulation of free cholesterol in blood. The activity of this enzyme, therefore, is important in the metabolism of cholesterol. Under different experimental condi-tions, the activity of this enzyme is either reduced, or increased by feeding *trans* fatty acids to animals (Takatori, Phillips and Privett, 1976; Privett *et al.*, 1977; Moore, Alfin and Aftergood, 1980a; Kritchevsky *et al.*, 1984; Chiang *et al.*, 1991). The effect, when present, is particularly associated to the *trans*-C18:2 family (Privett *et al.*, 1977). In view of possible effects of dietary *trans* fatty acids on the activity of LCAT, it would appear of interest to examine the influence of partially hydrogenated vegetable oils on blood cholesterol levels.

Some early experiments, as summarized by Brisson (1981), indicated that fatty acid *trans* isomers could increase blood cholesterol both in men and animals. In these experiments, however, the intake of *trans* fatty acid was equivalent to 37 g elaidic acid per day. Such a daily intake would appear to be the maximum level encounter in the general population (Enig *et al.*, 1990). Since then, experimental work has been carried out both in humans and animals.

Trans fatty acids had no effect on blood cholesterol in monkeys fed for one year diets in which near 14 % of dietary calories were from *trans* fatty acids (Kritchevsky *et al.*, 1984). In pigs, a diet high in *trans* fatty acids was compared to a diet rich in oleic acid, under conditions where about 12 % of dietary calories were from *trans*-C18:1 (Toda *et al.*, 1985). After a 4-month experimental period, serum cholesterol was the same in both the control and experimental groups. In a strain of mouse susceptible to hypercholesterolemia when fed atherogenic diet, *trans* fatty acids from partially hydrogenated vegetable oils did not appear to play a significantly different role than their *cis*-C18:1 isomer, with regard to plasma cholesterol levels (Walker, 1983). In rats, free and total serum cholesterol were actually decreased by feeding high *trans* fatty acid diets (Moore, Alfin and Aftergood, 1980a). But in rabbits, feeding high *trans* diets (near 12 % of dietary fat calories from *trans*) for 5 months elevated serum cholesterol by 90 %, compared to the control diet (Ruttenberg *et al.*. 1983).

In experiments with human subjects, diets in which *trans*-C18:1 fatty acids provided 7.7 % of total energy were compared to diets where 12.0 % of total energy came from linoleic acid (*cis,cis*-C18:2). The *trans* fatty acid diet, compared to the high linoleic acid diet, elevated total serum cholesterol by a factor of only 4 % in men and 2.9 % in women; the elevation in women was not statistically significant (Zock and Katan, 1992). In this work, an elevation of 6.8 % in LDL and a decrease of 8.5 % in HDL were also observed. It may be noted that, effectively, a diet in which 7.7 % of total calories is provided by *trans*-C18:1 may be encountered in the general population, but a diet in which 12.0 % of total calories is provided by linoleic acid is three to four times the recommended daily intakes (FAO, 1977; Gouvernement du Canada, 1983); such a level of dietary linoleic acid perhaps should be avoided (WHO, 1982). This data, therefore may not apply under normal food habits.

In an other experiment, a diet providing 11 % of energy intake as *trans*-C18:1 was compared to one providing 23 % of energy as oleic acid (Mensink and Katan, 1990). In this case, serum total cholesterol and LDL were higher in men and women consuming the *trans* fatty acid, when compared to those consuming the diet providing twice as much oleic acid. Serious questions have been raised with regards to the applicability of these observations under practical and normal food intake in human (Kritchevsky, 1991; Reeves, 1991).

High or low *trans* fatty acid margarines were consumed by women without effect on serum total cholesterol or LDL-cholesterol levels (Summa, Platt and Brosche, 1984). In more recent work, a hard margarine containing 29 % *trans* fatty acid was compared to a soft zero-*trans* margarine added at a level equivalent to 29 % of total calories to the diet of free-living men (Wood *et al.*, 1993). Daily intakes of *trans* fatty acids was 16 g. The hard margarine elevated total serum cholesterol by 5.6 % and LDL-cholesterol by 6.3 %, but HDL-cholesterol remained at identical levels with both types of margarines.

Considering all evidence, it appears that, under conditions of normal dietary habits, *trans* fatty acids, whatever the origin, are not an important factor regarding blood cholesterol levels in free-living people.

9 ATHEROSCLEROSIS

The role of *trans* fatty acids in the causation of atherosclerosis has been studied almost exclusively in animals. In one experiment with growing pigs a comparison was made between two types of fats, one considered high in *trans* fatty acids from partially hydrogenated soybean oil, the other one high in oleic acid (*cis*-18:1) from oleic acid-rich safflower oil. In this work, *trans* fatty acids provided about 12 % of calories supplied by dietary fat. After a 4-month experimental period, the degree of thickening of the coronary arteries was more severe in pigs fed the high *cis*-18:1 diet than in those fed the high *trans*-C18:1 diet (Toda *et al.*, 1985).

In other work, monkeys were fed diets in which up to about 14 % of dietary calories were from *trans* fatty acids; in the control diet, fat was supplied by olive oil and soybean oil. After a one year experimental period, there was no significant difference in aortic atherosclerosis or arteriosclerosis between the different groups (Kritchevsky *et al.*, 1984). In rabbits, feeding high *trans* diets (about 12 % of dietary fat calories from *trans*) for 5 months did not show atherogenicity compared to the control diet (Ruttenberg *et al.*, 1983).

Serum lipoprotein[a] is regarded as a strong risk factor for coronary heart disease. Short term experiments suggest that diets providing from 8 % to 10 % of total energy intake as *trans*-monounsaturated fatty acids significantly increased serum lipoprotein[a] in men (Mensink *et al.*, 1992). If these results are confirmed by other invertigations, it might become advisable to adjust dietary intake of *trans* fatty acids to less than 8 % of total calories.

Animal experiments suggest that dietary *trans* fatty acids may not be involved in the causation of atherosclerosis. But recent work in men indicated that further work is needed before a definite conclusion can be reached in this regard.

10 CANCER

Most of the increase in fat consumption during the 20th century, at least in North America, has been due to vegetable fats, a great proportion being partially hydrogenated and containing various amounts of *trans* fatty acids. Associations between dietary vegetable fat and cancer trends have been made (Enig, Munn and Keeney, 1978). It was suggested that the effects of *trans* fatty acids should be considered in studies of carcinogenesis (Keeney, 1981). The possible influence of *trans* fatty acids on cancer has been studied both in vivo using mice and rats, and in vitro using strains of *Salmonella typhimurium* following the method described by Ames *et al.* (1975) (Ames, McCann and Yamasaki, 1975).

In most of these trials, partially hydrogenated fat contained more than 40 % *trans* fatty acids, and no distinction was made between *trans*-monoenes and *trans*-dienes.

In two studies, feeding pure elaidic acid suggested that *trans* fatty acids found in partially hydrogenated oils may be promoter of tumor development (Awad, 1981; Hogan and Shamsuddin, 1984). These studies, however, could be criticized on the basis that the fatty acids in partially hydrogenated oils are in the form of triacylglycerols, and that non esterified *trans* fatty acids fed in the pure form may react differently from the metabolic point of view.

Other work carried out in mice showed that *trans* fatty acids in the form of dietary fat had the same effects as their *cis* counterpart, oleic acid, in promoting transplantable mammary tumor growth, but were less effective in promoting blood borne implantation and distant survival of the tumor cells (Erickson *et al.*, 1984). Explanation was based on the effectiveness of *trans* fatty acids in decreasing biosynthesis of prostaglandin precursors. Similarly, *trans* fat did not differ from *cis* fat in promoting mammary neoplasia (Selenskas, Ip and Ip, 1984; Watanabe and Sugano, 1986) or the incidence of DMH-induced colon tumors (Watanabe, Koga and Sugano, 1985) . In one of these investigations, polyunsaturated fatty acids fed as corn oil in a 20 % fat diet induced six to seven times more palpable mammary tumors than did *trans* and *cis* fatty acids (Selenskas, Ip and Ip, 1984). Furthermore, high fat diets containing various levels of *trans* fatty acids induced fewer liver and colon tumors in female rats than did a control diet based on corn oil, but more small intestinal tumors (Reddy, Tanaka and Simi, 1985). Therefore, it can be concluded that animal experiments to date suggest that *trans* fatty acids are not promoters of carcinogenesis.

Studies using *Salmonella typhimurium* strain TA 98, as described by Ames *et al.* (1975), indicated that mutagenecities, under different experimental conditions, are similar or significantly lower with the liver S-9 fraction from rats fed diets containing *trans* fatty acids than with the same liver fraction from rats fed control diets containing no *trans* fatty acids (Ostlund, Albanus and Croon, 1985; Ponder and Green, 1985; Schaub and Green, 1988).

Considering all evidence obtained to date, under different laboratory conditions, it would appear that *trans* fatty acids from partially hydrogenated vegetable oils are no more cancerogenic than their *cis* conterparts. In this regard, vegetable oils polyunsaturated fatty acids might be look at as greater risk factors than *trans* fatty acids. Much more work is needed, however, before definite statements can be made regarding the effective cancerogenecity of *trans* fatty acids, or lack of it, when applied to humans consuming normal diets.

11 CONCLUSION

The role of dietary *trans* fatty acids in the causation of disease in men remains unclear. In some people, the intake may reach a level where concern may be raised. This may be the case when dairy fat and dairy products in the diet are systematically substituted for food items containing partially hydrogenated vegetable oils and, consequently, unknown quantities of *trans* fatty acids.

REFERENCES

Adlof, R.O. & E.A. Emken. 1986. Distribution of hexadecenoic, octadecenoic and octadecadienoic acid isomers in human tissue lipids. *Lipids.* 21: 543-547.

Aitchison, J.M., W.L. Dunkley, N.L. Canolty & L.M. Smith. 1977. Influence of diet on *trans* fatty acids in human milk. *Am. J. Clin. Nutr.* 30: 2006-2015.

Alam, S.Q., A. Banerji & B.S. Alam. 1985. Membrane fluidity and adenylate cyclase activity in the lacrimal glands of rats fed diets containing *trans* fatty acids. *Cur. Eye Res.* 4: 1253-1262.

Alam, S.Q., Y.F. Ren & B.S. Alam. 1989. Effect of dietary *trans* fatty acids on some membrane-associated enzymes and receptors in rat heart. *Lipids.* 24: 39-44.

Ames, B.N., J. McCann & E. Yamasaki. 1975. Methods for detecting carcinogen and mutagens with the Salmonella microsome mutagenicity test. *Mutat. Res.* 31: 347-364.

Awad, A.B. 1981. *Trans* fatty acids in tumor development and the host survival. *J. Nat. Cancer Inst.* 67: 189-192.

Beare-Rogers, J.L. & E.A. Nera. 1976. Some nutritional aspects of partially hydrogenated oil. *J. Am. Oil Chem. Soc.* 53: 467A.

Bonaga, C., M.G. Trizzino, M.A. Pasquariello, & P.L. Biagi. 1980. Nutritional aspects of *trans* fatty acids. Note I. Their accumulation in tissue lipids of rats fed with normolipidic diets containing margarine. *Biochem. Exp. Biol.* 16: 51-54.

Booyens, J. & I.E. Katzeff. 1985. Evaluation of some South African margarines. *Sth. African Med. J.* 67: 399-400.

Brisson, G.J. 1981. *Lipids in Human Nutrition: An appraisal of Some Dietary Concepts.* Jack K. Burgess, Inc. Englewood, New Jersey, U.S.A.

Brisson, G.J. 1992. Fatty acid content of Canadian butter. Unpublished data.

Bruckner, G., S. Goswami & J.E. Kinsella. 1984. Dietary trilinoelaidate: effects on organ fatty acid composition, prostanoid biosynthesis and platelet function in rats. *J. Nutr.* 114: 58-67.

Brussaard, J.H. 1986. *trans* -Fatty acid content of the Dutch diet. *Voeding* 47: 108-111.

Carroll, K.K. 1989. Upper limits of nutrients in infant formulas: polyunsaturated fatty acids and *trans* fatty acids. *J. Nutr.* 119: 1810-1813.

Chiang, M.T., M.I. Otomo, H. Itoh, Y. Furukawa, S. Kimura & H. Fujimoto. 1991. Effect of *trans* fatty acids on plasma lipids, platelet function and systolic blood pressure in stroke-prone spontaneously hypertensive rats. *Lipids.* 26: 46-52.

Coll, H.L. & R.M. Gutierrez. 1989. Estimation of *trans*-unsaturated fatty acids in margarine and butter. *An. Kw Bromatologia.* 41: 115-128.

Craig-Schmidt, M.C., J.D. Weete, S.A. Faircloth, M.A. Wickwire & E.J. Livant. 1984. The effect of hydrogenated fat in the diet of nursing mothers on lipid composition and prostaglandin content of human milk. *Am. J. Clin. Nutr.* 39: 778-786.

Crawford, H.A., A.G. Hassam & P.A. Stevens. 1981. Essential fatty acid requirements in pregnancy and lactation with special reference to brain development. *Prog. Lipid Res.* 20: 31-40.

Croon, L.B. 1987. Results of 8 years of analytical work. Fatty acid composition of edible fats. *Var Foda* 39: 2-14.

De Schrijver, R. & O.S. Privett. 1982. Interrelatinship between dietary *trans* fatty acids and the 6- and 9-desaturases in the rat. *Lipids.* 17: 27-34.

De Schrijver, R.K. & O.S. Privett. 1984. Energetic efficiency and mitochondrial function in rats fed *trans* fatty acids. *J. Nutr.* 114: 1183-1191.

Enig, M.G., S. Atal, M. Keeney & J. Sampugna. 1990. Isomeric *trans* fatty acids in the U.S.diet. *J. Am. College Nutr.* 9: 471-486.

Enig, M.G., P. Budowski & S.H. Blondheim. 1984. *Trans*-unsaturated fatty acids in margarines and human subcutaneous fat in Israel. *Human Nutr.: Clin. Nutr.* 38C: 223-230.

Enig, M.G., R.J. Munn & M. Keeney. 1978. Dietary fat and cancer trends: a critique. *Fed. Proc.* 37: 2215-2220.

Enig, M.G., L.A. Pallansch, J. Sampugna & M. Keeney. 1983. Fatty acid composition of the fat in selected food items with emphasis on *trans* components. *J. Am. Oil Chem. Soc.* 60: 1788-1795.

Entressangles, B. 1986. Mise au point sur les isomères *trans* alimentaires. *Rev. Fran. corps gras.* Février: 47-58.

Erickson, K.L., D.S. Schlangaer, D.A. Adams, D.R. Fregeau & J.S. Stern. 1984. Influence of dietary fatty acid concentration and geometric configuration on murine mammary tumorigenesis and experimental metastasis. *J. Nutr.* 114: 1834-1842.

FAO. 1977. *Dietary Fats and Oils in Human Nutrition.* Report #3. FAO, Rome.

Gouvernement du Canada. 1983. *Apports nutritionnels recommandés pour les Canadiens.* Hawkins, W.W., ed. Ministère de la santé nationale et du bien-être social du Canada.

Hill, E.G., S.B. Johnson & R.T. Holman. 1979. Intensification of essential fatty acid deficiency in the rat by dietary *trans* fatty acids. *J. Nutr.* 109: 1759-1765.

Hogan, M.L. & A.M. Shamsuddin. 1984. Large intestinal carcinogenesis. 1. Promotional effect of dietary fatty acid isomers in the rat model. *J. Nat. Cancer Inst.* 73: 1293-1296.

Hundrieser, K.E., R.M. Clark & P.B. Brown. 1983. Distribution of *trans*-octadecenoic acid in the major glycerolipids of human milk. *J. Ped. Gastroentero. Nutr.* 2: 635-639.

Hwang, D.H. & J.E. Kinsella. 1979. The effects of *trans, trans* methyl linoleate on the concentration of prostaglandins and their precursors in rats. *Prostaglandins.* 17: 543-549.

Keeney, M. 1981. Comments on the effects of dietary *trans*-fatty acids in humans. *Cancer Res.* 41: 3743-3744.

Kinsella, J.E., G. Bruckner, J. Mai & J. Shimp. 1981. Metabolism of *trans* fatty acids with emphasis on the effects of *trans, trans*-octadecadienoate on lipid composition, essential fatty acid, and prostaglandins: an overview. *Am. J. Clin. Nutr.* 34: 2307-2318.

Kochhar, S.P. & T. Matsui. 1984. Essential fatty acids and *trans* contents of some oils, margarine and other food fats. *Food Chem.* 13: 85-101.

Koletzko, B., M. Mrotzek & H.J. Bremer. 1987. *Trans-fatty acids in human milk and infant plasma and tissue.* Vol. 3 of Human Lactation, pp 323-333. New York: Plenum Press.

Koletzko, B., M. Mrotzek & H.J. Bremer. 1988. Fatty acid composition of mature human milk in Germany. *Am. J. Clin. Nutr.* 47: 954-959.

Koletzko, B. & J. Muller. 1990. *Cis-* and *trans*-isomeric fatty acids in plasma lipids of newborn infants and their mothers. *Biol. Neonate.* 57: 3-4.

Kritchevsky, D. 1991. To the editor. *New England J. Med.* 324: 339.

Kritchevsky, D., L.M. Davidson, M. Weight, N.P.J. Kriek & J.P. du Plessis. 1984. Effect of *trans*-unsaturated fats on experimental atherosclerosis in Vervet monkeys. *Atherosclerosis.* 51: 123-133.

Lund, P. & F. Jensen. 1983. Isomeric fatty acids in milk fat. *Milchwissenschaft.* 38: 193-196.

Mahfouz, M. 1981. Effect of dietary *trans* fatty acids on the delta 5, delta 6 and delta 9 desaturases of rat liver microsomes in vivo. *Acta Biol. Med. Germanica.* 40: 1699-1705.

Mahfouz, M.M., T.L. Smith & F.A. Kummerow. 1984. Effect of dietary fats on desaturase activities and the biosynthesis of fatty acids in rat-liver microsomes. *Lipids.* 19: 214-222.

Mensink, R.P. & M.B. Katan. 1990. Effect of dietary *trans* fatty acids on high-density and low-density lipoprotein cholesterol levels in healthy subjects. *New England J. Med.* 323: 439-445.

Mensink, R.P., P.L. Zock, M.B. Katan & G. Hornstra. 1992. Effect of dietary *cis* and *trans* fatty acids on serum lipoprotein[a] levels in humans. *J. Lipid Res.* 33: 1493-1501.

Moore, C.E., S.R. Alfin & L. Aftergood. 1980a. Effect of *trans* fatty acids on serum lecithin: cholesterol acyltransferase in rats. *J. Nutr.* 110: 2284-2290.

Moore, C.E., S.R. Alfin & L. Aftergood. 1980b. Incorporation and disappearance of *trans* fatty acids in rat tissues. *Am. J. Clin. Nutr.* 33: 2318-2323.

Nutritional Consultative Panel. 1988. *Trans* fatty acids. *Nutrition Briefing.* U.K.

Ostlund, L.A., L. Albanus & L.B. Croon. 1985. Effect of dietary *trans* fatty acids on microsomal enzymes and membranes. *Lipids.* 20: 620-624.

Picciano, M.F. & E.G. Perkins. 1977. Identification of the *trans* isomers of octadecenoic acid in human milk. *Lipids*. 12: 407-408.

Ponder, D.L. & N.R. Green. 1985. Effects of dietary fats and butylated hydroxytoluene on mutagen activation in rats. *Cancer Res.* 45: 558-560.

Privett, O.S., R. Phillips, H. Shimasaki, T. Nozawa & E.C. Nickell. 1977. Studies of effects of *trans* fatty acids in the diet on lipid metabolism in essential fatty acid deficient rats. *Am. J. Clin. Nutr.* 30: 1009-1017.

Ratnayake, W., R. Hollywood & E. O'Grady. 1991. Fatty acids in Canadian margarines. *Can. Inst. Food Sci. Tech. J.* 24: 1-2.

Reddy, B.S., T. Tanaka & B. Simi. 1985. Effect of different levels of dietary *trans* fat or corn oil on azoxymethane-induced colon carcinogenesis in F344 rats. *J. Nat. Cancer Inst.* 75: 791-798.

Reeves, R.M. 1991. Effect of dietary *trans* fatty acids on cholesterol levels. *New England J. Med.* 324: 338-339.

Remmers, A.E., G.L. Nordby & F. Medzihradsky. 1990. Modulation of opioid receptor binding by *cis* and *trans* fatty acids. *J. Neurochem.* 55: 1993-2000.

Ren, Y.F., S.Q. Alam, B.S. Alam & L.M. Keefer. 1988. Adenylate cyclase and beta-receptors in salivary glands of rats fed diets containing *trans* fatty acids. *Lipids*. 23: 304-308.

Rosenthal, M.D. & M.A. Doloresco. 1984. The effects of *trans* fatty acids on fatty acyl delta 5 desaturation by human skin fibroblasts. *Lipids*. 19: 869-874.

Rosenthal, M.D. & M.C. Whitehurst. 1983. Selective effects of isomeric *cis* and *trans* fatty acids on fatty acyl delta 9 and delta 6 desaturation by human skin fibroblasts. *Biochimica Et Biophysica Acta*. 753: 450-459.

Ruttenberg, H., L.M. Davidson, N.A. Little, D.M. Klurfeld & D. Kritchevsky. 1983. Influence of *trans* unsaturated fats on experimental atherosclerosis in rabbits. *J. Nutr.* 113: 835-844.

Schaub, M. & N.R. Green. 1988. Effects of dietary *trans* fatty acids on mutagenesis of known carcinogens. *J. Food Protection*. 51: 117-120.

Selenskas, S.L., M.M. Ip & C. Ip. 1984. Similarity between *trans* fat and saturated fat in the modification of rat mammary carcinogenesis. *Cancer Res.* 44: 1321-1326.

Summa, J.D., D. Platt & T. Brosche. 1984. Effect of differing fat composition in the diet of elderly persons. *Munchener Medizinische Wochenschrift*. 126: 1233-1237.

Takatori, T., F. Phillips & O.S. Privett. 1976. Effects of dietary saturated and *trans* fatty acids on cholesteryl ester synthesis and hydrolysis in the testes of rats. *Lipids*. 11: 357-363.

Toda, T., Y. Toda, V.K. Yamamoto & F.A. Kummerow. 1985. Comparative study of the atherogenecity of dietary *trans*, saturated and unsaturated fatty acids on swine coronary arteries. *J. Nutr. Sci. Vitaminol.* 31: 233-241.

Walker, W.J. 1983. Changing U.S. life style and declining vascular mortality- A retrospect. *New England J. Med.* 308: 649-651.

Watanabe, M., T. Koga & M. Sugano. 1985. Influence of dietary *cis*- and *trans*-fat on 1,2-dimethyl-hydrazine-induced colon tumors and fecal steroid excretion in Fischer 344 rats. *Am. J. Clin. Nutr.* 42: 475-484.

Watanabe, M. & M. Sugano. 1986. Effects of dietary *cis*- and *trans*-monoene fats on 7,12-dimethyl-benz(a)anthracene-induced rat mammary tumors. *Nutr. Rep. Int.* 33: 163-169.

WHO. 1982. Technical Report Series, Report #678. World Health Organisation.

Wickwire, M.A., M.C. Craig-Schmidt, J.D. Weete & S.A. Faircloth. 1987. Effect of maternal dietary linoleic acid and *trans*-octadecenoic acid on the fatty acid composition and prostaglandin content of rat milk. *J. Nutr.* 117: 232-241.

Wood, R., D. Kubena, B. O'Brian, S. Tseng & G. Martin. 1993. Effect of butter, mono- and polyunsaturated fatty acid-enriched butter, *trans* fatty acid margarine, and zero *trans* fatty acid margarine on serum lipids and lipoproteins in healthy men. *J. Lipid Res.* 34: 1-11.

Zevenbergen, J.L. & E. Haddeman. 1989. Lack of effects of *trans* fatty acids on eicosanoid biosynthesis with adequate intakes of linoleic acid. *Lipids*. 24: 555-63.

Zock, P.L. & M.B. Katan. 1992. Hydrogenation alternatives: effects of *trans* fatty acids and stearic acid versus linoleic acid on serum lipids and lipoproteins in humans. *J. Lipid Res.* 33: 399-410.

Dairy Products in Human Health and Nutrition, Serrano Ríos et al. (eds) © 1994 Balkema, Rotterdam, ISBN 90 5410 359 0

Dairy products in liver disease

S. Hirsch
Human Nutrition and Alcoholism Unit, INTA, University of Chile, Chile

ABSTRACT: Liver cirrhosis is associated with metabolic changes involving protein and energy nutrition. As liver failure progresses, malnutrition becomes more common in patients with cirrhosis. Therefore, several approaches to improve nutritional status in these patients have been attepmted. A careful review of published reports shows that artificial aminoacid mixtures are not better than natural proteins. Among these, casein is well absorbed an does not worsen encephalopathy. Other milk component, namely lactose, has been successfully used in the treatment of hepatic encephalopathy.

Cirrhosis is one of the most common causes of death in developed and underdeveloped countries. It is the fifth individual leading cause of death in the Unites States (Smith 1982) and the third in Chile. Alcohol abuse is the most frequent cause of cirrhosis in the world. Mortality at one year ranges form 20 to 50%, depending on the degree of liver failure, etiology and persistence of alcohol abuse among alcoholics. The high mortality rate is usually ascribed to hepatic failure, gastrointestinal bleeding and infection but a common denominator is undernutrition (Nashrallah 1980, Marsano 1991). Undernutrition is clearly associated with morbidity and mortality in chronically ill noncirrhotic patients (Reinhardt GF 1980, Braga 1988, Kelsen 1986); this statement also applies to cirrhotic patients. The prevalence of protein malnutrition in chronic liver disease ranges from 10 to 100% (Mendenhall 1984, 1985,1986). Additionally Bollet (1973) found that alcoholic patients with liver disease had the worst nutritional status when compared with other hospitalized patients. In patients with primary biliary cirrhosis the prevalence of malnutrition is 40% and 12% in those with chronic hepatitis (Morgan 1981).

The cause of malnutrition in chronic liver disease is multifactorial. Negative nitrogen balance is a common finding. In a study of Fiaccardi(1981), 77% of patients had negative nitrogen balances, mostly related to poor nitrogen intakes. When protein ingestion is above 50g /day, positive nitrogen balances are obtain (Mueller 1983). Other studies have shown increased protein breakdown in these patients, leading to increased protein requirements. Studies measuring 3 methyl histidine excretion (Marchesine 1981) and $[N^{15}]$glycine turnover (Swart 1988) demonstrated that patients with decompensated liver disease had increased protein catabolism. There are several reports of leucine turnover in cirrhosis. Some did not found differences between healthy controls and cirrhotics (Mullen 1986, Shanghogue 1987, Petrides 1991), while others, that measured ketoisocaproate specific activity (McCullough 1992) or expressed turnover per unit of lean body mass, reported increased leucine turnover (McCullough 1992). Our group (1993) showed that those alcoholic cirrhotics that continued to drink had increased leucine flux and that abstinent cirrhotics were not different from controls.

Studies measuring energy expenditure in cirrhotics have shown normal (Owen 1983, John 1989, Schneeweiss 1990) or increased resting metabolic rate (Shanbhogue 1987). Invariably, these authors have found that there is an increase basal fat oxidation, similar to subjects adapted to prolonged starvation (Owen 1983, Merli 1990, Scheeweiss 1990). Infection, ascites and end stages of liver disease, further increase energy expenditure in these subjects (Müller 1992, Dolz 1991).

In addition to the metabolic disorders, the most important and potentially reversible factor that maintains a poor nutritional status in these patients is an inadequate protein and calories intake, specially in those with ascites. Anorexia, nausea, early satiety, malabsorption, encephalopathy, relative water intolerance and dietary restrictions result in the inability to ingest normal quantities of food . The efficacy of salt restriction to handle ascites is well known, but the role of protein restriction in the treatment of encephalopathy is not clear (Smith 1982).

The mechanisms that lead to the generation of encephalopathy are not fully understood. Ammonia traditionally has been considered the principal inducer of this state. Blood ammonia levels increase in cirrhosis due to portal systemic shunting, inhibition of urea cycle and overproduction by colonic bacteria. Further elevations are associated to gastrointestinal bleeding, intestinal bacterial overgrowth and animal proteins ingestion. Bacterial degradation of dietary nitrogen is the major source of ammonia in the body. The different amino acid composition of proteins influences blood ammonia concentrations and the development of encephalopathy (Jones 1986).

Bessman (1958) reported that, when equinitrogenous amount of whole blood and casein were given to patients with liver failure, the blood meal induced higher levels of blood ammonia and provoked central nervous system symptoms. Later, Fenton (1966) observed that a milk and cheese diet administered to cirrhotics, was better tolerated than mixed animal proteins, improved mental function and was associated with a drop in blood ammonia. Condon (1971) found that dogs with Eck fistulas had less encephalopathy and survived longer when milk rather than meat was the protein source. The explanation for the beneficial effect of this diet is that, either the proteins themselves undergo less putrefactive degradation and ammonia production before being absorbed, or that there is a change in the intestinal bacterial flora which resulted in a reduction in the number of ammonia-producing organisms. The later change could occur if the proteins or other constituents of the diet favored the induction of new balance among colonic bacterial species (Fenton 1966). McGhee (1983) demonstrated that casein was associated with an increased nitrogen balance and did not worsen encephalopathy in cirrhotics, when compared to similar amounts of an artificial branched- chain amino acid (BCAA) mixture. Egberts (1985) reported in cirrhotics receiving either BCAA or a casein supplement, similar improvements in nitrogen balance and no changes in mean fasting plasma ammonia, without precipitating encephalopathy .Soberon (1987) observed that, using casein as a protein source, nitrogen absorption exceeded 90% and the potential ammonium load reaching the colon was minimal. Our group (1989), in a controlled trial, demonstrated that providing 80 g protein/day of a casein based formula supplementation to hospitalized patients with alcoholic liver disease, blood ammonia did not increase and there was no deterioration in encephalopathy.

As mentioned before, blood ammonia levels are highly influenced by changes in intestinal flora. Its blood concentration can increase as a consequence of excess production due to changes in colonic pH or bacterial overgrowth.

Lactulose and lactitol, are synthetic disaccharides that can not be broken nor absorbed by the small intestine, because the lack of enzymes (Morgan 1987). In lactase deficient people, specially among Latin Americans, lactose behaves like lactulose and lactitol (Uribe 1980). The administration of these poorly absorbed disaccharides may have important beneficial effects on nitrogen metabolism within the colon. When these disaccharides reach the colon, they are metabolized by the intestinal flora into organic acids. The exact mechanism of action of non absorbable disaccharide is unknown. However, its useful effects could be ascribed to: 1) a lowering in colonic pH, thereby suppressing the absorption of unionized ammonia. 2) A suppression of bacterial and intestinal ammonia generation; 3) A stimulation of ammonia incorporation into bacterial protein; 4) A decrease in intestinal transit time because of its cathartic properties and hence reduction of the available time for the production and absorption of toxins and 5) An increase in fecal nitrogen excretion (Morgan 1987).
Whatever the mechanism, several clinical trials have demonstrated the efficacy of lactulose in the treatment of hepatic encephalopathy, even when compared to non absorbable antibiotics (Orlandi 1981). Welch (1974) reported that lactose effectively treated encephalopathy in a lactose- deficient

individuals. Controlled trials by Uribe (1980) demonstrated the effectiveness of oral lactose in acute and chronic encephalopathy in lactase deficient mexican patients. Later, the same group (1981) described the usefulness of lactose enemas in both lactose intolerant and lactose tolerant patients. An important advantage of this natural disaccharide is its low price.

Other authors suggest that mercaptan derived from the intestinal breakdown of methionine are important in the pathogenesis of hepatic encephalopathy. It has been demonstrated that loads higher than 8g/day given orally, induced encephalopathy in marginally compensated cirrhotics, whereas comparable doses of methionine given parenterally do not (Phear 1956). Greenbeger (1977), in a controlled, randomized and blinded trial, demonstrated that a vegetable diet (low methionine) given to 3 patients with postnecrotic cirrhosis and chronic hepatic encephalopathy resulted in clinical improvement, decrease in encephalopathy and arterial ammonia levels. Others authors confirmed this finding (Uribe 1982, Brujin 1983)

Later investigations have suggested that the development of encephalopathy is related to alterations in plasma amino acid pattern, consisting in an increase in the aromatic amino acids (phenylalanine, tyrosine, and tryptophan) and in methionine and decreases in the branched chain amino acids (valine, leucine, isoleucine). It has been postulated that, as a result of this imbalance, cerebral uptake of aromatic amino acids rises since they successfully compete against the depleted branched amino acids at the blood brain barrier. This excess, in turn, causes overproduction of normally minor metabolites of phenylalanine and tyrosine degradation, such as octopamines and tyramine. These "false neurotransmitter" displace the putative neurotransmitter from their receptors, resulting in the induction of hepatic encephalopathy. This hypothesis predicts that the correction of amino acids abnormalities with especial parenteral or enteral formulas will ameliorate encephalopathy (Jones 1986). However, most trials using enriched BCAA parenteral or enteral mixtures did not demonstrate their benefits, compared to traditional formulas (Naylor 1989, Eriksson 1988). Furthermore, Christie (1985) found that casein based supplements had, as well as enriched BCAA formulas, a good tolerance without inducing or worsening encephalopathy.

Malnutrition has been demonstrated as an independent risk factor for predicting clinical outcome in patients with chronic liver disease (Orrego 1983, Garrison 1984). Child (1964) used nutritional status as a prognostic factor in the Child-Turcotte classification, for estimating mortality in patients undergoing portocaval shunt surgery. A poor nutritional status also has prognostic value in patients undergoing liver transplantation or other abdominal operations (Abad 1987). An epidemiologic study by Qiao (1988) has described the importance of malnutrition as a prognostic factor in nonsurgical patients with liver disease. Galambos (1980) was the first who proved that an intravenous amino acid supplementation could decrease mortality in patients with alcoholic hepatitis. Our group (1989) in a short-term controlled study, provided 2707 calories and 80 g/proteins/day provided by a casein based formula for 3 weeks, to hospitalized malnourished alcoholic cirrhotic patients and compared the evolution with controls receiving a standard diet, that supplied 1813 calories and 47 g/protein. Mortality was less in experimentals than in controls (11% vs

26%), p=0.066. In a similar study, Cabre (1990), using a branched-chain amino acid enriched formula as nutritional supplementation, reduced mortality at a p value=0.065 in the experimental group. In a long term controlled trial on nutritional supplementation with a casein based formula, in outpatients with decompensated alcoholic liver disease, we (1993) observed a mortality rate of 24% in controls and 8% in the supplemented group. However this difference did not reach statistical significance, probably due to the small sample size (n=51,p=0.06).

Malnutrition is associated with diverse complications in different diseases, such as infections and delayed wound healing. These constitute the so called "nutritional associated complications". Patients with liver disease have a high rate of lung, urinary tract infection and spontaneous bacterial peritonitis (Nashrallah 1980). One contributing factor is a deterioration of humoral and cellular immunity (Ledesma 1990). Our above mentioned long-term study (1993) demonstrated an early improvement in nutritional status, along with a reduction in the need of hospitalization, attributed to a lower incidence of life threatening infections This beneficial effect, is related with a decrease in nutrition-associated complications and allow an improvement in life quality in patients with liver diseases.

Nutritional support to patients with liver disease, may improve liver function. Galambos (1980) found in a controlled study, that patients with parenteral nutrition improved ascites, bilirubin and albumin more than controls. Cabre (1990) showed recovery of serum albumin and Child's score in the supplemented patients. Kearns (1992) found that in patients receiving tube feeding with a casein based formula, antipyrine clearance and serum bilirubin had a better improvement than patients receiving a regular diet.

In summary, there is no doubt that nutritional support in liver disease reduces the incidence of nutrition associated complications. Also, there is some evidence that it could improve liver function, without inducing iatrogenic complications such as encephalopathy. Casein and lactose, nutrients derived from milk, appear to be beneficial for the nutritional support of patients with liver disease.

REFERENCES

Abad A, Cabre E, Gonzalez-Huix F. 1987. Influence of the nutritional status in the prognosis and clinical outcome of hospitalized patients with liver cirrhosis. Preliminary report. J Clin Gastroenterol 2:63-68.

Bessman AN, Mirck GS, Hawkins R. 1958.Blood ammonia levels following the ingestion of casein and whole blood. J clin invest 37: 900-904.

Bollet AJ, Owen S. 1973. Evaluation of nutritional status of selected hospitalized patients. Am J Clin Nutr 26:931-938.

Braga M, Baccari P, Scaccabarozzi S, Fiacco E, Radaelli G, Gallus G, DiPalo S, DiCarlo V, Cristallo M. 1988. Prognostic role of preoperative nutritional and immunological assessment in the surgical patient. JPEN 12:138-142.

Brujin KM, BlendisLM, Zilm DH, Carlen PL, Anderson GH. 1983. Effect of dietary protein manipulations in subclinical portal-systemic encephalopathy. Gut 24:53-60.

Bunout D, Aicardi V, Hirsch S, Petermann M, Kelly M, Silva G, Garay P, Ugarte G, Iturriaga H. 1989. Nutritional support in hospitalized patients with alcoholic liver disease. Eur.J.Clin. Nutr. 43:615-621.

Cabre E, Gonzalez-Huix F, Abad-La Cruz A, Esteve M, Fernandez-Banares F, Xiol X, Gassull MA. 1990. Effect of total enteral nutrition on the short-term outcome of severely malnourished cirrhotics: a randomized controlled trial. Gastroenterology 98;715-720.

Condon RE. 1971: Effect od dietary protein on symptoms and survival in dogs with Eck fistula. Am J Surg 121:107-114.

Child CGIII, Turcotte JG. 1964. Surgery and portal hypertension in : Child CG(ed): The liver and portal hypertension. Philadelphia, WB Saunders Co, 50-64.

Christie M, Sack D, Pomposelli J, Horst D. 1985. Enriched branched-chain amino acid formula versus a casein base supplement in the treatment of cirrhosis. JPEN 9:671-678.

D'Amico G, Morabito A, Pagliaro L, Marubine E, and the liver study group of Cervello Hospital. 1986. Survival and prognostic indicators in compensated and decompensated cirrhosis. Dig Dis Sci 31:468-475.

Dolz C, Ranrich JM, Ibanez J, Obrados P, Marse P, Gaya J.1991. Ascitis increases the resting energy expenditure in liver cirrhosis. Gastroenterology 100:738-744.

Egberts AH, Schomerus H, Manster W, Jurgens P.1985. Branched chain amino acids in the treatment of latent portosystemic encephalopathy. Gastroenterology 88:887-895.

Eriksson LJ, Conn HO. 1989. Branched-chained amino acids in the management of hepatic encephalopathy: an analysis of variance. Hepatology 10:228-246.

Fenton JCB, Knight EJ, Humpherson PL. 1966. Milk and Cheese in portal-systemic encephalopathy. Lancet 22:164-166.

Fiaccardi F, Ghinelli F, Pedretti G, Pelosi G, Sacchini D, Spandini G. 1981. Negative Nitrogen Balance in Cirrhotics. La Ricerca in Clinica e in Laboratorio 11:259-268.

Garrison RN, Cryer HM, Howard DA. 1984. Clarification of risk factors for abdominal operations in patients with hepatic cirrhosis. Ann Surg 199:648-655.

Greenberger NJ, Carley J, Schenker S, Bettinger I, Samnes C, Beyer P. 1977. Effect of vegetable and animal protein diets in chronic hepatic encephalopathy. Dig Diseases 22:845-855.

Hadengue A, Moreau R, Lee S, Gaudin C, Rueff B, Lebrec D. 1988. Liver hypermetabolism during alcohol withdrawal in humans. Gastroenterology 94:1047-1052.

Hirsch S, de la Maza MP, Petermann M, Iturriaga H, Ugarte G, Bunout D. 1992. Protein turnover in abstinent and non abstinent patients with alcoholic liver disease. Hepatology 16:232A (Abstract 750).

Hirsch S, Bunout D, de la Maza MP, Iturriaga H, Petermann M, Icaza G, Gattas V, Ugarte G. 1993. Controlled trial on nutritional in outpatients symptomatic alcoholic cirrhosis. JPEN March.

John WS, Philips R, Otto L, Adams LS, McClain CJ. 1988. Resting Energy expenditure in patients with alcoholic hepatitis. JPEN 13:124-127.

Jones A, Basset M, Mullen K. 1986. Hepatic encephalopathy. In The Liver Annual 5. Arias IM, Frenkel M, Wilson JHP eds. Elsevier.

Kearns PJ, Young H, Garcia G, et al. 1992. Accelerated improvement of alcoholic liver disease with enteral nutrition. Gastroenterology 102,200-205.

Kelsen SG. 1986.The effects of undernutrition on the respiratory muscles. Clinics in Chest Medicine 7:1.

Ledesma F, Echevarria S, Casafont F, Losano JL, Pons-Romero F. 1990. Natural killer cell activity in alcoholic cirrhosis: influence of nutrition. Eur.J.Clin.Nutr. 44:733-740.

Marchesini G, Zoli M, Angiolini A, Dondi C, Bianchi F, Pisi E. 1981. Muscle protein breakdown in liver cirrhosis and the roll of carbohydrate metabolism. Hepatology 1:294-299.

Marsano L, McLain CJ. 1991. Nutrition and alcoholic liver disease. JPEN 1991;15:337-344.

McCcullough AJ, Mullen KD, Tavill AS, Kalhan SC. 1992. In vivo differences between the turnover rates of leucine and leucine's keto-acid in stable cirrhosis. Gastroenterology 103:571-578.

McCcullough AJ, Mullen KD, Kalhan SC. 1992. Body cell mass and leucine metabolism in stable cirrhosis. Gastroenterology 102: 1325-1333.

McGhee A, Henderson JM, Millikan WJ, Bleier JC, Vogel R,Kassouny M,Rudman D. 1983. Comparison of the effects of hepatic-aid and a casein modular diet on encephalopathy, plasma aminoacids, and nitrogen balance in cirrhotic patients. Ann.Surg 197: 288-293.

Medenhall CL, Anderson SH, Weesner RE, Goldberg SJ, Crolic KA. 1984. Protein-caloric malnutrition associated with alcoholic hepatitis. Am.J. Med 76:211-222.

Medenhall CL, Tosch T, Weesner RE. VA Cooperative study on alcholic Hepatitis II. 1986. Prognostic significance of protein-calorie malnutrtion. Am J Clin Nutr 42:213-218.

Mendenhall C, Bongiovanni G, Goldberg S, Miller B, Moore J, Rouster S, Schneider D, Tamburro C, Tosch T, Weesner R, and the VA Cooperative Study Group on Alcoholic Hepatitis. VA Cooperative Study on Alcoholic Hepatitis III. 1985. Changes in protein-calorie malnutrition associated with 30 days of hospitalization with and without enteral nutrition therapy. JPEN 9:590-596.

Merli M, Riggio O, Romiti A, Franco A, Mango L, Pinto G, Savioli M, Capocaccia L. 1990. Basal energy production rate and substrate use in stable cirrhotic patients. Hepatology 12:106-112.

Morgan M,Hawley K. 1987. Lactitol vs Lactulosa in the treatment of acute encephalopathy in cirrhotic patients: A double-blind, randomized trial. Hepatology 7:1278-1284.

Morgan MY. 1981. Enteral nutrition in chronic liver disease. Acta Chir Scand 507(suppl).81-90.

Mueller Kf, Crosby LO, Oberlander JL 1983. Estimation of fecal nitrogen in patients with liver disease. JPEN 7:266-269.

Mullen KD; Denne Sc, McCullough AJ, Savin SM, Bruno D, Tarill AS, Kalhan SC. 1986. Leucine metabolism in stable cirrhosis. Hepatology 6:622-630.

Müller M, Lautz H, Plogmann B, Bürger M, Körber J, Schmidt F. 1992. Energy expenditure and substrate oxidation in patients with cirrhosis:The impact of cause, clinical staging and nutritional state. Hepatology 15:782-794.

Nasrallah JM, Galambos JT. 1980. Amino acid Therapy of alcoholic hepatitis. Lancet 2:1276-1277.

Naylor CD, O'Rourke K, Detsky AS, Baker JP. 1989. Parenteral nutrition with branched chain aminoacids in hepatic encephalopathy. A meta analysis. Gastroenterology 97:1033-1042.

Orlandi F, Freddara U, Candelares MT. 1981. Comparison between neomycin and lactulose in 173 patients with hepatic encephalopathy. Dig Dis Sci 26:498-506.

Orrego H, Israel Y, Blake JE, Medline A. 1983. Assessment of prognostic factors in alcoholic liver disease. Toward a global quantitative expression of severity. Hepatology 3:896-905.

Owen OE, Trapp VE, Reichard A, Mozzoli MA, Moctezuma J, Paul P, Skutches CL, Boden G. 1983. Nature and quantity of fuels consumed in patients with alcoholic cirrhosis. J.Clin.Invest 72:1821-1832.

Petrides A, Luzi L, Reuben A, Riely C, DeFronzo RA. 1991. Effect of insulin on plasma amino acid concentration on leucine metabolism in cirrhosis. Hepatology 14:432-441.

Phear EA, RuebnerB, Sherlock S. 1956. Methionine toxicity in liver disease and its prevention by chlortetracycline. Clin Sci 15:93-117.

Qiao Zk, Halliday ML, Coates RA. 1988. Relationship between liver cirrhosis death rate and nutritional factors in 38 countries. Int J Epidemiol 17:414-418.

Reinhardt GF, Myscofsky JW, Wilkens DB. 1980. Incidence and mortality of hipoalbuminemic patients in hospitalized veterans. JPEN 4:357-359.

Schneeweiss B, Graninger W, Ferenci P, Eichinger S, Grimm G, Schneider B, Laggner A, Lenz K, Kleinberger G. 1990. Energy metabolism in patients with acute and chronic liver disease. Hepatology 11:387-393.

Shanbhogue RL, Bistrian BR; Jenkins RL; Jones C, Benotti P, Blackburn Gl. 1987. Resting energy expenditure in patients with end-stage liver disease and in normal population. JPEN 11:305-308.

Smith J, Horowitz J, Henderson JM, Heymsfield S 1982. Enteral hyperalimentation in undernourished patients with cirrhosis and ascitis. Am J Clin Nut 35:56-72.

Soberon S, Pauley MP, Duplantier R, Fan A, Halsted CH 1987. Metabolic effects of enteral formula feeding in alcoholic hepatitis. Hepatology 7:1204-1209.

Swart GR, van den Berg JWO, Wattimena JLD, Rietveld T, van Vuure, Frenkel M 1988. Elevated protein requirements in cirrhosis of the liver investigated by whole body protein turnover studies. Clinical Science 75:101-107.

Uribe M, Berthier JM. Lewis H 1981. Lactose enemas plus placebo tablets plus starch enemas in acute portal-systemic encephalopathy. A double-blind randomized controlled study. Gastroenterology 81:101-106.

Uribe M. Treatment of chronic portal-systemic encephalopathy with lactose in lactase deficient patients. Dig Dis Sci 1980;25:924-928.

Uribe M, Marquez MA, Ramos GG 1982. Treatment of chronic portal-systemic encephalopathy with vegetable and animal protein diets: A controlled crossover study. Dig Dis Sci 27:1109-1116.

Welch JD, Cassidy D, Prigatono GP, Gunn CG 1974. Chronic hepatic encephalopathy treated with oral lactose in patient with lactose malabsorption. N Engl J Med 291:240-241.

5 Nutrition, immunity and carcinogenesis

Dairy Products in Human Health and Nutrition, Serrano Ríos et al. (eds) © 1994 Balkema, Rotterdam, ISBN 90 5410 359 0

Dairy products, calcium, and colon cancer

M.J.Wargovich
*Department of Gastrointestinal Medical Oncology and Digestive Diseases, The University of Texas, M.D.
Anderson Cancer Center, Houston, Tex., USA*

ABSTRACT: Population studies examining the relationship of calcium intake
to colon cancer risk have suggested a protective relationship when daily
intake is at the level of 1500-2000 mg elemental calcium. A mechanism for
the possible protective role of calcium has emerged from laboratory
research: calcium interacts with potential tumor promoters in the colon
rendering these promotors less active biologically. Supplementation of the
diet with enriched sources of calcium may be one route to cancer
prevention and is the current focus of ongoing chemoprevention efficacy
trials in subjects at increased risk for colon cancer.

CALCIUM AND COLON CANCER

The customary diet associated with
Western Europe, the United Kingdom,
Australia, New Zealand, Canada, and
the United States has long been
considered as a source of risk
factors for cancer of the colon
(Waterhouse, J., et al., 1976). In
the United States, colon cancer
remains a major health problem with
incident cases accumulating at a
rate of 160,000 per year;
mortalities from this disease are
about half of the incidence rate
(Boring, et al., 1993). Current
hypotheses suggest that the
probability of developing colon
cancer increases with the number of
genetic mutations in colonic
epithelial cells. Environmental
factors, from the diet, may confer
extraordinary risk, or attenuate
risk for the disease. For instance,
it is well established that the
inherited syndrome of familial
polyposis and it variants greatly
increase an individual's
susceptibility for colon cancer
(Burt, 1991). The presence of
defects in regions of certain
chromosomes has also been associated
with colon cancer (Fearon et. al.,
1990; Hollstein et al., 1991;
Kinzler et al., 1991; Peltomaki et.
al.,1991; ; Vogelstein et al.,
1988). Added to a probable

background of genetic commonalities
for colon cancer is considerable
evidence that excess dietary fat and
protein in concert with deficiencies
in fiber, natural anticarcinogens,
vitamins, and minerals increases
risk for colon cancer. The most
striking evidence in support of the
dietary environment as a mitigant of
colon cancer risk are the studies of
migrant populations. When
individuals move from a low risk
country to that with an increased
prevalence for colon cancer, they
and their descendants rapidly
acquire the high risk profile of
their new homeland. The Japanese
migration to the United States since
World War II clearly illustrates the
risk associated with the assumption
of a Western-style diet and an
increased risk for colon cancer
(Schottenfeld & Winawer, 1992).
Moreover, the current generation of
Japanese living in Japan have a
greatly increased probability of
developing colon cancer as Western
foods and cooking patterns become
more commonplace in their lifestyle
(Lee, 1976).

In man, various factors in the diet
have been studied as causes of the
disease: mutagenic fecapentaenes,
toxic products of fecal microflora,
and thermolysed proteins have been
postulated to initiate DNA damage,

whereas colonic bile acids and fatty acids are postulated to induce hyperproliferation of the colonic mucosa (Greenwald, 1992; Reddy et al., 1987; Zhang et al., 1992). These combine to increase the opportunity for expression of mutated cells. The proliferative nature of the colonic epithelium affords the opportunity for expression and expansion of damaged cells (Newmark et al., 1991). In animals, many components of the human diet have been investigated for single and interactive effects in colon carcinogenesis. However, for the purposes of examining and explaining the role of dietary calcium and dairy products as inhibitors of colon cancer, this discussion will be limited to dietary fat. From animal experiments it is clear that the type and the amount of dietary fat influence both the initiation and promotional phases of carcinogenesis (Reddy, 1992; Reddy et al., 1991; Kumar et al., 1990; Reddy et al., 1987). Selected data are summarized in the table below:

Table 1. Dietary Fat in Colon Carcinogenesis

Fat Type	Animal Model	Tumor Effect
Beef	DMH*	⇑
Fish	AOM	⇓
Vegetable	AOM	⇑

* DMH, Dimethylhydrazine
  AOM, Azoxymethane

While it is difficult to simplistically generalize from animal experiments to man, it is clear that under certain conditions (related to changes in colonic pH and to the percent of calories as fat) some dietary lipids act as tumor promoters within the colon. Several mechanisms have been suggested to explain how high fat diets promote colon cancer. Digestion of dietary fats may increase the levels of fecal diacyl gycerol, a trigger for protein kinase: this interrupts normal cell signaling (Morotomi et al., 1990). Some secondary bile acids, notably deoxycholic acid, have been shown to be mitogenic for the colon as well

as efficient tumor promoters (Buset et al., 1990). Other lipids may stimulate the activation of the ras oncogene, mutated in high prevalence in human colon cancers (Jacoby et al., 1992). The last mechanism impacts on the possibility of dietary calcium as a preventive for colon cancer. Some lipids act to destabilize colonocyte cell membranes causing damage to crypt epithelial cells. This cell loss is signaled by an, as yet, poorly understood pathway to initiate compensatory hyperproliferation. Recently a few reports have suggested that the same mechanism could apply to man.

Dairy products and colon cancer

There have been several attempts to link the consumption of dairy products with increased risk for colon cancer, since this dietary food group is a rich source of animal fat (Bostick et al., 1993; Negri et al., 1990; Steinmetz & Potter, 1993; Stemmermann, Nomura & Chyou, 1990). These and other epidemiological studies have, however, more consistently found a negative relationship. Individuals who consume higher levels of dietary calcium were found to have the lowest incidence of colon cancer. When calcium supplements are considered (i.e., non-dairy, mineral preparations) the same relationship has been observed (Heilbrun et al., 1986, Peters et. al., 1992; Slattery et al., 1988; Sorenson et al., 1988). Increased calcium consumption appears to retard the development of colon cancer. Just how calcium interacts with dietary lipids has been the focus of intensive basic research. Newmark and colleagues (1984, 1992) were the first group to articulate an hypothesis stating that calcium could sequester certain tumor promoting lipids in the human colon and that intestinal pH was a governing factor in the resulting chemistry that inactivated these lipids. It had been known for some time that primary and secondary bile acids increased the frequency of tumors and their pathological severity in animals treated with chemical carcinogens. In early experiments, Wargovich et al. (1988;1990;1991) demonstrated an apparent protective effect when calcium concentrations where increased in animal diets, thereby reducing the proliferation-inducing aspects of two dietary lipids and lessening the invasive potential of colon cancers. A series of experiments followed to show that bile acid and fatty acid induced hyperproliferation and that tumor promotion could be lessened by an increase in levels of dietary calcium. More recent experiments have shown that even when diets are enriched in fat, tumor promotion is ablated by adequate intakes of dietary calcium (Appleton et al., 1987; Behling et al., 1990). In the last several years, the work of Van der Meer and colleagues have been instrumental in substantiating the sequestration hypothesis (Lapre et al., 1993; Lapre & Van der Meer, 1992; Lapre et al., 1992; Van der Meer, Kleibeuker & Lapre, 1991; Van der Meer, Termont & De Vries, 1991). Work from this group has established a possible role for calcium from milk, interacting with secondary bile acids and other lipids, to strongly deter their ability to interact with colon cell membranes, thus reducing subsequent epitheliolysis and compensatory cell replication. In a very recent study, the observed protection for calcium was extended to dairy calcium in an experiment where rats were fed a lactase-treated milk diet designed to mimic the range of calcium consumed in man (Govers et al, in press). In other words, calcium and phosphate sequestered the toxic elements of lipid digestion implicated in inducing abnormal cellular proliferation, a potential risk factor for colon cancer. Ongoing experiments continue to explore in greater depth the molecular mechanisms for calcium's effect. In a recent rat carcinogenesis study (Sitrin et al., 1991) it was shown that calcium supplementation could reverse oncogene activation. With the wealth of evidence supporting a possible preventive role for calcium, a series of small scale clinical trials have been reported investigating dose and type of calcium supplements as putative chemopreventive agents for colon cancer.

Human studies effect of calcium supplementation

In a population study of calcium intake and colon cancer, Garland et al.(1985; 1991) associated the least probability for developing colon cancer with an intake in the range of 1500-2000 mg per day. Intervention studies have chosen a wider range (1000-2000 mg/d) to test the effect of supplementation on the recurrence of colonic premalignancies and/or intermediate biological endpoints (Barsoum et. al., 1992; Bartram et. al., 1993; Cross et. al., 1992; Lipkin et. al.,1985, 1993; Rozen et al., 1989; Stern et al., 1990; Wargovich et al., 1992; Welberg et al., 1993) For the most part, human studies have utilized calcium carbonate as the source of calcium as it provides the greatest calcium content per gram. Other formulations are being tested, however, including calcium citrate and calcium lactate. In general, these studies tend to show that calcium supplements can reduce proliferation in the human colon, but not all studies have found a beneficial effect. Phase 1 chemoprevention trial data at the M.D. Anderson Cancer Center have established that a dose of 3000 mg/d is the upper limit of possible calcium intake without toxic manifestations. In the United States and Europe, several Phase III clinical trials are underway to test whether calcium in doses of 1000-2000 mg daily can inhibit the recurrence of adenomatous polyps in subjects with a history of these premalignancies for the colon.

Summary

It is likely to be several years before adequate data are in to recommend whether Western diets should be supplemented with additional calcium in a effort to prevent colon cancer. While mineral supplements have been tested in the clinical studies using dairy products as a source of extra calcium in man, trials have yet to be implemented to allow contrast with the effects of calcium salts. It is interesting to note that Paleolithic man averaged 1500-3000 mg of calcium daily in a foraging environment where intakes of fat were very low (Eaton et al, 1988). Since that time man, at least in countries with a high incidence for colon cancer, has greatly increased dietary fat intake while calcium and fiber intakes have fallen to borderline adequacy levels. Are these then some of the important clues that predispose us to colon cancer?

REFERENCES

Appleton, G.V.N., P.W. Davies, J.B. Bristol & R.N.C. Williamson 1987. Inhibition of intestinal carcinogenesis by dietary supplementation with calcium. Br. J. Surg. 74:523-525.

Barsoum, G.H.,C. Hendrickse, M.C. Winslet, et al. 1992. Reduction of mucosal crypt cell proliferation in patients with colorectal adenomatous polyps by dietary calcium supplementation. Br. J. Surg. 79:581-583.

Bartram, H.P., W. Scheppach, H. Schmid, et al., 1993. Proliferation of human colonic mucosa as an intermediate biomarker of carcinogenesis: effects of butyrate, deoxycholate, calcium, ammonia, and pH. Cancer Res. 53:3283-3288.

Behling, A.R., S.M. Kaup & J.L. Greger 1990. Changes in intestinal function of rats initiated with DMH and fed varying levels of butterfat, calcium, and magnesium. Nutr. Cancer. 13:189-199.

Boring, C.C., T.S. Squires, & T. Tong 1993. Cancer statistics. CA. 43:7-26.

Bostick, R.M., J.D. Potter, T.A. Sellers, D.R. McKenzie, L.H. Kushi & A.R. Folsom 1993. Relation of calcium, vitamin D, and dairy food intake to incidence of colon cancer among older women. The Iowa Women's Health Study. Am.J Epidemiol. 137:1302-1317.

Burt, R. 1991. Polyposis syndromes. Textbook of Gastroenterology, 1674-1696. New York: J.B. Lippincott.

Buset, M., P. Galand, M. Lipkin, S. Winawer & E. Friedman 1990. Injury induced by fatty acids or bile acid in isolated human colonocytes prevented by calcium. Cancer Lett. 50:221-226.

Cross, H.S., M. Pavelka, J. Slavik & M. Peterlik 1992. Growth control of human colon cancer cells by vitamin D and calcium in vitro. J Natl. Cancer Inst. 84:1355-1357.

Eaton, S.B., M. Konner & M. Shostak 1988. Stone agers in the fast lane: chronic degenerative diseases in evolutionary

perspective. Am. J. Med. 84:739-749.

Fearon, E.R.& B. Vogelstein 1990. A genetic model for colorectal tumorigenesis. Cell 61:759-767.

Garland, C., R.B. Shekelle,E. Barrett-Conner, M.H. Criqui, A.H. Rossof & O. Paul 1985. Dietary vitamin D and calcium risk of colorectal cancer: a 19 year prospective study in men. Lancet. 1:307-309.

Garland, C.F., F.C. Garland & E.D. Gorham 1991. Can colon cancer incidence and death rates be reduced with calcium and vitamin D? Am. J. Clin. Nutr. 54:193S-201S.

Greenwald, P. 1992. Colon cancer overview. Cancer 70:1206-1215.

Heilbrun, L.K., J.H. Hankin, A.M.Y. Nomura & G.N. Stemmerman 1986. Colon cancer and dietary fat, phosphorus, and calcium in Hawaiian-Japanese men. Am. J. Clin. Nutr. 43:306-309.

Hollstein, M., D. Sidransky, B. Vogelstein & C.C. Harris 1991. p53 mutations in human cancers. Science 253:49-53.

Jacoby, R.F., R.J. Alexander, R.F. Raicht & T.A. Brasitus 1992. K-ras oncogene mutations in rat colon tumors induced by N-methyl-N-nitrosourea. Carcinogenesis 13:45-49.

Kinzler, K.W., M.C. Nilbert, L.K. Su, et al 1991. Identification of FAP locus genes from chromosome 5q21. Science 253:661-665.

Kumar, S.P., S.J. Roy, K. Tokumo & B.S. Reddy 1990. Effect of different levels of calorie restriction on azoxymethane-induced colon carcinogenesis in male F344 rats. Cancer Res. 50:5761-5766.

Lapre, J.A., D.S. Termont, A.K. Groen & R. Van der Meer 1992. Lytic effects of mixed micelles of fatty acids and bile acids. Am. J Physiol. 263:G333-G337.

Lapre, J.A., H.T. De Vries, J.H. Koeman & R. Van der Meer 1993. The antiproliferative effect of dietary calcium on colonic epithelium is mediated by luminal surfactants and dependent on the type of dietary fat. Cancer.Res. 53:784-789.

Lapre, J.A.& R. Van der Meer 1992. Diet-induced increase of colonic bile acids stimulates lytic activity of fecal water and proliferation of colonic cells. Carcinogenesis. 13:41-44.

Lee J.A.H 1976. Recent trends of large bowel cancer in Japan compared to the United States and England and Wales. Int. J. Epidemiol. 5:187-194.

Lipkin, M.& H.L. Newmark 1985. Effect of added dietary calcium on colonic epithelial cell proliferation in subjects at high risk for familial colon cancer. New. Engl. J. Med. 313:1381-1384.

Lipkin, M.& H. Newmark 1993. Supplemental dietary calcium and inhibition of colon cancer. Eur. J. Cancer Prev. 2:83-84.

Morotomi, M., J.G. Guillem, P. LoGerfo & I.B. Weinstein 1990. Production of diacylglycerol, an activator of protein kinase C, by human intestinal microflora. Cancer Res. 50:3595-3599.

Negri, E., C. La Vecchia, B. Davanzo & S. Franceschi 1990. Calcium, dairy products, and colorectal cancer. Nutr. Cancer. 13:255-262.

Newmark, H.L., M.J. Wargovich, and W.R. Bruce 1984. Colon cancer and dietary fat, calcium, and phosphate: an hypothesis. J. Natl Cancer Inst. 72:1323-1325.

Newmark, H.L. & M. Lipkin 1992. Calcium, vitamin D, and colon cancer. Cancer Res. 52:2067s-2070s.

Newmark, H.L., M. Lipkin & N. Maheshwari 1991. Colonic hyperproliferation induced in rats and mice by nutritional-stress diets containing four components of a human Western-style diet (series 2). Am. J. Clin. Nutr. 54:209S-214S.

Peltomaki, P., P. Sistonen, J.P. Mecklin, et al. 1991. Evidence supporting exclusion of the DCC gene and a portion of chromosome 18q as the locus for susceptibility to hereditary nonpolyposis colorectal carcinoma in five kindreds. Cancer Res. 51:4135-4140.

Peters, R.K., M.C. Pike, D. Garabrant & T.M. Mack 1992. Diet and colon cancer in Los Angeles County, California. Cancer Causes Control 3:457-473.

Reddy, B.S. 1987. Dietary fat and colon cancer: animal models. Prev. Med. 16:460-467.

Reddy, B.S. & S. Sugie 1988. Effect of different levels of omega-3 and omega-6 fatty acids on azoxymethane-induced colon carcinogenesis in F344 rats. Cancer Res. 48:6642-6647.

Reddy, B.S., C. Burill & J. Rigotty 1991. Effect of diets high in omega-3 and omega-6 fatty acids on initiation and postinitiation stages of colon carcinogenesis. Cancer Res. 51:487-491.

Reddy, B.S. 1992. Dietary fat and colon cancer: animal model studies. Lipids 27:807-813.

Reddy, B.S., C. Sharma, B. Simi, et al. 1987. Metabolic epidemiology of colon cancer: effect of dietary fiber on fecal mutagens and bile acids in healthy subjects. Cancer Res. 47:644-648.

Rozen, P.,Z. Fireman, N. Fine, Y. Wax & E. Ron 1989. Oral calcium suppresses increased rectal epithelial proliferation of persons at risk of colorectal cancer. Gut 30:650-655.

Schottenfeld D., S.J. Winawer 1992. Large Intestine. Cancer: Epidemiology and Prevention: 703-709. Philadelphia: WB Saunders.

Sitrin, M.D., A.G. Halline, C. Abrahams & T.A. Brasitus 1991. Dietary calcium and vitamin D modulate 1,2-dimethylhydrazine-induced colonic carcinogenesis in the rat. Cancer Res. 51:5608-5613.

Slattery, M.L., A.W. Sorenson & M.H. Ford 1988. Dietary calcium intake as a mitigating factor in colon cancer. Am. J. Epidemiol. 128:504-513.

Sorenson, A.W., M.L. Slattery & M.H. Ford 1988. Calcium and colon cancer: a review. Nutr. Cancer. 11:135-145.

Steinmetz, K.A. & J.D. Potter 1993. Food-group consumption and colon cancer in the Adelaide Case-Control Study. II. Meat, poultry, seafood, dairy foods and eggs. Int. J. Cancer. 53:720-727.

Stemmermann, G.N., A. Nomura & P.H. Chyou 1990. The influence of dairy and nondairy calcium on subsite large-bowel cancer risk. Dis. Colon Rectum. 33:190-194.

Stern, H.S., R.C. Gregoire, H. Kashtan, J. Stadler & R.W. Bruce 1990. Long-term effects of dietary calcium on risk markers for colon cancer in patients with familial polyposis. Surgery 108:528-533.

Van der Meer, R., J.H. Kleibeuker & J.A. Lapre 1991. Calcium phosphate, bile acids and colorectal cancer. Eur. J Cancer.Prev. 1 Suppl 2:55-62.

Van der Meer, R., D.S. Termont & H.T. De Vries 1991. Differential effects of calcium ions and calcium phosphate on cytotoxicity

of bile acids. Am. J. Physiol.
260:G142-G147.

Vogelstein, B., E.R. Fearon, S.R.
Hamilton, et al 1988. Genetic
alterations during colorectal-
tumor development. N. Engl. J.
Med. 319:525-532.

Wargovich, M.J., A.R. Baer, P.J. Hu
& H. Sumiyoshi 1988. Dietary
factors and colorectal cancer.
Gastroenterol Clin. North Am.
17:727-745.

Wargovich, M.J., D. Allnutt, C.
Palmer, P. Anaya & L.C. Stephens
1990. Inhibition of the
promotional phase of azoxymethane-
induced colon carcinogenesis in
the F344 rat by calcium lactate:
effect of simulating two human
nutrient density levels. Cancer
Lett. 53:17-25.

Wargovich, M.J., P.M. Lynch & B.
Levin 1991. Modulating effects of
calcium in animal models of colon
carcinogenesis and short-term
studies in subjects at increased
risk for colon cancer. Am. J.
Clin. Nutr. 54:202S-205S.

Wargovich, M.J., G. Isbell, M.
Shabot, et al. 1992. Calcium
supplementation decreases rectal
epithelial cell proliferation in
subjects with sporadic adenoma.
Gastroenterol. 103:92-97.

Waterhouse, J., C. Muir, P. Correa,
et. al. 1976. Cancer Incidence in
the Five Continents, Vol III,
Lyon: Internatinonal Agency for
Research on Cancer.

Welberg, J.W., J.H. Kleibeuker, R.
Van der Meer, et al. 1993.
Effects of oral calcium
supplementation on intestinal bile
acids and cytolytic activity of
fecal water in patients with
adenomatous polyps of the colon.
Eur..J. Clin. Invest 23:63-68.

Zhang, X.M., D. Stamp, S. Minkin, et
al 1992. Promotion of aberrant
crypt foci and cancer in rat colon
by thermolyzed protein. J Natl
Cancer Inst. 84:1026-1030.

Dairy Products in Human Health and Nutrition, Serrano Ríos et al. (eds) © 1994 Balkema, Rotterdam, ISBN 90 5410 359 0

Nutrition and immunity: An overview

F.Ortiz Maslloréns
Fundación Jiménez Díaz, Madrid, Spain

ABSTRACT: Because of the nutritional effort required for the development and maintenance of the body defenses, malnutrition in its various forms is a common cause of immunodeficiency, in developing countries as well as in affluent societies. Cell-mediated immune mechanisms are more severely affected by malnutrition than the humoral responses; non-specific effector mechanisms are also impaired. The detriment of the defensive forces of the body becomes manifest in an increased susceptibility to infections, that are often caused by opportunistic microorganisms; infections in turn aggravate the nutritional status of the host. Immune factors, on the other hand, contribute to the normal performance of nutritional processes. Secretory IgA protects the intestine from colonization by infectious agents; its presence in maternal milk and colostrum assures such protection to the neonate. Immune mechanisms assist in controlling the absorption of antigenic substances; even non-antigenic ones can be subjected to immune actions, at least under pathological circumstances.

The close relationship existing between the nutritional status and the immune performance of the host is clearly reflected in the highly increased susceptibility to infectious diseases in malnourished populations. As pointed out by Scrimshaw et al. (1959) almost fourty years ago, nutrition and immunity interact synergistically in determining hos resistance to infection; their association is not merely additive. The bidirectional character of this synergism becomes manifest in the fact that malnutrition is responsible for many cases of immunodeficiency, as well as in the involvement of immune factors in the process of nutrition.

1 MALNUTRITION AS CAUSE OF IMMUNODEFICIENCY

At the present time, malnutrition is the most frequent cause of immunodeficiency all over the world (Chandra 1992). The number of human beings dying and suffering because of failures in their immune mechanisms overtly exceeds that of patients suffering or dying from infectious (AIDS), congenital, or any other form of immunodeficiency. This is easy to understand considering that the maintenance of the non-specific barriers to infections, of the tissues, cells and molecules of the immune system, and of the ensemble of effector and amplification mechanisms involved in host defense, requires an important nutritional effort. Metabolic rates for immunoglobulins, complement system components and other immunological proteins (receptors, cytokines, etc.) are very high, amounting to a daily synthesis of not less than 10 grams of protein for an average sized adult. In addition, cell populations participating directly or indirectly in immune phenomena are kept at normal levels through very active replication processes. The whole population of lymphocytes (T and B cells) of the body ranges in the order of 10^{12} cells, a mass of approximately 1 kilogram. Of this, not less than 10^9 cells, or about 1 gram of cell mass are destroyed and renewed every day.

For all these reasons, nutritional deficits usually lead to immunodeficiency states that, as it is always the case, result in an increase in the frequency and severity of infections, quite often due to "opportunistic" microbes. This situation is of common occurrence in developing countries, where it is responsible, to a considerable degree, for the high rates of morbidity and case fatality due to infectious agents, characteristic of those countries. In them, malnutrition concurs with many other factors (economic, social, cultural) to yield the final situation (Gershwin, Beach & Hurley 1985). Nutritionally caused immunodeficiency is not, however, restricted to Third World communities; it also occurs significantly in the well developed societies of the western nations. In these, the most frequently affected population groups include hospitalized or asyled patients, elderly people living or not with their families (Chandra 1989 & 1991; Antognaci et al. 1992), and, with increasing frequency, persons following arbitrary diets, not rarely self-imposed or lacking adequate professional control, for slimming purposes. Emphasis should be also made on deficient nutrition, ending in a failure of defense mechanisms, that results from inappropriate medical intervention ("iatrogenic" malnutrition).

Negative nutritional balance, responsible for immune deficit, can be due to an insuficient intake or to an increased requirement of nutrients; not seldom, both occur at the same time. Undernourishment can adopt any of the known forms of protein-energy malnutrition, including marasmus or kwashiorkor, or consist of selective deficits of single nutrients (Beisel 1983; Hwang 1989), vitamins (Bendich 1987; Bendich & Cohen 1988; Rigby 1988; West, Howard & Sommer 1989; Ross 1992) minerals (Ogra 1984) or oligoelements (micronutrients) (Phillips & Baetz 1981; Dallman 1987; Bendich & Chandra 1990), not less necessary for the normal development and function of the immune system. Most often, the cause is multifactorial, and it is not easy to ascertain which of several nutrients absent from or deficient in the diet is involved in the pathogenesis of the immune ailment (Mims, 1987). Much as the mechanisms of defense are interwoven, so the causes leading to their defective functioning are complex.

Before considering the pathogenetic ways by which malnutrition can lead to an increased susceptibility to infections, it might be useful to remember the various kinds of mechanisms involved in defense against bacteria, viruses, fungi and parasites. They can be grouped into three categories:

(1) Non-specific "barriers" (physical, chemical, physiological or biological in nature), such as the integrity of the skin and mucous membranes, the low pH of the contents of the stomach, the presence of fatty acids on the skin surface, of lysozyme in tears, saliva and many other secretions, the permeability of natural orifices and ducts, allowing for the unimpeded flow of secretions, and the presence and activity of components of the normal microbial flora in such body locations as the airways or the intestinal tract.

(2) Non-specific responses to infection, including phagocytosis, cytokine production, fever, synthesis and release of acute phase proteins, complement activation, and the inflamatory response. Many of these mechanisms are related to each other and to members of the third category, for which they very often serve as effector mechanisms or amplification cascades.

(3) Specific responses, that is, the immune response proper, with two main components: the humoral response (the synthesis of various classes of antibody, different in function and distribution in the body) and the cellular response (the generation of effector T lymphocytes, endowed with pro-inflammatory, phagocytosis-enhancing or cytolytic properties). The complex regulatory mechanisms of the specific immune response, that make it finely tuned to the changing requirements of every moment, are essential for the fulfilment of its defensive functions. Also, "immune memory", the ability to respond in a quicker, stronger and more efficient manner to repeated stimuli, must be kept intact if the immune response is to take a significant part in the defense against infection.

The mechanisms in the three above categories are related to each other, and all of them are liable to become affected by malnutrition. Beginning with barrier mechanisms, avitaminosis A or C is accompanied by damage to the integuments, thus opening potential portals of entry to infectious agents (Mims 1987). Levels of lysozyme in secretions and of transferrin in blood are decreased in severe protein-energy malnutrition; lysozyme is effective in combating many superficial infections of the mucosae, and cooperates with the membrane attack complex (MAC) of the complement system to bring about lysis of several bacterial species. Transferrin, in turn, competes with transport molecules of microorganisms for the available iron resources. Changes in the intestinal flora related to unbalanced diets may alter the metabolism of bile salts, thus impairing fat absorption through the gut mucosa (Mims 1987).

Non-specific responses are affected, not only as defense mechanisms of their own, but also in their task as effector or amplificator systems for specific immune factors (Gershon, Beach & Hurley 1985). Phagocytes (neutrophil polymorphonuclear leukocytes and the mononuclear phagocytes of the monocyte-macrophage lineage) can be severely affected, not so much with respect to their capacity to engulf opsonized microbes, as in what concerns intracellular killing activities, especially because of a diminished oxidative burst following particle ingestion. The serum levels of complement whole activity and of various complement components have also been found to be lowered in undernourished people, C3 having received most attention in this respect because of ease of quantitation. Excessive complement consumption by the frequent infective episodes, as well as diminished synthesis of complement proteins, are responsible for these findings. Increases in endotoxins, C-reactive-protein, circulating immune complexes, etc., resulting from the frequent occurrence of clinical or subclinical infections, are findings that reflect the enhanced burden imposed on the normal non-specific responses of the body under such circumstances.

The effect of malnutrition on specific immune mechanisms deserves special consideration (Chandra 1992). Humoral immunity may remain relatively unaffected for long periods. B cells are often normal in numbers, whereas serum immunoglobulin levels either remain normal or are even increased. This last finding cannot be regarded as indicative of stronger humoral immune responses, but rather as the expression of the altered regulation of the response as a whole, resulting from damage to T lymphocytes, as commented below; a similar situation can also be found in other forms of predominantly cellular immunodeficiency (AIDS, for instance). IgA is usually decreased in many secretions, even in the presence of normal or elevated levels in serum, not so much because of diminished synthesis in the mucosa-associated lymphoid tissue (MALT), but rather as a consequence of functional defects in the mucosae, which interfere with the normal transport mechanism across the epithelial lining. The antibody responses to specific antigens vary, according to the degree of T-dependence of the particular antigens involved(Gershwin, Beach & Hurley 1985).

The impact of malnutrition is generally greatest on cell-mediated immune mechanisms (Woodward, Woods & Crouch 1992). When it is severe and prolonged, a reduction in size of all the lymphatic organs ensues, accompanied by structural disorganization involving mainly the T-dependent areas of the spleen, lymph nodes and other lymphatic territories (Woodward, Dwivedi & Nangpal 1992). In children, the reduction in the size of the thymus, by comparison with normally fed infants of the same age, can be considered as a marker of the degree of nutritional imbalance. By 1925, well before the true role of the thymus in immunity became known, this organ was apostrophized as the "barometer of nutrition" (Jackson 1925). T cells, especially of the CD4+ phenotype, that includes the helper population, are reduced in number, ability to divide, and functional activity (responsiveness to various stimuli). Production of cytokines is diminished, and this results in a worsened communication among cell types, with a fialure in the regulation of the immune responses, both cellular and humoral. A reduced synthesis and release of thymic hormones is one of the mechanisms responsible for these cellular defects; the increase in plasma cortisol, so often found in undernourished patients, as well as other endocrine imbalances, also contribute to the final immune disorder.

The severity of the effects of malnutrition on the immune capacity of the host depends on how long nutrient deprivation is maintained, and is the greater the earlier is the time of life at which malnutrition starts (intrauterine period, at birth, during growth, or in adult life (Gershwin et al. 1985). Defective nutrition of the mother can block the ontogenic development of the immune system of the fetus. A particularly crucial moment is weaning, when the infant passes from breast feeding to an insuficient diet; in fact, although maternal malnutrition may deteriorate the quality of the milk secreted, this can be kept in a relatively good state for long periods, in the face of profound alterations in other functions. It has been said that, at least under experimental conditions, the effect of malnutrition onb the immune system may still become apparent in the second generation (Chandra 1975), although the mechanisms leading to this effect, if ti is true, are not easily understood. In clinical practice, recovery of immune function, once re-nutrition is instituted, may be slow and difficult to attain completely, especially when malnutrition has been long lasting and has begun at an early age. The capacity to give anamnestic responses upon repeated immunization may be deficient for very long periods; this is an important point to bear in mind when designing vaccination campaigns in undernourished population groups.

Although it has been the subject of much less study, excess of nutrients in the diet can also have deleterious consequences on immune function (Levy 1982). It has been observed mainly in patients suffering from obesity, diabetes or hyperlipidemias, as well as in those receiving grossly unbalanced diets (Chandra 1991). The implication of excessive alimentary regimes on autoimmunity and cancer, to which attention has been paid from an experimental point of view, has in turn given way to some therapeutic trials (Gershwin et al. 1985).

2 IMMUNE FACTORS IN NUTRITION

Not only nutritional defects can affect the structure and function of the immune system; also normal or altered immune mechanisms are involved in the complex process of nutrition. My comments on this latter aspect of the mutual relationship between nutrition and immunity will turn around three issues: (1) immune mechanisms at mucosal surfaces, (2) absorption of antigenic substances through the intestinal epithelium, and (3) immune control of the absorption of non-antigenic nutrients.

2.1 Immune mechanisms at mucosal surfaces

Mucosal surfaces constitute the main portal of entry for a multitude of infectious agents and antigenic substances from the environment. For that reason, they are endowed with immune mechanisms controlling which substances can be admitted to or must be excluded from the internal milieu (Ogra 1984; Bird & Calvert 1988; Hanson & Brandtzaeg 1989). If this is true for mucosal surfaces generally, the importance of these mechanisms becomes paramount in the case of the intestine, as its surface is charged with the task of absorbing large amounts of nutrients, and its lumen is laden with the greatest burden of microorganisms in the normal microbial flora of the whole body. Immunoglobulin A (IgA), present in secretions of the digestive tract, acts as a "protective varnish", that controls the qualitative and quantitative composition of the intestinal flora, and prevents the indiscriminate access to the body of a large variety of potentially antigenic substances.

Intestinal IgA is of the secretory modality, composed of a dimer of this immunoglobulin isotype (4 alpha-1 or alpha-2 heavy chains, 4 kappa or lambda light chains, 1 J chain), to which an additional peptide, the "S" component, is added during the process of being taken by epithelial cells and getting transported through them to the external surface of the mucous membrane (French 1986; Strober & Brown 1988). The additional S component gives the ensemble of the secretory molecule an increased resistance to enzymatic cleavage, necessary for it to survive and devlop function in the adverse environment, with plenty of proteolytic enzymes of microbial or digestive origin, of the gut lumen. The IgA dimers contributing to secretory IgA may come from the general immune system of the body, but for the most part are locally produced by B lymphocytes of the gut-associated lymphoid tissue (GALT). This is a specialized division of the lymphatic system, mainly involved in regional immune responses (Klein 1990), not necessarily parallelling the systemic immune responses of the host. Secretory IgA in the intestinal contents, therefore, displays a spectrum of antibody specificities more adapted to the array of antigens it is to encounter locally.

The ontogenic development of the capacity to synthesize IgA deserves some attention, because of the impact it has on nutrition (Bird & Calvert 1988). Serum levels of IgA are very low, almost negligible, at birth, since the fetus is unable to synthesize significant amounts of this protein, which in addition cannot be transferred from the maternal to the fetal circulation across the placenta. Neither is IgA syntehsized in sufficient amounts in the mucosa-associated lymphoid tissue (MALT) of the fetus, so that the "protective varnish" is absent from the mucosal surfaces at the time of birth. Breast feeding affords a considerable supply of secretory IgA to the intestinal lumen of the neonate, thanks to the high concentration of this protein, first in calostrum and then in milk (Strober & Brown 1988). A sort of local passive immunization is thus provided by the mother to the infant for all the length of lactation, that allows for the acquisition and development of the microbial intestinal flora to be kept under control. Actually, microbiological examination of the stools of the suckling is a reliable method to ascertain whether he or she is receiving natural or artificial nutrition. In fact, no artificial dietary product can substitute for the presence of secretory IgA in maternal milk, since milks of animal origin forming the basis of artificial formulae have a quite different composition as far as immunoglobulins are concerned, as a reflection of the notable inter-species differences in the mechanisms of transfer of humoral immunity from mother to offspring. The protection afforded by antibodies (and cells) in maternal milk (Ogra 1984), partly as a result of local immune responses occurring in mammary gland lymphoid tissue, does not only become manifest in changes in the microbial flora, but also in the increased frequency of infections and diarrhoea and the higher incidence of food allergies in children that are not breast-fed.

2.2 Intestinal absorption of antigenic substances

In connection with the above, it should be borne in mind that the intestinal mucosa does not constitute an absolute barrier to the absorption of antigenic substances. Proteins in the diet are not completely degrades in the intestinal lumen down to single amino acids that are as such transferred to the internal milieu, to constitute the elementary building blocks for the proteins of the individual. Rather, small peptides, sufficient in size and complexity to work as antigenic epitopes, pass through the digestive epithelium to reach lymph or blood and be transported to distant destinations in the body. This view is supported by the following facts.

(1) Food allergies can display not only local (digestive tract), but also distant or systemic clinical manifestations (Doe 1982; Kettelhut & Metcalfe 1988); this suggests the arrival of antigenic fragments of the offending food to remote target tissues. Food allergies occur more frequently in patients suffering from IgA deficiency (Buckley & Dees 1969; Buckley 1988), which speaks in favour of a physiological role of this protein in controlling the absorption of eventually antigenic substances (Soothill et al. 1976).

(2) The challenge of a passive transfer (P.K.; Prausnitz-Küstner 1926) test for ana-

phylactic antibodies to food allergens can be carried out by the oral route (Bennich et al. 1977). In other words, the intradermal injection of serum from a patient sensitive to, let us say, cow milk into the skin of a normal subject, followed 24 to 48 hours later by the ingestion of the offending food (a glass of milk, in our example) by the recipient, results in less than an hour in the characteristic wheal-and-flare reaction at the passively sensitized skin site, in the absence of any reaction in the rest of the skin of the recipient or in skin sites passively sensitized with sera from atopic patients of other specificities. This experimental design rules out the possibility that the above mentioned occurrence of food allergies with extradigestive manifestations be due to an abnormal permeability of the intestinal epithelium in atopic individuals.

(3) Significant increases in the levels of circulating immune complexes occur, even in normal individuals, during the asorption phase following a meal. The magnitude of the increase keeps a close correlation with the amount and the nature of the food ingested. Obviously, antigen-antibody complexes could not be formed under such circumstances unless some dietary constituents would pass the epithelial barrier of the inestine and enter the bloodstream while still keeping their antigenic properties.

On the other hand, non-nutritional components of the diet are important for the normal development of detoxifying mechanisms, as well as for the defense against tumours; they exert some sort of continuous "training" of the immune system in order to maintain the homeostasis of the body.

2.3 Immune control of the absorption of non-antigenic nutrients

A suggestive instance of the immune control of the absorption of non-antigenic nutrients is found in patients with pernicious anemia. In this autoimmune disease, abnormal responses to constituents of the own body form the basis for many of the pathological findings (aclorhidria, deficient secretion of gastric hormones or peptides, atrophic gastritis, etc.) (Brown & Strober 1988). In advanced stages of the disease, failure of the gastric mucosa to secrete "intrinsic factor" causes the lack of absorption of vitamin B12, since this must be conjugated to intrinsic factor for transport across the intestinal mucosa. Before that point, intrinsic factor secretion can be conserved to a degree that may be dificult to reconcile with the severity of the signs and symptoms of cobalamine deprivation. In such instances, the presence of autoantibodies to intrinsic factor in the contents of the stomach explains the impairment in vitamin B12 absorption. At least two varieties of antibody have been identified (Doe 1982; Doniach et al. 1982; Gleeson & Toh 1991). Antibodies of the first variety act by blocking the vitamin-binding site on the intrinsic factor molecule, thus precluding formation of the complex, and consequently the access of vitamin B12 to the body. Autoantibodies of the second variety, without impeding vitamin B12-intrinsic factor complex formation, prevent the absorption of the formed conjugate, by blocking the site on the intrinsic factor that must be recognized by epithelial cells before activation of the transport mechanism.

Although the above findings have been defined for a pathological condition, it does not seem unreasonable to think that the antibodies to intrinsic factor found in patients with pernicious anemia could be the counterpart of something occurring also in the normal individual. There is growing evidence that the high titers of autoantibodies (rheumatoid factor, autoantibodies to erythrocyte antigens, to hormone receptors, etc.) characteristically found in some autoimmune diseases are just the expression of a considerable increase in the amount and affinity of antibodies that under normal circumstances play important roles in the regulation of a number of physiological functions ("positive" autoimmunity) (Smith & Steinberg 1983; Schwartz 1986; Bird & Calvert 1988; Marcos et al. 1989). Such findings open a field of great interest for future studies.

REFERENCES

Antonaci, S., A. Polignano, C. Tortorella, M.T. Ventura, E. Jirillo & L. Bonomo 1992. Immunocompetence and nutrient deficiency in the elderly. Biomed. Lett. 47: 289-300.
Beisel, W.R. 1983. Single nutrients and immunity. Am. J. Clin. Nutr. 35: 417-468.
Bendich, A. 1987. Vitamin C and immune responses. Food Technol. 41: 112-114.
Bendich, A. & M. Cohen 1988. B vitamins: effects on specific and nonspecific immune responses. In: Nutrition and Immunology (ed. Chandra, R.K.). New York: Alan R. Liss.
Bendich, A. & R.K. Chandra 1990. Micronutrients and immune functions. New York: New York Academy of Sciences.
Bennich, H., U. Ragnarson, S.G.O. Johansson, K. Ishizaka, T. Ishizaka, D.A. Levy & L.M. Lichtenstein 1977. Failure of the putative IgE pentapeptide to compete with IgE for receptors on basophils and mast cells. Int Arch. Allerg. Appl. Immunol. 45: 30-39.
Bird, G. & J.E. Calvert 1988. B lymphocytes in human disease. Oxford: Oxford University Press.
Brown, W.R. & W. Strober 1988. Immunological

diseases of the gastrointestinal tract. In: Immunological diseases (ed. Samter, M.) pp. 1995-2034. Boston: Little, Brown and Company.

Buckley, R.H. & S.C. Dees 1969. Correlation of milk precipitins with IgA deficiency. N. Engl. J. Med. 281: 465-470.

Buckley, R.H. 1988. Immunologic deficiency and allergic disease. In: Allergy. Principles and practice (eds. Middleton, E., C.E. Reed, E.F. Ellis, N.F. Adkinson & J.W. Yunginger) pp. 295-311. St. Louis: Mosby.

Chandra, R.K. 1975. Antibody response in the first and second generation of nutritionally deprived rats. Science 190: 189-190.

Chandra, R.K. 1989. Nutritional regulation of immunity and risk of infection in old age. Immunology 67: 141-147.

Chandra, R.K. 1991. Nutrition and immunity. In: Clinical immunology (eds. Brostoff, J. G.K. Scadding, D. Male & I.M. Roitt) pp. 25.1-25.11. London: Gower Medical Publishing.

Chandra, R.K. 1992. Nutrition and the immune system. In: Encyclopedia of immunology (eds. Roit, I.M. & P.J. Delves) pp. 1173-1175. London: Academic Press.

Dallman, P.R. 1987. Iron deficiency and the immune response. Am. J. Clin. Nutr. 46: 329-334.

Doe, W.F. 1982. Immunological aspects of the gut. In: Clinical aspects of immunology (eds. Lachmann, P.J. & D.K. Peters) pp. 985-1010. Oxford: Blackwell Scientific Publications.

Doniach, D., G.F. Botazzo & D.K. Drexhage 1982. The autoimmune endocrinopathies. In: Clinical aspects of immunology (eds. Lachmann, P.J. & D.K. Peters) pp. 903-937. Oxford: Blackwell Scientific Publications.

French, M.A.H. 1986. Immunoglobulins in health and disease. Lancaster: MTP Press Limited.

Gershwin, M.E., R.S. Beach & L.S. Hurley 1985. Nutrition and immunity. Orlando: Academic Press.

Gleeson, P.A. & B-H. Toh 1991. Molecular targets in pernicious anaemia. Immunol. Tod. 12: 233-238.

Hanson, L.A. & P. Brandtzaeg 1989. The mucosal defense system. In: Immunologic disorders in infants and children (ed. Stiehm, E.R.) pp. 116-155. Philadelphia: W.B. Saunders Company.

Hwang, D. 1989. Essential fatty acids and immune response. FASEB J. 3: 2052-2061.

Jackson, C.M. 1925. Cited by Gershwin, Beach and Hurley (1985).

Kettelhut, B.W. & D.D. Metcalfe 1988. Adverse reactions to food. In: Allergy. Principles and practice (eds. Middleton, E., C.E. Reed, E.F. Ellis, N.F. Adkinson & J.W. Yunginger) pp. 1481-1502. St. Louis: Mosby.

Klein, J. 1990. Immunology. Boston: Blackwell Scientific Publications.

Levy, J.A. 1982. Nutrition and the immune system. In: Basic and clinical immunology (eds. Stites, D.P., J.D. Stobo, H.H. Fudenberg & J.V. Wells) pp. 297-305. Los Altos: Lange Medical Publications.

Marcos, M.A.R., A. Sundblad, A. Grandien, F. Huetz, S. Avrameas & A. Coutinho 1989. The physiology of autoimmune reactivities. In: Progress in immunology VII (eds. Melchers, F.) pp. 793-804. Berlin: Springer-Verlag.

Mims, C.A. 1987. The pathogenesis of infectious disease. London: Academic Press.

Ogra, P.L. 1984. Neonatal infections. Nutritional and immunological interactions. Orlando: Grune & Stratton.

Phillips, M. & A. Baetz 1981. Diet and resistance to disease. New York: Plenum Press.

Prausnitz, C. & H. Küstner 1926. Studien über der Ueberempfindlichkeit. Zbl. Bakt. 86: 160-174.

Rigby, W.F.C. 1988. The immunobiology of vitamin D. Immunol. Tod. 9: 54-58.

Ross, A.C. 1992. Vitamin A status: relationship to immunity and the antibody response Proc. Soc. Exp. Biol. Med. 200: 303-320.

Schwartz, R. 1986. Autoantibodies and normal antibodies. In: Progress in Immunology VI (eds. Cinader, B. & R.G. Miller) pp. 478-482. Orlando: Academic Press.

Scrimshaw, N.S., C.E. Taylor & J.E. Gordon 1959. Interactions of nutrition and infection. Am. J. Med. Sci. 237: 367-374.

Smith, H.R. & A.D. Steinberg 1983. Autoimmunity – A perspective. Ann. Rev. Immunol. 1: 175-210.

Soothill, J.F., C.R. Stokes, M.W. Turner, A. P. Norman & B. Taylor 1976. Predisposing factors and the development of reaginic allergy in infancy. Clin. Allergy 6: 305-314.

Strober, W. & W.R. Brown 1988. The mucosal immune system. In: Immunological diseases (ed. Samter, M.) pp. 79-139. Boston: Little, Brown and Company.

West, K.P. G.R. Howard & A. Sommer 1989. Vitamin A and infection: public health implications. Ann. Rev. Nutr. 9: 63-86.

Woodward, B., A. Diwedi & A. Nangpal 1992. Mechanisms of thymic epithelial involution in weaning protein-energy malnutrition. Nutr. Res. 12: 1253-1264.

Woodward B.D., J.W. Woods & D.A. Crouch 1992. Direct evidence that primary acquired cell-mediated immunity is less resistant than is primary thymus-dependent humoral immunity to the depressive influence of wasting protein-energy malnutrition in weaning mice. Am. J. Clin. Nutr. 55: 1180-1185.

Dairy Products in Human Health and Nutrition, Serrano Ríos et al. (eds) © 1994 Balkema, Rotterdam, ISBN 90 5410 359 0

Malnutrition and the immune response

R. M. Suskind, C. L. Lachney & J. N. Udall Jr
Department of Pediatrics, Louisiana State University Medical Center, School of Medicine, New Orleans, La., USA

ABSTRACT: Malnutrition is a major health threat to millions of children worldwide. In addition to the estimated 100 million undernourished children in developing countries, there are millions of children suffering from secondary malnutrition (failure to thrive) in the developed world. Children with congenital heart disease, chronic renal disease, cancer, chronic infections, and other primary diseases may be secondarily malnourished. Most children with severe primary or secondary malnutrition are immunocompromised. Diseases of overnutrition, including obesity and diabetes, also affect the immune response. While early studies noted the relationship between malnutrition and compromised immunity in children suffering from severe protein-energy malnutrition, recent studies have also recognized that mild-to-moderate undernutrition, as well as specific deficiencies of vitamins, minerals, or trace elements, compromise the immune response.

Protein-energy malnutrition, which includes deficiencies of calories, protein, vitamins, minerals, and trace elements, affects several aspects of the immune response, including cell-mediated immunity, the humoral immune response, leukocyte function, and the complement system. Specific effects such as impairment of delayed cutaneous hypersensitivity to antigens, reduced numbers of peripheral T lymphocytes, reduction in secretory IgA, and lowered concentration and activity of several complement components, are commonly observed in children suffering from protein-energy malnutrition.

Evidence for the effects of certain vitamins and trace elements on specific phases of the immune response has come both from human and animal studies. It has been observed that iron deficiency significantly impairs the cellular immune response. Zinc deficiency in patients with acrodermatitis enteropathica also causes depression of the cellular immune response, while selenium deficiency decreases the antibody response to specific antigens and phagocytic bactericidal activity. Vitamin deficiencies are rare in industrialized nations, but are frequently associated with malnutrition in developing countries. Vitamin A deficiency results in impairment of the cellular immune response and increases susceptibility to infection. Adequate concentrations of vitamin E, an important antioxidant, are necessary for an optimal immune response. The B vitamins, which are involved in a wide range of metabolic reactions, are required for an adequate immune response. Pyridoxine deficiency, for example, profoundly affects immune function, causing lymphoid tissue atrophy as well as decreased cellular and humoral immune responsiveness.

The decreased immunity that often accompanies undernutrition increases the vulnerability of the child to recurrent infections, which further compromise the child's nutritional and immune status. These immune deficits are reversible with nutritional intervention. Understanding the relationship between nutritional status and the immune response is essential if one is dealing with either the primarily or secondarily malnourished child.

INTRODUCTION

Malnutrition is the most common cause of secondary immunodeficiency. Primary protein-calorie malnutrition, secondary protein-calorie malnutrition from such disease states as cancer, AIDS, chronic renal disease, and congenital heart disease (Table 1), as well as specific vitamin and mineral deficiencies have a significant impact on the immune system.

The general consequences of malnutrition on the immune system include deficits in cell-mediated immunity, the antibody response to certain antigens, mucosal

Table 1. Disease states often associated with secondary protein-energy malnutrition in children.

Low birth weight	Mucosal disease:
Short bowel syndrome	Celiac disease
Cystic fibrosis	Milk protein enteropathy
Chronic liver disease	Infectious enteritis
Inflammatory bowel disease	Soy protein enteropathy
Chronic renal disease	Tropical sprue
Congenital heart disease	Allergic gastroenteritis
Burns and trauma	Intractable diarrhea
Anorexia nervosa	Immune deficiency disorders
Cancer	

Table 2. Effects of protein-energy malnutrition on host defense.

CELL-MEDIATED IMMUNITY	
In vivo	DECREASED
In vitro	
T cell number	DECREASED
Mitogenic response	DECREASED
IMMUNOGLOBULIN SYNTHESIS	
Serum immunoglobulin	INCREASED
Antibody response	DECREASED
Secretory antibody response	DECREASED
POLYMORPHONUCLEAR	
LEUKOCYTE FUNCTION	
In vivo chemotaxis	NORMAL
In vitro migration	DECREASED
Phagocytosis	NORMAL
Oxidative burst	NORMAL
Killing function	NORMAL OR DECREASED
COMPLEMENT	
C1-C9	DECREASED
CH50	DECREASED
Anticomplement activity	PRESENT

secretory antibody response, and the complement system (Table 2) (Chandra, 1992a). Infectious diseases resulting from immune dysfunction can lead to further nutritional impairment, thereby exacerbating the clinical consequences.

The immune system

The immune system comprises a network of organs and cells that defends the body against invasion by pathogens and against development and metastasis of malignant tumors. This defense is effected by the lymphoid system, consisting of thymus and bone marrow (the primary lymphoid tissues), and the lymph nodes, spleen, and gut-associated lymphoid tissue, working in cooperation with the mononuclear phagocyte system. The latter includes macrophages, monocytes, fixed tissue histiocytes, and Kupffer cells, which, while found in all tissues, are found in the greatest numbers in the lymph nodes and spleen. By complex processes involving genetic rearrangement, hormonal influences, and antigen stimulation in the primary and secondary lymphoid tissues, hemopoietic stem cells give eventual rise to mature lymphoid and myeloid cells including T and B lymphocytes, monocytes, platelets, granulocytes, mast cells, macrophages, and neutrophils (Weir, 1983; Bellanti, 1985; Paul, 1989a,b; Roitt et al., 1989; Vo and Luster, 1989).

Host defense is effected by two broad systems. The first line of defense, the innate or nonspecific immune response, is activated when host surface barriers (skin, mucous membranes, and mucus and cilia of epithelial surfaces) are breached by microorganisms, and is comprised of the polymorphonuclear leukocyte system and the inflammatory response (activation of the complement, kinin, fibrinolytic, and clotting enzyme systems).

Polymorphonuclear leukocytes (PMN) phagocytose invading bacteria. Competence of phagocytic function can be assessed by measurement of chemotaxis (directed movement of PMN), phagocytosis (attachment and internalization of invading bacteria), bactericidal activity, and metabolic changes resulting from phagocytic activity (Bellanti, 1985). Activation of the complement system entails the coordinated synthesis of a cascade of plasma proteins and glycoproteins which interact to regulate the inflammatory response, to opsonize invading particles thereby "tagging" them for phagocytosis, and to effect cytotoxic activities against foreign organisms (deShazo et al., 1987).

The second line of defense is the adaptive (specific) immune response, initiated when the innate immune defense is penetrated. The response is specific to the invading pathogen by virtue of antigen-specific antibodies produced by mature plasma cells of the B-lymphocyte series (the humoral immune response), and by the cell-mediated immune response of the T lymphocytes. T cells of the CD4 or T4+ subpopulation are helper or inducer cells, whereas T cells of the CD8 or T8+ subpopulation are suppressor or cytotoxic cells. These subpopulations of T cells work in concert to modulate and regulate the immune response, e.g. to facilitate antibody production by plasma cells, to modulate immune responsiveness through the release of lymphokines, or to down-regulate the activities of other aspects of the immune response.

The traditional in vivo assessment of the competence of the cell-mediated immune response is through the delayed-type-hypersensitivity (DTH) intradermal test, which can measure prior or de novo sensitization. At least 80% of normal individuals respond to the intradermal injection of small amounts of antigen (e.g. mumps, *Candida*, streptococcal, or fungal antigens, or purified protein derivative [PPD]) with both erythema and induration within 48 h (Bellanti, 1985). In vitro tests assess the number of lymphocytes and the strength of antigen- or mitogen-induced lymphoproliferative (transformation, proliferation, and replication) response, and monoclonal antibody assays allow the quantitation of T-cell subsets. This information is used to evaluate the competence of immune regulation. The humoral immune response is assessed by measurement of circulating and secretory antibodies, determination of the number of B lymphocytes, and assessment of antibody response to antigenic stimulation (Bellanti, 1985).

Because deficiencies in nutrition have a high degree of correlation to immune impairment (Chandra and Scrimshaw, 1980; Chandra, 1981b; Puri and Chandra, 1985), these tests of immunocompetence have been used as indices of functional nutritional status (Calloway, 1982; Solomons and Allen, 1983; Solomons, 1985; Gibson, 1990;). For example, an anergic (absence of) response to DTH testing in the nutritionally compromised surgical candidate may identify that patient as being at risk of postoperative sepsis or death (Chandra and Scrimshaw, 1980; Casey et al., 1983; Chandra, 1983b). The patient's age, the use of drugs, or the presence of infection or disease are complicating factors in the use of immune status as an indicator of nutritional status.

Immunity and nutrition

The general relationship of nutritional adequacy to immunocompetence is that a decrease in the former is usually accompanied by a decrease in the latter -- as evidenced by the historical association between famine and epidemic (Chandra, 1992b). It is only comparatively recently that specific immune defects can be traced to nutritional factors, and that the significant cofactors of patient age, degree and type of malnutrition, or presence of infection or disease have been taken into consideration in these studies.

Infants and elderly adults are both vulnerable to infection, due to developmental immaturity or progressive loss of immunocompetence, respectively (Weksler, 1986; Bellanti et al., 1987). Nutritional deficiencies that do not impair adult health may cause serious problems such as stunted growth, learning disorders, or immunocompromise in infants and young children, who are more susceptible to nutritional deficits due to increased metabolic demands for growth and development. Compromised immunity has been well documented in several studies of children with protein-energy malnutrition (Seth and Chandra, 1972; Tanphiachitr et al., 1973; Chandra, 1975b; Suskind, 1977; Chandra, 1983b; Watson, 1984). Perinatal malnutrition can so impair the critical early development of the immune system that the damage is prolonged or permanent (Aref et al.,

1970; Ghavami et al., 1979; Chandra and Matsumura, 1979; Gershwin et al., 1985). Deficits in the cell-mediated immune response have been reported to persist up to several years in infants who suffered intrauterine growth retardation as a result of maternal malnutrition or infection (Chandra, 1975b; Chandra, 1984a; Ferguson et al., 1974), whereas the immune response is usually normal in 3 to 4 months in preterm, appropriate for gestational age infants (Chandra, 1981a; Fletcher et al., 1988).

While the deleterious effects of undernutrition on the immune response in infants and children have been well established, the relationship is not as well characterized in the elderly, who are especially at risk of depressed cell-mediated immunity (Weksler, 1986). Such a relationship is not unlikely, since even in industrialized nations large numbers of older adults are poorly nourished (up to one-third of the elderly living independently in the United States (Scrimshaw, 1989; USDHEW, 1972)), and since the age-related degeneration of cell-mediated immunity, T-cell number, and thymic factor activity is similar to that found to occur in protein-energy malnutrition (Chandra, 1985; Chandra, 1989a). Comparatively few studies have explored the effects of nutrition on immunocompetence in the aged population.

Malnutrition and the immune response

The spectrum of malnutrition ranges from the severe, third-degree marasmus or kwashiorkor in developing countries (Figures 1-3), to subclinical deficiencies of selected nutrients, to diseases of overnutrition such as obesity and diabetes. Mild to moderate nutritional deprivation, which is a significant health threat in both developing as well as industrialized nations (UNEP, 1990), is often overlooked; indeed, growth failure and small stature in young children are considered to be within normal range in certain countries. Similar undernutrition affects the elderly, the poor, and the chronically ill in developed countries. There is increasing evidence that mild to moderate undernutrition can impair the immune response (Chandra, 1972; 1974; 1981c; Ziegler and Ziegler, 1975). Obesity may also be associated with compromised cell-mediated immunity, phagocyte bactericidal activity, and antibody response to T-dependent antigens (Chandra, 1981c; 1983b; 1988). Specific nutrient deficiencies such as iron deficiency are common in humans, and may occur in the elderly, the obese, the pregnant woman, those who have chronic blood loss, or those who are on an inadequate intake. Controlled studies using laboratory animals indicate that single-nutrient deficiencies can compromise immune

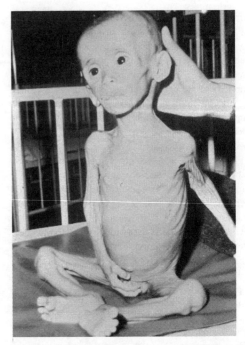

Figure 1A. The clinical effects of childhood malnutrition. This two-year-old child had marasmus, which is the predominant form of malnutrition in infancy. Marasmus is characterized by severe weight loss, gross wasting of muscle and subcutaneous tissue, and marked stunting, but no edema.

response (Gershwin et al., 1985; Beisel, 1982; Beisel et al., 1981; Bendich et al., 1990; Chandra, 1983a; Chandra and Puri, 1985; Gershwin et al., 1983; Gross and Newberne, 1980).

Protein-energy malnutrition broadly modifies both the nonspecific and the specific immune response. Generally reduced serum concentrations of almost all complement components, which are responsive to nutritional rehabilitation (Figure 4), have been described (Coovadia et al., 1974; Neumann et al., 1975; Sirisinha et al., 1973). In malnourished children, depressed hemolytic complement activity may result from the anticomplement activity of endotoxin or immune complexes (Figures 5-7) (Sirisinha et al., 1977). Klein and colleagues found that as many as 55% of malnourished children had circulating endotoxin at the time of admission to hospital (Figure 8) (Klein et al., 1977). The effects of malnutrition on PMN and macrophage function are subtle: in vitro leukocyte chemotaxis apparently is not different in malnourished children with or without infection from that in well nourished children

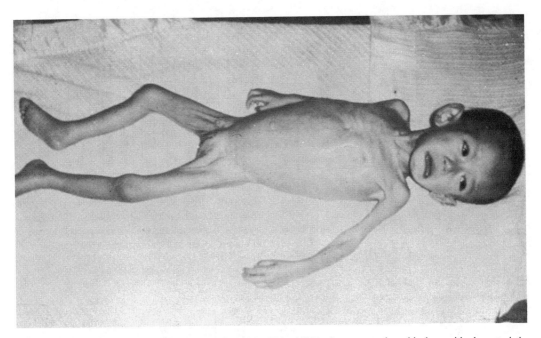

Figure 2. The clinical effects of childhood malnutrition. This child had marasmus-kwashiorkor, with characteristic edema, gross wasting, stunting, and with some fatty infiltration of the liver.

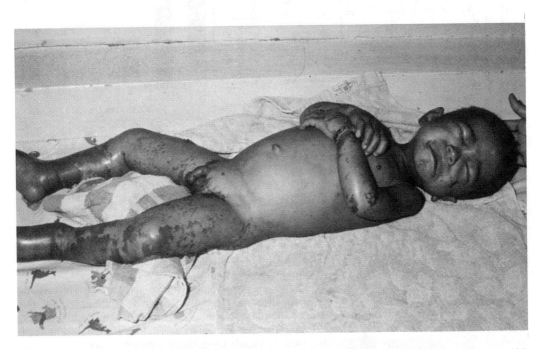

Figure 3. The clinical effects of childhood malnutrition. This two-and-a-half-year-old child had kwashiorkor, which is more frequent in older infants and young children. Kwashiorkor is characterized by edema, skin lesions, changes in the hair, enlarged fatty liver, and decreased serum albumin. From Suskind et al., 1990.

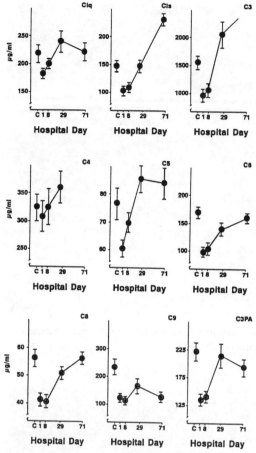

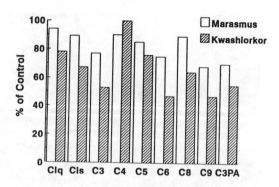

Figure 5: Serum levels of nine complement proteins upon hospital admission in 10 children with marasmus and 10 children with kwashiorkor, expressed as percent of control levels of 19 normal children. From Sirisinha et al., 1977.

Figure 4. Changes (connected points) in serum concentrations of nine complement proteins over the interval of hospitalization and nutritional intervention in 20 Thai children with protein-calorie malnutrition. The mean ± SEM values for normal children are shown in isolated vertical bars. The data were published in Sirisinha et al., 1973.

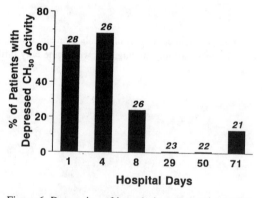

Figure 6. Depression of hemolytic complement activity in children with protein-calorie malnutrition during hospital stay and nutritional intervention. The numbers of patients tested are above the bars. From Sirisinha et al., 1977.

with or without infection. However, Edelman and colleagues found decreased in vivo macrophage chemotaxis (Figure 9) (Edelman et al., 1977). In both groups of children with infection, however, the chemotactic response is less than that in uninfected children (Rosen et al., 1975). Phagocytosis of particles by the circulating neutrophils of malnourished children is normal, while the intracellular bactericidal capacity of PMN is often decreased (Figure 10) (Douglas and Schopfer, 1977; Leitzmann et al., 1977), and the postphagocytic activity of leukocytes is also reduced (Selvaraj and Bhat, 1972).

The specific immune response is also broadly affect-ed by protein-energy malnutrition. Involution of the anatomic structures of the lymphoid system associated with undernutrition was noted early in this century (Jackson, 1925). The thymus, lymph nodes, tonsils, and spleen are atrophic in malnourished children, and thymus-dependent areas of the lymph nodes are depleted of lymphoid cells (Mugerwa, 1971). Reduction in tonsil size can be used as a clinical indicator of malnutrition (Smythe et al., 1971).

The depressed cell-mediated immune response in the malnourished child is a phenomenon that was first described in 1958, when it was noted that children with

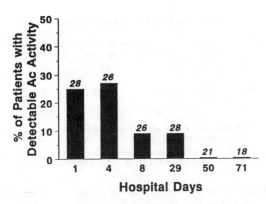

Figure 7. Presence of anticomplement activity in children hospitalized and treated for protein-calorie malnutrition. The numbers of patients tested are above the bars. From Sirisinha et al., 1977.

Endotoxemia in Protein-Calorie Malnutrition

Prevalence Day 1-4	Tested 24	Positive 11	% Positive 46%

Characteristics	Positive	Negative
UTI	6/11 (55%)	5/13 (38%)
Stool pathogens	5/11 (45%)	3/13 (23%)
Pneumonia	4/11 (35%)	3/11 (23%)
Ascaris	6/11 (55%)	3/13 (8%)

Figure 8. Prevalence and origin of endotoxemia in children admitted to hospital with protein-calorie malnutrition. The data were published in Klein et al., 1977.

protein-energy malnutrition had a decreased frequency of positive tuberculin skin tests (Jayalakshmi and Gopalan, 1958). Malnourished children could neither be sensitized to new antigens nor develop a normal inflammatory response to skin-test irritants (Harland, 1965). These depressed responses improve rapidly as nutritional status is improved (Figure 11) (Edelman et al., 1973). Other studies describe this anergic response to a wide range of antigens (Chandra, 1972; Feldman and Gianantonio, 1972; Law et al., 1973; Work et al., 1973), and to similar or lesser extent in moderately undernourished patients (Ziegler and Ziegler, 1975; McMurray et al., 1981).

The number of circulating T lymphocytes is reduced in protein-energy malnutrition (Figure 12) (Kulapongs et al., 1977). In particular, T4+ helper cells are more

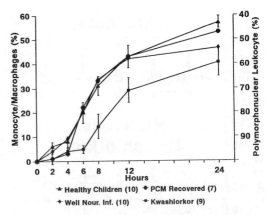

Figure 9. In vivo macrophage and polymorphonuclear leukocyte chemotactic response in children of different nutritional status. Leukocyte mobilization was assessed from Rebuck skin windows as described in Edelman et al., 1977. PCM recovered, children successfully treated for protein-calorie malnutrition; well nour. inf., clinically well nourished children suffering from febrile illnesses resulting from various bacterial infections. The numbers of patients tested are shown in parentheses.

depleted than T8+ suppressor cells, which significantly decreases the helper/suppressor ratio (Chandra, 1983e; Chandra et al., 1982). Peripheral blood lymphocytes of malnourished children have a diminished response to mitogen stimulation (Figure 13) (Chandra, 1975b; Smythe et al., 1971; Law et al., 1973; Work et al., 1973; Kulapongs et al., 1977; Sellmeyer et al., 1972). There is evidence that some factor or factors present in the serum of malnourished children can inhibit in vitro lymphocyte transformation (Chandra, 1974; Smythe et al., 1971; Moore et al., 1974). The effects of malnutrition on the production of cytokines (soluble mediators released by monocytes and macrophages -- monokines, or lymphocytes -- lymphokines) are varied: e.g. the monokine interleukin 1 production and activity appear to be depressed, while those of the lymphokine interleukin 2 appear to be normal (Hoffman-Goetz, 1988).

While protein-energy malnutrition generally depresses the cell-mediated immune response, its effects on the humoral immune response are more equivocal. Circulating immunoglobulins are present in normal or elevated concentrations (Figure 14) (Aref et al., 1970; Neumann et al., 1975; Chandra, 1977; Johansson et al., 1968; Keet and Thom, 1969; Suskind et al., 1977). B cells are present in normal or elevated numbers (Kulapongs et

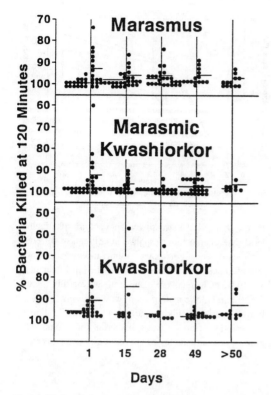

Figure 10. In vitro phagocytosis and killing function by leukocytes collected form children hospitalized and treated for three forms of protein-calorie malnutrition. Bacterial killing function was assessed from viability counts of *Escherichia coli* added to leukocyte-enriched plasma fractions as described in Leitzmann et al., 1977. Values below 88% are considered abnormal.

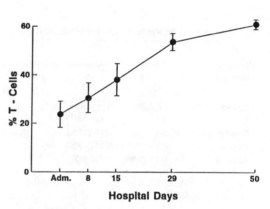

C. albicans Skin-Test Recall Response

Day tested	No. of patients	Skin-test response * Positive	Negative	Accumulated % positive
1	14	2	12	14
29	12	8[+]	4	72
70	4	3[+]	1	92

* Skin tests read 2 days after 0.1 ml 1/100 antigen injected intradermally; positive = 5 mm induration.

[+] Significantly different from proportion on day 1: $X^2 = 6.12$, $p \leq 0.02$ for day 29; $X^2 = 9.1$, $p < 0.01$ for day 70.

Figure 11. Skin-test recall response to injected *Candida albicans* antigen in children hospitalized and treated for protein-calorie malnutrition. Data are from admission and two points during the nutritional intervention, as reported in Edelman et al., 1973.

Figure 12. Increase in T-cell percentage during nutritional intervention in children hospitalized and treated for protein-calorie malnutrition. T-cell percentage in a control group of children was 57.3 ± 3.7%. From Kulapongs et al., 1977.

al., 1977). It is probable that increased exposure of the malnourished child to infectious agents causes elevated immunoglobulin production, or that suppression of the T-suppressor cells results in uncontrolled nonspecific antibody production (Suskind et al., 1977).

Antibody response to stimulation by various antigens is varied in malnourished children: responses to some antigens, e.g. vaccines for yellow fever, influenza, and typhoid, are reduced (Figure 15) (Sirisinha et al., 1975); responses to measles, polio virus, tetanus, and diphtheria toxoid appear to be adequate (Brown and Katz, 1966; Jose et al., 1970; Reddy and Srikantia, 1964; Scrimshaw et al., 1968). The presence of infection further suppresses antibody synthesis (Jose et al., 1970). The antibody response improves with nutritional repletion.

Protein-energy malnutrition depresses mucosal immunity (Chandra, 1977; 1983c; 1983d; 1989b; Suskind et al., 1977). The concentration of secretory IgA is decreased in nasopharyngeal and salivary secretions of malnourished children (Figure 16) (Sirisinha et al., 1975; Chandra, 1975a; Reddy et al., 1976) and its response to live attenuated measles and polio vaccines is reduced (Chandra, 1975a). It is possible that IgA synthesis is compromised or that mucosal secretion is impaired. Secretory component, which protects IgA from proteolysis, may be affected in malnutrition (Darip et al., 1979; Watson et al., 1985). Other gastrointestinal

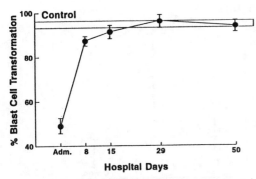

Figure 13. Increase of in vitro lymphocyte mitogenic response to phytohemagglutinin (PHA) during nutritional intervention in children hospitalized and treated for second- and third-degree protein-calorie malnutrition. From Kulapongs et al., 1977.

changes accompanying malnutrition that may compromise intestinal immune protection include gut wall atrophy, reduction in digestive enzymes, and an altered hepatic reticuloendothelial system (Chandra, 1977).

Single nutrient deficiencies

Many studies have demonstrated that single nutrient deficiencies have deleterious effects on immune function (Gershwin et al., 1985; Beisel, 1982; Beisel et al., 1981; Bendich et al., 1990; Chandra, 1983a; Chandra and Puri, 1985; Gershwin et al, 1983; Gross and Newberne, 1980). Such nutritional deficiencies are most often found in pregnant women, the elderly, premature, or obese, or those with chronic illness. General malnutrition also encompasses many specific nutritional deficiencies, whose individual effects on immune function are only recently being distinguished (Suskind, 1992).

Because iron is essential to several metabolic processes, a deficiency in this element affects many tissues, as well as several immune reactions. Iron deficiency is the most frequently occurring isolated nutritional deficiency; pregnant or lactating women, infants, adolescents, and the elderly are most at risk of developing iron deficiency. Lymphocyte proliferation in response to antigens or mitogens is reduced in iron-deficient patients (Chandra, 1983b; Beisel, 1982; Bhaskaram, 1988). The intracellular bactericidal activity of phagocytic cells is also decreased (Arbeter et al, 1971; Chandra, 1973; Macdougall et al., 1975). Serum immunoglobulin and complement appear to be relatively unaffected by iron deficiency (Beisel et al., 1981).

The importance of adequate zinc to immune function is evidenced by immune abnormalities and greater vulnerability to infection in persons with low serum zinc concentrations (Sandstead et al., 1976). Acrodermatitis enteropathica is characterized by impaired intestinal absorption of zinc, leading to zinc deficiency which is accompanied by multiple immunodeficiencies and greater susceptibility to infection. Treatment with supplemental zinc restores immune function (Hambridge, 1977). Alterations in immune tissues and responses associated with zinc deficiency include lymphoid atrophy, reduction in mitogen-stimulated lymphocyte proliferation, impaired delayed cutaneous hypersensitivity, fewer lymphocytes, reduced T4+ helper proportions, and diminished phagocytic activity (Allen et al., 1981; Chvapil et al., 1977; Cunningham-Rundles et al., 1979; Frost et al., 1977; Pekarek et al., 1979). Excessive zinc also disrupts immune function (Chandra, 1984b), an observation which suggests a role for zinc in immune regulation.

Selenium is essential to the activity of the antioxidant glutathione peroxidase; it is also an activator of vitamin E in cell membranes. Selenium deficiency is rare in humans, but can occur after prolonged intravenous hyperalimentation without selenium supplementation. In certain regions of China and New Zealand, the selenium content of the soil is very low, and the populations in those areas may suffer from selenium deficiency. In these persons antibody production, phagocytic bactericidal capacity, and thymic hormone activity are impaired (Fletcher et al., 1988).

Vitamins

Isolated vitamin deficiencies are also rare in developed nations, but may be found in association with malnutrition in developing areas. This is the case with vitamin A, where the deficiency is accompanied by increased vulnerability to infection (Vyas and Chandra, 1984). Experimental animals deprived of vitamin A are susceptible to viral infections from which there is a significant mortality (Bang et al., 1975).

The dietary requirement for vitamin E is linked to the quantity of dietary oxidizable fatty acids (RDA, 1980). It functions as an antioxidant in the intracellular milieu as well as among the lipids of cell membranes, where it protects against lipid peroxidation. The necessity of vitamin E for lymphocyte and mononuclear cell function has been demonstrated in experimental animals (Bendich, 1988), and vitamin E supplements enhance

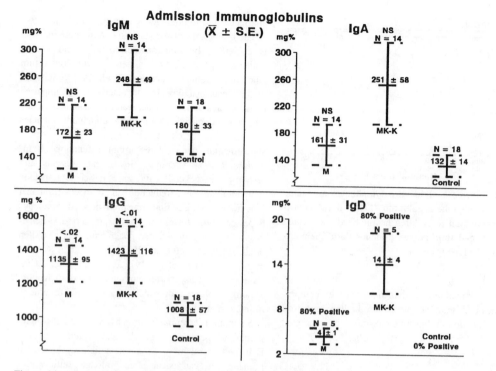

Figure 14. Admission levels of serum immunoglobulins in children hospitalized for marasmus (M), or marasmus-kwashiorkor or kwashiorkor (MK-K, pooled values), as compared to clinically well nourished children hospitalized for various viral or bacterial infections (control). From Suskind et al., 1977.

immune function. As with zinc, excessive vitamin E supplementation may depress the immune response (Beisel, 1982).

Deficiencies of B vitamins disrupt a wide range of immune reactions, reflecting the critical role of these nutrients in nutrient metabolism and nucleic acid synthesis. There is a reduced antibody response to vaccination in persons with deficiencies of thiamin, riboflavin, pantothenic acid, and biotin (Beisel, 1982; Hodges et al., 1962). A deficiency of pyridoxine, which is essential to both nucleic acid and protein synthesis, causes lymphoid tissue atrophy and impairment of cell-mediated and humoral response to test antigens (Beisel, 1982). Similarly, folic acid and vitamin B12 deficiencies also reduce cell-mediated and humoral immune responsiveness (Beisel, 1982).

Antioxidant nutrients

Antioxidant nutrients counteract the damaging oxidative effects on macromolecules and biological membranes

exerted by highly reactive oxygen free radicals (Bendich et al., 1990; Parke, 1982). These nutrients include vitamins A, C, and E, the provitamin ß-carotene, and the trace elements copper, and -- combined with antioxidant enzymes -- zinc, iron, manganese, and selenium (Bendich, 1990). The immune response, involving rapid cell division as well as intracellular communication by means of membrane receptors, is highly sensitive to oxidative membrane damage by free radicals (Bendich, 1990). In addition, controlled generation and release of oxygen free radicals by macrophages and neutrophils (the oxidative burst) is an important part of host defense, as is generation by free radical reactions of the inflammatory mediators prostaglandins and leukotrienes. Antioxidant enzymes and vitamins are critical to the delicate balance between effective host protection and membrane damage. Impairment of phagocytic function, cell-mediated immune reactions, and humoral immune response are associated with dietary deficiency of antioxidant nutrients, and supplementation with these nutrients consistently enhances immunocompetence in experimental animal models (Bendich, 1990).

Typhoid H- Antibody Response

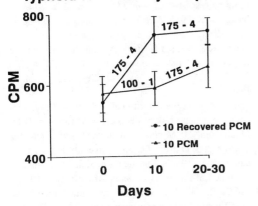

Figure 15. Humoral antibody response in counts per minute to intradermally injected killed typhoid antigen in children hospitalized and treated for protein-calorie malnutrition (PCM) as compared to children recovered from PCM. Baseline H-antibody titers were measured and children were immunized with antigen on admission (day 0). The children were nutritionally rehabilitated with either 100 or 175 calories/kg body weight/day plus 1 or 4 g protein/kg body weight/day, as shown above the lines. From Suskind et al., 1977.

Composition of Nasal Washing

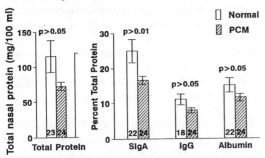

Figure 16. Proteins present in nasal washings of mal-nourished (PCM) and well nourished (normal) children. The numbers of children measured are at the bottoms of the bars. Secretory IgA (SIgA) is the predominant protein present in nasal washings of both groups, and is the only protein significantly decreased in children with PCM. From Sirisinha et al., 1975.

SUMMARY

Protein-energy malnutrition as well as single nutrient deficiencies can seriously compromise the host's immune system. The resulting infection and disease in turn increase the nutritional deficits. This cycle of malnutrition, increased host susceptibility to infection, and disease is responsible for staggering morbidity and mortality in the developing world, and insidious secondary immunodeficiency in the industrial world. Recognizing the interaction between nutrient deficiency and the immune response is an important first step in dealing with most significant causes of secondary immunodeficiency.

REFERENCES

Allen J.L., N.E. Kay & C.J. McClain 1981. Severe zinc deficiency in humans: Association with a reversible T-lymphocyte dysfunction. *Ann. Intern. Med.* 95: 154.

Arbeter A., L. Echeverri, D. Franco et al. 1971. Nutrition and infection. *Fed. Proc.* 30: 1421.

Aref G.H., K. El-Din & A.J. Hassan 1970. Immunoglobulins in kwashiorkor. *J. Trop. Med. Hyg.* 73: 186.

Bang F.B., B.G. Bang & M. Foard 1975. Acute Newcastle virus infection of the upper respiratory tract of the chicken. II. The effect of diets deficient in vitamin A on the pathogenesis of the infection. *Am. J. Pathol.* 78: 417.

Beisel W.R. 1982. Single nutrients and immunity. *Am. J. Clin. Nutr.* 35 [Suppl]: 417.

Beisel W.R., R. Edelman, K. Nauss et al. 1981. Single-nutrient effects on immunologic functions *J. Am. Med. Assoc.* 245: 53.

Bellanti J.A. 1985. *Immunology III.* Philadelphia: W.B. Saunders

Bellanti J.A., A.L. Boner & E. Valletta 1987. Immunology of the fetus and newborn. In Avery G.B. (ed.) *Neonatology* 3rd ed: 850. Philadelphia: J.B. Lippincott.

Bendich A. 1988, Antioxidant vitamins and immune responses. In Chandra R.K. (ed.) *Nutrition and Immunology*: 125. New York: Alan R. Liss.

Bendich A. 1990. Antioxidant micronutrients and immune responses. *Ann. N.Y. Acad. Sci.* 587: 168.

Bendich A., M. Phillips & R.P. Tengerdy eds. 1990. *Antioxidant Nutrients and Immune Functions*, New York: Plenum Press.

Bhaskaram P. 1988, Immunology of iron-deficient subjects. In Chandra R.K. (ed.) *Nutrition and Immunology*: 149. New York: Alan R. Liss.

Brown R.E. & M. Katz 1966. Failure of antibody production to yellow fever vaccine in children with kwashiorkor. *Trop. Geogr. Med.* 18: 125.

Calloway D.H. 1982. Functional consequences of malnutrition. *Rev. Infect. Dis.* 4: 736.

Casey J., W.R. Flinn & J.S.T. Yao 1983. Correlation of immune and nutritional status with wound complications in patients undergoing vascular operations. *Surgery* 93: 822.

Chandra R.K. 1972. Immunocompetence in undernutrition. *J. Pediatr.* 81: 1194.

Chandra R.K. 1973. Reduced bactericidal capacity of polymorphs in iron deficiency. *Arch. Dis. Child.* 48: 864.

Chandra R.K. 1974. Rosette-forming T lymphocytes and cell-mediated immunity in malnutrition. *Br. Med. J.* 3: 608.

Chandra R.K. 1975a. Reduced secretory antibody response to live attenuated measles and poliovirus vaccine in malnourished children. *Br. Med. J.* 2: 583.

Chandra R.K. 1975b. Fetal malnutrition and postnatal immunocompetence. *Am. J. Dis. Child.* 129: 450.

Chandra R.K. 1977. Immunoglobulins and antibody response in protein-calorie malnutrition. In R.M. Suskind (ed.) *Malnutrition and the immune response:* 155. New York: Raven Press.

Chandra R.K. 1981a. Serum thymic hormone activity and cell-mediated immunity in healthy neonates, pre-term infants and small-for-gestational-age infants. *Pediatrics* 67: 407.

Chandra R.K. 1981b. Immunocompetence as a functional index of nutritional status *Br. Med. Bull.* 37: 89.

Chandra R.K. 1981c. Immunodeficiency in undernutrition and overnutrition. *Nutr. Rev.* 39: 225.

Chandra R.K. 1983a. Trace elements and immune responses. *Immunol. Today* 4: 322.

Chandra R.K. 1983b. Nutrition, immunity, and infection: Present knowledge and future directions. *Lancet* 1: 688.

Chandra R.K. 1983c. Nutritional regulation of immunity and infection in the gastrointestinal tract. *J. Pediatr. Gastroenterol. Nutr.* 2(Suppl 1): S181.

Chandra R.K. 1983d. Mucosal immune responses in malnutrition. *Ann. N. Y. Acad. Sci.* 409: 345.

Chandra R.K. 1983e. Numerical and functional deficiency in T helper cells in protein-calorie malnutrition. *Clin. Exp. Immunol.* 51: 126.

Chandra R.K. 1984a. Nutritional regulation of immune function at the extremes of life: in infants and in the elderly. In P.L. White & N. Selvey (eds.) *Malnutrition: determinants and consequences:* 245. New York: Alan R. Liss.

Chandra R.K. 1984b. Excessive intake of zinc impairs immune responses. *J. Am. Med. Assoc.* 252: 1443.

Chandra R.K 1985. *Nutrition, immunity and illness in the elderly.* New York: Pergamon Press.

Chandra R.K. 1988. Effects of overnutrition on immune responses and risk of disease. In R.K. Chandra (ed.) *Nutrition and immunology:* 315. New York: Alan R. Liss.

Chandra R.K. 1989a. Nutritional regulation of immunocompetence and risk of disease. In A. Horwitz, D.M. Macfadyen, H. Munro et al. (eds.) *Nutrition in the elderly:* 203. Oxford: Oxford University Press.

Chandra R.K. 1989b. Nutritional modulation of intestinal mucosal immunity. *Immunol. Invest.* 18: 119.

Chandra R.K. 1992a. Nutrition and immunoregulation. Significance for host resistance to tumors and infectious diseases in humans and rodents. *J. Nutr.* 122: 754.

Chandra R.K. 1992b. Protein-energy malnutrition and immunological responses. *J. Nutr.* 122: 597.

Chandra R.K & T. Matsumura 1979. Ontogenic development of the immune system and effects of fetal growth retardation. *J. Perinat. Med.* 7: 279.

Chandra R.K. & S. Puri 1985. Trace element modulation of immune responses and susceptibility to infection. In R.K. Chandra (ed.) *Trace elements in nutrition of children:* 87. New York: Raven Press.

Chandra R.K. & N.S. Scrimshaw 1980. Immunocompetence in nutritional assessment. *Am. J. Clin. Nutr.* 33: 2694.

Chandra R.K., S. Gupta & H. Singh 1982. Inducer & suppressor T-cell subsets in protein-energy malnutrition: analysis by monoclonal antibodies. *Nutr.Res.* 2: 21.

Chvapil M., L. Stankova, P. Weldy et al. 1977. The role of zinc in the function of some inflammatory cells. In E.J. Brewer & A.S. Prasad (eds.) *Zinc metabolism: current aspects in health and disease:* 103. New York: Alan R. Liss.

Coovadia H.M., M.A. Parent, W.E.K. Loening et al. 1974. An evaluation of factors associated with the depression of immunity in malnutrition and in measles. *Am. J. Clin. Nutr.* 27: 665.

Cunningham-Rundles C., S. Cunningham-Rundles, J. Garafolo et al. 1979. Increased T lymphocyte function and thymopoietin following zinc repletion in man. *Fed. Proc.* 38: 1222.

Darip M.D., S. Sirisinha & A.L. Lamb 1979. Effect of vitamin A deficiency on susceptibility of rats to *Angiostrongylus cantonensis. Proc. Soc. Exp. Biol. Med.* 161: 600.

deShazo R.D., M. Lopez & J.E. Salvaggio 1987. Use and interpretation of diagnostic immunologic laboratory tests. *J. Am. Med. Assoc.* 258: 3011.

DHEW: U.S. Department of Health Education and Welfare 1972. Ten State Nutrition Survey 1968-1970. Publications 72: 8131, 8132, 8133. Atlanta: Centers for Disease Control.

Douglas S.R. & K. Schopfer 1977. The phagocyte in protein-calorie malnutrition. In R. Suskind (ed.) *Malnutrition and the immune response*: 231. New York: Raven Press.

Edelman R., P. Kulapongs, R.M. Suskind & R.E. Olson 1977. Leukocyte mobilization in Thai children with kwashiorkor. In R.M. Suskind (ed.) *Malnutrition and the immune response*: 265. New York: Raven Press.

Edelman R., R.M. Suskind & R.E. Olson 1973. Mechanisms of defective delayed cutaneous hypersensitivity in children with protein-calorie malnutrition. *Lancet* 1: 506.

Feldman G. & C.A. Gianantonio 1972. Aspectos immunologicos de la desnutricion en el nino. *Medicina* 32: 1.

Ferguson A., G. Lawlor, L. Neumann et al. 1974. Decreased rosette-forming lymphocytes in malnutrition and intrauterine growth retardation. *Trop. Pediatr.* 85: 717,

Fletcher M.P., M.E. Gershwin, C.L. Keen et al. 1988. Trace element deficiencies and immune responsiveness in human and animal models. In R.K. Chandra (ed.) *Nutrition and immunology*: 215. New York: Alan R. Liss.

Frost P., J.C. Chem, I. Rabbani et al. 1977. The effect of zinc deficiency on the immune response. In G.J. Brewer & A.S. Prasad (eds.) *Zinc metabolism: current aspects in heath and disease*: 143. New York: Alan R. Liss.

Gershwin M.E., R. Beach & L. Hurley 1983. Trace metals, aging and immunity. *J. Am. Geriatr. Soc.* 31: 374.

Gershwin M.E., R.S. Beach & L.S. Hurley 1985. *Nutrition and immunity*. Orlando: Academic Press.

Ghavami H., W. Dutz, M. Mohallatee et al. 1979. Immune disturbances after severe enteritis during the first six months of life. *Isr. J. Med. Sci.* 15: 364.

Gibson R.S. 1990. *Principles of nutritional assessment*. Oxford: Oxford University Press.

Gross R.L. & P.M. Newberne 1980. Role of nutrition in immunologic function. *Physiol. Rev.* 60: 188.

Hambridge K.M. 1977. The role of zinc in the pathogenesis and treatment of acrodermatitis enteropathica. In G.J. Brewer & A.S. Prasad (eds.) *Zinc metabolism: current aspects in health and disease*: 329. New York: Alan R. Liss.

Harland P.S.E.B. 1965. Tuberculin reactions in malnourished children. *Lancet* 2: 719.

Hodges R.E., W.B. Bean, M.A. Ohlson et al. 1962. Factor affecting human antibody response. V. Combined deficiencies of pantothenic acid and pyridoxin. *Am. J. Clin. Nutr.* 11: 187.

Hoffman-Goetz L. 1988. Lymphokines and monokines in protein-energy malnutrition. In R.K. Chandra (ed.) *Nutrition and immunology*: 9. New York: Alan R. Liss.

Jackson C.M. 1925. *The effects of inanition and malnutrition upon growth and structure*. London: P. Blakiston's Son.

Jayalakshmi V.T. & C. Gopalan 1958. Nutrition and tuberculosis I. An epidemiological study. *Indian J. Med. Res.* 46: 87.

Johansson S.G., T. Melbin & B. Vahlquist 1968. Immunoglobulin levels in Ethiopian preschool children with specific reference to high concentration of immunoglobulin E(IgND). *Lancet* 1: 1118.

Jose D.G., J.S. Welch & R.L. Doherty 1970. Humoral and cellular immune responses to streptococci, influenza, and other antigens in Australian Aboriginal school children. *Aust. Paediatr. J.* 6: 192.

Keet M.P. & H. Thom 1969. Serum immunoglobulins in kwashiorkor. *Arch. Dis. Child.* 44: 600.

Klein K., R.M. Suskind, P. Kulapongs, G. Mertz, R.E. Olson 1977. Endotoxemia, a possible cause of decreased complement activity in malnourished Thai children. In R.M. Suskind (ed.) *Malnutrition and the immune response*: 321. New York: Raven Press.

Kulapongs P., R. Suskind, V. Vithayasai et al. 1977. In vitro cell-mediated immune response in Thai children with protein-calorie malnutrition. In R. Suskind (ed.) *Malnutrition and the immune response*: 99. New York: Raven Press.

Law D.K., S.J. Dudrick & N.I. Abdou 1973. Immunocompetence of patients with protein-calorie malnutrition. The effects of nutritional repletion. *Ann. Intern. Med.* 79: 545.

Leitzmann C., V. Vithayasai, P. Windecker, R.M. Suskind, R.E. Olson 1977. Phagocytosis and killing function of polymorphonuclear leukocytes in Thai children with protein-calorie malnutrition. In R.M. Suskind (ed.) *Malnutrition and the immune response*: 253. New York: Raven Press.

Macdougall L.G., R. Anderson, G.M. McNab et al. 1975. The immune response in iron-deficient children: Impaired cellular defense mechanisms with altered humoral components. *J. Pediatr.* 86: 833.

McMurray D.N., S.A. Loomis, L.J. Casazza et al. 1981. Development of impaired cell-mediated immunity in mild and moderate malnutrition. *Am. J. Clin. Nutr.* 34: 68.

Moore D.L., B. Heyworth & J. Brown 1974. PHA-induced lymphocyte transformation in leukocyte cultures from malarious malnourished and control Gambian children. *Clin. Exp. Immunol.* 17: 647.

Mugerwa J.W. 1971. The lymphoreticular system in kwashiorkor. *J. Pathol.* 105: 105.

Neumann C.G., G.J. Lawlow, M.E. Stiehm et al. 1975. Immunologic responses in malnourished children. *Am. J. Clin. Nutr.* 89: 104.

Parke D.V. 1982. Mechanisms of chemical toxicity -- a unifying hypothesis. *Regul. Toxicol. Pharmacol.* 2: 267.

Paul W.E. 1989a. *Fundamental Immunology*. 2nd ed. New York: Raven Press.

Paul W.E. 1989b. The immune system: an introduction. In W.E. Paul (ed.) *Fundamental immunology*. 2nd ed: 3. New York: Raven Press.

Pekarek R.S., H.H. Sandstead, R.A. Jacob et al. 1979. Abnormal cellular immune responses during acquired zinc deficiency. *Am. J. Clin. Nutr.* 32: 1466.

Puri S. & R.K. Chandra 1985. Nutritional regulation of host resistance and predictive value of immunologic test in assessment of outcome. *Pediatr. Clin. North Am.* 32: 499.

RDA, Committee on Dietary Allowances, Food Nutrition Board, National Research Council: 1980. Recommended Dietary Allowances, 9th ed., National Academy Press, Washington.

Reddy V. & S.G. Srikantia 1964. Antibody response in kwashiorkor. *Indian. J. Med. Res.* 53: 1154.

Reddy V., N. Raghuramulu, C. Bhaskaram 1976. Secretory IgA in protein-calorie malnutrition. *Arch. Dis. Child.* 51: 871.

Roitt V., J. Brostoff & D. Male 1989. *Immunology*. London: Gower Medical Publishing.

Rosen E.U., J. Geefhuysen, R. Anderson et al. 1975. Leukocyte function in children with kwashiorkor. *Arch. Dis. Child.* 50: 220.

Sandstead H.H., K.P. Vo Khactu & N.W. Solomons 1976. Conditioned zinc deficiencies. In A.S. Prasad (ed.) *Trace Elements in Human Health and Disease*: Vol 1: 33. New York: Academic Press.

Scrimshaw N.S. 1989. Epidemiology of nutrition of the aged. In A. Horwitz, D.M. Macfayden, H. Munro et al. (eds.) *Nutrition in the elderly*: 3. Oxford: Oxford University Press.

Scrimshaw N.S., C.E. Taylor & J.E. Gordon 1968. Interactions of Nutrition and Infection. WHO Monograph Series 57, WHO: Geneva.

Sellmeyer E., E. Bhettay, A.S. Truswell et al. 1972. Lymphocyte transformation in malnourished children. *Arch. Dis. Child.* 47: 429.

Selvaraj R.J. & K.S. Bhat 1972. Metabolic and bactericidal activities of leukocytes in protein-calorie malnutrition. *Am. J. Clin. Nutr.* 25: 166.

Seth V. & R.K. Chandra 1972. Opsonic activity, phagocytosis, and bactericidal capacity of polymorphs in undernutrition. *Arch. Dis. Child.* 47: 282.

Sirisinha S., R. Edelman, R. Suskind et al. 1973. Complement and C3-proactivator levels in children with protein-calorie malnutrition and effect of dietary treatment. *Lancet* 1: 1016.

Sirisinha S., R. Suskind, R. Edelman et al. 1975. Secretory and serum IgA in children with protein-calorie malnutrition. *Pediatrics* 55: 166.

Sirisinha S., R. Suskind, R. Edelman et al. 1977. The complement systems in protein-calorie malnutrition. In R. Suskind (ed.) *Malnutrition and the immune response*: 309. New York: Raven Press.

Smythe P.M., G.G. Brereton-Stiles, H.J. Grace et al. 1971. Thymolymphatic deficiency and depression of cell-mediated immunity in protein-calorie malnutrition. *Lancet* 2: 939.

Solomons N.W. 1985. Assessment of nutritional status: Functional indicators of pediatric nutriture. *Pediatr. Clin. North. Am.* 32: 319.

Solomons N.W. & L.H. Allen 1983. The functional assessment of nutritional status: Principles, practice and potential. *Nutr. Rev.* 41: 33.

Suskind R. 1977. *Malnutrition and the immune response*. New York: Raven Press.

Suskind R.M. 1992. Immunologic mechanisms and the role of nutrition. In A.B Tarcher (ed.) *The principles and practice of environmental medicine*: 159. New York: Plenum Medical Book Company.

Suskind R., S. Sirisinha, R. Edelman et al. 1977. Immunoglobulins and antibody response in Thai children with protein-calorie malnutrition. In R. Suskind (ed.) *Malnutrition and the immune response*: 185. New York: Raven Press.

Suskind D., K.K. Murthy & R.M. Suskind 1990. The malnourished child: An overview. In R.M. Suskind & L. Lewinter-Suskind (eds.) *The malnourished child*. Nestlé Nutrition Workshop Series, vol. 19: 1. New York: Raven Press.

Tanphiachitr P., V. Meknanandha & A. Valyasevi 1973. Impaired pla/sma opsonic activity in malnourished children. *J. Med. Assoc. Thai.* 56: 118.

UNEP: United Nations Environmental Programme and United Nations Children's Fund. *Children and the environment: the state of the environment*. New York: United Nations.

Vos J.C. & M.I. Luster 1989. Immune alterations. In R.D. Kimbrough & A.A. Jensen (eds.) *Halogenated biphenyls, terphenyls, naphthalenes, dibenzodioxins and related products.* 2nd ed: 275. Amsterdam: Elsevier.

Vyas D. & R.K. Chandra 1984. Vitamin A and immunocompetence. In R.R. Watson (ed.) *Nutrition, disease resistance, and immune function*: 325. New York: Marcel Dekker.

Watson R.R. 1984. *Nutrition, disease resistance, and immune function*. New York: Marcel Dekker.

Watson, R.R., D.N. McMurray, P. Martin et al. 1985. Effect of age, malnutrition and renutrition on free secretory component and IgA in secretions. *Am. J. Clin. Nutr.* 42: 281.

Weir D.M. 1983. *Immunology*. 6th ed. Edinburgh: Churchill Livingstone.

Weksler M.E. 1986. Biological basis and clinical significance of immune senescence. In I. Rossman (ed.) *Clinical Geriatrics*. 3rd ed: 57. Philadelphia: J.B. Lippincott.

Work T.H., A. Ifewunigwe, D.B. Jelliffe et al. 1973. Tropical problems in nutrition. *Ann. Intern. Med.* 79: 701.

Ziegler H.D. & P.B. Ziegler 1975. Depression of tuberculin reaction in mild and moderate protein calorie malnourished children following BCG vaccination. *Johns Hopkins Med. J.* 137: 59.

6 Diet, atherosclerosis and cardiovascular risk factors

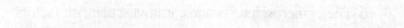

Dairy Products in Human Health and Nutrition, Serrano Rios et al. (eds) © 1994 Balkema, Rotterdam, ISBN 90 5410 359 0

Genetic and environmental factors: Effects on plasma lipoproteins

J.M.Ordovas
Lipid Metabolism Laboratory, USDA Human Nutrition Research Center on Aging at Tufts University, Boston, Mass., USA

ABSTRACT: Individual responses to dietary factors vary depending upon the individual's genetic makeup. It has been shown that genetic variation at several candidate genes, namely apolipoprotein A-I, A-IV, B, and E, have a significant effect on plasma lipid levels and dietary response. Knowledge in this important area will allow in the future a more individualized approach to the treatment of dyslipidemias and prevention of coronary heart disease. Until more complete information is available, the current recommendations regarding a prudent diet in the general population appear reasonable.

INTRODUCTION

The study of the interaction between genetic an environmental factors and the effect on plasma lipoproteins is attracting increased attention from basic and clinical scientists.

Genetic mutations affecting the primary protein structure have been found in most human plasma apolipoproteins, low density lipoprotein (LDL) receptor, lipolytic enzymes and transfer proteins. Some of these mutations are rare, and although they may have a great impact on the development of hyperlipidemia and coronary artery disease (CAD) for an individual, they have little impact in the population. For the most part, common mutations have a relatively small effect in the individual, but because of their high frequency, they may affect significantly the prevalence of the disease in the general population.

Many other mutations have been detected in candidate genes that do not affect the sequence of the translated gene product. Some of these polymorphisms have been associated with variable strength to different lipid abnormalities and or coronary artery disease risk.

Here we will focus on the impact of some common polymorphisms on lipid and lipoproteins levels and how the effect of these variants may be modulated by environmental factors.

APOLIPOPROTEIN A-I

ApoA-I is the major protein component of plasma high density lipoproteins (HDL). In addition to its role as a carrier of lipids in plasma, apoA-I is an activator of the enzyme lecithin:cholesterol acyltransferase (LCAT) and plays a key role in reverse cholesterol transport. Low levels of HDL and apoA-I, or apoA-I absence, have been associated with premature atherosclerosis.

ApoA-I is polymorphic in humans; a number of structural variants have been identified by isoelectric focusing. Their characterization has contributed to our knowledge of structure-function relationships and the role of apoA-I in the mechanisms leading to dyslipidemia and atherosclerosis.

Several studies in the last 10 years have examined the association of restriction fragment length polymorphisms (RFLPs) in the apoA-I/C-III/A-IV gene cluster with lipid, lipoprotein and apolipoprotein levels as well as CAD risk (Ordovas et al.1991a). The S2 allele of the SstI RFLP 3' to the apoC-III gene has been found associated with higher triglyceride levels and sometimes higher CAD risk in most Caucasian populations. The molecular basis responsible for this quantitative variation has not been defined. This mutation is present in the noncoding region of the gene and consequently is not responsible by itself of changes in the primary structure of the gene product. However, it has been reported that the rare S2 allele is significantly associated with higher levels of apoC-III. This finding provides a mechanistic interpretation to the hyperlipidemia associated with the S2 allele, as apoCIII is an inhibitor of the enzyme lipoprotein lipase (Shoulders et al.1991). The different strength of this association reported in previous studies, as well as the apparent lack of effect observed in Oriental populations suggests that the impact of this genetic polymorphism may be affected by environmental variables. Other RFLPs at these loci have been also reported to affect lipid levels and CAD risk. However, the results are less consistent. Thus a PstI polymorphism 3' to the apoA-I gene has been associated with hypoalphalipoproteinemia and high CAD risk in some in studies but not in others (Ordovas et al.1986; Ordovas et al.1991b). Another interesting mutation is the A→G transition polymorphism in the apoA-I promoter region. It has been reported that the A allele is significantly associated with higher levels of apoA-I in men and women (Pagani et al.1990), although using a functional assay for this mutation, the molecular basis for this observation could not be substantiated (Smith et al.1992). An intriguing interaction between this polymorphism and smoking has been shown. The increase in HDL levels associated with the A allele was present in men who did not smoke but was totally abolished in smokers, and no effect was observed in females. This interaction gene-smoking may explain the discrepancies observed in some studies (Sigurdsson et al.1992).

APOLIPOPROTEIN A-IV

ApoA-IV is synthesized primarily in the intestine and secreted into the lymph as part of newly synthesized chylomicrons. The function of apoA-IV remains largely unknown. In vitro, apoA-IV activates the enzyme lecithin cholesterol acyl transferase (LCAT) and could have a regulatory effect on lipoprotein lipase. In addition, it has been hypothesized that apoA-IV could play an important role in reverse cholesterol transport. No mutants exclusively lacking apoA-IV have been described; however, in one kindred in which apoA-I, apoC-III and apoA-IV were missing in the proband, HDL was absent, and mild essential fatty acid and liposoluble vitamin deficiencies were observed (Ordovas et al.1989).

ApoA-IV is polymorphic in humans. Five different isoforms have been identified using one and two dimensional isoelectric focusing and immunoblotting. ApoA-IV-1 and apoA-IV-2 are the most frequent isoforms and have been found in all Caucasian populations studied, with allele frequencies of 0.9 and 0.08 respectively (Menzel et al.1990; Menzel et al.1988; de Knijff et al.1988). The molecular basis of this polymorphism has been elucidated, and it is due to a single point mutation which converts the glutamine at position 360 of the mature protein to a histidine. This mutation takes place in a region that is highly conserved among different species, namely mouse, rat and human (Lohse et al.1990; Lohse et al.1991).

ApoA-IV polymorphism has been shown to have a significant effect on plasma HDL cholesterol in Tyrolean and in Icelandic populations (Menzel et al.1990; Menzel et al.1988). These data suggest that apoA-IV polymorphism, whether by a direct physiological effect or by linkage disequilibrium of this locus with another locus, such as apoA-I or apoC-III, has a strong impact on HDL cholesterol levels, which may be independent of apoA-IV levels.

We have found in several diet studies that subjects carrying the A-IV-2 allele were less responsive to cholesterol lowering drugs than those homozygotes for the A-IV-1 allele. In addition HDL cholesterol levels in females carrying the A-IV-2 allele were greater than in females homozygotes for the A-IV-1 allele.

APOLIPOPROTEIN B

Genetic variation at the apoB gene locus was first identified using immunological techniques with alloantisera obtained from multiple transfused patients (Berg et al.1986). In addition, binding studies using monoclonal antibodies against various epitopes of apoB100 in patients with primary hypercholesterolemia have demonstrated low affinity for the LDL receptor due to a defective binding site (Innerarity et al.1987). Seventy-five nucleotide differences in the apoB sequence have been identified, 54 of which could result in amino acid substitutions. One of these variants arises from a G→A substitution at nucleotide 10699, which results in a glutamine for arginine substitution at amino acid residue 3500. This mutation has been associated with familial defective apoB100 (FDB), a genetic disorder characterized by moderate to severe hypercholesterolemia. The frequency of this mutation appears to be 1:500 (Innerarity et al.1990).

Numerous RFLPs of the apoB gene have been detected. Those detected with EcoRI, XbaI and PvuII have been associated with different degrees of hyperlipidemia and CAD risk and they may be related to dietary response (Genest et al.1990).

Tikkanen et al. (Tikkanen et al.1990b) have shown in 103 healthy subjects, participants in the North Karelian dietary intervention trial that the XbaI RFLP at this gene locus was not associated like in previous studies with elevated plasma cholesterol.. However after 6 weeks on a low fat, low cholesterol diet, total, LDL and HDL cholesterol decreased more in those subjects in which the XbaI cutting site was missing. This mutation does not affect the amino acid sequence of apoB, suggesting that this RFLP may be in linkage disequilibrium with a functionally important mutation. Another study in this population showed that an apoB RFLP detected with MspI was associated with diet induced changes on apoA-I levels (Miettinen et al.1988). Since this apoB polymorphism was found associated with changes in plasma apoA-I levels rather than apoB levels it is necessary to speculate that the MspI RFLP may be in linkage disequilibrium with some other polymorphic site.

APOLIPOPROTEIN E

ApoE is one of the most important proteins present on chylomicrons and very-low-density lipoproteins (VLDL). ApoE serves as the ligand for the receptor-mediated uptake of chylomicron and VLDL remnants by the liver. ApoE is polymorphic in humans and three of its common variants, E4, E3 and E2 can be identified by isoelectric focusing of the VLDL protein or by a combination of isoelectric focusing and immunoblotting of whole plasma. Other much less common isoforms, the E5, E7, E1, and some E2 and E3 variants, have been reported in population studies. The E3 allele is the most common in the population and codes for a protein with a cysteine residue at position 112 and an arginine at position 158. The E4 allele differs from E3 in a single point mutation, resulting in a cysteine by arginine substitution at position 112. The common E2 allele is the result of a cysteine arginine substitution at position 158. Presence of homozygosity for the E2 allele has been associated with familial dysbetalipoproteinemia due to impaired hepatic removal by the apoB,E and the apoE receptors of chylomicron and VLDL remnants containing this apoE variant (Davignon et al.1988).

In most population studies, apoE variation has been shown to affect total plasma and LDL cholesterol levels. In general, subjects carrying the E4 allele have higher total cholesterol and LDL cholesterol than those carrying the most common E3 allele. Conversely, the E2 allele has been associated with lower levels of these lipid parameters. However the magnitude of these effects varies dramatically among populations (see Figure 1).

These observations suggest that it may be an interaction between genetic variation at this locus and environmental factors such as diet, physical exercise, smoking or alcohol which differ significantly among the populations studied.

Tikkanen et al. (Tikkanen et al.1990a) determined the apoE phenotype in 110 subjects participating in the North Karelian dietary intervention study. These authors demonstrated that subjects homozygous for the E4 allele had significantly higher LDL cholesterol levels while consuming high fat, high cholesterol diets than any other phenotype. In addition these subjects were more responsive to the change to a low

AVERAGE APOE ALLELE EFFECT ON PLASMA CHOLESTEROL

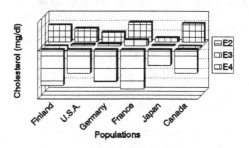

Figure 1

fat, low cholesterol diet. Miettinen et al. (Miettinen et al.1988) showed in 16 men, that those carrying the E4 allele were more responsive than those without E4. Manttari et al. (Manttari et al.1991) found a significant association between response to diet and apoE phenotype in 117 dyslipidemic men participating in the Helsinky Heart Study. The reductions in plasma total cholesterol were significantly greater in those subjects with an E4 allele than in those without.

In agreement with these investigators, we have found in several well controlled diet studies that subjects carrying the E4 allele were more responsive to cholesterol lowering drugs than those with homozygotes for the E3 allele.

These data indicate that the difference between E alleles is more evident when subjects are consuming high fat diets, but the differences are less noticeable when subjects are consuming low fat diets. This observation agrees with the epidemiological data (Figure 1) where it can be seen that the difference in plasma cholesterol levels in countries with high fat intake, such as Finland, is more pronounced than in countries with low dietary fat such as Japan.

CONCLUSIONS

Individual responses to dietary factors vary depending upon the individual's genetic makeup. In the past few years we have gained considerable understanding on how variation in certain genes affect plasma lipid levels and dietary response. However, much more research is needed in this area. Until more complete information is available, the current recommendations regarding a prudent diet in the general population appear reasonable.

REFERENCES

Berg, K., Powell, J.T., Wallis, S., Pease, R., Knott, T.J. and Scott, J. 1986.Genetic linkage between the antigenic group (Ag) variation and the apolipoprotein B gene: assignment of the Ag locus. *Proc Natl Acad Sci USA* 83:7367-7370.

Davignon, J., Gregg, R.E. and Sing, C.F. 1988.Apolipoprotein E polymorphism and atherosclerosis. *Arteriosclerosis* 8:1-21.

de Knijff, P., Rosseneu, M., Beisiegel, U., De Keersgieter, W., Frants, R.R. and Havekes, L.M. 1988.Apolipoprotein A-IV polymorphism and its effect on plasma lipid and apolipoprotein concentrations. *Journal of Lipid Research* 29:1621-1627.

Genest, J.J., Ordovas, J.M., McNamara, J.R., et al. 1990.DNA polymorphisms of the apolipoprotein B gene in patients with premature coronary artery disease. *Atherosclerosis* 82:7-17.

Innerarity, T.L., Weisgraber, K.H., Arnold, K.S., et al. 1987.Familial defective apolipoprotein B-100: low density lipoproteins with abnormal receptor binding. *Proceedings of the National Academy of Sciences of the United States of America* 84:6919-6923.

Innerarity, T.L., Mahley, R.W., Weisgraber, K.H., et al. 1990.Familial defective apolipoprotein B-100: A mutation of apolipoprotein B that causes hypercholesterolemia. *J Lipid Res* 31:1337-1349.

Lohse, P., Kindt, M.R., Rader, D.J. and Brewer, H.B.,Jr. 1990.Genetic polymorphism of human plasma apolipoprotein A-IV gene. *J Biol Chem* 265:10061-10064.

Lohse, P., Kindt, M.R., Rader, D.J. and Brewer, H.B.,Jr. 1991.Three genetic variants of human plasma apolipoprotein A-IV. Apoa-IV-1(Thr³⁴⁷--> Ser), Apoa-IV-0(Lys¹⁶⁷--> Glu, Glu³⁶⁰ --> His), and Apoa-IV-3(Glu¹⁶⁵--> Lys). *J.Biol.Chem.* 266:13513-13518.

Manttari, M., Kosninen, P., Enholm, C., Huttunen, J.K. and Manninen, V. 1991.Apolipoprotein E polymorphism influences the serum cholesterol response to dietary intervention. *Metabolism* 40:217-221.

Menzel, H.J., Boerwinkle, E., Schrangl-Will, S. and Utermann, G. 1988.Human apolipoprotein A-IV polymorphism: frequency and effect on lipid and lipoprotein levels. *Hum Genet* 79:368-372.

Menzel, H.J., Sigurdsson, G., Boerwinkle, E., Schrangl-Will, S., Dieplinger, H. and Utermann, G. 1990.Frequency and effect of human apolipoprotein A-IV polymorphism on lipid and lipoprotein levels in an Icelandic population. *Hum Genet* 84:344-346.

Miettinen, T.A., Gylling, H. and Vanhanen, H. 1988.Serum cholesterol response to dietary cholesterol and apoprotein E phenotype. *Lancet* 2:1261.

Ordovas, J.M., Schaefer, E.J., Salem, D., et al. 1986.Apolipoprotein A-I gene polymorphism associated with premature coronary artery disease and familial hypoalphalipoproteinemia. *N Engl J Med* 314:671-677.

Ordovas, J.M., Cassidy, D.K., Civeira, F., Bisgaier, C.L. and Schaefer, E.J. 1989.Familial apolipoprotein A-I, C-III and A-IV deficiency and premature atherosclerosis due to deletion of a gene complex on chromosome 11. *J Biol Chem* 264:16339-16342.

Ordovas, J.M., Civeira, F., Garces, C. and Pocovi, M. Genetic variation at the apolipoprotein A-I,C-III,A-IV gene complex. In: *DNA Polymorphisms as Disease Markers*, edited by Galton, D.J. Plenum Press, 1991a, p. 91-105.

Ordovas, J.M., Civeira, F., Genest, J.J., et al. 1991b.Restriction fragment length polymorphisms of the apolipoprotein A-I, C-III, A-IV gene locus: Relationships with lipids, apolipoproteins, and premature coronary artery disease. *Atherosclerosis*

Pagani, F., Sidoli, A., Giudici, G.A., Barenghi, L., Vergani, C. and Baralle, F.E. 1990.Human apolipoprotein A-I gene promoter polymorphism: Association with hyperalphalipoproteinemia. *J Lipid Res* 31:1371-1377.

Shoulders, C.C., Harry, P.J., Lagrost, L., et al. 1991.Variation at the apolipoprotein AI/CIII/AIV Gene Complex is associated with elevatedplasma levels of apoCIII. *Atherosclerosis* 87:239-247.

Sigurdsson, G.,Jr., Gudnason, V., Sigurdsson, G. and Humphries, S.E. 1992.Interaction between a polymorphism of the Apo A-I promoter region and smoking determines plasma levels of HDL and Apo A-I. *Arterioscler.Thromb.* 12:1017-1022.

Smith, J.D., Brinton, E.A. and Breslow, J.L. 1992.Polymorphism in the human apolipoprotein A-I gene promoter region. Association of the minor allele with decreased production rate in vivo and promoter activity in vitro. *J.Clin.Invest.* 89:1796-1800.

Tikkanen, M.J., Huttunen, J.K., Enholm, C. and Pietinen, P. 1990a.Apolipoprotein E4 homozygosity predisposes to serum cholesterol elevation during high fat diet. *A rteriosclerosis* 10:285-288.

Tikkanen, M.J., Xu, C.-F., Hamalainen, T., et al. 1990b.XbaI Polymorphism of the apolipoprotein B gene influences plasma lipid response to diet intervention. *Clin Genet* 37:327-334.

Dairy Products in Human Health and Nutrition, Serrano Ríos et al. (eds) © 1994 Balkema, Rotterdam, ISBN 90 5410 359 0

Coronary heart disease: Prevention and treatment by nutritional change

W.E.Connor & S.L.Connor

ABSTRACT: The principal goal of dietary prevention and treatment of coronary heart disease is the achievement of physiological levels of the plasma cholesterol, low density lipoprotein (LDL), triglyceride and very low density lipoproteins (VLDL). This is first accomplished by enhancing LDL receptor activity and at the same time depressing liver synthesis of cholesterol and triglyceride. Both dietary cholesterol and saturated fat decrease LDL receptor activity and inhibit the removal of LDL from the plasma by the liver. Saturated fat decreases LDL receptor activity especially when cholesterol is concurrently present in the diet. The total amount of dietary fat is of importance also. The greater the flux of chylomicron remnants into the liver the greater is the influx of cholesterol ester. In addition, factors which affect VLDL and LDL synthesis could be important. These include excessive calories (obesity) which enhance triglyceride and VLDL and hence LDL synthesis; and weight loss and omega-3 fatty acids which depress synthesis of both VLDL and LDL.

The optimal diet for the treatment of children and adults to prevent coronary disease has the following characteristics: cholesterol (100 mg/day), total fat (20% of kcalories, 6% saturated with the balance from omega-3 and omega-6 polyunsaturated and monounsaturated fat), carbohydrate (65% kcalories, two-thirds from starch including 11 to 15 grams of soluble fiber), and protein (15% kcalories). This low fat, high carbohydrate diet can lower the plasma cholesterol 18 to 21 percent. This diet is also an anti-thrombotic diet, thrombosis being another major consideration in preventing coronary heart disease. Dietary therapy is the mainstay of the prevention and treatment of coronary heart disease through the control of plasma lipid and lipoprotein levels.

Diet greatly affects many of the risk factors which cause coronary heart disease. In fact, nutrition itself must be listed as one of the major risk factors because of its tremendous modifying effects on the disease process, atherosclerosis. The most important risk factor in which diet plays the major role, both in causation and in treatment, is hyperlipidemia (see Figure 1).

Hyperlipidemia is important because it forms the basis for the excessive infiltration of lipid into the arterial intima with atherosclerosis an ultimate consequence. Stage 1 in the development of coronary heart disease is hyperlipidemia or, as depicted in the figure, hypercholesterolemia but this could indicate any abnormality of the plasma lipids-lipoproteins including cholesterol, LDL, VLDL, triglyceride, HDL and the remnants of chylomicrons and VLDL. If hyperlipidemia is not present, then atherosclerosis does not result. Should atherosclerosis be prevented,

then stage 3, coronary heart disease, the clinical expression of this underlying and silent disorder will not occur.

The cause of hyperlipidemia is clearcut for 1% or less of the population. Hyperlipidemia will result regardless of environmental factors because of genetic predisposition. Familial hypercholesterolemia is the classic example of genetic hyperlipidemia but there are many others. For the 99% of the population, dietary factors are crucial in the development of hyperlipidemia. Even dietary factors will affect the hyperlipidemia of genetically based disorders, but, in most instances, will probably not make the situation completely normal. Pharmaceutical agents will be required but these act synergistically with diet.

The second risk factor affected by diet is thrombosis, a critical event in the evolution of the atherosclerotic plaque to complete coronary occlusion. Certain nutritional factors are thrombogenic, others are antithrombogenic. In

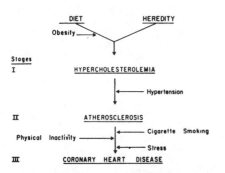

Figure 1. The stages and important factors in the development of coronary heart disease.

both hyperlipidemia and thrombosis, the amount and kind of dietary fat is important.

A third risk factor, one obviously important and affected by nutrition, is obesity, which influences in turn hyperlipidemia, thrombosis and hypertension. Overweight may develop when another risk factor is abolished (i.e. cigarette smoking). Finally, the important risk fctor, hypertension, is greatly affected by dietary electrolytes: sodium raises and potassium lowers blood pressure (Intersalt Cooperative Research Group 1988). Fortunately, from the point of view of therapeutic simplicity, the same dietary lifestyle can be used to modify all four of these coronary risk factors: hyperlipidemia, thrombosis, obesity and hypertension.

The goals of this paper are (1) to review the precise roles that nutritional factors play in the causation of the atherosclerotic plaque, which is the underlying lesion of coronary heart disease (Figure 1) and, (2) to delineate a practical approach to the dietary prevention and treatment of atherosclerosis. Attention will be given to the two components of the atherosclerotic plaque that lead to the development of overt coronary heart disease - namely, the lipid-rich, fibrous atheroma and the superimposed thrombotic lesion.

Dietary factors affect both the initiation and growth of the atherosclerotic plaque and the final thrombotic episode. The evidence about dietary factors and the genesis of atherosclerosis is best illustrated by the numerous experiments over the past 30 years carried out in sub-human primates. In these experiments dietary cholesterol and fat were the "sine qua non" components necessary to produce hypercholesterolemia and

atherosclerosis in many species of monkeys (Armstrong 1967,1970; Taylor 1959). The atherosclerosis produced was severe and complicated, culminating in some monkeys in myocardial infarction, stroke and gangrene of an extremity (Taylor 1959). These clinical features have reproduced the spectrum of the consequences of atherosclerotic disease in humans. In all of these experiments, diet exerted its effect on atherosclerosis by raising plasma lipid and lipoprotein concentrations.

The epidemiological evidence is likewise clearcut: populations consuming a low cholesterol, low-fat diet have little coronary heart disease, whereas in populations of the Western world, where the diet concentrates upon animal foods rich in cholesterol and saturated fat, the incidence of coronary heart disease is very high (Connor, W. 1972). Japan is a classic example of a country with modern technology and a high living standard and· yet a low incidence of coronary heart disease. The Japanese consume a low cholesterol, low fat diet and habitually have low plasma cholesterol levels. Here, again, the links between diet and clinical expression of coronary heart disease are the lifelong plasma cholesterol and LDL concentrations. In addition, populations with a low incidence of coronary heart disease and a low fat dietary background also have a low incidence of clinical thrombosis.

The review of information on the vital role of plasma lipid and lipoprotein concentrations in the development of atherosclerosis, raises a crucial question: Can dietary change lower elevated plasma lipid and lipoprotein concentrations in patients and in population subgroups of the Western world? The answer is an unequivocal yes. Experiments over the past 20 years have indicated which dietary components have an important effect upon plasma lipid and lipoprotein concentrations in humans. The major dietary factors to be considered include the following:

1 Cholesterol

2 Total fat
   Saturated fat
   Monounsaturated fat
   Polyunsaturated fat
   (omega-3 and omega-6)

3 Carbohydrate, fiber, starch and sugars

4 Protein

5 Other nutrients (calories, alcohol, lecithin, vitamins and minerals)

1 DIETARY CHOLESTEROL

Dietary cholesterol enters the body via the chylomicron pathway and is removed from the plasma by the liver as a component of chylomicron remnants. Only about 40 percent of ingested cholesterol is absorbed, the remaining 60 percent passing out in the stool. Dietary cholesterol is thus added to the cholesterol synthesized by the body since feedback inhibition of cholesterol biosynthesis in the body only partially occurs in man even when a large amount of dietary cholesterol is ingested (Lin 1981). Because the ring structure of the sterol nucleus cannot be broken down by the tissues of the body as does occur for fat, protein and carbohydrate, it must be either excreted or stored. Thus, it is easy to see how the body or a particular tissue, i.e. a coronary artery, can become overloaded with cholesterol if there are limitations in cholesterol excretion from the body and from certain tissues. Cholesterol is excreted in the bile and ultimately in the stool, either as such or as bile acids synthesized in the liver from cholesterol. Both of these pathways of excretion are limited and, furthermore, the very efficient enterohepatic reabsorption and circulation returns much of what is excreted into the bile back into the body.

Table 1. Effects of dietary cholesterol on LDL levels

1 Increased chylomicrons and remnants

2 Increased hepatic cell cholesterol
   Consequences:
   Decreased cholesterol biosynthesis
   Partial compensation in excretion of biliary cholesterol
      and bile acids to lessen hepatic cholesterol.
   Decreased synthesis of LDL receptors
   Increased plasma LDL

3 Increased plasma LDL
   Deposition of cholesterol into the arterial wall.

Dietary cholesterol does not directly enter into the formation of the lipoproteins synthesized in the liver, VLDL and LDL, since it is removed by the liver as a component of the chylomicron remnants. It can, however, profoundly affect the catabolism of LDL as mediated through the LDL receptor. Since dietary cholesterol ultimately contributes to the total amount of hepatic cell cholesterol, it can affect the biosynthesis of cholesterol and

modify LDL receptor activity in the liver. In particular, an increase in hepatic cell cholesterol will decrease of LDL receptor activity, and, subsequently cause an increase in the level of LDL cholesterol in the plasma (Spady 1985,1988; Kovanen 1981; Mahley 1981). Conversely, a drastic decrease in dietary cholesterol will increase the LDL receptor activity in the liver, enhance LDL removal, and, hence, lower plasma LDL levels. Table 1 lists the effects of dietary cholesterol.

Over the past thirty years some 26 separate metabolic experiments involving 196 human subjects and patients have shown decisive effects of dietary cholesterol upon plasma cholesterol and LDL levels (Beveridge 1960; Connor, W. 1961a,1964; Steiner 1962). Even patients with familial hypercholesterolemia also respond greatly to dietary cholesterol. Table 2 shows that the plasma cholesterol level decreased 18 and 21 percent in two patients with FH (homozygotes) in response to the removal of cholesterol from the diet. This is similar to the mean plasma cholesterol increase of 17 percent that occurred when 1000 mg dietary cholesterol was added to a cholesterol-free diet in 25 subjects (11 normal and 7 with type II-a mild, 5 with II-a severe, and 9 with type IV hyperlipidemia) (Connor, W. 1964) (Figure 2).

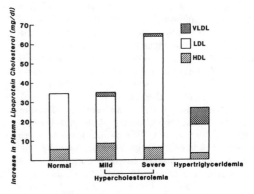

Figure 2. The effects of a 1,000 mg cholesterol diet on the content of cholesterol in the different lipoprotein (LP) fractions.

LDL increased very significantly in all groups, again showing indirectly the affects of dietary cholesterol upon the LDL receptor. These data further document the importance of dietary factors in hyperlipidemia of any phenotype or genotype. However, as pointed out years ago, however, the doubling or tripling of the amounts of dietary cholesterol will not necessarily increase the plasma levels if the initial amount of dietary cholesterol is already substantial, i.e. an increase to 950 mg per day from a previous intake of 475 mg per day (Connor, W. 1961a). Despite this earlier literature such attempts are still being carried out and are highly touted as showing that dietary cholesterol has no effect on the plasma cholesterol levels. There is a review for those who wish to explore the subject more fully (Roberts 1981).

Table 2. The effect of a cholesterol-free diet on the plasma cholesterol level in two patients with familial hypercholesterolemia (homozygotes)

Diet	Plasma Cholesterol (mg/dl)	
	DL	DC
Cholesterol, 250 mg/day	737	786
Cholesterol-free	578	644
Change	-21%	-18%
Hyperalimentation	401	418

The effects upon the plasma cholesterol as the amount of dietary cholesterol is gradually increased may be depicted in Figure 3, and are supported by both animal and human experiments. With a baseline cholesterol-free diet, the amount of dietary cholesterol necessary to produce an increase in the plasma cholesterol concentration is termed "the threshold amount". Then, as the amount of dietary cholesterol is increased, the plasma cholesterol increases likewise until the second important point on this curve is reached, which is termed "the ceiling amount". Further increases in dietary cholesterol do not lead to higher levels of the plasma cholesterol even though phenomenally high amounts may be fed. Each animal or human being probably has its own distinctive threshold and ceiling amounts. Generally speaking, however, and again based on the experimental literature, we would suggest that an average threshold amount for human beings would be 100 mg/day. An average ceiling amount of dietary cholesterol would be in the neighborhood of 300-400 mg/day. Further experiments will be necessary to provide more precise information about the ceiling. Thus, a baseline dietary cholesterol intake of 500 mg/day from two eggs would, for most individuals, already exceed the ceiling. The addition of two more egg yolks for a total

of 1,000 mg/day would not then further increase the plasma cholesterol concentration. Yet, beginning with a baseline very low cholesterol diet under 100 mg/day and adding the equivalent of two egg yolks, or 500 mg, to this baseline amount would produce a striking change in plasma cholesterol concentrations, perhaps 60 mg/dl as shown in many experiments.

Recent dietary surveys indicate that the average American intake of dietary cholesterol is about 400 mg/day for women and 500 mg/day for men (Gordon 1982). Decreasing these amounts of dietary cholesterol, as would take place in therapeutic and preventive diets to be amplified subsequently, would then have a profound effect on plasma cholesterol concentrations because operationally one would be on the descending limb of the curve as exemplified in Figure 3.

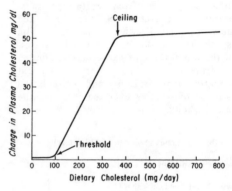

Figure 3. The effects upon the plasma cholesterol level of gradually increasing the amount of dietary cholesterol in human subjects whose background diet is very low in cholesterol content. See the text for discussion of the threshold and ceiling concepts.

There has been recent discussion about the wide distribution of individual response to change in dietary cholesterol intake (Katan 1986) although this finding is not new (Beveridge 1960; Connor, W. 1961a, 1961b, 1963, 1969a; Katan 1986; Flaim 1981). Further, variation in individual plasma cholesterol response occurs with other nutrients as well as with lipid-lowering drugs. Katan (1986) recently showed that 2 percent of their subjects had a negative or minimal response to dietary cholesterol feeding. Sixteen percent had responses less than half of the mean and eighty-four percent had a plasma cholesterol

312

increase greater than half the mean. Therefore, the majority of people could be expected to respond significantly to a decrease in dietary cholesterol from 400-500 mg/day to 100 mg/day or less. Unfortunately, studies to date do not provide a way to predict who would have less than a 10 percent decrease and who would have greater than 10 percent decrease in the plasma cholesterol level in response to maximal dietary changes. Studies are needed to provide a means by which one could correctly identify individuals with regard to plasma cholesterol response to decreases in dietary cholesterol and saturated fat intakes.

Also intriguing are the possible metabolic sequelae that could contribute to this individual variation in response such as the LDL receptor which dietary cholesterol has been shown to down-regulate (Spady 1988). Mistry, suggested that individual differences in plasma lipid and lipoprotein response to dietary cholesterol appear to be related in part to differences in the capacity of peripheral cells to catabolize LDL and to down-regulate cholesterol synthesis (1981). Recent data indicate that the various apolipoprotein E alleles may be involved with the E-2 isoform causing less binding to the LDL receptor (Mahley 1984) and the E-4 isoform possibly increasing VLDL catabolism independently of the LDL receptor (Gregg 1986).

2 FAT

2.1 The effects of dietary fats upon the plasma lipids and lipoproteins

The amount and kind of fat in the diet have a well documented effect upon the plasma lipid concentrations (Ahrens 1957; Keys 1957a). The total amount of dietary fat is important in that the formation of chylomicrons in the intestinal mucosa and their subsequent circulation in the blood is directly proportional to the amount of fat which has been consumed in the diet. A fatty meal will result in the production of large numbers of chylomicrons and will impart the characteristic lactescent appearance to post-prandial plasma observed some three to five hours after meal consumption. A typical American diet with 110 gm of fat would produce 110 gm of chylomicron triglyceride per day. "Remnant" production from chylomicrons is proportional to the number of chylomicrons synthesized. Chylomicron remnants are considered atherogenic particles (Zilversmit 1979a). Fat is

important in cholesterol metabolism since cholesterol is absorbed in the presence of dietary fat and is transported in chylomicrons.

However, the most important effect of dietary fat upon the plasma cholesterol level relates to the type of fat. Fats may be divided into three major classes identified by saturation and unsaturation characteristics. Long-chain, saturated fatty acids have no double bonds, are not essential nutrients, and may be readily synthesized in the body from acetate. Dietary saturated fatty acids have a profound hyper-cholesterolemic effect, increase the concentrations of LDL and have thrombogenic implications (Ahrens 1957; Keys 1957a). All animal fats are highly saturated (30% or more of the fat is saturated) except for those which occur in fish and shellfish, these latter being, contrastingly, highly polyunsaturated. The molecular basis for the effects of dietary saturated fat on the plasma cholesterol level is now well understood and rests upon its influence on the LDL receptor activity of liver cells, as described by Brown and Goldstein (1986). Dietary saturated fat suppresses hepatic LDL receptor activity, decreases the removal of LDL from the blood and thus increases the concentration of LDL cholesterol in the blood (Spady 1985). Cholesterol augments the effect of saturated fat by further suppressing hepatic LDL receptor activity and raising the plasma LDL cholesterol level (Spady 1988). Conversely, a decrease in dietary cholesterol and saturated fat increases the LDL receptor activity of the liver cells, enhances the hepatic pickup of LDL cholesterol and lowers the concentration of LDL cholesterol in the blood (Spady 1988). Metabolic studies suggest that one can expect an average plasma cholesterol lowering of 10-20% by maximally decreasing dietary cholesterol and saturated fat intake.

Attention has been called to the fact that some saturated fats are not hypercholesterolemic (see Table 3). Medium chain triglycerides (C8 and

Table 3. Effects of saturated fatty acids upon plasma cholesterol levels

C8, C10	-	Medium chain	Neutral
C12	-	Lauric	Increase
C14, C16	-	Myristic, palmitic	Increase
C18	-	Stearic	Neutral

C10 saturated fatty acids) are handled metabolically more like carbohydrate and are transported to the liver via the portal vein blood rather than as chylomicrons. These fatty acids do not elevate the plasma cholesterol concentration. Stearic acid, an 18 carbon saturated fatty acid, likewise has a limited effect upon the plasma cholesterol concentration. This is because the body resists the accumulation of stearic acid and the liver converts excessive stearic acid from the diet into oleic acid, a monounsaturated fatty acid by virtue of the action of a desaturase enzyme. Feeding animals large quantities of a fat such as cocoa butter containing a considerable percentage of its total fatty acids as stearic acid (33 percent) does not result in the deposition of stearic acid in the adipose tissue as would occur with mono and polyunsaturated fat feeding (Lin 1993). This again is because of the action of the desaturase enzyme.

The practical importance of these observations on certain saturated fatty acids is limited because they are not present to any appreciable extent in the diet. The equations developed for the prediction of plasma cholesterol change have been based upon the changes produced by a given fat including its concentration of stearic acid. Thus all of the information which has accumulated about the hypercholesterolemic and atherogenic properties of a given fat such as beef fat, butterfat, lard, palm oil, cocoa butter and coconut oil is completely valid. To be emphasized is the fact that palmitic acid which is the most common saturated fat found in our food supply is intensely hypercholesterolemic. It has 16 carbons; myristic acid and lauric acid at 14 and 12 carbon links are likewise intensely hypercholesterolemic. It is these fatty acids which are present in dietary fats and which cause their unfortunate effects. Amounts of stearic acid in the American diet are not great compared with palmitic acid.

The second class of dietary fats consists of the characteristic monounsaturated fatty acids present in all animal and vegetable fats. For practical purposes, oleic acid, having one double bond at the omega-9 position, is the only significant dietary monounsaturated fatty acid. In general, the effects of dietary monounsaturated fatty acids have been "neutral" in terms of their effects on the plasma cholesterol concentrations, neither raising nor lowering them (Becker 1983). However, reports that Mediterranean basin populations who consume olive oil in relatively large quantities have fewer heart attacks than people in this country has led to further investigations. Recent studies have shown that large amounts of monounsaturated fat, like polyunsaturated oils, lower plasma cholesterol and LDL levels when compared with saturated fat (Grundy 1986; Mattson 1986). Furthermore, unlike polyunsaturated oils, monounsaturated fat did not lower the plasma HDL cholesterol level. However, distinct from omega-3 fatty acids from fish oil, monounsaturated fat does not decrease the plasma triglyceride concentrations (Grundy 1986; Mattson 1985). Furthermore, monounsaturated fat has no known effect upon prostaglandin metabolism or upon platelet function. Omega-3 fatty acids are antithrombotic; monounsaturated fat has no such action.

There are serveral additional points to be made in regards to these recent studies: 1. The Mediterranean diet is also rich in fish, beans, fruit and vegetables, and is low in saturated fat and cholesterol. These could be the decisive factors which influence the lessened incidence of coronary disease and lower plasma cholesterol levels. 2. Olive oil is low in saturated fatty acids (which raise plasma cholesterol levels); this may be why the recent metabolic experiments have shown some cholesterol lowering from large amounts of monounsaturates in the diet. 3. Large amounts of any kind of fat should be avoided to lower the risk of other diseases such as colon or breast cancer and obesity. And all fats, after absorption, form large particles (remnants) which circulate in the blood and are atherogenic. One translation of the latest research on monounsaturated fats is to recommend that patients include them as part of a general lower fat eating style -- Use olive oil in salad dressing and Italian dishes. Use peanut oil for special stir-fried dishes. Avocado is delicious but high in fat, so use as a garnish only.

Polyunsaturated fatty acids, the third class of fatty acids, are vital constituents of cellular membranes and serve as prostaglandin precursors (Goodnight 1982). Because they cannot be synthesized by the body and are only obtainable from dietary sources, they are "essential" fatty acids. The two classes of polyunsaturated fatty acids are the omega-6 and omega-3 fatty acids (Figure 4). The most common examples of omega-6 fatty acids are linoleic acid, found in food, and arachadonic acid, 20 carbons in length with four double bonds, usually synthesized in the body from linoleic acid by the liver. Since the basic structure of omega-6 fatty acids cannot be synthesized by the body, up to 2-3% of total energy in the diet must be supplied as linoleic acid to meet the requirements of the body for the omega-6 structure, i.e. an essential fatty acid.

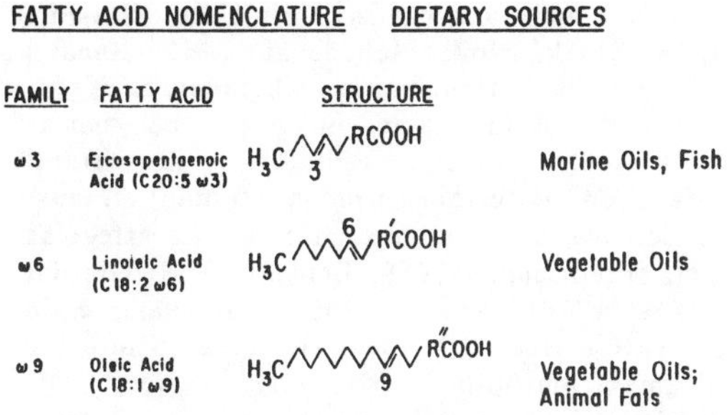

FATTY ACID NOMENCLATURE   DIETARY SOURCES

FAMILY	FATTY ACID	STRUCTURE	
ω3	Eicosapentaenoic Acid (C20:5 ω3)	H₃C⌇RCOOH	Marine Oils, Fish
ω6	Linoleic Acid (C18:2 ω6)	H₃C⌇R'COOH	Vegetable Oils
ω9	Oleic Acid (C18:1 ω9)	H₃C⌇R"COOH	Vegetable Oils; Animal Fats

Figure 4. Fatty acids can be organized into families according to the position of the first double bond from the terminal methyl group. Typical fatty acids from three common families are shown in this figure. Omega-3 fatty acids all have three carbons between the methyl end and the first double bond. Besides eicosapentaenoic acid (C20:5), other common omega-3 fatty acids are linolenic acid (C18:3) and docosahexaenoic acid (C22:6). Linoleic acid (C18:2) and arachidonic acid (C20:4) are the most important omega-6 fatty acids, while oliec acid (C18:1) is the commonest fatty acid in the omega-9 family.

Omega-3 fatty acids differ in the position of the first double bond counting from the methyl end of the molecule, this double bond being at the number 3 carbon. Omega-3 fatty acids are also an essential nutrient for human beings since the body is unable to synthesize this particular structure. Omega-6 and omega-3 fatty acids are not interconvertible. The dietary sources of omega-3 fatty acids are from plant foods - some, but not all, vegetable oils, and leafy vegetables which are especially rich in omega-3 fatty acids - and, in particular, fish and shellfish. Linolenic fatty acid, C18:3, is obtained from vegetable products. Eicosapentaenoic acid, C20:5, and docosahexaenoic acid, C22:6, are derived from fish, shellfish and phytoplankton (the plants of the ocean) and are highly concentrated in fish oils. Once either the omega-3 or omega-6 structure comes into the body as the 18 carbon linoleic or linolenic acid, the body can

synthesize the longer chain and more highly-polyunsaturated omega-6 or omega-3 fatty acids (20 and 22 carbons).

There are distinctly different functions in the body for omega-3 and omega-6 fatty acids. Both serve as substrate for the formation of different prostaglandins (Goodnight 1982) and are rich in phospholipid membranes. Both omega-3 and omega-6 fatty acids are particularly concentrated in nervous tissue. Omega-3 fatty acids are rich in the retina, spermatozoa, the gonads, and many other organs. Omega-6 fatty acids are concentrated in the different plasma lipid classes (cholesterol esters, phospholipids, etc.) and, in addition, are concerned with lipid transport.

Polyunsaturated fatty acids in large amounts, of either the omega-6 or omega-3 structure, depress plasma total and LDL cholesterol concentrations (Connor, W. 1969a; Becker 1983). Omega-3 fatty acids have a second additional action in lowering plasma triglyceride concentrations and, in particular, VLDL, chylomicrons and remnants (Harris 1980,1988).

Already stressed is the wealth of evidence from experimental animals about the important and sine qua non necessity of dietary cholesterol and fat being present in the nutrition of animals to produce atherosclerosis. Several important studies in regard to fish oil containing omega-3 fatty acids have indicated much less atherosclerosis developing when fish oil was present in the diet. The species studied to date have been pigs (Weiner 1986) and rhesus monkeys (Davis 1987). Both coronary and aortic atherosclerosis has been greatly reduced by fish oil. This reduction in experimental atherosclerosis from omega-3 fatty acids is not necessarily explainable by changes in the plasma lipid-lipoprotein concentration. Since these were lowered only partially or not at all during the experimental atherosclerosis period, other mechanisms, possibly prostaglandins, must be postulated to explain the anti-atherogenic effects of fish oil. Table 4 lists possible effects of omega-3 fatty acids from fish oil upon coronary heart disease.

It is not known exactly how the evidence about omega-3 fatty acids should translate in eating behavior. However, one study from The Netherlands showed that men who included fish in their diet twice a week had fewer deaths from heart disease (Kromhout 1985). Even very low fat seafood contains an appreciable amount of omega-3 fatty acids. Eating a total of 12 ounces of a variety of fish and shellfish each week would provide 1000 to 5000 milligrams of omega-3 fatty acids as well as protein, vitamins and minerals. The patient with hyperlipidemia could only be expected to have beneficial effects from following this dietary advice, especially if the fish replaced meat in the diet.

Table 4. The Cardiovascular effects of omega-3 fatty acids

1. Hypolipidemic: decrease plasma lipids-lipoproteins, cholesterol, triglycerides, LDL, VLDL, chylomicrons and remnants.

2. Anti-thrombotic and vasodilatory. Decrease platelet stickiness, increase bleeding time.

3. Lower blood pressure.

Most of the comparisons of the effects of saturated and polyunsaturated fat upon the plasma lipids have indicated that gram for gram, saturated fat is up to two times greater at raising plasma cholesterol than is polyunsaturated fat in depressing it (Hegsted 1965; Keys 1957b). Regression equations have been calculated to indicate the plasma cholesterol changes from dietary manipulations of saturated fat, polyunsaturated fat and cholesterol. These will be discussed later in the development of the Cholesterol-Saturated Fat Index of foods.

Many, but not all, of the currently marketed vegetable oils, shortenings, and margarines are only partially hydrogenated and thus retain the basic unsaturated characteristics of vegetable oils. Coconut oil, cocoa butter (the fat of chocolate) and palm oil are common "saturated" vegetable fats consumed in quantities; they have a hypercholesterolemic effect. The ratio of polyunsaturated to saturated fatty acids in a given fat or oil is termed the P/S value. Fats with a high P/S value of 2 and above, compared to 0.4 and less, are generally recognized as being hypocholesterolemic. The typical Western diet has a P/S value of 0.4. In the suggested low fat, high carbohydrate diet to prevent coronary disease, the P/S value is above 1.0.

2.2 Dietary fat and thrombosis

Table 5 lists possible dietary effects on thrombosis and platelet aggregation. These effects are based upon both experimental and epidemiological evidence. As may be appreciated, firm documentation in this arena may not always be possible and no clinical trials have been conducted to support the suggested relationships. However, both in vitro and in vivo, saturated fatty acids of a chain length C12 and above appear to be thrombogenic, activating the coagulation cascade and aggregating platelets (Haslam 1964; Hoak 1967; Mahadevan 1966; Renaud 1970). Any circumstance which elevates the levels of free fatty acids in the plasma such as starvation, diabetic acidosis, myocardial infarction, or certain hormonal stimulation must be considered as having a thrombotic effect as well (Fredrickson 1958; Beckett 1958; Gjesdal 1976a, 1976b; Kurian 1966) For example, in starvation free fatty acids are released into the plasma from adipose tissue triglyceride. The mechanism of this effect may occur from a level of free fatty acids exceeding the two tight binding sites on the albumin molecule, the usual transport form of free fatty acids (Connor, W. 1969b). This, then, allows the free fatty acids to interact with various coagulation proteins and with platelets.

Table 5. Dietary factors affecting thrombosis and platelet function

1. Thrombotic factors
   Saturated fatty acids
   Free fatty acids

2. Anti-thrombotic factors
   Low-fat, high CHO diet
   Polyunsaturated fat
      omega-6 fatty acids (linoleic)
         from vegetable oil
      omega-3 fatty acids (eicosapentaenoic)
         from fish oil

Polyunsaturated fat, in general, has an antithrombotic effect. This effect is best documented by dietary studies in human beings (Goodnight 1982) and by the epidemiological evidence in the Greenland Eskimos who have a low incidence of thrombotic disease (Bang 1980). They consume fish and seal, both rich in the omega-3 fatty acids, eicosapentaenoic and docosahexaenoic fatty acids (Bang 1973). The feeding of fish and fish oil to humans or their presence in a natural diet not only has a hypolipidemic effect but also increases the bleeding time and reduces platelet aggregation (Dyerberg 1979; Goodnight 1981). On the other hand, the ingestion of a low-fat diet high in carbohydrate and fiber is associated with a low incidence of thrombosis in certain population groups, such as the Ugandans (Burkitt 1972; Davies 1948; Latto 1981). These populations ingest a low fat diet and consume most of their fat in the form of polyunsaturated fatty acids with a very low intake of saturated fat.

Accordingly, an antithrombotic diet for human beings would be low in total fat and saturated fat and might contain fish. It should also be a high carbohydrate, high fiber diet. High circulating levels of the plasma free fatty acids should also be avoided. This is particularly important in obese patients with vascular disease who are given low calorie diets. Such diets should avoid ketosis which would be an indication that plasma free fatty acid concentrations are greatly increased. They should contain sufficient calories in general, about 700-1000 kcalories/day in which the chief sources of calories would be carbohydrate and protein.

3 CARBOHYDRATE

If the total fat content of an anti-coronary diet is reduced from the current American intake of 40% to 20% of the total calories and if protein is to be kept constant, then the difference in caloric intake between a high fat diet and a low fat diet must be made up by increasing the carbohydrate content of the diet. As already indicated, both the epidemiological evidence and experimental studies buttress this basic concept since populations ingesting a high carbohydrate diet, usually from complex carbohydrates, have a low incidence of coronary disease and other thrombotic conditions.

Over 25 years ago it was demonstrated that a sudden increase in the amount of dietary carbohydrate in Americans accustomed to a high fat diet would increase the plasma triglyceride concentration rather dramatically (Ahrens 1961). However, after many weeks adaptation occurs and the hypertriglyceridemia regresses (Stone 1963; Weinsier 1974). We regard this situation as metabolically normal since it is a universal occurrence in Americans given a high carbohydrate diet. It is analogous to the hyperglycemia which results in individuals who have previously been consuming a reduced number of calories or a low carbohydrate diet and are given a glucose load. In order to obtain a valid glucose tolerance curve an individual must eat a diet reasonably high in carbohydrate for at least three days before the test.

High carbohydrate diets have been used in diabetic patients over a long period of time without impairment of glucose tolerance and without the occurrence of hypertriglyceridemia (Stone 1963). Since any lasting dietary change is adopted gradually, as will be emphasized in the behavioral modification approach taken to educate patients about dietary change, it is highly unlikely that any patient with coronary disease asked to follow the low cholesterol, low fat, high carbohydrate diet would develop hypertriglyceridemia. There would be ample time for adaptation as he passes through the three or more phases of this dietary approach.

We recently increased the dietary carbohydrate intake gradually from 45% kcal to 65% kcal over a 28 day period in seven mildly hypertriglyceridemic subjects. There was a significant lowering of the mean plasma cholesterol level from 226 to 190 mg/dl, -16% (p<0.001) whereas the mean plasma triglyceride level remained constant, 217 mg/dl to 222 mg/dl (Ullmann 1988).

Studies in rats have indicated that sucrose and fructose have a hypertriglyceridemic effect in contrast to starch or glucose (Nikkila 1965). The evidence in human beings that even very large amounts of sucrose (over 50% of the total calories) produces hyperlipidemia is not completely convincing. However, even if large quantities of sucrose have a mild hypertriglyceridemic and perhaps also a hypercholesterolemic effect, this does not bear particularly upon the dietary design of the anti-coronary diet as envisioned. In the low fat, high carbohydrate diet the vast majority of the carbohydrate is in the form of cereals and legumes and not as sucrose. Americans commonly consume about 20% of the total calories as sucrose or about half of their carbohydrate intake. In the dietary changes being suggested, sucrose would fall to 10-15% of the total calories and so any effect from sucrose would be diminished rather than accentuated by the dietary change.

4 FIBER

Dietary fiber is a broad nondescript term which includes several carbohydrates thought to be indigestible by the human gut. These include cellulose, hemicelluloses, lignin, pectin and beta glucans. Dietary fiber is only found in plants and is commonly present in unprocessed cereals, legumes, vegetables and fruits. In ruminant animals, dietary fiber is completely digested by the microbial flora of the rumen, so that fiber provides a major source of energy for these animals. In man, however, dietary fiber contributes little to the caloric content of the diet, promotes satiety through its bulk, and affects colonic function greatly. A high fiber diet produces larger stools and a more rapid intestinal transit, factors which may prevent certain diseases of the colon (i.e., diverticulitis, colon cancer). A high fiber diet increases the emptying time of the stomach, thereby promoting slower absorption of nutrients, especially glucose.

Fiber experiments date back at least 30 years (Keys 1961; Grande 1965). Fiber added to semisynthetic diets fed to rats has usually had a plasma cholesterol lowering effect. In humans, feeding fiber predominantly in the insoluble form was not hypocholesterolemic (Raymond 1971). A study in which large amounts of soluble fiber (17 gms/2000 kcal) from oat bran and beans were fed to people produced a 20 percent lowering of the plasma total and LDL cholesterol levels (Anderson 1984). Other studies have produced similar results (Kay 1977; McLean 1983). Rich sources of soluble fiber include fruits, pectin being a soluble fiber, oats and other cereals, legumes and vegetables. One way soluble fiber acts is to bind bile acids in the gut, prevent their reabsorption and thus lower cholesterol levels much like the bile acid binding resins like cholestyramine.

A high fiber diet is integral to the dietary concepts for the treatment of hyperlipidemia. The consumption of more foods from vegetable sources will automatically mean a higher consumption of both total and soluble fiber.

5 PROTEIN

The dietary treatment of hyperlipidemia involves, in general, a shift from the consumption of protein derived from animal sources, such as meat and dairy products, to the consumption of more protein from plants. The nutritional adequacy of such protein shifts is assured because mixtures of vegetable proteins, plus the provision of ample low fat animal protein sources, provide abundantly for essential amino acid requirements. Ranges of protein intake from 25 to 150 grams have been tested over the years for effects upon blood lipids and have been found to have no effect within amounts commonly consumed by Americans. However, experiments in animals have suggested that an animal protein such as casein (from milk) is definitely hypercholesterolemic and a vegetable protein such as soy protein has the opposite effect. There have been few definitive experiments in humans to test the hypocholesterolemic effect of vegetable proteins vis a vis animal proteins. As might be expected, it is difficult to control all the variables, including the cholesterol and fat content. However, there are suggestions that the consumption of vegetable protein may have some hypocholesterolemic action. Thus, it may be postulated that a shift in protein intake to include more vegetable protein carries no harm and may confer some benefit to the hyperlipidemic individual.

6 CALORIES

Excessive caloric intake and adiposity can contribute also to both hypertriglyceridemia and hypercholesterolemia by stimulating the liver to overproduce VLDL. The plasma triglyceride and VLDL concentrations of hypertriglyceridemic patients greatly improve after weight reduction and are increased by the hypercaloric state (Galbraith 1966; Olefsky 1974; Schwartz 1981). There is little direct evidence, however, that the LDL receptor and plasma cholesterol and LDL concentrations are directly affected by caloric excess. Nonetheless it is known that obese individuals have a total body cholesterol production which is higher than in individuals of normal weight. Weight reduction and fasting which involve a decrease in the consumption of cholesterol and saturated fat from the diet could certainly upregulate the LDL receptor and could be expected to improve LDL levels in patients with familial hypercholesterolemia. It is, therefore, reasonable to advise caloric control and the avoidance of obesity in the dietary management of hyperlipidemia. The role of increased physical activity is most important in weight control.

7 ALCOHOL

Results from large population studies have shown that people who report consuming alcohol have a lower incidence of coronary heart disease than people who do not drink (Castelli 1977; St. Leger 1979). These studies, while indicating trends in large populations, need to be reinforced by the much stronger evidence provided by controlled experiments in which other factors that influence the plasma HDL cholesterol level such as body weight, smoking, exercise habits and diet are accounted for. Many such studies testing the effect of alcohol consumption on HDL cholesterol levels have been conducted. These studies have shown significant increases in HDL cholesterol after alcohol consumption ranging from an equivalent to 2 beers to 7 beers per day over 3 to 6 weeks compared to a similar abstention period. The type of alcohol given (beer, wine, spirits) did not appear to influence results. Alcohol appears to increase the HDL3 component of HDL which is less related to protection against coronary heart disease (Haskell 1984). It is HDL2, affected by exercise but not alcohol, which is more protective (Wood 1983). Because of these results and since the increased levels of HDL have been linked to lower rates of atherosclerosis, some drinkers have been tempted to drink more, claiming that alcohol is "good for the heart". Should alcohol consumption be encouraged to protect against coronary heart disease?

Specific recommendations are not easy to make because the effects of alcohol consumption are complex, affecting other components of the plasma in addition to HDL cholesterol. Most of the metabolic studies have involved people with plasma cholesterol values below 190 mg/dl, and these results may not translate directly to patients with hyperlipidemia. The effects of alcohol on the levels of HDL2 (linked to reduced coronary disease) and HDL3 (no relationship to coronary disease) are controversial. Alcohol is packed with calories. There are about 290 kcalories in two 12 ounce beers or two 6 ounce glasses of wine. On the average, up to 8 percent of calories consumed by adult Americans come from alcohol. This may be one of the reasons why so many people who drink heavily are overweight and have alcohol-related problems. Theoretically, the amount of alcohol it would take to increase a person's HDL cholesterol from below 30 to above 40 mg/dl is 5 to 6 drinks per day. Other consequences of alcohol consumption - admittedly when excessive - include cirrhosis of the liver, certain cancers, gastritis, mental deterioration, neuropathies and, of course, the personal and social ravages of chronic alcoholism.

We do not think that alcohol should be part of a daily diet, rather - for those who enjoy an occasional drink - we suggest a limit of 1 to 2 drinks on any given day and up to 4-5 drinks per week. The inclusion of alcohol in the diet to increase HDL cholesterol levels is not recommended.

8 LECITHIN

This phospholipid derived from soybeans is commonly sold in health food stores and is widely publicized as a popular remedy for hypercholesterolemia. Aside from its high content of linoleic acid, the consumption of lecithin has little or no effect upon lipid metabolism. Contrary to popular belief, lecithin is not absorbed as such from the digestive tract but is hydrolyzed into its constituent fatty acids and choline. Choline is a lipotrophic substance which was tested in the treatment of hypercholesterolemia 30 years ago and found to be of no value (Katz 1958). The plasma phospholipid levels have not been affected by the addition of lecithin in the diet; the circulating plasma phospholipids are largely synthesized by the liver. Parenthetically, high levels of plasma phospholipids are found in patients with familial hypercholesterolemia.

9 MINERALS AND VITAMINS

Under the assumption that the minimum daily requirements have been met in the diet, then there is no information to indicate that additional vitamins and minerals above and beyond the content of a nutritionally adequate diet will have any effect upon the plasma lipid concentrations. This comment applies equally to vitamin C (Peterson 1975) and vitamin E (Beveridge 1957), both enthusiastically consumed by the public without there being any proof of benefit. On the other hand, massive doses of vitamin A may produce liver damage (Connor, W. 1982). The sole exception is niacin, a B-vitamin used in massive doses for the treatment of hyperlipidemia.

10 DESIGN OF A DIETARY APPROACH FOR TREATING AND PREVENTING CORONARY HEART DISEASE

In view of the evidence about dietary factors, hyperlipidemia, thrombosis and coronary heart disease, it now should be possible to indicate the features of an appropriate and effective preventive diet against coronary heart disease in patients with hyperlipidemia and for the public at large. In general terms, such a diet from what has already been indicated in this chapter should be hypolipidemic and antithrombotic. It should be nutritionally adequate and meet the necessary nutritional requirements during childhood and adult life. This feature is essential because the dietary approach is less likely to succeed unless it is familial. Coronary heart disease occurs in families. Many in the family who have not yet developed overt symptomatology of coronary heart disease are undoubtedly at risk for subsequent coronary heart disease. Another criteria of the dietary approach is that it should be no more costly than the current Western diet. Finally, its use should be facilitated and supported by recipes and menu plans which should make it possible for interested patients and their families to incorporate the proposed dietary changes into their lifestyle after a suitable educational and training period. The dietary approach presented subsequently, i.e. the low fat, high carbohydrate diet is intended to produce a maximal lowering of plasma total and LDL cholesterol concentrations, to reduce excess body weight when this is present, and to fit all of the evidence concerning antithrombotic dietary factors. This diet can be used to treat all of the different types of hyperlipidemia. No longer is it necessary to have a different diet for each phenotype of hyperlipidemia. The same diet with slight modification can be used for any type of hyperlipidemia. This single diet concept has been delineated in detail elsewhere (Connor, W. 1982,1985).

10.1 The cholesterol-saturated fat index (CSI) of foods (Connor, S. 1986a)

The major plasma cholesterol elevating effects of a given food reside in its cholesterol and saturated fat content. To help understand the contribution of these two factors in a single food item and to compare one food with another we have computed a cholesterol-saturated fat index (CSI) for selected foods (Figure 5 and Table 6). This index was based on a modification of the regression equation used earlier to calculate the cholesterol index of foods (Zilversmit 1979b). Since the objective of the low fat, high carbohydrate diet is to maintain, but not to increase, the current intake of polyunsaturated fat, we chose not to include the polyunsaturated fat component of the equation in assessing an individual food item. The cholesterol index of foods was thus modified and is called the cholesterol-saturated fat index (CSI): CSI=(1.01 x gms. saturated fat) + (0.05 x mg. cholesterol), where the amounts of saturated fat and cholesterol in a given amount of a food item are entered into this equation.

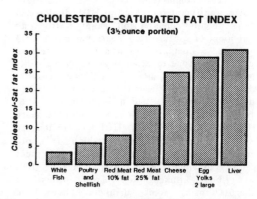

Figure 5. The cholesterol-saturated fat index (CSI) of 3 1/2 oz. of fish, poultry, shellfish, meat cheese, egg yolk, and liver. The CSI for poultry is the average CSI for cooked light and dark chicken without skin. The CSI for shellfish is the average CSI of cooked crab, lobster, shrimp, clams, oysters and scallops. The CSI for cheese is the average CSI of cheddar, Swiss and processed cheese.

In this context it is particularly instructive to compare the CSI of fish versus moderately fat beef. A 100 gm portion of cooked fish contains 66 mg of cholesterol and 0.20 gm of saturated fat. This contrasts to a 96 mg cholesterol content and 8.1 gm of saturated fat of 20 percent fat beef. The CSI for 100 gm (3.5 oz) fish is 4 while that of beef is 13. The caloric value of these two portions also differs greatly (91 for fish and 286 for beef). The CSI of cooked chicken and turkey (without the skin) is also preferable to beef and other red meats. Again the total fat content is quite a bit lower and the saturated fat per 100 gm is 1.3 with the cholesterol 87 mg. The CSI of poultry is 6. Table 6 lists the CSI for various foods.

Table 6. The cholesterol-saturated fat index (CSI) and kilocalorie content of selected foods

	CSI	kcalories
Fish, Poultry, Red Meat (3-1/2 ounces or 100 grams cooked)		
Whitefish-snapper, perch, sole, cod, halibut, etc.	4	91
Salmon	5	149
Shellfish(shrimp, crab, lobster)	6	104
Poultry, no skin	6	171
Beef, Pork and Lamb:		
10 per cent fat (ground sirloin,flank steak)	9	214
15 per cent fat (ground round)	10	258
20 per cent fat (ground chuck, pot roasts)	13	286
30 per cent fat (ground beef, pork, and lamb, steaks, ribs, pork and lamb chops, roasts)	18	381
Cheeses (3-1/2 ounces or 100 grams)		
Low-fat cottage cheese, tofu (bean curd), pot cheese,	1	98
Cottage cheese, Lite-Line, Lite 'n Lively, part-skim ricotta, reduced calorie Laughing Cow	6	139
Imitation Mozzarella, Cheezola, Min Chol, Hickory Farm Lyte, Saffola American*	6	317
Olympia Low Fat, Green River, (lower fat Cheddars), part-skim mozzarella, Neufchatel (lower fat cream cheese), Skim American,	12	256
Cheddar, roquefort, Swiss, brie, jack, American, cream cheese, Velveeta, cheese spreads (jars), and most other cheeses	26	386
Eggs		
Whites (three)	0	51
Egg Substitute (equivalent to two eggs)	1	91
Whole (two)	29	163
Fats 1/4 cup or 4 tablespoons)		
Peanut Butter	6	380
Mayonnaise	8	404
Most vegetable oils	6	491
Soft vegetable margarines	8	420
Soft shortenings	13	464
Bacon grease	20	464
Butter	36	409
Coconut oil, palm oil	38	491
Frozen Desserts (1 cup)		
Water ices	0	245
Sherbet or frozen yogurt	2	290
Ice milk	6	214
Ice cream, 10% fat	13	272
Rich ice cream, 16% fat	18	349
Specialty ice cream, 22% fat	34	768
Milk Products (1 cup)		
Skim milk (0.1% fat) or skim milk yogurt	<1	88
1% milk, buttermilk	2	115
2% milk or plain lowfat yogurt	5	144
Whole milk (3.5% fat) or whole milk yogurt	10	159
Liquid non-dairy creamers: Mocha Mix, Poly Rich	7	376
Liquid non-dairy creamers: store brands, Cereal Blend, Coffee Rich	22	344
Sour cream	39	468
Imitation sour cream (IMO)	43	499

* Cheeses made with skim milk and vegetable oils.

Shellfish have low CSIs because their saturated fat content is extremely low despite the fact that their cholesterol or total sterol content is 2.5 to 3 times higher than fish, poultry or red meat. This means that, when considering both cholesterol and saturated fat, shellfish have a CSI of 6, very much like poultry and is a better choice than even the leanest red meats. Salmon also has a low CSI and is preferred to meat.

10.2 The low-fat, high-carbohydrate diet

The relationship between nutrients and coronary heart disease presents both responsibility and opportunity. The challenge is to define dietary objectives in specific and very practical terms, relating to shopping, food preparation and eating (Connor, S. 1986b). One of the first low-cholesterol, low-fat cookbooks was produced by Dobbin (1957). Our own such diet plan and cookbook is called *The New American Diet* (Connor, S. 1986b). The first objective of all low-fat diets must be to reduce cholesterol consumption from 500 to less than 100 mg per day. This requires keeping egg yolk consumption to a minimum since 45 per cent of dietary cholesterol comes from egg yolk with approximately half from visible eggs and half

from eggs incorporated into foods (Figure 6) (Brewster 1978). Meat and poultry and fish are limited as well as the use of lower fat dairy products.

The second objective is to reduce fat intake by one-half from 40 to 20 percent of calories. This can be done by avoiding fried foods, reducing the fat used in baked goods by one-third and using low-fat dairy products. Added fat should be limited to three teaspoons per day for women and children and five teaspoons per day for teenagers and men. Peanut butter should be used as part of a meal and not as a snack, and nuts used sparingly as condiments.

Another objective is to decrease the current saturated fat intake by two-thirds, from 14 to 5-6 percent of calories. This requires eating red meat or cheese no more than twice a week, using lower-fat cheeses (20 percent fat or less), avoiding products containing coconut and palm oil, limiting ice cream and chocolate to once a month and using soft margarines and oils sparingly.

When people are advised to decrease the amount of fat in their diets, they usually think only of visible fat and are surprised to learn that fat added at the table represents only 22 percent of their fat intake (Figure 7) (Welsh 1982). Decreasing dietary fat would be very

Sources of Cholesterol

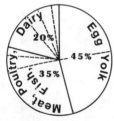

Figure 6. The sources of dietary cholesterol for people in the United States. Forty-five percent of the dietary cholesterol is derived from egg yolk, with half of that being from visible eggs (1-2 eggs per week) and half from eggs used in food preparation (the broken line in the egg yolk segment). Twenty-eight percent of the cholesterol is from red meats, poultry (4%), and fish (2%). Twenty percent is from dairy products: 8% from milk; 5% from cheese, 4% from butter, and 2% from ice cream.

Sources of Fat

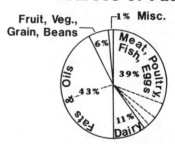

Figure 7. The sources of dietary fat for people in the United states. Thirty percent of the dietary fat is derived from red meats (30%), poultry (5%), eggs (3%), and fish (1%), as per the broken lines dividing that segment of the circle. Eleven percent is from dairy products. Forty-three percent is directly from fats and oils, 21.5% being from visible fat (spreads and dressings) and 21.5% from fat used in cooking and baking. Six percent is from fruits, vegetables, grains, and beans, and 1% is from miscellaneous sources.

322

difficult without knowing that 78 percent is invisible with the majority coming from red meat, cheese, ice cream and other dairy products and fat used in food preparation.

If dietary fat is reduced from 40 to 20 percent of calories and protein kept constant at 15 percent of calories to maintain weight, carbohydrate intake then must be increased from 45 to 65 percent of total calories. What this means practically is that at least two complex carbohydrate-containing foods should be eaten at each meal. For example, eating toast and cereal for breakfast, a sandwich (2 slices of bread) or bean soup and low fat crackers at lunch and 1-2 cups of rice, pasta, potatoes, corn, etc. with bread at dinner, in addition to selecting complex carbohydrate snacks such as popcorn or low fat crackers and low-fat cookies. This is a significant change as most Americans currently limit carbohydrate foods to no more than one per meal. To reach the increased carbohydrate objective, the patient must also eat two to four cups of legumes per week and two to four cups of vegetables per day. While research supports the value of a high carbohydrate diet, many people are reluctant to adopt it because "starchy" foods are falsely associated with gaining weight and are viewed as the food of the poor. Another objective is to eat three to five pieces of fruit per day with a concomitant decrease in refined sugar intake from 20 percent of calories to 10 percent. This means that sweets (pop or candy or desserts) must be limited to no more than one serving per day.

10.3 The phases of the low-fat, high-carbohydrate diet

Even well motivated patients do not make abrupt changes in their dietary habits that are maintained over time. It will take many months and even years to make permanent changes in food consumption patterns. Therefore, we suggest that the recommended changes be approached in a gradual manner, with each phase introducing more changes toward the low fat, high carbohydrate diet pattern (Connor, W. 1976, 1985; Connor, S. 1986b). The manner in which patients are guided through these phases can be individualized. An example of three phases is summarized in Table 7.

Phase I. The aim of phase I is to decrease the consumption of foods high in cholesterol and saturated fat (Table 6). This can be accomplished by deleting egg yolk, butterfat,

lard, and organ meats from the diet and by using substitute products when possible: soft margarine for butter, vegetable oils and shortening for lard, skim milk for whole milk, and egg whites for whole eggs. Many alternative foods can replace foods that contain large amounts of cholesterol and saturated fat. Increasing numbers of new products low in cholesterol and saturated fat are now marketed: low-fat cheeses, egg substitutes, soy meats, frozen yogurt, and many other products.

Many recipes currently in use can be easily altered. For example, most recipes, including baked items, can be made without egg yolks. Usually 1½ to 2 egg whites can be used successfully in place of 1 whole egg in making cakes, cookies, custards potato salad and many other products without changing their quality.

Phase II. The goal of Phase II is a reduction of meat and cheese consumption with a gradual transition from the Western ideal of up to a pound of meat a day to no more than 6-8 ounces per day (Table 7). The use of lean, well-trimmed meat will help to decrease greatly the amount of saturated fat. Fatter meats such as lunch meats, bacon, sausage, wieners, spareribs and others should be saved for very special occasions. Meat or cheese should be used no more than once a day. One significant point is the change in the composition of the traditional sandwich. Meat and cheese are not necessarily essential parts of a sandwich, nor is a sandwich always necessary for lunch. In addition, less fat and cheese should be used. Broiling, baking, steaming or braising should be the methods of cooking instead of frying foods. Fewer foods should be used which contain a lot of fat. Only cheeses with part or all skim milk (20 percent fat or less) should be selected for daily cooking. Cheeses made from whole milk should be used sparingly, one ounce of cheese being substituted for three ounces of lean meat.

At this time, new recipes will be needed to replace the recipes which cannot be altered to meet these new requirements. Recipes which are centered about meat or high-fat dairy products (cream cheese, butter, sour cream, cheese) can be replaced with recipes that use larger amounts of grains, legumes, vegetables and fruits. Furthermore, because of the worldwide concern for the conservation of natural resources and the use of economical foods and the current interest in gourmet cooking and exotic foods, a large number of new recipes can be found in current cookbooks, magazines and newspapers. Many of these stress the use of non-animal food products.

Table 7. Summary of the three phases of the low fat, high carbohydrate diet

Phase I Substitutions	This is accomplished by: avoiding egg yolks, butterfat, lard and organ meats (liver, heart, brains, kidney, gizzards);	trimming fat off meat and skin from chicken
	substituting soft margarine for butter;	choosing commercial food products lower in cholesterol and fat (low-fat cheeses, egg substitutes, soy meat substitutes, frozen yogurt, etc.)
	substituting vegetable oils and shortening for lard;	
	substituting skim milk and skim milk products for whole milk and whole milk products;	modifying favorite recipes by using less fat or sugar and vegetable oils instead of butter or lard;
	substituting egg whites for whole eggs;	
Phase II: New Recipes	This step involves: reducing amounts of meat and cheese eaten and replacing them with chicken and fish;	eating more grains, beans, fruit and vegetables;
	eating meat, chicken or fish only once a day;	when eating out, make low-fat, low-cholesterol choices;
	cutting down on fat; as spreads, in salads, cooking and baking;	finding new recipes to replace those which cannot be altered
Phase III: A New Way of Eating	The final phase means: eating meat, cheese, poultry and fish as "condiments" to other foods, rather than as main courses;	drinking 4-6 glasses of water per day;
	eating more beans and grain products as protein sources;	keeping extra meat, shellfish, regular cheese, chocolate, candy, coconut, and richer home-baked or commercially
	using no more than 3-5 teaspoons of fat per day as spreads, salad dressings, or in cooking and baking	prepared food for special occasions (once a month or less
	enjoying a wide variety of new food and repertoire of totally new and savory recipes	

Many other cultures have developed delicious meals which are low in cholesterol and are low-fat. A wide variety of spices and different products and foods from the cuisines of other countries can be used. Oriental dishes emphasize fresh vegetables and rice products; Mexican dishes make use of tortillas, peppers and beans. The Mediterranean countries (Greece, Italy and Spain) incorporate pastas and vegetable sauces. The cuisine of the Middle Eastern countries employs a variety of wheat products and legume dishes.

Phase III. In Phase III the endpoint goals of the low fat, high carbohydrate diet are attained. The cholesterol content of the diet is reduced to 100 mg per day and the saturated fat lowered to 5 to 6 percent of the total calories. These changes mean that consumption of meat and cheese, in particular, must be reduced. For most patients this will present a considerable challenge. We take an historical approach to the consumption of meat. Man has always eaten meat. What he has not done is to eat meat every day, let alone several times a day. Even today, daily meat consumption is only possible for the affluent minority of the world's population. It is not to our advantage, from the standpoints of either health or the wise use of resources, to consume large amounts of meat every day.

We propose, therefore, in Phase III, that meat, fish and poultry be used as "condiments" rather than "aliments." With this philosophy no longer will the meat dish occupy the center of the table. Instead, meat in smaller quantities will spice up vegetable-rice-cereal-legume based dishes, much as Oriental, Indian and Mediterranean cookery. The use of low fat, low cholesterol cheeses is also an important component of Phase III.

The total of meat, shellfish (shrimp, crab, lobster) and poultry should average three to four ounces per day. Poultry and especially fish should be stressed instead of meat because of their lower saturated fat content. In lieu of meat or poultry, fish and shellfish (clams, oysters, scallops) may be included in the diet in amounts up to six ounces per day because of the omega-3 fatty acids.

By this time new recipes will be emphasizing whole grains and legumes. In Phase II of the low fat, high carbohydrate diet lunch, the smaller meal of the day, was changed by using beans, grains and low-fat animal products in place of meat. In Phase III the larger meal of the day becomes very different. A large variety of new flavors and spices will be introduced. An example of entrees for dinner over a week include lean beef or pork for 1-2 days, poultry for 2-3 days, fish for 2-3 days, and meatless for 1-2 days. During Phase III, the transition from the current Western diet to the low fat, high carbohydrate diet will have been completed (Table 7). Sample menus for one week are provided in Table 8.

10.4 Special occasions: eating away from home, and entertainment

Many restaurants serve a variety of the foods recommended in Phase III of the low fat, high carbohydrate diet. Oriental, Italian, Mexican and Middle Eastern restaurants all have tasty foods to choose from. In the inevitable situation where the food choices are minimal, such as at parties or when eating in friends' homes, one can concentrate upon the salad,

vegetable, fruit and cereal foods and take small amounts of the animal foods to be used as condiments. Guests entertained at home can be introduced to a new way of eating which they will discover to be attractive, tasty and healthful. Obviously, meeting the goals for Phase III is very difficult when eating out of the home. Therefore, one needs to eat as low fat as possible to meet the goals at home. Then by being selective about the frequency of eating out and by making choices one can afford to have special occasions or feasts which include extra meat, cheese, chocolate and coconut.

10.5 Chemical and nutrient content

The chemical composition of the Western diet and the three phases of the low fat, high carbohydrate diet are given in Figure 8. The Western diet contains approximately 500 mg cholesterol per day. This is decreased in Phase I to 350 mg, in Phase II to 200 mg, and in Phase III to 100 mg per day. The fat content decreases from 40% of calories in the Western diet to 35% in Phase I, to 25% in Phase II, and to 20% in Phase III with special consideration given to the decrease of saturated fat. In order to have sufficient calories to meet body needs we propose a gradual increase in carbohydrate, with emphasis on the use of the fiber-containing complex carbohydrates contained in whole grains, cereal products and legumes. The increase in carbohydrate content to 65% in Phase III increases the bulk of the diet considerably, a feature which induces satiety sooner per unit of calories and helps to promote weight loss. The dietary fiber content of the low fat, high carbohydrate diet increases from 10 to 12 gms per day to 35 to 50gms per day. Increasing the complex carbohydrate as fruits,

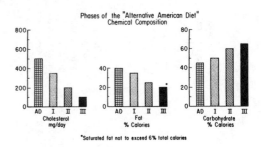

Figure 8. The cholesterol, fat, and carbohydrate content of the Western diet (AD) and the phases of the low fat, high carbohydrate diet (I, II, III).

Table 8. Low fat, high carbohydrate sample menus

Day 1	Day 2	Day 3	Day 4	Day 5	Day 6	Day 7
Cantaloupe Raisin bran cereal Skim milk English muffin with jam	Orange juice Whole wheat pancakes topped with unsweetened applesauce	Plain low-fat yogurt with banana Cereal Bran Muffins*	Berries Shredded wheat Skim milk Whole grain toast	Grapefruit half Potatoes (Hashbrowned with small amount of oil in non-stick pan) Whole grain toast with marmalade	Blueberries Hot whole grain cereal Skim milk English muffin	Fresh melon German oven pancakes*
Tuna sandwich (water-packed tuna mixed with Tangy Dressing* or imitation mayonnaise) Carrot sticks Fresh fruit	Chili Bean Salad* in whole wheat pocket bread Tomato soup (Low-sodium) Fresh fruit Graham crackers	Lentil Soup* Low-fat crackers Laughing cow reduced calorie cheese Fresh fruit	Bean burritos lettuce and sliced tomato Fresh fruit	Salad bar (greens topped with kidney beans, tomato, radishes, garbanzo beans, and cucumbers) Low-calorie commercial or Western Dressing* Bagel Fruit	Peanut butter and jelly sandwich Vegetable sticks (carrot, celery, etc) Fresh orange Whole wheat fig bar	Minestrone soup Wheat berry rolls Low-fat cottage cheese, Fresh fruit
Bean Lasagna* Tossed salad with Western Dressing* French bread Fresh berries	Cashew Chicken* Steamed rice Fresh pineapple slices Wheat berry rolls Hot Fudge Pudding Cake*	Easy Tuna Noodle Casserole* Steamed broccoli Confetti Apple-slaw* Wheat rolls Strawberry Ice*	Pizza Rice Casserole* Green peas Green salad with low-calorie dressing Sourdough rolls Gingersnaps	Baked Herbed Fish* Baked potato with Mock Sour Cream* Steamed zucchini Waldorf Salad* Caraway Puffs*	Corn Chips* with Bean Dip* Creamy Enchiladas* Meatless spanish rice Shredded lettuce & tomato Fresh fruit	Spaghetti with Marinara Sauce* Tossed salad with low-calorie dressing Steamed green beans, seasoned with lemon and pepper French bread Fresh fruit

* recipes from Connors (1986b)

vegetables, grains and beans will ensure that 30 percent of the fiber intake is soluble fiber (11 to 15 grams). Even though the total carbohydrate is increased, the refined sugar content is actually decreased, from 20 to 10% of calories and a greater emphasis is placed on eating more fruit.

10.6 Using the low-fat, high-carbohydrate diet for patients who are also hypertensive or diabetic

A persistent problem in the dietary treatment of disease has been the use of a separate and individual diet for each disease. A good example would be the hyperlipidemic patient who also has high blood pressure and has been advised to follow a low sodium, high potassium diet. Such a diet is completely compatible with the low fat, high carbohydrate diet which has incorporated into its design a phased approach to a low sodium and high potassium intake (Connor, W. 1976, 1982, 1985; Connor, S. 1986b). Should caloric reduction be required to treat obesity, the low fat, high carbohydrate diet in reduced calories can be utilized. This diet has also been used in the treatment of diabetic patients (Stone 1963). Its high intakes of complex carbohydrate and fiber are in keeping with the latest trends in diabetic diets.

10.7 Predicted plasma cholesterol lowering from the three phases of the low-fat, high-carbohydrate diet

As has been emphasized, both dietary cholesterol and saturated fat elevate plasma cholesterol levels, whereas polyunsaturated fat has a mild depressing effect. In stepwise fashion, the cholesterol and saturated fat of each phase of the low fat, high carbohydrate diet are progressively reduced, with Phase III providing for the lowest intakes. According to calculations derived from Hegsted and coworkers (1965), one would expect a 6 to 7 percent decrease, on the average, in the plasma total and LDL cholesterol level for each dietary phase (Table 9). If a patient were to reach phase III goals there would be, on the average, an 18 to 21 percent lowering of the plasma cholesterol level. Approximately one-half of the plasma cholesterol lowering would result from decreasing dietary cholesterol intake from 500 to 100 mg/day and one-half of the lowering would result from decreasing saturated fat intake from 14 to 5 percent of calories.

For example, a patient with a plasma cholesterol level of 300 mg/dl when consuming the typical Western diet would have a plasma cholesterol level of 237 to 246 mg/dl if phase III goals were to be achieved. Then a small dose of one of the hypocholesterolemic drugs would be used to further decrease the plasma cholesterol to below 200 mg/dl.

The scenario just described represents a mean plasma cholesterol response to dietary change. Based on the data from Katan (1986) one would estimate that 75 to 85 percent of people who achieved maximal dietary changes would have a plasma cholesterol decrease of 9 percent or greater and 50 percent of those people would have an 18 percent or greater reduction in the plasma cholesterol level. Extrapolation from the Lipid Research Clinics Primary Prevention Trial results which showed a 2 percent reduction in risk for coronary disease for every 1 percent reduction in plasma cholesterol (Lipid Research Clinics Programs 1984), one might then expect that 50 percent of individuals maximally reducing their plasma cholesterol level by diet would decrease their coronary risk by 36 percent and 75 to 85 percent of individuals having such reductions would decrease their coronary risk by 18 percent.

11 SUMMARY AND CONCLUSIONS

The dietary treatment and prevention of the atherosclerotic lesions underlying coronary heart disease have a logical and well established rationale which has been developed over the past three decades. The low fat, high carbohydrate diet for these purposes is designed to prevent and treat hyperlipidemia and to have an antithrombotic action. The proposed low cholesterol, low fat diet is safe, inexpensive, and can become habitual through the process of gradual change, practice and patience. It offers a practical means of dealing with some of the key risk factors in coronary heart disease, especially hyperlipidemia. Furthermore, the same dietary philosophy may be applied to hyperlipidemias of differing severity, of different etiologies and of different lipoprotein types.

This dietary approach may be used with therapeutic benefit at any stage in the development of coronary heart disease. Atherosclerosis is inevitably progressive but focal. The same coronary artery may have occlusive lesions in one location and in neighboring location only beginning lesions.

Table 9. Predicted plasma cholesterol lowering from the three phases of the low fat, high carbohydrate diet

	Total Fat*	Saturated Fat*	Poly-unsaturated Fat*	P/S	Cholesterol (mg/day)	Predicted total change in plasma cholesterol from Western Diet to each phase (percent)	Predicted change in plasma cholesterol from phase to phase (percent)
Western Diet	40	15	6	0.4	500		
Low Fat, High Carbohydrate Diet							
Phase I	35	14	9	0.6	350	- 6	- 6
Phase II	25	8	8	1.0	200	- 13	- 7
Phase III	20	5	8	1.3	100	- 1º	- 6

* per cent of the total calories

calculated per the formula of Hegsted, McGandy, Myers, and Stare (1965):

$$\text{Chol} = 2.16 \ S \ - \ 1.65 \ P \ + \ 6.77 \ C \ - \ 0.53$$

Where   Chol = the change in plasma cholesterol in mg/dl
S = the change in saturated fat as per cent of total calories
P = the change in polyunsaturated fat as per cent of total calories
C = the change in dietary cholesterol intake in decigrams/day

The baseline diet from which changes have been made is the Western Diet.

Likewise, in other coronaries the lesions may be minimal, severe or variable. Thus, the complete therapy of coronary heart disease must concentrate upon the removal or alleviation of those factors causing plaques to worsen and to enhancing those factors promoting regression of atherosclerosis.

The primary prevention of coronary heart disease is clearly the ultimate goal to deal most effectively with the current epidemic of coronary heart disease. The dietary changes suggested for the coronary patient are completely safe and are prudent measures to be followed by any population (i.e., Western) at serious risk for coronary disease. These nutritional changes should be instituted early in life when they will have the greatest impact. This is a familial disease and its control and treatment can best be approached on a family basis. The primary prevention of coronary heart disease is dependent upon the prevention of diet-induced hyperlipidemia.

12 ACKNOWLEDGEMENTS

First published in Connor, S.L. & Connor, W.E. 1990. Coronary Heart Disease: Prevention and Treatment by Nutritional Change. In: Carroll, K.K., ed., *Diet, Nutrition, & Health*. Montreal: McGill-Queen's University Press, p. 33-72. Reproduced by permission of McGill-Queen's University Press.

Special thanks are accorded to Robin W. Virgin and Karida C. Griffith for the meticulous preparation of this manuscript.

REFERENCES

Ahrens E.H., J. Hirsch, & W. Insull 1957. The influence of dietary fats on serum lipid levels in man. *Lancet*. 1:943-953.

Ahrens E.H., J. Hirsch, K. Oette, J.W. Farquhar, & Y. Stein 1961. Carbohydrate-induced and fat-induced lipemia. *Trans. Assoc. Amer. Phys.* 74:134-146.

Anderson J.W., L. Story, B. Sieling, W.J.L. Chen, M.S. Petro, & J. Story 1984. Hypocholesterolemic effects of oat-bran or bean intake for hypercholesterolemic men. *Am. J. Clin. Nutr.* 40:1146-1155.

Armstrong M.L., W.E. Connor, & E.D. Warner 1967. Xanthomatosis in rhesus monkeys fed a hypercholesterolemic diet. *Arch. Path.* 84:226-237.

Armstrong M.L., E.D. Warner, & W.E. Connor 1970. Regression of coronary atheromatosis in rhesus monkeys. *Circ. Res.* 27:59-67.

Bang H.O., J. Dyerberg, & N. Hjorne 1973. The composition of food consumed by Greenlandic Eskimos. *Acta. Med. Scand.* 200:69-73.

Bang H.O., & J. Dyerberg 1980. Lipid metabolism and ischemic heart disease in Greenland Eskimos. In: Draper H.H., ed. *Advanced nutrition research*, vol 3. New York: Plenum Press, 1-22.

Becker N., D.R. Illingworth, P. Alaupovic, W.E. Connor, & E.E. Sundberg 1983. Effects of saturated, monounsaturated, and omega-6 polyunsaturated fatty acids on plasma lipids, lipoproteins and apoproteins in humans. *Am. J. Clin. Nutr.* 37:355-360.

Beckett A.G., & J.G. Lewis 1960. Mobilization and utilization of body fat as an aetiological factor in occlusive vascular disease in diabetes mellitus. *Lancet.* 2:14-18.

Beveridge J.M.R., W.F. Connell, & G.A. Mayer 1957. The nature of the substances in dietary fat affecting the level of plasma cholesterol in humans. *Can. J. Biochem. and Physiol.* 35:257-270.

Beveridge J.M.R., W.F. Connel, G.A. Mayer, & H.L. Haust 1960. The response of man to dietary cholesterol. *J. Nutr.* 71:61-65.

Brewster L., & M.F. Jacobson 1978. *The Changing American Diet.* Washington, D.C.: Center for Science in the Public Interest.

Brown M.S., & J.L. Goldstein 1986. A receptor-mediated pathway for cholesterol homeostasis. *Science.* 232:34-47.

Burkitt D.P. 1972. Varicose veins, deep vein thrombosis, and hemorrhoids. *Brit. Med. J.* 2:556-561.

Castelli W.P., T. Gordon, M.C. Hjortland, A. Kagan, J.T. Doyle, C.G. Hames, S.B. Hulley, & W.J. Zukel 1977. Alcohol and blood lipids. *Lancet.* 2:153-155.

Connor S.L., S.M. Artaud-Wild, C.J. Classick-Kohn, J.G. Gustafson, D.P. Flavell, L.F. Hatcher, & W.E. Connor 1986a. The cholesterol-saturated fat index: an indication of the hypercholesterolemic and atherogenic potential of food. *Lancet.* 1:1229-1232.

Connor S.L., & W.E. Connor 1986b. *The New American Diet.* New York: Simon & Schuster.

Connor W.E., R.E. Hodges, & R.E. Bleiler 1961a. The serum lipids in men receiving high cholesterol and cholesterol-free diets. *J. Clin. Invest.* 40:894-900.

Connor W.E., R.E. Hodges, & R.E. Bleiler 1961b. The effect of dietary cholesterol upon the serum lipids in man. *J. Lab. Clin. Med.* 57:331-342.

Connor W.E., J.J. Rohwedder, & J.C. Hoak 1963. The production of hypercholesterolemia and atherosclerosis by a diet rich in shellfish. *J. Nutr.* 79:443-450.

Connor W.E., D.B. Stone, & R.E. Hodges 1964. The interrelated effects of dietary cholesterol and fat upon the human serum lipid levels. *J. Clin. Invest.* 43:1691-1696.

Connor W.E., D.T. Witiak, & D.B. Stone 1969a. Cholesterol balance and fecal neutral steroid and bile acid excretion in normal men fed dietary fats of different fatty acid composition. *J. Clin. Invest.* 48:1363-1375.

Connor W.E., J.C. Hoak, & E.D. Warner 1969b. Plasma free fatty acids, hypercoagulability and thrombosis. In: Sherry S., Brinkhous K.M., Genton E.D., Stengle J.M., eds. *Thrombosis.* Washington, D.C.: Nat. Acad. Sci., p. 355-373.

Connor W.E., & S.L. Connor 1972. The key role of nutritional factors in the prevention of coronary heart disease. *Prev. Med.* 1:49-83.

Connor W.E., S.L. Connor, M.M. Fry, & S. Warner 1976. *The Alternative Diet Book.* Iowa City: University of Iowa Press.

Connor W.E. & S.L. Connor 1982. The dietary treatment of hyperlipidemia: Rationale, technique and efficacy. In: Havel R.J., ed. Lipid disorders. *Medical Clinics of North America.* 66:485-518.

Connor W.E. & S.L. Connor 1985. The dietary prevention and treatment of coronary heart disease. In: Connor W.E., Bristow J.D., eds. Coronary heart disease: *Prevention, Complications and Treatment.* Philadelphia: Lippincott, p. 43-64.

Connor W.E. & S.L. Connor 1986. Dietary cholesterol and fat and the prevention of coronary heart disease: risks and benefits of nutritional change. In: Hallgren B., et al. (eds.), *Diet and Prevention of Coronary Heart Disease and Cancer.* New York: Raven Press, p. 113-147.

Davies J.N.P. 1948. Pathology of central African natives. IX cardiovascular diseases. *East African Med. J.* 25:454-467.

Davis H.R., R.T. Bridenstine, D. Vesselinovitch, R.W. Wissler 1987. Fish oil inhibits development of atherosclerosis in Rhesus monkeys. *Arteriosclerosis* 7:441-449.

Dobbin L.V., H.F. Gofman, L. Jones, L. Lyon, & C.B. Young 1957. *The Low Fat, Low Cholesterol Diet.* New York: Doubleday.

Dyerberg J., & H.O. Bang 1979. Hemostatic function and platelet polyunsaturated fatty acids in Eskimos. *Lancet.* 2:433-435.

Flaim E., L.F. Ferreri, F.W. Thye, J.E. Hill, & S.F. Ritchey 1981. Plasma lipid and lipoprotein cholesterol concentrations in adult males consuming normal and high cholesterol diets under controlled conditions. *Am. J. Clin. Nutr.* 34:1103-1108.

Fredrickson D.S.& R.S. Gordon Jr. 1958. Transport of fatty acids. *Physiol. Rev.* 38:585-630.

Galbraith W.B., W.E. Connor, & D.B. Stone 1966. Weight loss and serum lipid changes in obese subjects given low-calorie diets of varied cholesterol content. *Ann. Int. Med.* 64:268-275.

Gjesdal K. 1976a. Platelet function and plasma free fatty acids during acute myocardial infarction and severe angina pectoris. *Scand. J. Haematol.* 17:205-212.

Gjesdal K., A. Nordoy, H. Wang, H. Bernsten, & O.D. Mjos 1976b. Effects of fasting on plasma and platelet-free fatty acids and platelet function in healthy males. *Thromb. Haemost.* 36:325-333.

Goodnight S.H. Jr., W.S. Harris, & W.E. Connor 1981. The effects of dietary omega-3 fatty acids upon platelet composition and function in man: a prospective, controlled study. *Blood.* 58:880-885.

Goodnight S.H. Jr, W.S. Harris, W.E. Connor, & D.R. Illingworth 1982. Polyunsaturated fatty acids, hyperlipidemia and thrombosis. *Arteriosclerosis.* 2:87-113.

Gordon T., M. Fisher, N. Ernst, B.M. Rifkind 1982. Relation of diet to LDL cholesterol, VLDL cholesterol and plasma total cholesterol and triglycerides in white adults. *Arteriosclerosis.* 2:502-512.

Grande F., J.T. Anderson, & A. Keys 1965. Effect of carbohydrates of leguminous seeds, wheat and potatoes on serum cholesterol concentration in man. *J. Nutr.* 86:313-317.

Gregg R.E., H.B. Brewer, Jr. 1986. The role of apolipoprotein E in modulating the metabolism of apolipoprotein B-48 and apolipoprotein B-100 containing lipoporteins in humans. In: Angel, A., Frohlich J., eds., Lipoprotein deficiency syndromes. *Adv. Exp. Med. Biol.* 201:289-298.

Grundy S.M. 1986. Comparison of monounsaturated fatty acids and carbohydrates for lowering plasma cholesterol. *N. Eng. J. Med.* 314:745-748.

Harris W.S., & W.E. Connor 1980. The effects of salmon oil upon plasma lipids, lipoprotein and triglyceride clearance. *Trans. Assoc. Am. Phys.* 93:148-155.

Harris W.S., W. E. Connor, N. Alam, & D.R. Illingworth 1988. The reduction of postprandial triglyceridemia in humans by dietary n-3 fatty acids. *Journal of Lipid Research.* 29:1451-1460.

Haskell W.L., C. Camargo, P.T. Williams, K.M Vranizan, R.M. Krauss, F.T. Lindgren, & P.D. Wood 1984. The effect of cessation and resumption of moderate alcohol intake on serum high-density lipoprotein subfractions. *N. Engl. J. Med.* 310:805-810.

Haslam R.J. 1964. Role of adenosine diphosphate in the aggregation of human blood-platelets by thrombin and by fatty acids. *Nature.* 202:765-768.

Hegsted D.M., R.B. McGandy, M.L. Myers, & F.J. Stare 1965. Quantitative effects of dietary fat on serum cholesterol in man. *Am. J. Clin. Nutr.* 17:281-295.

Hoak J.C., E.D. Warner, & W.E. Connor 1967. Platelets, fatty acids and thrombosis. *Circ. Res.* 20:11-17.

Intersalt Cooperative Research Group 1988. Intersalt: an international study of electrolyte excretion and blood pressure. Results for 24 hour urinary sodium and potassium excretion. *Brit. Med. J.* 297:319-328.

Katan M.B., A.C. Beynen, J.H.M. De Vries, & A. Nobels 1986. Existence of consistent hypo- and hyper responders to dietary cholesterol in man. *Am. J. of Epidemiology.* 123:221-234.

Katz L.N., J. Stamler, & R. Pick 1958. *Nutrition and Atherosclerosis.* Philadelphia: Lea and Febriger, p. 98.

Kay R.M., & A.S. Truswell 1977. Effect of citrus pectin on blood lipids and fecal steroid excretion in man. *Am. J. Clin. Nutr.* 30:171-175.

Keys A., J.T. Anderson, & F. Grande 1957a. Serum cholesterol response to dietary fat. *Lancet.* 1:787.

Keys A., J.T. Anderson, & F. Grande 1957b. Prediction of serum-cholesterol responses of man to changes in fats in the diet. *Lancet.* 2:959-966.

Keys A., F. Grande, & J.T. Anderson 1961. Fiber and pectin in the diet and serum cholesterol concentration in man. *Proc. Soc. Exp. Biol. Med.* 106:555-558.

Kovanen P.T., M.S. Brown, S.K. Basu, D.W. Bilheimer, & J.L. Goldstein 1981. Saturation and suppression of hepatic lipoprotein receptors: a mechanism for the hypercholesterolemia of cholesterol-fed rabbits. *Proc. Natl. Acad. Sci. U.S.A.* 78:1396-1400.

Kromhout D., E.B. Bosschieter, & C.deL Coulander 1985. The inverse relation between fish consumption and 20-year mortality from coronary heart disease. *N. Engl. J. Med.* 312:1205-1209.

Kurien V.A., & M.F. Oliver 1966. Serum free fatty acids after myocardial infarction and cerebral vascular occlusion. *Lancet.* 1:122-127.

Latto C. 1981. Hemorrhoids, diverticular disease and deep vein thrombosis. In: Trowell HC, Burkitt DP, eds. *Western diseases: their emergence and prevention.* Cambridge, Mass: Harvard University Press. 421-424.

Lin D.S., & W.E. Connor 1981. The long-term effects of dietary cholesterol upon the plasma lipids, lipoproteins, cholesterol absorption, and the sterol balance in man: the demonstration of feedback inhibition of cholesterol biosynthesis and increased bile acid excretion. *J. Lip. Res.* 21:1042-1052.

Lin D.S., W.E. Connor & C.W. Spenler 1993. Monounsaturated and polyunsaturated fatty acids deposited to the same extent in adipose tissue of rabbits?. *Am. J. Clin. Nutr.* (In Press).

Lipid research clinics programs: The lipid research clinics coronary primary prevention trial results: I. Reduction in incidence of coronary heart disease. 1984. *J.A.M.A.* 251:351-364.

McLean Ross A.H., M.A. Eastwood, J.R Anderson, & D.M.W. Anderson 1983. A study of the effects of dietary gum arabic in humans. *Am. J. Clin. Nutr.* 37:368-375.

Mahadevan V., M.H. Singh, & W.O. Lundberg 1966. Effects of saturated and unsaturated fatty acids on blood platelet aggregation in vitro. *Proc. Soc. Exp. Biol. Med.* 121:82-85.

Mahley R.W., D.Y. Hui, T.L. Innerarity, & K.H. Weisgraber 1981. Two independent lipoprotein receptors on hepatic membranes of dog, swine and man. *J. Clin. Invest.* 68:1197-1206.

Mahley R.W., T.L. Innerarity, S.C. Rall, et al. 1984. Plasma lipoproteins: apolipoprotein structure and function. *J. Lipid Res.* 25:1277-1294.

Mattson F.H., & S.M. Grundy 1985. Comparison of effects of dietary saturated, monounsaturated and polyunsaturated fatty acids on plasma lipids and lipoproteins in men. *J. Lipid Res.* 26:194-202.

Mistry P., N.E. Miller, M. Laker, W.R. Hazzard, & B. Lewis 1981. Individual variations in the effect of dietary cholesterol on plasma lipoproteins and cellular cholesterol homeostasis in man. *J. Clin. Invest.* 67:493-502.

Muenter M.D., H.O. Perry, & L. Jurgen 1971. Chronic vitamin A intoxication in adults. *Amer. J. Med.* 50:129-136.

Nikkila E.A., & K. Ojala 1965. Induction of hypertriglyceridemia by fructose in the rat. *Life Sci.* 4:937-943.

Olefsky J., G.M. Reaven, & J.W. Farquhar 1974. Effects of weight reduction on obesity. *J. Clin. Invest.* 53:64-76.

Peterson V.E., P.A. Crapo, J. Weininger, H. Ginsberg, & J. Olefsky 1975. Quantification of plasma cholesterol and triglyceride levels in hypercholesterolemic subjects receiving ascorbic acid supplements. *Am. J. Clin. Nutr.* 28:584-587.

Raymond T.L., W.E. Connor, D.S. Lin, S. Warner, M.M. Fry, & S.L. Connor 1971. The interaction of dietary fibers and cholesterol upon the plasma lipids and lipoproteins, the sterol balance, and bowel function in human subjects. *J. Clin. Invest.* 60:1429-1437.

Renaud S., R.L Kinlough, & J.F. Mustard 1970. Relationship between platelet aggregation and the thrombotic tendency in rats fed hyperlipemic diets. *Lab. Invest.* 22:339-343.

Roberts S.L., M. McMurry, & W.E. Connor 1981. Does egg feeding (i.e. dietary cholesterol) affect plasma cholesterol levels in humans? The results of a double-blind study. *Am. J. Clin. Nutr.* 34:2092-2099.

St. Leger A.S., A.L. Cochrance, & F. Moore 1979. Factors associated with cardiac mortality in developed countries with particular reference to the consumption of wine. *Lancet.* 1:1017-1020.

Schwartz R.S., & J.D. Brunzell 1981. Increase of adipose tissue lipoprotein lipase activity with weight loss. *J. Clin. Invest.* 67:1425-1430.

Spady D.K., & J.M. Dietschy 1985. Dietary saturated triacylglycerols suppress heaptic low density lipoprotein receptor activity in the hamster. *Proc. Natl. Acad. Sci. U.S.A.* 82:4526-4530.

Spady D.K., & J.M. Dietschy 1988. Interaction of dietary cholesterol and triglycerides in the regulation of heptic low density lipoprotein transport in the hamster. *J. Clin. Invest.* 81:300-309.

Steiner A., E.J. Howard, & S. Akgun 1962. Importance of dietary cholesterol in man. *J. Am. Med. Assoc.* 181:186-190.

Stone D.B., & W.E. Connor 1963. The prolonged effects of a low cholesterol, high carbohydrate diet upon the serum lipids in diabetic patients. *Diabetes.* 12:127-132.

Taylor C.B., D.E. Patton, & G.E. Cox 1959. Atherosclerosis in rhesus monkeys. VI. Fatal myocardial infarction in a monkey fed fat and cholesterol. *Arch. Path.* 76:404-412.

Ullmann D., W.E. Connor, L.F. Hatcher, S.L. Connor, & D.P. Flavell 1988. The absence of carbohydrate-induced hypertriglyceridemia during a phased high carbohydrate diet. *Abstract. Circulation.* 78(suppl):II73.

Weiner B.H., I.S. Ockene, P.H. Levine, et al. 1986. Inhibition of atherosclerosis by cod liver oil in a hyperlipidemic swine model. *N. Engl. J. Med.* 315:841-846.

Weinsier R.L., A. Seeman, M.G. Herrera, J.P. Assul, J.S. Soeldner, & R.G. Gleason 1974. High and low carbohydrate diets in diabetes: study of effects on diabetic control, insulin secretion and blood lipids. *Ann. Int. Med.* 80:332-341.

Welsh S.O., & R.M. Marston 1982. Review of trends in food use in the United States, 1909 to 1980. *J. Amer Dietet. Assoc.* 81:120-125.

Wood P.D., W.L. Haskell, S.N. Blair et al. 1983. Increased exercise level and plasma lipoprotein concentrations: a one-year randomized, controlled study in sedentary middle-aged men. *Metabolism.* 32:31-39.

Zilversmit D.B. 1979a. Atherogenesis: a postpradial phenomenon. *Circulation.* 60:473-485.

Zilversmit, D.B. 1979b. Cholesterol index of foods. *J. Amer. Dietet. Assoc.* 74:562-565.

Dietary fatty acids and serum lipids

D. M. Hegsted
New England Regional Primate Research Center, Harvard University, Southborough, Mass., USA

ABSTRACT: Analyses of the total experimental data on the effects of dietary fat modification on serum cholesterol and lipoprotein levels in groups of human subjects confirm the general conclusions reached 25-30 years ago, namely, that the saturated fatty acids (S) raise serum cholesterol, the polyunsaturated fatty acids (P) actively lower serum cholesterol and the monounsaturated fatty acids (M) have no statistically significant effect. The saturated fatty acids are the most important determinants of serum cholesterol but it does not appear to be possible to accurately quantitate the relative potency of S and P. Given the mass of data now available, additional studies are most unlikely to modify these conclusions. The effects on LDL-C are roughly similar to those on total serum cholesterol. The data suggest that all three classes of fatty acids tend to elevate HDL-C but the prediction of the change expected is poor and we believe that the physiologic significance of such changes is unknown.

1. INTRODUCTION

It is unfortunate that our understanding of the effects of various fatty acids upon serum lipids and lipoproteins has been confused in recent years by isolated studies in which the cholesterol-lowering ability of oils high in monounsaturated and polyunsaturated fats appeared to be no different. The commercial interests in oils high in monounsaturated fatty acids became active, of course, to promote their products. The result has been numerous studies, costing millions of dollars, which have yielded inconsistent results. The public is more confused, rather than educated, particularly since every paper that appears on the modification of serum lipids by dietary manipulation is treated in the public press as though it were the final word.

It is now time to put this issue to rest. There are now available two independent evaluations of the data available on the effects of dietary fat modification upon serum cholesterol and lipoprotein levels in groups of human subjects. Both of these studies confirm what was concluded 25-30 years ago, namely that the saturated fatty acids (S) elevate serum cholesterol, the polyunsaturated fatty acids (P) actively lower serum cholesterol and the monounsaturated fatty acids (M) have no significant effect.

2. TOTAL DATA ON CHANGE IN SERUM CHOLESTEROL

Mensink and Katan (1992) evaluated the data from 27 different trials reported since 1972 in which the dietary fat was modified but the dietary cholesterol level was maintained constant. We (Hegsted, et al, 1993) have analyzed the total data on the effects of modifying S, M, and P, as well as dietary cholesterol (C). We have also evaluated a more limited data set - studies done in more recent years - in which the lipoprotein levels were reported. Only those studies in which the foods were prepared and fed to the experimental subjects have been included. It should be emphasized, however, that in many studies the subjects were free-living and only some of the meals were fed under supervision. We do not know the degree of dietary compliance under these conditions. In the studies we evaluated, we also excluded data obtained with "formula diets".

The data have been evaluated by multiple regression analysis and these show the predicted changes in serum cholesterol or lipoprotein cholesterol, expressed as mg/dl, due to modification of the intake of the 3 classes of fatty acids. The fatty acids are expressed percent of energy intake and dietary cholesterol is in mg/1000 kcals. The several predictive equations are as follows:

$$\delta SC = 1.15\delta S - 0.12\delta M - 0.56\delta P \quad R^2 = 0.89$$
Mensink & Katan (1992)

$$\delta SC = 2.10\delta S - 1.16\delta P + 0.067\delta C \quad R^2 = 0.84$$
Hegsted et al 1993

$$\delta SC = 2.08\delta S - 0.82\delta P + 0.054\delta C \quad R^2 = 0.86$$
Hegsted et al, 1993. Recent data

In the Mensink and Katan equation, the coefficient of δM was included even though it was not statistically significant. In neither of the data sets that we analyzed was the coefficient of δM significant so it was not included. The equations may be compared to the equations published by Keys et al (1957) and by Hegsted et al (1965)

$$\delta SC = 2.74\delta S - 1.32\delta P$$
Keys et al 1957

$$\delta SC = 2.16\delta S - 1.65\delta P + 0.17\delta C$$
Hegsted et al 1965

In all of the data sets it is apparent that the coefficient of δS is positive, ie S raises serum cholesterol, while that of δP is negative and lowers serum cholesterol. In none of the data sets can δM be shown to have a statistically significant effect. Hence, while individual studies may fail to distinguish between the effects of M and P, these appear to be aberrant results when compared to the mass of data now available.

It is also apparent that the relative potency of S and P vary substantially depending upon which data set one analyzes. The coefficient of δS is always larger than that of δP but the ratio of activity, $\delta S/\delta P$, varies from 1.3 to 2.6. The reason for this is apparent if one examines the standard errors of the regression coefficients. For example, Mensink and Katan found that, based on the 95% confidence interval, while the mean value is 1.51, the true value may fall between 1.2 and 1.8. All of the coefficients in these equations show similarly large error terms. These are obviously due to the substantial variation in the distribution of the data points around the regression lines. Hence, even though these regression equations account for a very large proportion of the variance - 85 to 90% - very similar studies do yield quite different results as can be seen from Figure 1.

It should be emphasized that in the original data of Keys et al (1957) and Hegsted et al (1965) this was also true. One can easily select values in either of these data sets which are not well predicted by the general equation. The merit of these studies was

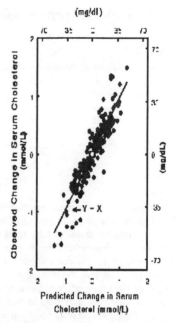

Figure 1. Observed versus predicted changes in SC by the equation, $\delta SC = 2.108\ \delta S - 1.16\delta P + 0.067\delta C$ (Hegsted et al 1993). A total of 248 values from the literature.

simply that in both a fairly large number of fats and oils were studied and this allowed some generalization. It is clear that if only a few fats or oils had been investigated, any number of conclusions might have been reached.

The message ought to be clear, namely, that you cannot generalize from data generated by data from 2 or 3 comparisons. Unfortunately, practically all of the data presented in the past decade or so is of this kind ie limited studies of a very few fats or oils.

An important question, of course, is why data obtained in different laboratories, or even in the same laboratory, yield discordant results when similar changes in fat composition are compared. We can rarely identify the specific causes in any particular study but here are a multitude of reasons why this may occur. We know that individuals vary in their response so the results depend, in part, upon the characteristics of the subjects chosen for study. It is not easy to accurately describe either the change in serum cholesterol or the absolute composition of the diet. Calculations made from food composition tables may differ considerably from analyzed values. As already noted, the cost of well-controlled metabolic studied have become so outrageous in recent years that practically all investigators have been forced to rely upon free-living subjects. However well they are managed, it is certain that some subjects fail to comply rigorously and the degree of compliance is not known. In addition, it is becoming increasingly clear that there area number of dietary components other than fatty acids and dietary cholesterol which affects the serum lipid levels. These include the plant sterols, dietary fiber, protein, and unknown materials. We have very little idea about the quantitative importance of these kinds of materials compared to the fatty acids and cholesterol and we do not know whether these kinds of materials affect the serum lipid response to fatty acids. We are sure, however, that different sample of oils and fats, even though they have the same name and content of fatty acids, vary in their composition of various materials. No sample of olive oil, for example, has the same composition as all samples of olive oil. The basal diets which have been used also vary greatly in their content of these materials. There is no basal diet that is representative of all diets.

There are some lessons we should learn. The major one is that one cannot generalizer from small studies. The second is that while the fatty acids are major determinants of the serum cholesterol response, other things do affect the response. But it should be clear that there are now available a tremendous amount of data of these kinds- data on over 400 diets have been reported- and simply adding another few data points is not going to change the general conclusions.

3. CHANGES IN LIPOPROTEINS

It is reasonably clear, as would be expected since low density lipoproteins carry most of the serum cholesterol, that dietary-induced changes in low density lipoprotein cholesterol (LDL-C) are quite similar to those of total serum cholesterol and I will not discuss this. There is now, however, a great interest in the changes in high density lipoproteins (HDL-C). The epidemiologic data obtained within communities where the diet is generally similar, such as in Framingham (Castelli et al, 1986), show that low HDL-C levels increases risk of heart disease. I wish to argue, however, that we do not know how to interpret changes in HDL-C induced by changes in dietary fat and cholesterol. It is of interest that in both the data analyzed by Mensink and Katan and Hegsted et al, the best predicative equations have positive coefficients for each of the 3 classes of fatty acids suggesting that all three tend to elevate HDL-C with S being the most

effective. However, the best predictive equations can account for only 40-60% of the variance. That is, the errors in prediction are relatively large, probably because the changes in HDL-C are relatively small and the errors in measurement relatively large. More disturbing. however, is the fact that low fat diets lower HDL-C levels. If there is anything that we know, it is that very low fat diets protect against heart disease. Obviously, what we are interested in is reducing risk of heart disease, not HDL-C levels per se. The explanation may be that as Brinton et al (1990) reported, when HDL-C is lowered by dietary means, the metabolism of HDL is different from that in individuals who have naturally low HDL levels. Hence, while many have concluded that lowering HDL levels by dietary manipulation is disadvantageous, this may not be true.

I would add, however, that the elevation of HDL-C levels by modest alcohol consumption or by exercise or estrogen does appear
to be of definite benefit.

4. FUTURE STUDIES

There are a number of areas of practical importance which need resolution. There is substantial evidence that not all saturated fatty acids are equally hypercholesterolemic. In particular, there is considerable evidence that stearic acid has little or no effect. However, when we (McGandy et al, 1970) attempted to evaluate the effects of specific saturated fatty acids, we could not show that they have different effects. We added similar amounts of lauric, myristic, palmitic and stearic acid to samples of olive oil and of safflower oil and then transesterified the mixture producing fats in which the fatty acids were randomly distributed in the triglycerides. Each these tranesterified fats had substantially the same effect on serum cholesterol. If the data available are correct, that stearic acid is usually not hypercholesterolemic and our studies are also correct, then it would appear that the triglyceride structure may be important. If substantial amounts of fat are absorbed as monoglycerides and these are re-synthesized into the circulating triglycerides, then the structure of the dietary triglycerides may be important.

We (Hegsted et al, 1965) originally concluded that myristic acid was the most hypercholesterolemic of the saturated fatty acids. Whether this is true remains to be seen but our original studies were flawed. In those studies the saturated fats that ere varied were primarily butterfat and coconut oil. Since both of these are relatively high in myristic acid, it is not surprising that myristic acid appeared to be the most hypercholesterolemic.

I believe that we have about exhausted our capacity to examine the effects of fatty acids upon serum lipids in human subjects primarily because of excessive costs and other restrictions on the use of human subjects. Further studies are most unlikely to be productive or change what we now know. I believe that the most productive areas which now present themselves are the study of all of those other materials in diets or fats which influence serum lipids and risk of coronary heart disease. We need quantitative data comparable to the data we have with the fatty acids. The other area which needs extensive research is on the effects of materials, like the n-3 fatty acids, which appear to be important but through systems other than the serum lipids.

REFERENCES

Brinton, E. A., Eisenberg, S. & Breslow, J. L. 1990. A low-fat diet decreases high density lipoprotein (HDL) cholesterol by decreasing HDL apolipoprotein transport rates. J. Clin. Invest. 85: 155-151.

Castelli, W. P., Garrison, R. J., Wilson, P. W., Abbott, R. D., Kalousian, S. & Kannel, W. B. 1986. Incidence of coronary heart disease and lipoprotein cholesterol levels. The Framingham Study. J, Am. Med. Assoc. 256: 2835-2838.

Hegsted, D. M., McGandy, R. B., Myers, M. L. & Stare, F. J. 1965. Quantitative effects of dietary fat on serum cholesterol in man. Am. J. Clin. Nutr. 17: 281-295.

Hegsted, D. M., Ausman, L. M., Johnson, J. A. & Dallal, G. E. 1993. Dietary fat and serum lipids: an evaluation of the experimental data. Am. J. Clin. Nutr. In press.

Keys, A., Anderson, J. T. & Grande, F. 1957. Prediction of serum-cholesterol responses of man to changes in fats in the diet. Lancet 2: 959-966.

McGandy,R. B., Hegsted, D. M. & Myers, M. L. 1970. Use of synthetic fats on determining effects of specific fatty acids on serum lipids in man. Am. J. Clin Nutr. 23: 1288-1298.

Mensink, R. P. & Katan, M. B. 1992. Effect of dietary fatty acids on serum lipids and lipoproteins. Arterio Thrombosis 12: 911-919.

Dairy Products in Human Health and Nutrition, Serrano Ríos et al. (eds) © 1994 Balkema, Rotterdam, ISBN 90 5410 359 0

Effects of monounsaturated fatty acids on serum lipoproteins

R.P.Mensink
Department of Human Biology, Limburg University, Maastricht, Netherlands

ABSTRACT: Low-density lipoprotein (LDL) cholesterol levels are positively, and high-density lipoprotein (HDL) cholesterol levels are negatively related to coronary heart disease. Changes in dietary fatty-acid intake affect the distribution of cholesterol over LDL and HDL. Lauric, myristic and palmitic acid and *trans* fatty acids elevate the serum total and LDL-cholesterol when compared with isoenergetic caloric amounts of carbohydrates. Other saturated fatty acids do not influence the serum cholesterol level. Linoleic and probably also oleic acid have a small LDL cholesterol lowering effect. Replacement of carbohydrates by fat increases the level of HDL cholesterol. *Trans* fatty acids, however, might be an exception and may lower the level of HDL cholesterol relative to other fatty acids. It seems that - as far as lipoproteins are concerned - a reduction in the intake of saturated fatty acids is more important for lowering the risk of coronary heart disease than a reduction in total fat intake per se.

INTRODUCTION

Lipoproteins are particles that transport cholesterol and triglycerides through the blood vessels. In man about 60 to 70 percent of the total serum cholesterol levels is transported by the low-density lipoproteins (LDL), and 30 to 40 percent by the high-density lipoproteins (HDL). Another lipoprotein particle, the very-low density lipoprotein (VLDL), carries mainly triglycerides, but also small amounts of cholesterol. Epidemiological studies have shown that the risk for coronary heart disease is positively related to LDL cholesterol levels, but negatively to that of HDL cholesterol (Gordon 1989). High serum triglyceride levels may also be an independent risk factor for coronary heart disease. Lipoprotein cholesterol and triglyceride levels can be modified by dietary means and diet is therefore an important tool for lowering the risk of coronary heart disease. Here the effects of dietary fatty-acid composition on serum HDL and LDL cholesterol, and triglycerides concentrations are discussed.

EFFECTS OF FATTY ACIDS ON SERUM TOTAL AND LDL CHOLESTEROL

A fatty acid is hypercholesterolemic when the serum total cholesterol concentration increases, if this fatty acid replaces carbohydrates in the diet. The amount of energy provided by the fatty acid and carbohydrates should be the same. Otherwise body-weight will be affected, which will result in a change in the serum total cholesterol concentration (Dattilo 1992). Consequently, effects of changes in dietary fatty-acid composition on serum lipids cannot be separated from those of changes in weight.

Saturated fatty acids

Table 1 shows the fatty-acid composition of some edible fats and oils. Fats - which are solid at room temperature - have high levels of saturated fatty acids, while the liquid oils are rich in unsaturated fatty acids. Thus, butter fat has a relatively high level of saturated fatty acids, while olive oil is rich in oleic acid (C18:1), and sunflower oil in linoleic acid (C18:2). A diet is composed of many different types of fats and oils, and contains many different fatty acids.

To describe the effects on serum total cholesterol levels, it is useful to categorize the saturated fatty acids into three different classes. The first category consist of fatty acids with less than 12 carbon atoms. These are call short and medium chain saturated fatty acids and are found in coconut fat, palm kernel oil and butter fat. The second category consists of lauric acid (C12:0), myristic acid (C14:0) and palmitic acid (C16:0), and the

Table 1. Pattern of fatty acids in some edible, non-hydrogenated, fats and oils.

Fat or oil	<12	LA	MA	PA	SA	OA	LLA	LNA
	gram per 100 gram of fatty acids							
Coconut	11	41	17	9	3	12	7	0
Palm kernel	7	46	17	10	3	15	4	0
Butter	10	3	10	27	12	23	1	1
Palm	0	0	1	41	7	40	10	0
Rapeseed	0	0	0	5	2	59	2	10
Olive	0	0	0	11	3	76	8	1
Sun flower	0	0	0	6	5	23	64	0
Soy-bean	0	0	0	11	4	23	55	6
Linseed	0	0	0	5	3	19	16	56

<12 = less than 12 carbon atoms; LA, C12:0 = lauric acid; MA, C14:0 = myristic acid; PA, C16:0 = palmitic acid; SA, C18:0 = stearic acid; OA, C18:1 = oleic acid; LLA, C18:2 = linoleic acid; LNA, C18:3 = linolenic acid

third category of stearic acid (C18:0). These three classes of saturated fatty acids contributes to a different extent to daily energy intake. Although some variation does exist between the Western countries, the short chain saturated fatty acids provide in general less than 6 percent of total saturated fat intake, lauric, myristic and palmitic acid between 60 and 70 percent, and stearic acid between 20 and 25 percent.

Short and medium-chain fatty acids

A mixture of short and medium chain saturated fatty lowers the serum total cholesterol level relative to butter fat (Hashim 1960) and effects are thought to be similar to those of carbohydrates. Whether these fatty acids have an effect on the distribution of cholesterol over the various lipoproteins is not known.

Lauric-, myristic-, and palmitic acid

Lauric-, myristic- en palmitic acid (C12:0, C14:0 and C16:0) increase the serum total cholesterol level. Keys, Anderson and Grande (1965) estimated that the serum total cholesterol increases by 0.62 mmol/L [24 mg/dL], when 10 percent of energy in the diet provided by carbohydrates is replaced by a mixture of these saturated fatty acids. These three saturated fatty acids, however, are not equally hypercholesterolemic. From a series of experiments with natural fats and oils Hegsted and co-workers (1965) found that myristic acid was the most hypercholesterolemic. This conclusion was not supported by experiments with synthetic fats and oils. McGandy et al (1970) reported that myristic and palmitic acid increased the serum total cholesterol level to a greater extent than lauric acid did. In contrast, Vergroesen and de Boer (1971) found that lauric and myristic acid were more hypercholesterolemic that palmitic acid. Whether these discrepant findings can be explained by the different nature of the fat - natural fats in the study of Hegsted at al (1975) versus synthetic fats in the other studies (McGandy 1979; Vergroesen 1971) - is not known. However, these three saturated fatty acids definitively increases the serum total and LDL cholesterol levels compared to isoenergetic caloric amounts of carbohydrates.

Stearic acid

Keys et al (1965) concluded that stearic acid has no effect on serum total cholesterol levels. This conclusion was supported by a study from Grande et al (1970), who found that the serum total cholesterol level increased by 0.60 mmol/L [23 mg/dL] when 10 percent of total energy from stearic acid was replaced by an equal amount of palmitic acid.

Monounsaturated fatty acids

Oleic acid is the most abundant monounsaturated fatty acid in the human diet. Although olive oil probably is the most well-known source of oleic acid, the contribution of animal fats to total intake is of much more importance. Also, the consumption of other oils like the low-erucic rapeseed oil and the high-oleic acid sunflower oil may become important as well.

Oleic acid

The serum total and LDL cholesterol level are similar when iso-energetic amounts of carbohydrates are replaced by oleic acid (Mensink 1987). In addition, the effects of oleic acid on serum total and LDL cholesterol may be comparable with those of stearic acid. This has recently been shown again by Bonanome and Grundy (1988): exchanging 16 percent of energy from oleic acid for stearic acid did not change significantly serum total or LDL cholesterol levels.

Thus, oleic acid is not hypocholesterolemic as compared with carbohydrates, but is hypocholesterolemic as compared with saturated fatty acids.

Polyunsaturated fatty acids

Polyunsaturated fatty acids can be divided into the (n-6)- and (n-3)-fatty acids. The nomenclature is based on the position of the first double bond at the methyl end of the fatty acid molecule. About 80 to 90 percent of the total level of polyunsaturated fatty acids in the diet is provided by linoleic acid (C18:2, n-6) from vegetable oils like sunflower oil, corn oil and soy-bean oil. Important (n-3) polyunsaturated fatty acids are α-linolenic acid (C18:3,n-3), as found in rapeseed and soy bean oil, and the very long chain fatty acids eicosapentaenoic acid (EPA; C20:5, n-3) and docosahexaenoic acid (DHA; C22:6, n-3) from fish oils.

(N-6)-polyunsaturated fatty acids

Linoleic acid was thought to be hypocholesterolemic as compared with carbohydrates and monounsaturated fatty acids. Keys et al (1965) concluded from their studies that replacement of 10 percent of total energy intake from carbohydrates by linoleic acid decreases the serum total cholesterol level by 0.31 mmol/L [12 mg/dL]. Recently, however, we have carried out an experiment in which 6.5 percent of daily energy intake from saturated fatty acids was substituted by oleic acid plus linoleic acid (oleic-acid diet) or by linoleic acid alone (Mensink 1989). The intake of linoleic acid was 7.7 percent on the oleic-acid diet and 12.6 percent of energy on the linoleic-acid diet. Surprisingly, the decrease in serum total and LDL cholesterol on the oleic-acid and the linoleic-acid diet was similar. Other, more recent, studies also found that linoleic acid was not hypocholesterolemic relative to oleic acid (Valsta 1992). At present there is no unequivocal explanation for the discrepancy between these results and those of Keys and co-workers (1965).

Due to these discrepant findings, we decided to analyze results from 27 well-controlled trials that met specific inclusion criteria (Mensink 1992). These trials yielded 65 data points, which were analyzed by multiple regression analyses using is-energetic exchanges of saturated, monounsaturated, and (n-6)-polyunsaturated fatty acids against carbohydrates as the independent variables. Diets specifically enriched in stearic acid, fish-oils or trans fatty acids were excluded. As expected, saturated fatty acids markedly increased the LDL cholesterol level as compared with carbohydrates (Figure 1). It was estimated that replacing one percent of energy from carbohydrates by linoleic acid lowered the serum total cholesterol level by only 0.015 mmol/L [0.60 mg/dL], which was substantially lower than the effect of 0.031 mmol/L [1.20 mg/dL] as estimated by Keys et al (1965) and of 0.048 mmol/dL [1.87 mg/dL], as predicted Hegsted et al (1965). Oleic acid itself also had a small LDL cholesterol-lowering

effect of 0.006 mmol/L [0.24 mg/dL].

(N-3)-polyunsaturated fatty acids

The effects of α-linolenic acid on the serum total and LDL cholesterol levels are comparable to those of linoleic acid (Singer 1986).

Keys, Anderson and Grande were among the first to study the effects of fish oils on serum total cholesterol levels (1958). They concluded that the hypocholesterolemic effect of fish oils is similar to that of linoleic acid. However, data from more recent studies suggest that a daily intake of EPA and DHA up to 5 grams in the form of fish oil capsules increases the LDL cholesterol level (Beynen 1989). These fatty acids, however, do lower serum triglycerides and the level of cholesterol in the VLDL. The opposite effects on VLDL and LDL explains why fish oils do not change the serum total cholesterol level.

Trans fatty acids

Because of the double bond in the molecule, unsaturated fatty acids may exist as either cis or trans isomers. Double bonds, both in monounsaturated and in polyunsaturated fatty acids, do mostly have the cis configuration. However, during hydrogenation of unsaturated fatty acids cis double bonds are partly converted to trans double bonds. In addition, the position of a double bond may change, and after hydrogenation a complex mixture of many different cis and trans fatty acids is formed. These mixtures can be used for the production of certain types of margarines, frying fats, and foods prepared with these fats. The average consumption of trans fatty acids is around 2 to 5 percent of total daily energy intake.

Although many studies have been carried out with trans fatty acids, the effects of these fatty acids on cholesterol metabolism in man are largely unknown. The intake of trans fatty acids was not the only difference between the experimental diets, so that effects on cholesterol or lipoprotein levels could not be specifically ascribed to the presence of trans fatty acids.

Trans-monounsaturated fatty acids

Only three studies have compared side-by-side the effects of oleic acid, a cis-monounsaturated fatty acids, with those of trans-monounsaturated fatty acids with the same chain length. Results were contradictory. Mattson et al (1975) found similar serum total cholesterol levels on a diet high in cis or trans fatty acids. Vergroesen et al (1972), however, concluded that trans fatty acids are hypercholesterolemic, which has recently been

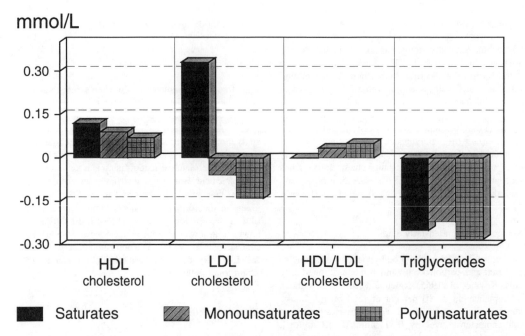

mmol/L

Figure 1. Predicted changes in serum lipids and lipoproteins when 10% of energy as carbohydrates is replaced by fatty acids of a particular class (Mensink 1992). Saturated fatty acids include the contribution of the non-cholesterol-raising saturated fatty acids, while monounsaturated fatty acids mainly refer to oleic acid, and polyunsaturated fatty acids to linoleic acid.

confirmed (Mensink 1991). In that study 59 volunteers received three different diets. The composition of the diet was similar, except for 10 percent of energy, that was provided by either oleic acid, *trans* isomers of oleic acid, or by lauric plus myristic plus palmitic acid, the cholesterol-raising saturated fatty acids. It was found that serum LDL cholesterol levels were the lowest on the diet high in oleic acid, and increased with 0.37 mmol/L [14 mg/dL] on the *trans* fatty-acid rich diet and with 0.47 mmol/L [18 mg/dL] on the saturated-fat diet. These results clearly show that *trans* fatty acids may have an unfavorable effect on serum LDL cholesterol. However, more studies should be carried out to examine whether our results may be extended to other types of *trans* fatty acids, to lower intakes, and to other groups of volunteers.

EFFECTS OF FATTY ACIDS ON HDL

Using results from epidemiological studies Katan (1984) estimated that the serum HDL cholesterol decreases by about 0.10 mmol/L [4 mg/dL] if fat intake decreases by 10 percent of energy intake and is replaced by carbohydrates. This estimate has been confirmed by controlled dietary experiments.

The effects on HDL cholesterol of the different fatty acids, however, are not identical. Mattson and Grundy (1985) found that the HDL cholesterol level decreased by 0.11 mmol/L [4 mg/dL], when as much as 23 percent of energy from oleic acid was replaced by linoleic acid. Although all fatty acids increase HDL-cholesterol relative to carbohydrates, this effect decreases with increasing unsaturation of the fatty acid (Figure 1; Mensink 1992). *Trans* fatty acids, however, may lower HDL cholesterol. In our study (Mensink 1991) the HDL cholesterol levels was 0.17 mmol/L [7 mg/dL] higher on the oleic-acid on saturated-fat diet. Several studies also suggest that stearic acid lowers HDL cholesterol relative to other saturated and *cis*-unsaturated fatty acids (Zock 1992; Mensink 1993).

EFFECTS OF FATTY ACIDS ON SERUM TRIGLYCERIDES

According to our meta-analysis a mixture of saturated fatty acids, and monounsaturated and (n-6)-polyunsaturated fatty acids from vegetable oils lower the serum triglyceride level (Figure 1; Mensink 1992) relative to carbohydrates. This effect was similar for all fatty acids. (N-3)-polyunsaturated fatty acids from fish oil, however, have very powerful triglyceride-lowering effect (Harris 1983). Some studies suggest that stearic acid and *trans* fatty acids have a slight triglyceride-elevating effect relative to other fatty acids (Mensink 1991; Zock 1992), but this needs further study.

CONCLUSION

A decrease in the consumption of lauric, myristic and palmitic acid is the most effective way to reduce the serum LDL cholesterol level. When these fatty acids are replaced by carbohydrates the decrease in LDL cholesterol will be accompanied by a decrease in HDL cholesterol, and an increase in the serum triglyceride concentration. The slight serum total-cholesterol lowering effect of polyunsaturated fatty acids over monounsaturated fatty acids is caused by lowering of both HDL and LDL cholesterol levels. *trans* fatty acids do have a very unfavorable effect on the serum lipoprotein profile. It should be emphasized, however, that - although diet rich in unsaturated fatty acids with the *cis* configuration may be helpful for optimizing serum lipoprotein level -, an overall reduction in total fat intake seems advisable in view of the possible positive association between dietary fat intake with obesity, and other welfare diseases.

REFERENCES

Beynen, A.C. & M.B. Katan 1989. Impact of dietary cholesterol and fatty acids on serum lipids and lipoproteins in man. In: Vergroesen A.J. & M.A. Crawford, eds. *The role of fats in human nutrition.* London: Academic Press Limited, 237-286.

Bonanome, A. & S.M. Grundy. 1988 Effect of dietary stearic acid on plasma cholesterol and lipoprotein levels. *N Engl J Med* 318:1244-1248.

Dattilo, A.M. & P.M. Kris-Etherton 1992. Effects of weight reduction on blood lipids and lipoproteins: a meta-analysis. *Am J Clin Nutr* 56:320-326.

Gordon, D.J. & B.M. Rifkind 1989. High-density lipoprotein - The clinical implications of recent studies. *N Engl J Med* 321:1311-1316.

Grande, F., J.T. Anderson & A. Keys 1979. Comparison of effects of palmitic and stearic acids in the diet on serum cholesterol in man. *Am J Clin Nutr* 23:1184-1193.

Harris, W.S., W.E. Connor & M.P. McMurry 1983. The comparative reductions of the plasma lipids and lipoproteins by dietary polyunsaturated fats: salmon oil versus vegetable oils. *Metabolism* 32:179-184.

Hashim, S.A., A. Arteaga & T.B. Van Itallie 1960. Effect of a saturated medium-chain triglyceride on serum-lipids in man. *Lancet* i:1105-1108.

Hegsted, D.M., R.B. McGandy, M.L. Myers & F.J. Stare 1965. Quantative effects of dietary fat on serum cholesterol in man. *Am J Clin Nutr* 17:281-295.

Katan, M.B. 1986. Diet and HDL. In: Miller G.J. & N.E. Miller, eds. *Metabolic aspects of cardiovascular disease. Vol 3. Clinical and metabolic aspects of high-density lipoproteins.* Oxford: Elsevier, 1984:103-132.

Keys, A., J.T. Anderson & F. Grande 1958. Prediction of serum-cholesterol responses of man to changes in fats in the diet. *Lancet* 1958:ii;959-966.

Keys, A., J.T. Anderson & F. Grande 1965. Serum cholesterol response to changes in the diet. IV. Particular saturated fatty acids in the diet. *Metabolism* 1965;14:776-787.

Mattson, F.H., E.J. Hollenbach & A.M. Kligman 1975. Effect of hydrogenated fat on the plasma cholesterol and triglyceride levels of man. *Am J Clin Nutr* 1975;28:726-731.

Mattson, F.H. & S.M. Grundy 1985. Comparison of effects of dietary saturated, monounsaturated, and polyunsaturated fatty acids on plasma lipids and lipoproteins in man. *J Lipid Res* 1985;26:194-202.

McGandy, R.B., D.M. Hegsted & M.L. Myers 1970. Use of semisynthetic fats in determining effects of specific dietary fatty acids on serum lipids in man. *Am J Clin Nutr* 1970;23:1288-1298.

Mensink, R.P. & M.B. Katan 1987. Effect of mono-unsaturated fatty acids versus complex carbohydrates on high-density lipoproteins in healthy men and women. *Lancet* i:122-125.

Mensink R.P. & M.B. Katan 1989. Effect of a diet enriched with monounsaturated or polyunsaturated fatty acids on levels of low-density and high-density lipoprotein cholesterol in healthy women and men. *N Engl J Med* 321:436-441.

Mensink R.P. & M.B. Katan 1991. Effect of dietary *trans* fatty acids on levels of high-density and low-density lipoprotein cholesterol in healthy subjects. *N Engl J Med* 323:439-445.

Mensink, R.P. & M.B. Katan 1992. Effect of dietary fatty acids on serum lipids and lipoproteins. A meta-analysis of 27 trial. *Arterioscler Thromb* 12:911-919.

Mensink R.P. 1993. Effects of the individual saturated fatty acids on serum lipids and lipoprotein concentra-tions. *Am J Clin Nutr,* in press.

Singer P., L. Berger, M. Wirth, W. Gödicke, W. Jaeger & S. Voigt 1986. Slow desaturation and elongation of linoleic and α-linolenic acids as a rationale of eicosapentaenoic acid-rich diet to lower blood pressure and serum lipids in normal, hypertensive and hyperlipemic subjects. *Prostaglandins Leukotr Med* 24:173-193.

Valsta, L.M., M. Jauhiainen, A. Aro, M.B. Katan & M. Mutanen 1992. Effects of a monounsaturated rapeseed oil and a polyunsaturated sunflower oil diet on lipoprotein levels in man. *Arterioscler Thromb* 12:50-57.

Vergroesen, A.J. & J. de Boer 1971. Quantitative und qualitative Effekte mehrfach ungesättigter und anderer Fettsäuren in der menschlichen Diät. *Wissenschaftliche Veröffentlichungen der Deutschen Gesellschaft für Ernährung* 22:76-89.

Vergroesen A.J. 1972. Dietary fat and cardiovascular disease: Possible modes of action of linoleic acid. *Proc Nutr Soc* 31:323-329.

Zock, P.L. & M.B. Katan 1992. Hydrogenation alternatives: effects of *trans* fatty acids and stearic acid versus linoleic acid on serum lipids and lipoproteins in humans. *J Lipid Res* 33:399-410.

Dairy Products in Human Health and Nutrition, Serrano Ríos et al. (eds) © 1994 Balkema, Rotterdam, ISBN 90 5410 359 0

Micronutrients, antioxidants and general mechanisms of disease

N.W. Solomons

Center for Studies of Sensory Impairment, Aging Metabolism (CeSSIAM), Guatemala

ABSTRACT: Increasing knowledge and understanding in basic biochemistry as well as gains in pathophysiology, epidemiology and human ecology have raised an general question about the relation of health with antioxidants in general, and micronutrients from the diet with antioxidant properties in particular. We review the general mechanisms of disease in both the pathological and the ecological context. Definitions and examples of biological oxidation mechanisms and micronutrient antioxidants are provided. The epidemiological observations relating intake of antioxidant micronutrients alone or in combination to human health and well-being, and the assumptions underlying the operation. The translation of epidemiological hypotheses to "chemoprevention" trial design is addressed. The potential adverse and toxicological consequences of elevated and unbalanced intakes of dietary micronutrients are discussed. Prudent reservations and restrained optimism, rather than unbridled and uncritical enthusiasm, are needed as we continue to evaluate the implications of oxidation for ill health and the potential of antioxidants from the diet to counteract their negative effects.

1 OXIDANTS IN THE NEWS

The topical nature of the theme of "Micronutrients, Antioxidants and the General Mechanisms of Disease" is no better exemplified than in recent communications in such premier scientific journals as Science and Nature. The issue of March 4, 1993 of Nature, the British science journal, provided evidence for (Rosen et al., 1993) -- and commentary on (McNamara & Fridovich, 1993) -- a linkage between the crippling neuromuscular disease, amyotrophic lateral sclerosis (ALS), also known as Lou Gerhig's disease for its association with the legendary New York Yankees baseball player, and a mutation in chromosome 21 which misencodes the cytosolic variety of superoxide dismutase (SOD). It is speculated that toxic O_2^- radical, generated by the action of xanthine oxidase, can damage motor neurons selectively (McNamara & Fridovich, 1993). The optimistic aspect of this finding is the possibility of directing exogenous SOD to the neurons or of using drugs to regulate free-radical generation (Rosen et al., 1993).

2 THE CONSEQUENCES OF LIVING IN AN AEROBIC ENVIRONMENT

All life began in the primeval sea under anaerobic conditions. When living species emerged onto the land and into the air, evolution accepted the need to live in an oxygen-rich environment and to be vigilant against the adverse effects of oxidation (Jukes, 1992). The conventional concept of disease is based on the medical passion to classify lesions that can be detected and recognized in pathology. However, the roots of the word (dys - ease), i.e. not at ease, conveys a broader individual concept of subjective discomfort and a collective concept of suboptimal physical or social functioning. In the sense of human ecology, this is a more reasonable context.

Molecular oxygen is the centerpiece of oxidation, and most of the free radicals that propagate oxidative reactions contain one or more oxygen atom. The forces for oxidation come from normal intrinsic sources (energy metabolism, host defense) and from extrinsic sources (chemicals, ionizing radiation, meta- bolites of invading pathogens). Compatibility with aerobic life meant the evolution of antioxidant mechanisms in the cells and the circulations. These include: chain-breaking of lipid peroxidation in membrane; glutathione peroxidase with glutathione and its reducing enzyme; superoxide dismutase and catalase; and circulating ceruloplasmin and skin pigmentation. A number of micronutrients and dietary constituents are considered to be the oxidant in nature, e.g. ionic iron, zinc, copper. On the other hand, the constituents of the anti-oxidant system require micronutrients.

One of the components of the topic is "disease," but its relation to the other components -- "antioxidants" and "micronutrients" -- must be taken in a definitional and philosophical context.

3 DISEASE AS PATHOLOGY

There are two ways to look at disease: 1) from the point of view of the physician; and 2) from that of the sufferer. The process of developing a mechanistic,

TABLE 1. GENERAL MECHANISMS OF SOMATIC DISEASE IN A CLASSIC PATHOLOGIC AND SYSTEMS CONCEPT

- Deformity and Mutilation

- Deprivation

- Degeneration

- Proliferation

- Hormonal Imbalance

- Inflammation/Immune Disorders

- Infections

physical concept of pathology began with the physicians of antiquity and culminated with the enormous animus of 19th century pathologists such as Rudolf Virchow. Table 1 develops a system of classification of disease mechanism according to this author, but based on the concepts of classic pathology.

The system deals with somatic categories omitting psychological and psychiatric issues. The categories in the table are not mutually exclusive. The emphasis is on processes more than on specific lesions.

By deformity, we mean include those structural abnormalities of organs of congenital origin or those acquired issues such as amputations or mutilating injuries produced by accidents, surgery, radiation or chemicals. Tooth loss would be in this class. Various types of scarring would belong to this category.

Nutritional deficiency diseases would be classified under deprivation, but so would other deficits such as acute asphyxia (deprivation of oxygen) and acute dehydration (deprivation of fluid and electrolytes).

By degeneration, we mean the loss of tissue integrity or the loss of optimal consistency. Atrophic conditions such as osteoporosis, retinopathies and periodontal disease, and various neuro-myo-dystrophies, and even skin depigmentation, would represent cases of degenerative disorders. In general, exposure to toxic chemicals and heavy metals in the environment produces degeneration of tissues.

Proliferation covers dysplastic and neoplastic processes, both benign and malignant, that lead to solid tumors and blood dyscrasia in humans. This category could also embrace infiltrations, and hence atherosclerotic plaques would fall into this group. Nutritional excess, specifically energy overload and adiposity, would also represent proliferation.

Hormonal imbalances cover all of the ailments that would be considered in metabolism, endocrinology and hypertension medical subspecialties and relate to glandular secretions.

Inflammation and immune disorders are, in fact, hormonal to the extent that the cytokine mediators are messengers. Arthritis and ulcerative colitis would be examples of inflammatory conditions whereas celiac disease and multiple sclerosis could be considered to be immune disorders.

Infectious diseases are based on interactions between the host and a pathogenic agent. The latter can

unicellular organisms such as viruses, Chlamydia, bacteria or protozoa, or multicellular such as yeast, fungi, and helminths. With respect to antioxidants and oxidants, oxidizing free radicals are liberated by white cells in the process of killing micro-organisms. Given that infectious diseases have specific infective agents, they can be controlled (as with brucellosis, leprosy, protozoal diseases) or even eradicated (e,g, small pox).

4 DISEASE AS "DYS - EASE"

We have a penchant for the dichotomization of "health" and "disease." Health is seen as the absence of disease; disease is contradictory to a state of complete good health. In the previous section, disease was seen in the context of organic pathology, as deviance from normal, i.e. with an identifiable and classifiable infirmity. Moreover, based on the Declaration of Alma Ata, health is considered to include social, psychic and economic well-being in addition to freedom from disease. Thus, contemporary public health thinking reaches to more holistic concepts.

Thus, disease can also be seen is its elemental components as "dys - ease," or not being at ease. This values the perception, not from the pathologist's microscope, but from the feelings and perspective of the individual. The question is modified from what does one have to how does one feel. And how does one feel must be taken in the context of one's surroundings and one's expectations. The issue of harmony and balance within the individual and of the individual with his or her external context. Life-style, diet and the physical, climatic elements of the environment define this external context.

5 IS NORMAL AGING A DISEASE?

Recently, I attended a discussion on carotenes in human health (Canfield et al., 1993) where more than one of the speakers projected slides with a long list of "diseases" that might be amenable to anti-oxidant therapy. "Aging" was included on these lists which raises the question of whether normal aging is a "disease." Can be meaningfully draw a distinction between "senescence" and "pathology." Grimley-Evans (1988) asserts that what we recognize as aging is the accumulation of the effects of disease. If one could remain disease-free, one would not age. Others (Kirkwood, 1988) believe that aging is a genetically-programmed phenomenon. The linkage of antioxidants and aging may come from a series of theories that suggest that oxidant free radicals mediate -- if not cause -- aging (Harman, 1956).

Researchers have looked at the blood lipid peroxide levels across age in Dannish women (Schafer & Thorling, 1990). Older women had greater lipid peroxidation. Neither selenium nor vitamin E status nor a 3-mo placebo-controlled supplementation trial with vitamin E and selenium correlated with lipid peroxidation; only blood lipid variables explained the extent of peroxidation. Thus, the primary role of aging in peroxidation of circulating lipids may be in characterizing the lipid pattern. Of note, however, was a decreasing selenium status with advancing age noted in the older group. The aging process in an animal model of the Fischer 344 aged rat found a mixed picture of reduction in some antioxidant enzymes, stability in others and improvement in others (Rikans et al., 1992).

6 INTERACTIONS AMONG HOST, AGENT AND ENVIRONMENT REGARDING OXIDANTS AND ANTIOXIDANTS

If one steps back from the strict pathological classification to the more ecological perspective, one can take the epidemiological formulation of host, agent and environment to analyze the influence of oxidants on human health. This synthesis is outlined in Table 2. With respect to host factors, the genetic constitution of the individual comes into play. There may be genetically-determined interindividual variability in susceptibility or resistance of tissues to the effect of oxidants. Similarly, variation in the handling of antioxidants -- making them more or less effective against oxidizing processes -- may obtain in populations. It is more likely to be specific to a specific antioxidant mechanism than to be general. Finally, behavioral traits of the host can play a role. The practices of avoiding radiation exposure, not smoking, avoiding areas of volatile chemicals, etc., can make a difference at the level of contact with oxidizing species.

Substances such as molecular oxygen, oxidant chemicals and oxidizing promotors such as light and ionizing radiation in the environ-ment represent agent factors. These factors, however, must have a medium for transmission to the host; this is dependent, in turn, on how conducive is the environment to the production or conduction of natural and artificial oxidants and how much natural protection from oxidants are provided.

6.1 OXIDATION FOR NUTRIENT SYNTHESIS

In the case of one essential nutrient, vitamin D^3, photo-oxidation of 7-dehydro-cholesterol to produce cholecalciferol in the skin (Holick, 1985). This is a precursor of the vitamin D hormones that serve as messengers to control genetic transcription in the nucleus of cells. In fact, photo-oxidation is also the process that acts on a natural plant sterol, ergosterol, to produce vitamin D_2, the fortification form in milk.

7 OXIDANTS AND CHEMICAL OXIDATION

Organic oxidation is based primarily on the action of free radicals, and to a lesser extent on singlet oxygen. Halliwell et al. (1992) define as "any species capable of independent existence that contains one or more unpaired electrons, an unpaired electron being one that is alone in an orbital." One of the features of free radicals is propagation or chain reactions in which one radical begets another. Only when to radicals interact is the reaction terminated. Singlet oxygen and hydrogen peroxide are not free radicals themselves, but are involved in the oxidation process as "reactive oxygen species."

Free radical oxidation can consist of three processes as defined by Halliwell et al. (1992): 1) addition, in which a radical joins a nonradical; 2) electron donation, in which the unpaired electron passes to another species forming a radical; or 3) electron removal, in which a radical extracts an electron from a nonradical species to create a radical of the latter. In biological terms, the hydroxyl radical, $OH^{\bullet}$, which is generated in reactions of hydrogen peroxide (H_2O_2) with transition metals such as manganese, copper and iron.

TABLE 2. INTERACTIVE DETERMINANTS OF EFFECTS OF OXIDANTS ON HEALTH IN A HUMAN, ECOLOGICAL PERSPECTIVE

Host Factors
- Genetic Constitution
    Susceptibility or resistance to oxidants

- Genetic Constitution
    Metabolism of antioxidants

- Behavioral Practices
    Promoting or opposing adverse exposures

Agent Factors
- Molecular Oxygen

- Chemical Oxidants

- Oxidizing Processes

Environmental Factors
- Natural AntiOxidants

- Protection against Oxidizing Processes

TABLE 3. CLASSES OF ENVIRONMENTAL OXIDANTS

- Oxidant Nutrients

- Ozone

- Ionizing Radiation

- Photo Radiation (Light)

- Complex Chemicals

- Drugs

TABLE 4. THE OXIDANT NUTRIENTS

- Oxygen

- Iron

- Zinc

- Copper

Table 3 lists categories of substances, natural or synthetic, that can produce oxidation directly or generate oxidizing free radicals. Of greatest pertinence to nutritionist are the oxidant nutrients. Table 4 enumerates those nutrients that result in oxidation. Oxygen heads the list. The lungs are, logically, the organs most exposed to environmental oxygen, and hence the most susceptible to oxygen damage. Interest in oxidation and anti-oxidants in pulmonary tissue has centered on bronchopulmonary dysplasia, a lung disorder common in very-low-birth-weight infants treated in environments with oxygen a high barometric pressures. The lungs are too immature to oxygenate the body well (hence the need for high levels of oxygen) but also too immature to defend themselves against oxygen damage (hence the vicious cycle of tissue damage).

Iron has been recognized for almost a century as an organic oxidant from the observations of Fenton (1894), working in concert with hydrogen peroxide to produce a potent oxidant, later to be provisionally identified by Haber and Weiss (1934) as the hydroxyl radical. In vivo, we know that the oxidation of xanthine, catalyzed by xanthine oxidase, produces a superoxide radical from molecular oxygen as uric acid is produced. Hypotheses related to reactive oxygen species and oxygen radicals in the genesis of asbestos induced pulmonary damage (Kamp et al., 1992) and the inflammatory damage in ulcerative colitis (Babbs, 1992). This notion has been extended to the gamut of intestinal diseases, especially ischemic injury (van der Vlliet & Bast, 1992). Iron is posited to play a role in both, and the leukocyte-generated radical species involved in the inflammatory reactions.

Zinc and copper ionized in salts are capable of influencing electrons to the point of oxidation. In the normal course of events, antioxidant nutrients such as tocopherol and ascorbic acid become oxidants: tocopheroxyl radical and dehydroascorbic acid, respectively. The tripeptide, glutathione is enzymatically converted to its oxidized, dimeric form (via glutathione oxidase) and to its reduced, monomeric form (via glutathione reductase).

Ozone is an oxidizing stimulus which is prevalent in the smog of urban metropolises. It can initiate lipid peroxidation, but the reaction of ozone with biological molecules generates singlet oxygen in abundance (Karnofsky & Sima, 1991). Both ionizing radiation such as Xrays or gamma radiation and photo radiation (sunlight, artificial lights) can unleash a chain of oxidation. Interest in oxidation biology has also focused on another form of energy: sound. At least in in vitro models, ultrasound, used extensively in diagnostic and therapeutic procedures, produces hydroxy radicals in aqueous media (Reisz & Kondon, 1992). The implication of this finding, for example, for patients undergoing lithotripsy therapy for stones.

Not only nutrients but other complex chemicals, both natural and artificial, including drugs are oxidants. The antimalarial drug, primaquine, and members of its class are prime examples. The traditional Chinese anti-malarial drug, qinghaosu, acts againt malaria by generating free radicals that presumably attack parasitized red blood cells (Levander, 1992).

There are 10^{15} organic radicals in each puff od cigarette smoke (Pryor, 1992). Specific interest has been directed to nitric oxide which decomposes to peroxynitrous acid in aqueous solutions yield hydroxy radicals (Yang et al., 1992).

8 MICRONUTRIENTS WITH ANTIOXIDANT FUNCTIONS

Table 5 lists the roster of nutrients commonly mentioned as having an antioxidant function. Krinsky (1992) defines an antioxidant as: "compounds that protect biological systems against the potentially harmful effects of processes or reactions that can cause excessive oxidations." They are divided into those that function in a free-standing manner and those that are related to enzyme systems. The enzymes mentioned in Table 5 constitute the system of "antioxidant enzymes" of mammalian tissues.

Retinol or vitamin A is listed as an antioxidant nutrient. Of all of the nutrients listed in Table 5, Current understanding of the physiological function of this nutrient focuses on its role in regulating cell proliferation (Darmon, 1990; Chytil, 1992) based on a role as a nuclear hormone. It may indeed be true that, by regulating the proliferation of cells, retinol and retinoic acid exercise an antineoplastic function, and thereby compliment the action of more specific antioxidants. Some confusion may have derived from the association between preformed vitamin A and provitamin A retinols in recording dietary data and converting it to a common expression of retinol equivalents for vitamin A. At present, although listed, we do not recognize any free radical interaction or

TABLE 5. THE ROSTER OF ANTIOXIDANT NUTRIENTS

Free-Standing

- Retinol

- Carotenoids

- Vitamin E

- Vitamin C

System-Related

- Selenium in Glutathione Peroxidase

- Riboflavin with Glutathione Reductase

- Copper in Ceruloplasmin

- Zinc and Copper in cytosolic Superoxide Dismutase

- Manganese in mitochondrial Superoxide Dismutase

- Iron in Catalase

singlet-oxygen quenching functions for retinol and must reserve judgement as to its appropriateness in the roster of antioxidant nutrients.

There are over 600 distinct carotenoids in nature. Carotenes are not, strictly speaking, nutrients, but some are legitimate precursors of the essential nutrient, vitamin A. A fraction of carotenoids have provitamin A activity, and can be converted by enzymatic processes into retinoid precursors of retinol or retinoic acid. A feature common to carotenoids are their long, double-bond-laden chains. The important issue of carotenoids are their singlet-oxygen quenching capacity (Olson & Kobayashi, 1992). In this way, they are postulated to reduce or eliminate tissue damage from the generation of singlet oxygen (Krinsky, 1992). Carotenes are of plant origin. They represent the deep yellow, orange and red pigments in yellow and orange fruits and vegetables. They are also abundant in dark green leafy herbs, but their color is overwhelmed by the intense color of chlorophyll. It is well established that the function of carotenoids in plants is as a natural antioxidant. Photosynthesis requires the exposure of plants to sunlight and the capture of light energy by the chloroplasts for carbohydrate production. But plants are exposed at the same time to the radiation damage from the light energy. As singlet-oxygen quenchers, carotenoids serve as a type of "phyto sun screen."

Beta-carotene, the symmetrical molecule with the greatest theoretical yield of vitamin A is the best known and most commonly discussed of the carotenoids. It is synthesized in its pure, chemical form and abundant in both chemical research, medicine and nutrition. Other carotenoids, such as lycopene, the reddish pigment in tomatoes and watermelon and canthaxanthine in paprika and peppers, may, in fact have greater singlet-oxygen quenching capacity.

The roles of vitamin E, which includes   It is the major chain-breaking antioxidant in membranes. By virtue of the unsaturated fatty acids and lipids incorporated into membranes of cells and cellular organelles, they are susceptible to forming peroxides and epoxides. Tocopherols and tocotrienols, the lipids that constitute vitamin E activity, are inserted into the membranes' lipid bilayers and terminate radical-generated reactions, many of which originate in the more metabolically active cytosolic or intra-organelle spaces (Packer, 1992).
- Vitamin C or ascorbic acid is a reducing agent in classical, organic redox reactions. In the context of antioxidant protection, ascorbic acids are capable of scavenging radicals and singlet oxygen (Krinsky, 1992).

The so-called "antioxidant enzyme" system is comprised of glutathione peroxidase and glutathione reductase which are compartmen-talized in the cytosolic compartment of the cell. They act in concert to reduce hydrogen peroxide, and probably organic peroxides formed in the aqueous phase, using the tripeptide, glutathione as the electron donor/acceptor moiety. Selenium plays its antioxidant role as an essential component of the metalloenzyme, glutathione oxidase and riboflavin works in antioxidant processes as the coenzyme for glutathione reductase.

Another important aqueous phase in the body is the extracellular one, comprising plasma, lymph and interstitial fluid. Evidence has been provided that the copper transport protein, ceruloplasmin, is an effective antioxidant. Krinsky (1992) has listed a host of minor extracellular antioxidants such as albumin, haptoglobin, hemopexin, lactoferrin, transferrin and uric acid as adding the biological antioxidant process by scavenging radicals or binding transition metals.

The cations, zinc, copper, manganese and iron, operate in a system that eliminates superoxide radicals and their derivative oxidant product, hydrogen peroxide. Three superoxide dismutases (SOD) are recognized (Fridovich & McNamara, 1993). That which is present in the cytosol and that in the intercellular spaces is a metalloenzyme containing zinc and copper. The SOD in the mitochondria is a manganese metalloenzyme. The superoxide radicals generated by the oxidation of xanthine is dismutated to hydrogen peroxide. This latter product can be transformed to water and ground-state oxygen by catalase, and iron-containing metalloenzyme. It should be noted that the oxidative killing of micro-organisms in phagocytic white blood cells and macrophages involves the operation of this oxidant-antioxidant system.

8.1 ADDITIONAL ANTIOXIDANT MECHANISMS RELATED TO HUMAN NUTRITION AND METABOLISM

Yet another mechanism of anti-oxidant action relates to polyunsaturated fatty acids (PUFAs), dispersed in the cytosolic compartment of the cell. PUFAs are, of course, the focus of lipid peroxidation. However, the chemical reactions that give rise to free radicals occur in the aqueous phase, and Dormandy (1969) proposed that, while floating in the cytosol, the double bonds in PUFAs could represent a non-propagating sink for free radicals, in fact preventing the oxidant products from reaching membranes.

Since iron is such a dangerous tissue oxidant, it has been proposed that the storage protein, ferritin, plays the role of protecting cells, themselves, from the adverse effects of this mineral (Balla et al., 1992). With respect to thionein, the sulfhydryl-group-rich protein that binds zinc, copper, mercury and cadmium (Kagi et al., 1990), one could postulate that its sequestering zinc and copper as metallothionein also provides intracellular, antioxidant protection.

As increasing analytical chemistry is performed on traditional medicines, a better understanding of the biochemical nature and in vitro and in vivo functions of the compounds is developed. Widely used Chinese herbal medicines contain organic antioxidants (Hong et al., 1992).

9 OXIDANT DAMAGE OF TISSUES

Basic science experiments and careful clinical observations are producing detailed findings on the mechanisms of interaction between oxidants and tissue and among oxidants, tissue damage and the mitigating effects of antioxidants both in the form of micro-nutrients and as synthetic or natural antioxidant drugs. The synthesis of this information leads to some specific relationships of oxidation and health and some more general models of the ways that oxidation injures tissue.

Only a few of these recent observations can be reviewed in this section.

After ischemic injury to the myocardium or intestine, additional damage is done during reperfusion by oxygen radicals (superoxide radical, hydroxyl radical). Cell membrane permeable scavengers of oxygen metabolites hold promise for salvage of ischemic tissue preventing completed infarction with tissue death.

Interest has grown in the theory that oxidation of low-density lipoproteins (LDL) plays a role in atherogenesis and development of coronary artery plaques (Regnstrom, J. et al. 1992; Salonen, J.T. et al., 1992). This oxidation can take place in the circulation or in the endothelial cells, themselves, and iron is thought to be a mediator. The fact that beta-carotene reduced the rate of fatal myocardial infarctions in a prospective chemoprevention trial in high-risk middle-age physicians (Hennekens et al., 1993) lends credence to the LDL-oxidation mechanism. A consensus panel commission of the National Institutes of Health of the U.S.A. has concluded that the evidence on hand merits the evaluation of chemoprevention using micronutrient supplementation (Steinberg, 1992)

The whole series of anti-oxidant enzymes are involved in protecting the lungs (Frank, 1992). By virtue of their role in oxygenation of the body, the lung alveolar cells are exposed to a high concentration of O_2. The premature infant, who needs oxygen to survive, is exposed to toxicity by the high concentrations provided. Trials of various antioxidant nutrients have been tried for the protection of lung and ocular tissues from oxygen damage; vitamin E has been generally unsuccessful in protecting the premature's tissue from injury (Frank, 1992; Mino, 1992). Vitamin A is the only micronutrient that has been protective against broncho-pulmonary dysplasia of the premature newborn (Chytil, 1992).

In a process that cannot be termed other than a vicious cycle, primary tissue damage -- of whatever cause -- leads secondarily to the activation of free radical release which, in turn propagates the damage. Reviews that characterize this with case examples have been provided recently by Halliwell et al. (1992) and Strain (1991).

10 DIETARY INTAKE OF FOODS AND MICRONUTRIENTS AND RISK OF ILLNESS

As reviewed above, the enzymatic and non-enzymatic elements of the antioxidant system require micronutrients, such as tocopherol, retinol, riboflavin, selenium, manganese, zinc, copper, and ascorbic acid while evidence exists for antioxidant properties of certain carotenoids. Willett (1990) has set the tone for the contemporary analysis of usual dietary intake and chronic illness risk in his textbook. Within the variance of human intake of the "antioxidant" nutrients, epidemiological studies have observed variation in risk of specific pathological processes such as cataract, lung cancer, ischemic heart disease. The current debate is whether supplemental and supradietary amounts of antioxidant micronutrient conveys added protection beyond the highest intakes provided by a natural diet. It is clear that, in pharmacological doses, dietary

substances that have functions as nutrients can be true physiological antioxidants in vivo. This aspect is worthy of discussion. We also know that some nutrients exercise their nutritional and metabolic functions as part of (or in support of) the intrinsic antioxidant mechanisms of an organism in an aerobic environment. Deficiency states of certain nutrients, hence, can weaken physiological antioxidant protection.

What is of some considerable interest is the degree to which variation within the range of the extremes of natural human dietary intakes can enhance protection against dysfunction and pathological variation comes from epidemiological studies of either an ecological (across-geography comparisons) or case-control (across-individual comparisons) (Willett, 1990).

The examples of clear or promising associations between higher intakes of nutrients from the diet and lower rates of a disease or disorder are numerous, especially with respect to retarding malignant neo-plastic disease (Chen et al., 1992; Henderson et al., 1991; Rogers & Longneker, 1988).

A classical example of this is the study of men working in the 1950's at the Western Electric plant outside of Chicago. Lung cancer rates among smokers were 7 to 8 times higher in those who were in the lowest fourth of the distribution for consumption of vitamin A than in the those in the highest quartile (Shekelle et al., 1981). This has been interpreted over timr to have bern provitamin A sources or carotenoids, and in fact, tomato soup was probably driving the relationship. Since that time, there have been a number of studies showing a similar relationship between intake of provitamin A (carotenoid)-rich foods and lung cancers among smokers. The apparent carotene protective effect for lung tumors has been seen consistently in epidemiological studies (Block et al., 1992). In all of the studies, dietary carotenes were provided by foods and beverages commonly consumed. The higher levels of carotene intake within a distri-bution and/or higher circulating levels of carotenes have also been associated with lower risks of angina pectoris (Riemersma et al., 1991), cataract (Jacques et al., 1991; Hankinson et al., 1992), and dysplasia of the uterine cervix (Singh & Gaby, 1991).

Intake of another putative antioxidant nutrient, riboflavin, has been associated with the level of risk of cataract (Taylor, 1989). This conclusion derives from observations in Alabama where individuals with superior riboflavin status had lower age-adjusted rates of cataract occurrence.

For the same degenerative process of the crystalline lens of the eye, the habitual and spontaneous intake of vitamin C both in food forms and as vitamin supplements has recently been associated inversely with cataract occurrence (Jacques et al., 1988; Hankison et al., 1992) This is supported by substantial animal and in vitro research on lens opacification and ascorbic acid (Taylor 1990). Gastrointestinal cancer incidence, notably of the stomach and esophagus, is inversely associated with consumption of vitamin C-rich foods, specifcally of the citrus fruit variety (NRC, 1989).

Packer (1992) has reviewed the epidemiological associations of vitamin E intake and various disorders. Given the putative therapeutic role of this vitamin, much more experiencve exists in therapeutic trials than in population-based surveys. The only strong epidemiological associations revealed was an inverse association of angina pectoris with circulating vitamin E levels, after adjustment for known risk factors (Riemersma et al., 1991).

With respect to selenium, inverse associations between habitual selenium intake or prior selenium levels and cancer outcomes (incidence of specific tumors, overall cancer mortality) has been reported (NRC, 1989). In general, the relationship hinged on levels in the deficient range providing increased risk with adequacy the protective state. Enhanced selenium status does not yet figure in epidemiogical studies related to this trace element.

10.1 IF SOME IS GOOD, A LOT MORE IS BETTER

The logic that, "if some is good, a lot more is better" seems to have dominated the transition from epidemiological observations to clinical trials. Two firm conclusions about the studies in free-living populations are: 1) the protection for the low-risk group(s) was achieved within the dietary range; and 2) the majority of intake of the micronutrients of interest came from food and beverage sources. When it comes to designing chemoprevention trials, however, not foods (but pills) and not dietary amounts (but pharmacological doses) have been the prospective studies in normal or at-risk populations.

It is clear that one can get greater amounts of a micronutrient into one's body with increasing levels of consumption. It is also generally the rule, however, that the efficiency of uptake of substances from the alimentary tract into the body decreases with increasing concentrations of the substance of interest. That is, one absorbs proportionally more of a nutrient at moderate doses. The final, and most crucial issue, however, is the identity of the specific micronutrient or the specific combination of micronutrients responsible for the decreased disease risks observed in epidemiological studies (Block, 1992; Block et al., 1992; Ziegler, 1991; 1993). It is obvious that both carotenoids and vitamin C occur in the same food items. Riboflavin is also found in dark green leaves. Similarly, riboflavin and vitamin E share some common sources. Selenium in foods is more a consequence of the soils in which the plants are grown and over which the livestock are grazed, but selenium-bearing foods are also rich in other micronutrients, and often of oxidants as well. Given this complex relationship among nutrients in the foods that have shown protective effects against specific chronic diseases, it is a major leap of speculation to decide that an one nutrient or another was the source of the dominant effect, and then to isolate it in purified form for supplementation trials of chemoprevention. The soundness of the inferences across the intellectual gap from epidemiological observations related to foods and health-promoting effects from specific nutrients in those foods, supplemented alone, will determine the success with developing positive chemoprevention trials with the present experimental paradigms.

10.2 TAILORING ANTIOXIDANTS TO THE PATHOGENESIS OF DISEASE

We know enough about the mechanisms of illness to suggest that an oxidizing process may be operating, and that antioxidants, including selected nutrients, may be of benefit. We know sufficiently little about the interactions of oxidants and antioxidants, their tissue specificity and cellular penetration to predict what will benefit where. For this reason, the justification for the efficacy of antioxidants in a given condition are usually retrospective, based on epidemiological observations.

In the case of photosensitivity disorders, such as erythrocytic porphyria (Mathews-Roth, 1982), however, a tolerable substance with singlet-oxygen quenching capacity was prospectively prescribed, based on the pathophysiology of the disease. Beta-carotene was postulated as a possible remedy, and oral doses of 180 mg daily allowed porphyria patients to receive outdoor light exposure without skin reactions. Whether other carotenoids with even greater in vitro singlet oxygen quenching would be even more effective has yet to be explored.

11 ADVERSE CONSEQUENCES OF HIGH DOSES OF ANTIOXIDANT NUTRIENTS

There are two potential adverse consequences of high intakes of specific anti-oxidant nutrients. The first level is that of toxic manifestations, damage to the integrity or function of tissues. A second level is that of inhibitory interactions making other essential substances less available. In the case of one family of compounds, carotenoids, aesthetic considerations come into play. Assorted adverse consequences of high doses of the antioxidant nutrients are listed in Table 6.

Retinol or preformed vitamin A is potentially the most toxic, and most diversely toxic of the nutrients we have classified as antioxidant. For the somatic manifestations, it is believed that the accumulation of circulating retinyl esters act as membrane destroying detergents. It produces elevation in intracranial pressure. hepatic damage that can lead to fibrosis, and ascites. Retinol and its retinoid analogues are also potent teratogenic agents, producing malformations in gestating fetuses of pregnant women.

Carotenoids are generally regarded as non-toxic. The intestine has a homeostatic mechanism that prevents conversion to vitamin A above the needs of the body; hence, hypervitaminosis A cannot result from high intakes of provitamin A carotenoids. Yellowish skin pigmentation or carotenodermia can result from prolonged high intakes of carotene-rich foods such as carrot juice and papaya or supplemental forms of beta-carotene or other carotenoids (Mathews-Roth, 1986). With respect to what we are considering in this review, however, there are other adverse aspects to consider, namely, carotenoid-carotenoid interactions. Evidence for mutual antagonism among carotenoids is beginning to emerge (Erdman et al., 1993). Use of high doses of one carotenoid, e.g. beta-carotene, may counteract a positive effect from a more physiologically-useful compound in the family.

As a fat soluble vitamin, vitamin E is stored for prolonged periods in body tissue stores. There is experience with voluntary ingestion of large amounts of this vitamin in manifold excesses of the recommended levels. In adults, however, no adverse consequences are known. Mino (1992) narrates the experience of toxic consequences for premature children, including 40

TABLE 6. TOXIC OR ADVERSE RESPONSES IN HUMANS TO ANTIOXIDANT NUTRIENTS

- Retinol (preformed vitamin A)
    Hepatic lesions
    Increased intracranial pressure
    Ascites
    Teratogenesis

- Carotenoids
    Yellowish skin pigmentation
    Inhibition of other carotenoid

- Vitamin E
    Toxicity from Additive in Preparation

- Vitamin C
    Hypoglycemia
    Induced Hyperuricosuria
    Laxative effect/Diarrhea
    Inhibition of vitamin B_{12}
    Dependency with Withdrawal Syndrome

- Riboflavin
    Not defined

- Selenium
    Not defined

- Zinc
    Gastric erosion
    Copper deficiency

- Copper
    Nausea and vomiting

- Manganese
    Parkinson's like neurological symptoms

fatalities, from a parenteral vitamin E preparation (Ferol-E). The deaths were ascribed to the emulsifying agents, rather than the vitamin, itself. In vitro research by Mino (1992) show that megadosing of vitamin E increases white cell superoxide radical generation. The consequences for human health are not defined.

By virtue of the manifold claims of beneficial effects of large doses of vitamin C, massive (gram) amounts of ascorbic acid have commonly been consumed by humans. Adverse manifestations include hypoglycemia, uric acid wastage in urine, and a laxative effect that can reach overt diarrhea. In persons with tendency to form oxalate stones, excessive intake of ascorbic acid enhances stone formation (Sauberlich, 1990). Herbert (1990) claims that megadoses of vitamin C converts vitamin B_{12} to inactive cobalamin analogues. Unlike other water-soluble vitamins, the prolonged, chronic ingestion of supra-requirement levels of vitamin C leads to a dependency, and a rebound effect of scurvy-like manifestations occur with abrupt withdrawal (Omaye et al., 1986). A tapering of the dose must be instituted after long-term high-dose supplementation with ascorbic acid.

The issue of supplementary excess of micronutrients is somewhat moot in the instances of those nutrients that function as part of the antioxidant nutrients. There is no evidence for induction of the enzymes by extra intakes of the cofactors or components, and simply maintaining nutritional adequacy and normal body stores should ensure maximal enzyme activities. However, since excessive intakes of some of the micronutrient components is problematic, as shown in the table, the net effect is a disadvantage to increased intake. Iron is not even considered in the table, as its role as an oxidant outweighs its antioxidant role as part of catalase. Adverse and toxic effects of excessive riboflavin intakes have not been defined.

Debate exists regarding the short- or long-term consequences of extra intake of selenium in either inorganic or organic dietary forms. Hyperselenoisis has been described due to high levels in soil. The putative consequences were dental caries, abnormality of integument (hair loss; nail deformity; skin lesions) (Yang et al., 1983). The same signs as well as nausea, vomiting, irritability, fatigue and peripheral neuropathy (Levander & Burk, 1990). It has been speculated that excessive selenium intake can be carcinogenic (NRC, 1989), and it is well documented that acute intoxication with massive amounts of selenium salts can produce fatalities.

High oral doses of zinc can produce gastric erosions. Since a competitive interaction exist between zinc and copper, high intakes of the former have led to overt copper deficiency anemia (Patterson et al., 1985).

Copper deposition in hepatic tissues as occurs in Wilson's disease or Indian childhood cirrhosis leads to severe damage, and hemolytic anemia can result from acute massive release of copper with hepatic necrosis in Wilson's disease or from ingestion of gram amounts of copper. With medicinal or nutritional supplementation none of these toxic complications are ever to be seen. At doses of 2 to 5 mg, copper is an emetic. Although inhibitory interactions of copper with other transition elements has been demonstrated (Hill & Matrone, 1970), dietary and supplemental levels of the metal are unlikely to influence the body economy of the competitive elements.

Manganese toxicity has been seen with industrial contact, rather than in the dietary context. The primary toxicity manifestation is a neurological syndrome reminiscent of Parkinson's disease. Finally, it is logical to consider that, as with copper, zinc and selenium, one cannot induce or drive the SOD system beyond the point of total-body manganese adequacy. Only with a condition that interfered with the bioavailability or utilization of any of the antioxidant trace elements would intakes beyond requirement levels be of theoretical advantage for enhancing antioxidant protection in vivo.

12 CONCLUSIONS

The living beings and the inanimate and inorganic substances on the Earth are sharing the same planet and, hence, an interaction. A major watershed was reached in evolution when organisms left the anaerobic environment of the sea to live on the land in the oxygen-rich atmosphere (Jukes, 1992).

The natural imperative of the species is the survival of that species. Throughout the eons of humankind's existence, evolution and change have generally been slow. The diet has been constant, as has the physical environment. Major changes in the life-style have been provoked by modifications in climate (ice-ages, droughts), by migrations of humans (across continents, across oceans) or changes or their co-habitant species. The pace of change accelerated greatly in the past century with the emergence of technology. The latter has done more to influence both diet and the chemical nature of the environment than any other factor. These changes have not placed homo sapiens in danger as a species, but have influenced the ways that individual men and women experience health, illness and death.

As we have evolved and shaped our environment over the eons, we have included substances in the diet that have antioxidant functions while at the same time ingesting items that are oxidant. The radiation in the environment and the chemicals we breathe and touch can also be oxidant. Generation of oxidizing radicals is attendant to the interaction of hosts with infective pathogens. The consequence of oxidation are changes in DNA that promote cancer and modification of lipoproteins that favor formation of atherosclerotic plaques to name a few. However, there are limits to the ability of antioxidant nutrients to prime antioxidant processes and limits in antioxidant processes to counteract oxidation. Hence, reliance on diet for protection from advancing environmental oxidant challenge is unwarranted and unwise.

If promoting well-being and the harmony between humans and their physical and chemical environment has emerged here as a consideration, the threat from major imbalances will be appreciated. Self-supplementation with antioxidant nutrients runs the risk of producing some specific toxicities but also has the potential to interfere with the storage and metabolism of other nutrients. The theme remains topical by virtue of what we do still do not know about micronutrients as antioxidants and human performance and well-being. Genetic factors that condition the interaction, and how to identify them, would be high on the list for investigation. The words of Olson and Kobayashi (1992) in an overview to a symposium on antioxidants in health and disease sum up a coherent position: "...one must retain perspective. Panaceas don't exit. ... Antioxidants clearly are important in cellular regulation, but the appropriate balance between oxidative and antioxidative processes in cells under various conditions still needs to be defined. The investigator also must retain a proper balance between enthusiam and constraint."

13 IMPLICATIONS FOR THE DAIRY INDUSTRY

Since this is a volume dedicated to the I World Dairy Congress, it is worth adding a word of "epilogue" regarding the implications of antioxidants, micronutrients and general mechanisms of disease for the dairy industry. The comments are mostly speculative, but can serve to provoke multidisciplinary consideration and discussion and provide a template for new directions in research.

In the evolutionary focus that has been brought to this discussion, we can see the consumption of milk from cows and other dairy animals as a derivative of the evolution of human culture with the domestication of dairy animals (Simoons, 1981). From a food that would only have been available to the nursing infant in

the first year or two of life, the advent of dairying made milk and its nutrient content part of the life-long diet for all ages of the population. There is even a suggestion that, among dairying societies, the presence of milk in the diet exerted a selective pressure favoring the survival of individuals carrying the lactase-persistence gene. To the extent that other genes relevant to the handling of oxidant stress or metabolism of antioxidant nutrients are closely associated with and the lactase gene.

A number of questions related to technology, behavior and the environment come together in this consideration of the implications for the dairy industry and possible avenues for research. To what extent do dairying practices bring more or fewer oxidizing chemicals to the environment? What is the antioxidant micronutrient and food-oxidant content in milk? What is the net effect on antioxidant micronutrients intake, antioxidant balance, and food-oxidant consumption of the displacement of other traditional foods by diary products in the evolution of dietary practices. What is the potential for milk and dairy products to serve as vehicles for delivery of increased amounts of dietary antioxidants?

With respect to the extent that dairying practices bring more or fewer oxidizing chemicals to the environment, the first step would be to make an inventory of the chemicals used in the care of milk- producing animals and in production and storage of their feeds? The key description would be concentrations of residues in the environment of dairy farms and processing centers, and through risk assessment inferences, the oxidant exposure for personnel in the industry could be estimated. The profile of oxidant exposure for dairy and dairy food workers would of course be evaluated, in occupational health, in comparison to workers in other industries. This question must be considered a dynamic -- rather than a static one -- as technological advances, such as the wider use of bovine somatotrophic hormone or returns to original, less chemical-dependent farming practices, would set off a cascade of effects that would inevitably alter the description. Once contemporary patterns of oxidant exposure in the environments of dairy industry centers are defined, serial monitoring and surveillance would be in order.

What are the elements of judgement to examine the antioxidant micronutrient and food-oxidant content in milk? Having defined the antioxidant micronutrients and dietary substances with antioxidant functions, as well as the pro-oxidant dietary elements in the body of the text, one could reflect upon our contemporary knowledge of the chemical composition of milk and dairy products, its variation, and the determinants of variation, to forge a profile of exposure both to potentially beneficial compounds and potentially noxious ones. Beyond chemical food composition, however, is the context of levels of usual consumption of milk and dairy products as well as the dietary context in which these products are eaten in various cultures. At a superficial level, we know that bovine milk is a relatively iron-poor food. This feature which makes it problematic for a risk of anemia in children, may favor it to the extent that controlling excessive tissue storage is a positive strategy to limit tissue oxidation. Milk is naturally rich in riboflavin, one of the antioxidant micronutrients, and is often fortified with vitamin A, another member of our list (Table 5). Its selenium content is the casual consequence of the selenium content of fodder and grazing soils. Similarly, both the pattern and content of carotenoids in milk will vary with the food consumed by the dairy animals, and possibly with the evolution of the lactation cycle. Large regional variations in carotenoid content of bovine milk have been documented in the few publications available. Most date back to an age of less sophisticated analytical chemical techniques.

With respect to the pro-oxidant issue, to the extent that unsaturated fatty acids in membranes are more susceptible to lipid oxidation, the fatty acid content of milk is largely saturated. The influence of full-fat milk on cholesterol levels, but most specifically in the LDL lipoproteins, has been discussed (A.M.A., 1993). Popularization of use of milks and cheeses of lower fat content has modified the intake of both the saturated fats and the cholesterol for large segments of the informed consumer population in industrialized countries.

With respect to the net effect on antioxidant micronutrients intake, antioxidant balance, and food-oxidant consumption of the displacement of other traditional foods by diary products in the evolution of dietary practices, anthropological research -- both contemporary and historical -- would be required to address the question. The foregoing paragraphs discussed the safe generalities about antioxidant and pro-oxidant content of milk and diary foods, but a similar consideration of the mixture and balance of these foods in the rest of the diet is needed to complete the panorama. What foods did populations eat before the introduction of dairying? What was its chemical composition. What foods declined in intake as milk, cheese and derivative products were introduced into the diet? What was the balance-sheet effect on anti- and pro-oxidant compounds? These are some of the relevant questions, and it is important to consider dietary changes as a dynamic and continuing process, especially in the so-called "transitional" nations such as Costa Rica and Chile in the Americas and Malaysia and Indonesia in Asia, in which urbanization and economic development are fostering changes in purchasing patterns and dietary intake. These nations represent living "laboratories" for learning about this process of displacement and replacement of foods as influenced by the dairy sector and the consequences for macro- and micronutrient intake patterns. We should not neglect, moreover, the dietary context in which milk and dairy products are consumed, i.e. with what other foods in the meal and with what preparatory and cooking processes. Many chemical compounds can be created and destroyed both in the creation of mixed dishes and in the actual passage through the levels of the alimentary tract. Concern for the ingestion of preformed oxidants from foods that induce lipid peroxidation has recently been reviewed (Kubow, 1992).

Food technology for the processing, modification and "improvement" of milk and dairy products is a major topical concern of this Congress. To the extent that this involves modification of the dairy animals' diets or direct fortification of foods, we confront the issue of the potential for milk and dairy products to serve as vehicles for delivery of increased amounts of dietary

antioxidants? Collaborative research among laboratories in Guatemala, Minnesota and Arizona (Savaiano ét al., 1991), with which CeSSIAM has been associated, suggests that the bioavailability of beta-carotene (and potentially other carotenoids) may be enhanced when consumed with milk or yoghurt. On the other hand, iron fortification of milk-based infant formulas has become popular in recent decades. One must consider carefully the pros and cons of any extension of this technology to the milk supply available to the older segments of the population, balancing the issues of formation of radicals and oxidized products with the nutritional benefits for improving iron reserves in an anemia-endemic population.

As implied in the conclusions above, the gaps in our knowledge about the antioxidant micronutrients and well-being are large. The human population is an evolving species, with technology having accelerated the rate of change in the forces that motivate evolution. The implication of milk and dairy products as important foods in a changing human food supply raise a host of questions and issues including, and extending beyond, those considered in the preceding paragraphs. Research and surveillance activities, focused on this issues, should be supported and encouraged by the dairy industry. The benefits have potential for answering basic questions about the theme as a whole as well as resolving those specific questions relevant to the lives and health of those that produce, process and consume the food and beverage principal products provided from the world's dairies.

REFERENCES

American Medical Association. 1993. Diet and cancer: Where do we stand? Report of the Council on Scientific Affairs. Arch. Intern. Med. 153:50-56.

Balla, G., Jacob, H.S., Balla, J., Rosenberg, M., Nath, K., Apple, F., Eaton, J.W. & Vercellotti, G.M. 1992. Ferritin. A cytoprotective antioxidant strategem of endothelium. J. Biol. Chem. 267:18148-18153.

Block, G. 1992. The data support a role for anti-oxidants in reducing cancer risk. Nutr. Rev. 50: 204-213.

Block, G., Patterson, B. & Subar, A. 1992. Fruit, vegetables, and cancer prevention: A review of the epidemiological evidence. Nutr. Cancer 18:1-29.

Bunce, G.E., Kinoshita, J & Horowitz, J. 1990. Nutritional factors in cataract. Annu. Rev. Nutr. 10: 233-254.

Canfield, L.M., Forage, J.W. & Valenzuela, J.G. 1992. Carotenoids as cellular antioxidants. Proc. Soc. Exp. Biol. Med. 200:260-265.

Canfield, L.M., Krinsky, N.I. & Olson, J.A., eds, 1993. Carotenoids in Human Health. New York, New York Academy of Science.

Chen, J., Geissler, C., Parpia, B., Li, J. & Campbell, T.C. 1992. Antioxidant status and cancer mortality in China. Int. J. Epidemiol. 21:625-635.

Chytil, F. 1992. The lungs and vitamin A. Am. J. Physiol. 262:L517-L527.

Darmon, M. 1990. The nuclear receptors of retinoic acid. J. Lipid Mediators 2:247-256.

Dormandy, T.L. 1969. Biological rancidification. Lancet 2:684-685.

Erdman, J.W. Jr., Bierer, T. & Gugger, E.T. 1993. In: L.M. Canfield, N.I. Krinsky & J.A. Olson, eds. Carotenoids in Human Health. New York, N.Y. Acad, Sci. (in press).

Fenton, H.J.H. 1894. Oxidation of tartaric acid in presence of iron. J. Chem. Soc. 65:899-910.

Frank, L. 1992. Antioxidants, nutrition, and bronchopulmonary dysplasia. Clin. Perinatol. 19:541-562.

Grimley-Evans, J. 1988. Ageing and disease. In: D. Evered & J. Whelan, eds., Research and the Ageing Population. Chichester, John Wiley & Sons, 38-47.

Haber, F. & Weiss, J. 1934. The catalytic decomposition of hydrogen peroxide by iron salts. Proc. Roy. Soc. (London, Ser. A.) 147: 332-351.

Halliwell, B., Gutteridge, J.M.C. & Cross, C.E. 1992. Free radicals, antioxidants, and human disease: Where are we now? J. Lab. Clin. Med. 119:598-620.

Hankinson, S.E., Stampfer, M.J., Seddon, J.M., Colditz, G.A., Rosner, B., Speizer, F.E. & Willett, W.C. 1992. Nutrient intake and cataract extraction in women:a prospective study. BMJ 305:335-339

Harmon, D. 1956. Aging: a theory based on free radical and radiation chemistry. J. Gerontol. 11:298-300.

Henderson, B.E., Ross, R.U. & Pike, M.C. 1991. Toward the primary prevention of cancer. Science 254:1131-1138.

Hennekens, C.H. 1993. Beta-carotene and risk of cardiovascular disease. In: L.M. Canfield, N.I. Krinsky & J.A. Olson, eds., Carotenoids in Human Health. New York, N.Y. Acad, Sci. (in press).

Herbert, V. 1990. Vitamin B-12. In: M.L. Brown, ed., Present Knowledge in Nutrition. Sixth Edition Washington, D.C., I.L.S.I.: 171-172.

Hill, C.H. & Matrone, G. 1970. Chemical parameters in the study of in vivo and in vitro interactions of transition elements. Fed. Proc. 29:1474-1481.

Holick, M.F. 1985. The photobiology of vitamin D and its consequences for humans. Ann. N.Y. Acad. Sci. 453:1-13.

Hong, Y-L., Pan, H-Z., Scott, M.D. & Meshnick, S.R. 1992. Activated oxygen generation by a primaquine metabolite: Inhibition by antioxidants derived from Chinese herbal remedies. Free Rad. Biol. Med. 12:213-218.

Jacques, P.F., Chylack, L.T., McGandy, R.B. & Hartz, S.C. 1988. Antioxidant status in persons with and without senile cataract. Arch. Ophthalmol. 106:337-340.

Jukes, T.H. 1992. Antioxidants, nutrition and evolution. Prev. Med. 21:270-276.

Kagi, J.H.R., Hunziker, P. & Vasak, M. 1990. Metallothionein: Biochemistry and spatial structure. In: H. Tomita, ed., Trace Elements in Clinical Medicine. Tokyo, Springer-Verlag:395-403.

Kamp, D.W., Graceffa, P., Pryor, W.A. & Weitzman, S.A. 1992. The role of free radicals in asbestos-induced diseases. Free Rad. Biol. Med. 12:293-315.

Karnofsky, J.R. & Sima, P. 1991. Singlet oxygen production from the reactions of ozone with biological molecules. J. Biol. Chem. 266: 9039-9042.

Kirkwood, T.B.L. 1977. Evolution of ageing. Nature (Lond.) 270:301-304.

Krinsky, N.I. 1992. Mechanisms of action of biological antioxidants. Proc. Soc. Exp. Biol. Med. 200:248-254.

Kubow, S. 1992. Routes of formation and toxic consequences of lipid oxidation products in foods Free Rad. Biol. Med. 12:63-81.

Lesnefsky, E.J. 1992. Reduction of infarct size by cell-permeable oxygen metabolite scavengers. Free Rad. Biol. Med. 12:429-446.

Levander, O.A. 1992. Selenium and sulfur in antioxidant protective systems:Relationships with vitamin E and malaria. Proc. Soc. Exp. Biol. Med. 200:255-259.

Levander, O.A. & Burk, R.F. 1990. Selenium. In: M.L. Brown, ed., Present Knowledge in Nutrition. Sixth Edition. Washington, D.C., I.L.S.L.: 268-273.

Mathews-Roth, M. 1982. Beta-carotene therapy for erythropoietic and other photosensitivity diseases. In: J.D. Regan & J.A. Parish, eds., The Science of Photomedicine. New York, Plenum Press: 409-440.

McNamara, J.O. & Fridovich, I. 1993. Did radicals strike Lou Gehrig? Nature 362:20-21.

Mino, M. 1992. Clinical uses and abuses of vitamin E in children. Proc. Soc. Exp. Biol. Med. 200:266-270.

National Research Council.. 1989. Diet and Health: Implications for Chronic Disease Risk. Washington, D.C., National Academy of Sciences.

Olson, J.A. & Kobayashi, S. Antioxidants in health and disease:Overview. Proc. Soc. Exp. Biol. Med. 200:245-247.

Omaye, S.T., Skala, J.H. & Jacob, R.A. 1986. Plasma ascorbic acid in adult males: Effects of depletion and supplementation. Am. J. Clin. Nutr. 44:257-264.

Packer, L. 1992. Interactions among antioxidants in health and disease:Vitamin E and its redox cycle. Proc. Soc. Exp. Biol. Med. 200:271-276.

Patterson, W.P., Winkelmann, M. & Perry, M.C. 1985. Zinc-induced copper deficiency: megamineral sideroblastic anemia. Ann. Intern. Med. 103:385-386.

Pryor, W.A. 1992. Biological effects of cigarette smoke, wood smoke, and the smoke from plastics: The use of electron spin resonance. Free Rad. Biol. Med. 13:659-676.

Regnstrom, J., et al. 1992. Susceptibility to low-density lipoprotein oxidation and coronary atherosclerosis in man. Lancet 339:1183-1186.

Reif, D.W. 1992. Ferritin as a source of iron for oxidative damage. Free Rad. Biol. Med. 12:417-427.

Reisz, P. & Kondo, T. 1992. Free radical formation induced by ultrasound and its biological implication Free Rad. Biol. Med. 13:247-279.

Riemersma, R.A., Wood, D.A., Macintyre, C.C., Elton, R.A., Gey, K.Y. & Oliver, M.W. 1991. Risk of angina pectoris and plasma concentrations of vitamin A, C, and E and carotene. Lancet 337: 1-5.

Rikans, L.E., Snowden, C.D. & Moore, D.R. 1992. Effect of aging on enzymatic antioxidant defenses in rat liver mitochondria. Gerontology 38:133-138.

Rogers, A.E. & Longnecker, M.P. 1988. Biology of disease: dietary and nutritional influences on cancer: a review of epidemiologic and experimental data. Lab. Invest. 59:729-759.

Rosen, D.R., Siddique, T., Patterson, D., et al. 1993. Mutations in Cu/Zn superoxide dismutase

353

gene are associated with familial amyotrophic lateral sclerosis. Nature 362:59-62.

Salonen, J.T. et al. 1992. Autoantibody against oxidised LDL and progression of carotid atherosclerosis. Lancet 339:883-887.

Sauberlich, H.E. 1990. Ascorbic acid. In: M.L. Brown, ed., Present Knowledge in Nutrition, Sixth Edition. Washington, D.C., I.L.S.I.:132-141.

Savaiano, D.A., Martini, M.C.., Solomons, N.W., Guerrero, A-M., Zepeda, E., Valenzuela, J.G. & Canfield, L.M. 1991. Beta-carotene bioavailability FASEB J. 5:A1323 (abst.)

Schafer, L. & Thorling, E.B. 1990. Lipid peroxidation and antioxidation supplementation in old age. Scand. J. Clin. Lab. Invest. 50:69-75.

Shekelle, R.B., Lepper, M., Liu, S., Maliza, C., Raynor, W.J., Rossof, A.H., Paul, O., Shryock, A.M. & Stamler, J. 1981. Dietary vitamin A and risk of cancer in the Western Electric study. Lancet 2: 1186-1190.

Simoons, F. 1981. Geographic patterns of primary adults lactose malabsorption: A further interpretation of evidence for the Old World. In: D.M. Paige & T.M. Bayless, eds., Lactose Intolerance: Clinical and nutritional implications. Baltimore, Johns Hopkins University press:23-48.

Singh, V.N. & Gaby, S.K. 1991. Premalgnant lesions: Role of antioxidant vitamins and beta-carotene in risk reduction and prevention of malignant transformation. Am. J. Clin. Nutr. 53:368S-390S.

Steinberg, D. 1992. Antioxidants in the prevention of human atherosclerosis. Circulation 85:2337-2344.

Strain, J.J. 1991. Disturbances of micronutrient and antioxidant status in diabetes. Proc. Nutr. Soc. 50: 591-604.

Taylor, A. 1989. Associations between nutrition and cataract. Nutr. Rev. 47:225-234.

Taylor, A. 1990. Role of nutrients in delaying < cataracts. In: H.E. Sauberlich & L.J. Machlin, eds., Beyond Deficiency: New Views on the Function and Health Effects of Vitamins. Ann. N.Y. Acad. Sci. 669:111-123.

Willett, W.C. 1990. Nutritional Epidemiology. Oxford Press.

Yang, G., Candy, T.E.G., Boaro, M., Wilkin, H.E., Jones, P., Nazhat, N.B., Saadalla-Nazhat, R.A. & Blake, D.R. 1992. Free radical yields from the homolysis of peroxynitrous acid. Free Fad. Biol. Med. 12: 327-300.

Yang, G.Q., Zhu, L., Liu, S., Qian, P., Huang, J. & i ", M. 1983. Endemic selenium intoxication of humans in China. Am. J. Clin. Nutr. 37:872-881.

Ziegler, R.G. 1991. Vegetables, fruits and carotenoids and the risk of cancer. Am. J. Clin. Nutr. 53:251S-259S.

Ziegler, R.G. 1993. Carotenoids, vegetables and fruits, and risk of cancer. In: L.M. Canfield, N.I. Krinsky & J.A. Olson, eds. Carotenoids in Human Health. New York, N.Y. Acad, Sci. (in press).

354

Dairy Products in Human Health and Nutrition, Serrano Rios et al. (eds) © 1994 Balkema, Rotterdam, ISBN 90 5410 359 0

Early dietary habits, cholesterolemia and coronary artery disease

J.M.Ordovas
Lipid Metabolism Laboratory, USDA Human Nutrition Research Center on Aging at Tufts University, Boston, Mass., USA

ABSTRACT: Coronary artery disease starts in childhood and it continues to develop into adulthood. Thus, every effort should be put in identifying adequate preventive measures to reduce CAD risk starting in the childhood. This is specially important in countries with high prevalence of CAD, and those in which a rise has been observed. Dietary recommendations should focus primarily on reducing saturated fat intake. Low-fat, low-cholesterol diets should not be used in children under 2 years of age. A gradual transition towards the dietary guidelines should be implemented as children grow older. Treatment of high-risk children should always be under the guidance of a team of experts (physician, dietitian, nurse). Careful monitoring should be instituted to achieve a normal lipid profile, while maintaining proper growth and nutritional intake.

CORONARY ARTERY DISEASE

Coronary artery disease (CAD), the major cause of death in the United States and other industrialized countries, is the final outcome of atherosclerosis, a process by which the lumen of an artery is gradually narrowed by focal areas of lipid deposition, smooth muscle cell proliferation, enhanced collagen formation, and occasionally calcification. The first stage in atherosclerosis is development of the fatty streak composed mainly of foam cells beneath the endothelial cell layer The second stage in this process is the formation of a fibrous plaque consisting of a central necrotic core containing intracellular lipid within macrophages as well as some extracellular lipid, with a fibrous cap above it, this fibrous plaque may remain stable for many years. The final stage in atherosclerosis is the formation of a complex lesion, consisting, in addition to the fibrous plaque, of areas of hemorrhage, calcification, ulceration and thrombosis. A thrombus is usually the terminal event that leads to arterial occlusion (Ross, 1986).

Autopsies performed in young adults during the Korean and Vietnam Wars have shown the presence of fibrous thickening within the coronaries and advanced lesions with coronary occlusions of up to 70% (Strong, 1986). More recent studies have shown that over 50% of children aged 10-14 years had lesions associated with the first stage of atherosclerosis, and about 8% had more advanced lesions with larger accumulations of extracellular lipid in coronary arteries (Stary, 1989). These findings clearly demonstrate that the genesis of atherosclerosis takes place early in life.

Elevated plasma levels of low density lipoprotein cholesterol and dyslipidemia have been shown to be a major coronary artery disease (CAD) risk factor. These levels are determined by the combination of modifiable and nonmodifiable factors among which diet has a preeminent role (The Expert Panel, 1988) (see table 1).

This review will summarize the current recommendations regarding infant and child nutrition and our knowledge on how early nutrition may affect CAD risk during the adult years.

Table 1. Factors Affecting LDL Cholesterol Levels

Nonmodifiable	Modifiable
Age	Diet
Gender	Exercise
Race	Smoking
Heredity	Obesity
	Medications
	Alcohol

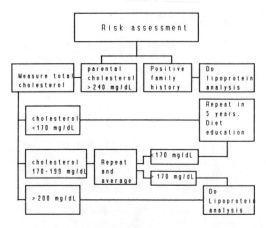

Figure 1

Table 2. Characteristics of the Step-One Diet for Lowering Blood Cholesterol Levels	
Nutrient	Recommended Intake
Total fat	Average of no more than 30% of total calories
Saturated fatty acids	Less than 10% of total calories
Polyunsaturated fatty acids	Up to 10% of total calories
Monounsaturated fatty acids	Remaining total fat calories
Cholesterol	Less than 300 mg/day
Carbohydrates	About 55% of total calories
Protein	About 15%-20% of total calories
Calories	To promote normal growth and development and to reach or maintain desirable body weight

PLASMA CHOLESTEROL LEVELS DURING EARLY INFANCY

Plasma total cholesterol in the newborn ranges between 50 and 100 mg/dl, independently of race and sex, and unlike the lipoprotein pattern found in adults, the cholesterol is evenly distributed between low- and high density lipoproteins (Berenson et al.1983; Davis et al.1982; Dharmady et al.1972; Rosenthal et al.1983). These lipid levels and distribution are similar in most animal species, despite the interspecies differences observed in the adult state (Innis, 1989). In healthy term newborn infants, total cholesterol increases about twofold during the first days after birth, mainly due to increases in low density lipoprotein (LDL) cholesterol. LDL cholesterol levels continue to gradually increase during the 3-4 years of childhood and then remain stable until adolescence, when they continue to increase until adult levels are reached.

The mean plasma cholesterol levels of American children and adolescents (1 to 19 years of age) is about 160 mg/dL. and the mean LDL cholesterol levels is about 100 mg/dL. The 75th and 95th percentile for total cholesterol are roughly 170 and 200 mg/dL, while for LDL cholesterol these percentiles are 110 and 130 mg/dL respectively.

Compared to children in many other countries, US children have higher plasma cholesterol levels and higher intakes of saturated fatty acids and cholesterol. Some studies have shown that the levels of plasma cholesterol during infancy are a good predictor of the levels later in life, this phenomenon is known as "tracking" (Newman et al.1986). In addition, plasma cholesterol levels in children of different societies are positively correlated with the incidence of adult mortality from CAD in that society (Knuiman et

al.1980). In view of this evidence, it is reasonable to speculate that early dietary intervention in children to reduce total cholesterol, and more specifically LDL cholesterol levels will be the most efficacious preventive measure to reduce morbidity and mortality in populations at high risk for CAD. However, this issue is subject to fervent controversy and some key questions must be addressed.

In the first place, it is necessary to determine what to measure in order to determine individual risk. Based on population studies, involving mainly middle age subjects, tests that may predict the presence of atherosclerosis and CAD risk include total cholesterol, LDL cholesterol, HDL cholesterol, apolipoproteins AI and B, fibrinogen and more recently DNA analysis. For practical reasons, total cholesterol is accepted as the first screening procedure. The second question is the type of screening: selective versus universal. According to the National Cholesterol Education program (NCEP), selective screening should include children and adolescents with a positive family history of CAD before age 55 or the presence of a parent with cholesterol levels >240 mg/dl (Figure 1). However, there is evidence that selective screening in those children with family history of CAD will fail to detect 30-40% of all children with abnormal lipid profile, consequently universal screening is favored by those advocating early screening, between 4-7 years of age (Dysart et al.1992).

Table 3. Diets of children and adolescents (% of Energy, unless otherwise indicated) (Kersting et al., 1992)		
	Present (1-14y)	Proposed (>2y)
protein	13	13
animal: vegetable protein	66:33	50:50
fat	39	35
Linoleic	4	7
Saturated	18	13
P:S ratio	0.28	0.63
cholesterol (mg/1000Kcal)	170	100
carbohydrates	48	52
sucrose	14	8
fiber	8	16

Opponents of the concept of selective or universal cholesterol screening of children maintain that although a child with an elevated plasma cholesterol has a three times greater risk of having a high levels as an adult, there are many children with high cholesterol levels who will have normal levels as an adult. This could lead to "labeling" of children that could result in unnecessary anxiety in the children and their parents. In addition, total cholesterol is not predictive of LDL cholesterol. Once reliable, and readily available tests for LDL cholesterol are available, screening will be more selective (Weidman, 1992; Hulley et al.1992).

CHILDHOOD DIET AND SERUM LIPIDS

As we have previously indicated, nutritional factors are major determinants of plasma lipids and lipoproteins at any stage of development, and may account for the higher cholesterol levels observed in children from urban industrial societies when compared to children in rural, developing areas. The effect of dietary fat on plasma lipid levels in infants and children are similar to those found in adults.

Today's parents face major challenges in feeding infant and young children. The availability of different types of infant feeding and the eating behavior of children have contributed to parents'

anxiety about feeding young children adequately, while keeping up with an overwhelming amount of information regarding "good" and "bad" foods.

The current recommendations for feeding infants, indicate that breast milk continues to be the ideal nutrient for the first 6 to 12 months. It is obvious to think that the nutritive composition of breast milk is perfectly suited to meet the needs of infants. The best alternative to breast milk are the commercially prepared iron-fortified infant formulas. Cow's milk is not recommended during the first year of life.

Plasma cholesterol levels are lower in those infants fed formulas rich in polyunsaturated fatty acids (PUFA) than in those fed breast milk that contains a higher proportion of saturated fatty acids (SAT). Consequently, it is possible that the feeding of the infant could influence the development of obesity and cardiovascular disease later in life. However this has to be proven, and in general most health organizations agree that fat, cholesterol, and calories should not be restricted for children under 2-3 years of age. Above that age, children should reduce their dietary fat intake to no more than 30 percent of total calories, and saturated fatty acids should account for less than 10% of total calories. Dietary cholesterol should be less than 300 mg/day (NCEP Expert Panel, 1992; Committee on Nutrition, 1992). Such diet can support normal growth and development during childhood (see Table 1). However, careful food selection has to be made and nutrient-rich foods such as meat and dairy products have to be included in the diet.

While in Eastern societies, children have traditionally consumed well-balanced diets low in fat, in Western societies children are used to consume high fat diets. According to surveys in the United States, children 1-to-5 years of age consume more than 35% of their total calories as fat, 14% from saturated fat, 6% from polyunsaturated fat, and 233 mg cholesterol per day. In order to achieve the current recommendations it will need a considerable change in dietary habits, that will require elimination or reduction of foods that are familiar to children in industrialized societies. The situation is even more dramatic in other industrialized countries where the fat consumption in children amounts to roughly 40% of total energy (Mann, 1992; Kersting et al.1992). For these reasons, it has been suggested that this goal should be relaxed to 30-35% of total calories (See Tables 3 and 4) (Lifshitz, 1992; Kersting et al.1992). Above all, the specific needs of the growing child should take priority over hypothetical risks later in life, and the energy intake should be adequate to support growth and development and to reach and maintain desirable body weight.

A recent survey of students from 9 to 13 years of age, showed that 83% of children believe in avoiding

357

Table 4. Proposed consumption by food groups in a balanced diet [g(ml)/day] (Kersting et al., 1992)	Children 4-6 years
Milk, milk products	350
Lean meat	50
Saltwater fish	100
Eggs/week	2
visible fats and oils	20
Bread (>50% wholegrain)	150
Cereals (wholegrain)	20
Potatoes	120
Vegetables	180
Fruit	180
Cake, biscuits	<40
Sugar, jams	<25
Beverages	700
Energy content,Kcal/d	1500

"high-fat foods" and 71% of them worry about fat and cholesterol. These data brings the positive aspect of the awareness by young children that intake of cholesterol and fat may be detrimental to the health. However, children could impose on themselves dietary restrictions, often unsupervised, that could result in energy or micronutrient deficiencies with potentially harmful consequences. The diets consumed by these children maybe similar to the "prudent diet" recommended by many experts, but insufficient for normal growth.

We should keep in mind that physical inactivity is another important modifiable factor (See table 1) associated with higher cholesterol levels and increased CAD risk. It has been reported that excessive television viewing was an strong predictor for high cholesterol levels in children. We should keep in mind that excessive television viewing is associated with certain dietary and physical activity habits and may prove to be a useful, global marker for several life-style factors predisposing children to hypercholesterolemia (Wong et al.1992).

As result of the NCEP recommendations for the general population, a change in dietary habits is taking place in the United States. Since the early seventies, the per capita consumption of milk and ice cream has declined by 20% and butter by 30%. Intake of animal fats and eggs during this period declined by 12 and 28% respectively, while the vegetable oil intake has increased by 55%. During this time mortality from CAD has declined significantly, however we should remember that in addition to changes in dietary habits, other changes in lifestyle such as increased physical activity and reduced smoking have contributed to these changes in CAD morbidity and mortality.

DIET AND DRUG TREATMENT

Diet therapy is the primary approach to treating children with elevated plasma cholesterol levels. The borderline values established by the NCEP for LDL cholesterol are between 110 and 129 mg/dL. Above 129 is considered high LDL cholesterol. The ideal goal is to lower the LDL cholesterol below 110 mg/dL.

The diet therapy is prescribed in two steps. First, the Step-One diet (see Table 2) should be followed under the monitoring of a physician, registered dietitian or other qualified nutrition professional. If careful adherence to this diet for at least 3 months fails to achieve the goals, the Step-Two diet should be initiated. This represents an additional reduction of the saturated fatty acid intake to less than 7%, and of the cholesterol intake to less than 200 mg/dL. This diet requires a very careful supervision to ensure adequacy of all nutrients.

If after and adequate trial of diet therapy (6 month to 1 year) the LDL cholesterol remains above 190 mg/dL (or 160 mg/dL) in the presence of other CAD risk factors), then drug treatment should be implemented in children more than 10 years of age. Bile acid sequestrants such as cholestyramine and cholestypol are the only drugs recommended by the American Academy of Pediatrics, because of the limited experience in the use of other cholesterol-lowering agents in children. Even the bile acid sequestrants must be used with caution because they all have potential for interfering with growth as well as producing significant side effects.

CONCLUSIONS

Coronary artery disease starts in childhood and it continues to develop into adulthood. Thus, every effort should be put in identifying adequate preventive measures to reduce CAD risk starting in the childhood. This is specially important in countries with high prevalence of CAD, and those with a rise in this disease.

Dietary recommendations should focus primarily on

reducing saturated fat intake, and for these recommendations to be generally accepted, the particular country's cultural and dietary habits should be taken into consideration.

Low-fat, low-cholesterol diets should not be used in children under 2 years of age. A gradual transition towards the dietary guidelines should be implemented as children grow older.

Treatment of high-risk children should always be under the guidance of a team of experts (physician, dietitian, nurse). Careful monitoring should be instituted to achieve a normal lipid profile, while maintaining proper growth and nutritional intake.

REFERENCES

Berenson, G.S. and Epstein, F.H. 1983.Conference on blood lipids in children: optimal levels for early prevention of coronary artery disease. *Prev. Med.* 12:741-797.

Committee on Nutrition, 1992.Statement on cholesterol. *Pediatrics* 90:469-473.

Davis, P.A. and Forte, T.M. 1982.Neonatal umbilical cord blood lipoproteins. Isolation and characterization of intermediate density and low density lipoproteins. *Arteriosclerosis* 2:37-43.

Dharmady, J.M., Fosbrooke, A.S. and Lloyd, J.K. 1972.Prospective study of serum cholesterol levels during first years of life. *Br.Med.J.* 2:685-688.

Dysart, J. and Strong, W.B. 1992.The `pros' of cholesterol screening of children. *J.Am.Coll.Nutr.* 11 Suppl.:16S-17S.

Hulley, S.B. and Newman, T.B. 1992.Cholesterol screening in children is not indicated, even with positive family history. *J.Am.Coll.Nutr.* 11 Suppl.:20S-22S.

Innis, S.M. 1989.Changes in plasma cholesterol density distribution of rats fed a high fat and cholesterol diet following early induction of HMG CoA reductase activity. *J.Nutr.* 119:373-379.

Kersting, M. and Schöch, G. 1992.Achievable guidelines for food consumption to reach a balanced fat and nutrient intake in childhood and adolescence. *J.Am.Coll.Nutr.* 11 Suppl.:74S-78S.

Knuiman, J.T., Hermus, R.J.J. and Hautvast, J.G.A.J. 1980.Serum total and high-density lipoprotein cholesterol concentrations in rural and urban boys from 16 countries. *Atherosclerosis* 36:529-537.

Lifshitz, F. 1992.Children on adult diets: Is it harmful? Is it healthful. *J.Am.Coll.Nutr.* 11 Suppl.:84S-90S.

Mann, J. 1992.Nutrition options when reducing saturated fat intake. *J.Am.Coll.Nutr.* 11 Suppl.:82S-83S.

NCEP Expert Panel, 1992.National Cholesterol Education Program (NCEP): Highlights of the report of the expert panel on blood cholesterol levels in children and adolescents. *Pediatrics* 89:495-501.

Newman, W.P., Freeman, D.S., Voors, A.V., et al. 1986.Relation of serum lipoprotein levels and systolic blood pressure to early atherosclerosis: The Bogalusa Heart Study. *N Engl J Med* 314:138-144.

Rosenthal, M., Van Biervliet, J.P., Bury, J. and Vinaimont, N. 1983.Isolation and characterization of lipoprotein profiles in newborns by density gradient ultracentrifugation. *Pediatr.Res.* 17:783-794.

Ross, R. 1986.The pathogenesis of atherosclerosis. *N Engl J Med* 314:488-500.

Stary, H.C. 1989.Evolution and progression of atherosclerosis lesions in coronary arteries of children and young adults. *Arteriosclerosis* 9 (Suppl 1):I-19-I-32.

Strong, J.P. 1986.Coronary atherosclerosis in soldiers. A clue to the natural history of atherosclerosis in young. *JAMA* 256:2863-2866.

The Expert Panel, 1988.Report of the National Cholesterol Education Program Expert Panel on Detection, Evaluation, and Treatment of High Blood Cholesterol in Adults. *Arch.Intern.Med.* 148:36-69.

Weidman, W.H. 1992.The `cons' of cholesterol screening of children. *J.Am.Coll.Nutr.* 11 Suppl.:18S-19S.

Wong, N.D., Hei, T.K., Qaqundah, P.Y., Davidson, D.M., Bassin, S.L. and Gold, K.V. 1992.Television viewing and pediatric hypercholesterolemia. *Pediatrics* 90:75-79.

Dairy Products in Human Health and Nutrition, Serrano Ríos et al. (eds) © 1994 Balkema, Rotterdam, ISBN 90 5410 359 0

Dietary fats and blood lipids as cardiovascular risk factors in the general population: A critical overview

U. Ravnskov
Lund, Sweden

SUMMARY: Although changes of the amount and character of dietary fat may raise the serum cholesterol level, and a high level is associated with an increased risk of coronary heart disease in men, other findings contradict the idea that the mentioned association is causal. A correlation has never been found between intake of animal fat, or saturated or polyunsaturated fatty acids, and degree of atherosclerosis; if anything coronary patients eat more polyunsaturated fatty acids than non-coronary controls; a correlation between the serum cholesterol level and degree of atherosclerosis has never been found in unbiased studies; mortality from cardiovascular disease in various populations and their mean serum cholesterol concentration do not covariate; and coronary and total mortality cannot be lowered by reduction of the serum cholesterol concentration. As an overview of all controlled trials has shown a significant increase of non-cardiovascular deaths after intervention there are obvious reasons to stop the cholesterol campaign.

INTRODUCTION

For several decades, research on the causation of atherosclerotic vascular disease, especially coronary heart disease (CHD), has been dominated by epidemiologists. Their main instrument has been to identify risk factors, eg. factors which are statistically associated with an increased risk of dying from coronary heart disease. Almost 300 risk factors, or, more correctly, risk markers, are known; for instance smoking, obesity, hypertension, lack of exercise, psychological stress, baldness, snoring, and eating too much or too little of a steadily increasing number of various food ingredients. Although statistical associations do not prove causality, no matter how strong they are or how plausible they may seem, altering risk markers has more and more been considered a way to diminish coronary heart disease.

Two risk markers are of special interest for this meeting, the diet and the serum cholesterol concentration. According to the diet-heart idea it is the amount and the character of dietary fat which mainly determine the blood cholesterol concentration, and a high cholesterol concentration is the main cause of atherosclerosis and coronary heart disease. Prestigious committees have declared that the evidence for this chain of events from food to heart is strong and consistent and that scepticism is unwarranted (National Research Council 1989, Gotto & al 1990). As a consequence, general diet recommendations have been intro-

duced in many countries, and population screening to identify individuals with a high serum cholesterol has been proposed and even effectuated.

A great number of observations and experiments are incompatible with the mentioned ideas, however (Stehbens 1988, Smith 1991, Gurr 1992), but let me start with some facts which are generally accepted.

THE UNDISPUTED FACTS

Diet and cholesterol concentration.

An exchange of certain saturated with certain polyunsaturated fatty acids in the diet may lower the serum cholesterol level in many people. This has been convincingly demonstrated in small trials or in trials performed in institutions. Compared with control individuals a net decrease of serum cholesterol of 8-14 percent was reached in these trials.

It is unlikely however, that the extreme diets which were used are adoptable in population strategies. In larger trials where a more palatable diet was used the effect on the cholesterol level was only marginal in spite of great educational efforts. Part of the explanation is probably that factors other than diet have a stronger influence on the serum cholesterol level. Thus, although they eat gargantuan amounts of animal fat primitive African tribes have a lower mean serum cholesterol concentration than has any population in the western world (Shaper 1962; Lapiccirella & al 1962; Mann & al 1964). Their low cholesterol is **not a** genetic trait because when Maasai people **for** instance migrated to a modern urban environment their cholesterol rose to western levels (Day & al 1976). Also, the serum cholesterol concentrations of Polynesians increased after migration although they halved their consumption of saturated fatty acids (Stanhope & al 1980).

Serum cholesterol as a risk marker

It is accepted generally that there is a statistical association between a high blood cholesterol concentration and an increased risk of death from coronary heart disease. This has been demonstrated again and again in a great number of populations around the world.

The increased risk is much smaller than is generally believed, however; in the largest meta-analysis of 68406 deaths in 23 cohort studies from Europe, Israel, Japan and the US (Jacobs & al 1992) the rate ratio for total cardiovascular mortality after >5 years was only 1.48 (in the MR.FIT study 1.86) for men in the highest cholesterol quartile. In the 30-year follow-up of the Framingham population no association was found either for men above the age of fifty, and a decreasing, not an increasing cholesterol level was associated with a higher coronary and total mortality (Anderson & al 1987).

For those who have used the rising curve for coronary mortality at high cholesterol levels as an argument for intervention there are two major problems. No increased risk was seen for women; and at the low range (the first cholesterol quartile) there was an increased risk of digestive, respiratory, cancer and traumatic death for both sexes. The resulting curve for total mortality for men appeared as a symmetric U; and for women the rising curve in the low cholesterol range had no counterpart in the high range (Jacobs & al 1992).

Most authors consider the association to noncardiovascular death in the first cholesterol quartile as a result of confounding, and they may be right, but they ignore that the same explanation may be valid for the association found in the other end of the cholesterol scale. Factors such as stress (Dimsdale & Herd 1982), low physical activity (Naito 1976), overweight (Dattilo & Kris-Etherton 1992), and to a lesser degree smoking (Craig & al 1989) may predispose to vascular death by other mechanisms and at the same time raise the serum cholesterol level.

In recent years great attention has been devoted to the cholesterol fractions transported by low density and high density lipoproteins (LDL and HDL); a high level of LDL- and a low level of HDL-cholesterol are said to increase the risk of coronary heart disease.

Again, the statistical associations found

are indirect evidence only. It should be recalled that a "beneficial" balance between LDL and HDL cholesterol is induced for instance by weight reduction and exercise, and it has never been proved which of these factors, the higher HDL/LDL ratio itself, or the weight reduction or the exercize, that are cardioprotective. If concentrations of HDL are corrected for body weight, smoking, age, and LDL concentration its predictive power decreases considerably, and for serum triglycerides, another lipid risk marker, it disappears totally (Gordon & al 1989).

Thus, these two risk markers, the diet and the high blood cholesterol concentration, are important only if it can be proved by other means that an imbalance of dietary fatty acids and a high blood cholesterol level lead to atherosclerosis and coronary heart disease, and if a lowering of blood cholesterol can prevent these disorders without harm. Evidence for these prerequisites is hard to find.

THE COUNTER-EVIDENCE

Diet and atherosclerosis

If an imbalance between dietary fatty acids leads to a high blood cholesterol, and if hypercholesterolemia leads to atherosclerosis, the dietary habits should predict the degree of atherosclerosis at autopsy.

In the International Atherosclerosis Project the degree of atherosclerosis and the dietary habits were compared between twelve localities on four continents (Scrimshaw and Guzmán 1968). Although mean degree of atherosclerosis in a locality was correlated to mean intake of fat (r = 0.67) it was not correlated to mean intake of animal fat (r = 0.07). Similar results were achieved in a study between individuals in the New Orleans branch of the same project (Moore & al 1976). A weak correlation was found to intake of total fat but not to intake of animal or vegetable fat; if anything those with a high percentage of raised coronary lesions had eaten more vegetable fat than the others.

Intake of nutrients was also reported in the Honolulu Heart Program, but no association was found with the atherosclerosis scores between individuals at autopsy (Reed & al 1987).

Diet and coronary heart disease

In an early study a positive correlation was found between coronary mortality and national consumption data of animal fat. To use this correlation as an argument for causality is premature because it is specific neither for dietary fat nor for mortality from coronary heart disease (Yerushalmy & Hilleboe 1957) and secular comsumption trends do not follow trends in vital statistics (Marmot & al 1982). And in a recent comparison between 23 cohorts in various countries no correlation between consumption of saturated fatty acids and coronary mortality was found for women and the correlation coefficient for men was only 0.25 (Jacobs & al 1992).

Migration studies, especially those which concerned Japanese emigrants, are also used as argument. The CHD mortality figures for such emigrants in Hawaii, and especially in the US, were much higher than in Japan and close to those found in their new homeland. This was said to be due to the high-fat western diet.

It is rarely mentioned that while coronary mortality increased after migration, stroke mortality decreased just as much and total mortality much more (Worth & al 1975). Besides, Marmot & Syme (1976) found that the cultural upbringing of the emigrant was far more important than the diet. Thus, the prevalence of coronary heart disease for Japanese-Americans who preferred the lean Japanese diet but had been brought up non-traditionally was more than four times higher than for Japanese-Americans who preferred the fat western diet but had otherwise been brought up in the traditional Japanese way.

It may be argued that dietary information was based on a regular 24-hour dietary recall for a subsample only; the rest were asked to indicate which of a number of traditional Japanese and typically western food items they had eaten the previous 24 hours, obviously an imprecise measure.

At least eleven studies however, have reported dietary intakes in coronary patients and non-coronary control individuals based on re-gular recall interviews (table 1). Contrary to what was expected only one study found that coronary patients had consumed more saturated fatty acids than controls, and in the same population and in a further three coronary patients had also consumed more fatty acids of the polyunsaturated variety.

An objection to these studies may be that even such information is unreliable, or that the consumption during a single or a couple of 24-hours periods is not representative for the diet of a whole lifetime. This may be correct; the point is, however, that these unsupportive studies are widely used as evidence of the diet-heart idea, even by some of their directors.

Familial hypercholesterolemia

The combination of a very high serum cholesterol concentration and severe, premature atherosclerosis found in individuals with familial hypercholesterolemia is generally considered as the best evidence for a high serum cholesterol concentration being the direct cause of atherosclerosis.

However, in many contributions Stehbens (1988) has argued that homozygous familial hypercholesterolemia, like experimental "atherosclerosis", is a generalized lipid storage disease, whereas atherosclerosis is confined to arteries, has great topographical variations and is often followed by intimal tears, plaque fissuring, ulceration, thrombosis and aneurysm formation, changes which are never seen in homozygous familial hypercholesterolemia. In its heterozygous form the vas-

Table 1. Consumption of saturated and polyunsaturated fatty acids (per cent of energy if nothing else is stated) in coronary patients and non-coronary controls.

		Saturated Fatty Acids		Polyunsaturated Fatty Acids	
		CHD	Controls	CHD	Controls
Zukel & al 1959	r	18.7	18.9	3.6	3.6
Paul & al 1963	p	59[a]	59[a]	13.2[a]	14[a]
Finegan & al 1968	r	19	18	4	4
Bassett & al 1969	r				
Hawaiian men		13.3	13.2	5.4	5.9
Japanese men		10.7	11.1	6.3	6.3
Kannel & Gordon 1970	p	28.9[b]	27.9[b]	10.8[c]	10.6[c]
Yano & al 1978	p	13	12	7	6
Garcia-Palmieri & al 1980	p				
urban		13.6	13.5	6.7**	5.9
rural		13.1	12.6	3.9	3.9
Gordon & al 1981	p				
Framingham		15.3	14.9	5.8	5.4
Puerto Rico		13.5	13.3	6.0**	5.3
Honolulu		12.7	12.3	6.7**	6.0
McGee & al 1984	p	12.7*	12.3	6.3*	6.0
Kromhout & Coulander 1984	p	17.7	17.6	5.9	5.9
Kushi & al 1985	p	17.4	16.9	2.6	2.7

p=prospective; r=retrospective; a=gram per day; b=animal fat; c=vegetable fat; * p<0.05; ** p<0.01

cular changes are more or less an admixture of those seen in the homozygous form and those of atherosclerosis.

Thus, although an extremely high cholesterol concentration may worsen atherosclerosis in patients with familial hypercholesterolemia by inducing a diffuse storing of cholesterol in the vessel walls this is no proof that atherosclerosis itself is caused by an elevated cholesterol concentration, neither that a moderately elevated cholesterol level causes a storing of cholesterol in the vessels of normal human beings. Unfortunately, few studies have distinguished between individuals with familial hypercholesterolemia and others, a serious bias because although rare, it is heavily overrepresentated among young and middle-aged patients with coronary heart disease.

Serum cholesterol and atherosclerosis

If a high serum cholesterol concentration were a causal factor there should evidently be a positive correlation between the serum cholesterol concentration and the degree of atherosclerosis, both in the coronary vessels and elsewhere. This is also what has been claimed in numerous papers. However, all studies in which a correlation was found have included mainly young and middle-aged patients with coronary heart disease, or coronary patients have been heavily overrepresented, which means that patients with familial hypercholesterolemia have been overrepresented also. When such patients are analysed together with ordinary people with great variations in serum cholesterol and great variations in degree of atherosclerosis a correlation is automatically created even if there is no correlation in the two populations studied separately (Ravnskov 1991). Nevertheless no correlation was found in the studies of Nitter-Hauge & Enge (1973) or Cabin & Roberts (1982); in the rest the correlation coefficient rarely exceeded 0.35, and usually it was much smaller (Ravnskov 1991).

Also disturbing is the fact that degree of atherosclerosis in Japan, where the mean serum cholesterol is low (and the diet lean) is just as great as in the US (Gore & al 1959; Resch & al 1969).

But most important studies of unselected individuals found no correlation at all between the lipid content of the artery walls or the degree of vascular atherosclerosis, and the serum cholesterol concentration. Such studies included individuals who had died suddenly from non-medical causes (Landé & Sperry 1936, Mathur & al 1961), or institutionalized individuals whose cholesterol had been measured regularly during many years (Paterson & al 1963).

A study of unselected young individuals did show a close positive correlation between

degree of atherosclerosis in the aorta (but not in the coronary vessels) and the serum cholesterol concentration. The correlation was with fatty streaks however, not to raised lesions, (Newman & al 1986) and it has never been proved that fatty streaks are the forerunners of raised lesions. That serum cholesterol concentrations correlate with fatty streaks but not with raised lesions in fact indicates that these two entities are induced by different mechanisms.

Several angiographic follow-up studies have failed to demonstrate an association between the serum cholesterol concentration and the development of coronary atherosclerosis (Ravnskov 1991). In three of them secular changes in cholesterol concentration were recorded also, and were in many cases as great as can be seen after treatment with cholesterol-lowering drugs. Progress of atherosclerosis was seen whether the initial cholesterol concentration was high or low; or whether it increased or decreased during the observation period (Bemis & al 1973, Shub & al 1981, Kramer & al 1983).

Although these findings are in obvious conflict with the results from the cholesterol lowering trials using angiographic changes as end-point they are never mentioned in the trial reports.

Serum cholesterol and coronary heart disease. Epidemiological evidence.

It is often claimed that the mean serum cholesterol and coronary mortality in populations correlate with each other. The evidence comes from the "Seven Countries" study (Keys 1970). However, although mean blood cholesterol and coronary mortality correlated between countries coronary mortality varied greatly between different populations in some of the countries in spite of almost identical mean cholesterol concentrations (Table 2). Keys himself erroneously thought that future research would clarify these discrepancies.

Table 2. Mean serum cholesterol and five-year incidence of coronary heart disease (rates per 10,000, age standardized) in three of the "Seven countries." From Keys 1970.

	Serum cholesterol mg%	Coronary Heart Disease
West Finland	253	367
East Finland	265	942
Dalmatia	186	163
Slavonia	198	313
Crete	202	12
Corfu	198	201

Results from the ongoing WHO study MONICA, which includes far more countries, do not support Keys however. An analysis of the data has not yet been published, but the raw figures alone revealed lack of covariance between the mean serum cholesterol concentration and coronary mortality (WHO MONICA Project 1989a, 1989b).

Serum cholesterol and coronary heart disease. Evidence from trials.

From the above it can be concluded that you can eat excessive amounts of animal fat and yet have a low cholesterol level in your blood; and atherosclerosis and coronary heart disease may develop whether your diet is fat or lean, and whether your cholesterol is high or low. It is therefore unlikely that atherosclerosis and coronary heart disease can be prevented by dietary changes or by lowering blood cholesterol; a human trial, the ultimate proof for causality, seems doomed to failure.

THE CHOLESTEROL-LOWERING TRIALS

There are many potential ways a trial designed to prevent coronary heart disease may be biased. I shall here shortly mention only two of the most important ones, confounding and unblindedness.

Confounding

To get a fair impression of the effect of preventive measures, important risk markers for coronary heart disease should be equally distributed in treatment and control group. By randomizing a sufficient number of test individuals to each group chance will hopefully lead to the result desired.

To avoid confounding, the number of risk markers in each group is usually compared by a X^2 test and the variance is accepted if it lies within the 95 per cent confidence interval. But even such small differences may bias the result because most of the differences in end-points did not reach statistical significance either.

As an example selected data from The Veterans Administration's dietary trial are given in table 3. It is obvious that a 6 per cent surplus of heavy smokers seriously confounds the result as the difference in coronary mortality was only 2.2 per cent. The difference between heavy smokers was also statistically significant and should exclude this study from overviews. But also the 2.2 per cent non-significant difference between the number of old individuals is important because age is the most important risk factor for coronary heart disease.

Table 3. End-points and some risk markers in the Veterans Administration's dietary trial (Dayton & al 1969).

	Treatment Group (n=424)		Control Group (n=422)		Difference; per cent
	n	(%)	n	(%)	
CHD deaths	41	(9.7)	50	(11.9)	2.2 NS
Total deaths	174	(41.0)	177	(41.9)	0.9 NS
>20 cig/day	45	(10.6)	70	(16.6)	6.0*
>80 years	12	(2.8)	21	(5.0)	2.2 NS

*p=0.01   NS= Not significant.

Non-significant, but nevertheless important differences between risk markers were seen in most trials and probably explain the great variability in outcome which was seen in the small trials (Ravnskov 1992).

To improve the randomization the participants in some of the trials were stratified according to the risk markers considered the most important. In Upjohn's Colestipol trial for instance (Dorr & al 1978) the participants were stratified for presence or absence of diabetes mellitus, and for high and low triglyceride concentrations. Curiously, the serum triglyceride concentrations for men differed much more between treatment and control group than any other laboratory value in any trial not using stratification (Colestipol-group: 284 mg/dl, Placebo-group: 229 mg/dl). As an elevated cholesterol concentration combined with a normal triglyceride concentration is typical for familial hypercholesterolemia, such patients were admittedly overrepresented in the control group, but no information was given about their number.

Counfounding is present if preventive measures against risk markers other than a high cholesterol concentration have been used. In the Oslo trial (Hjermann & al 1981), one of the trials most cited in support of the diet-heart idea, lowering of blood cholesterol by diet was combined with smoking advice. Multivariate analysis showed that the major part of the effect was achieved by a lowering of cholesterol. However, some of the individuals in the treatment groups were also advised to reduce weight and the whole treatment group also had a mean reduction of body mass index (weight/height^2) of 2.37 kg/m^2 corresponding to a net mean reduction of about 7 kg. To claim that the observed effect on morbidity and mortality was due mainly to the reduction of the serum cholesterol level therefore seems unjustified.

Almost all major confounding bias seems to have favoured the treatment groups with one exception. In one of the subgroups in the Coronary Drug project (The Coronary Drug Project Research Group 1972) dextrothyroxine was used as cholesterol lowering agent. The trial was discontinued after three years because of an excess of cardiovascular deaths in the treatment group (14.7% versus 12.2%; corresponding to a relative percentage of 20.5).

It is possible that the cause was an unfavour-able effect of the drug, but a chance result of an unsuccesful randomization cannot be excluded because the difference between all suspect or definite cardiovascular events was relatively much smaller (68.0% versus 64.8%; relative percentage 4.9).

Confounding is also present in several over-views because they have excluded mainly trials with an unfavourable outcome (Ravnskov 1992). In most overviews trials using oestrogen as lipid-lowering agent have been excluded be-cause this hormone is claimed to be cardio-toxic. This statement has no scientific sup-port; a subgroup in one of the trials and a double-blind trial reported a beneficial ef-fect of estrogen (Ravnskov 1992), and post-menopausal estrogen therapy is associated with a decreased risk of coronary heart disease (Stampfer & al 1991).

Unblindedness

An early overview of eleven trials (Corn-field & Mitchell 1969) demonstrated that out-come depended on the design of the trial. Thus, four of six open trials reported a beneficial effect, two were inconclusive; whereas one of five blinded trials reported a harmful effect of intervention, three were inconclusive and one was beneficial.

These figures should be kept in mind when it comes to an evaluation of the more recent trials because blinding of dietary trials is impossible in freely living individuals, and there are also great problems connected with blinding of drug trials. Most of the lipid lowering drugs which have been used have fre-quent and easily recognizable side effects, and the laboratory records may also add infor-mation about group affiliation, especially when the modern, highly effective cholesterol-lowering drugs are used.

Overviews of trials

Taking all possible bias in consideration, few studies satisfy usual criteria for a scienti-fically acceptable clinical trial. This means that authors of overviews may come to diffe-rent conclusions depending on which criteria they consider crucial for acceptance of a trial. Since the number of trials with a bene-ficial and an unsuccesful outcome is almost equal authors of other papers may choose the trials they like to support their view. Conse-quently, trials claimed to be supportive are cited 5-6 times more often than unsupportive trials (Ravnskov 1992).

An overview of all trials using the inclu-sion of a control group as the only criterion for participation gave the following result (Table 4).

Table 4. Overall result of 26 controlled cho-lesterol lowering trials. The number of indi-viduals in the two calculations are not iden-tical because a few trials gave only coronary mortality, or total mortality (After Ravnskov 1992). The unsupportive result of the largest secondary trial of fat advice (Burr & al 1989) is not included for technical reasons.

	Treatment groups	Control groups
Number of individuals	60,456	53,958
Total mortality; percent	6.1	5.8
Number of individuals	60,824	54,403
CHD mortality; percent	2.9	2.9

Clearly, coronary mortality was unaffected by cholesterol reduction, and more sophisti-cated analyses did not change the picture (Ravnskov 1992).

Total mortality was greater in the treat-ment groups but the difference was not sta-tistically significant. However, mortality from non-medical causes (violence and sui-cide) was significantly higher in the treat-ment groups, thus confirming previous fin-dings by Muldoon & al (1990). This was not due to the drug treatment because the number of violent deaths was identical in diet and drug trials. In a subsequent analysis of the data Smith (1992) found that non-coronary mortality was also significantly greater in the treatment groups.

If a lowering of the serum cholesterol level prevents coronary heart disease, the preventive effect should of course be propor-tional to the degree and the duration of such lowering, which it was not. In 14 trials a relationship between individual cholesterol changes and outcome had been sought by the investigators. In four of the trials the cor-relation was weak and unsystematic, in nine it was totally absent. Neither correlated net cholesterol reduction and outcome between trials; and if anything the net mean dif-ference between end-points in the long trials was more unfavourable than the difference in the short ones (Ravnskov 1992).

Even supporters of the diet-heart idea admit that an effect of cholesterol lowering on coronary or total mortality has not been demonstrated, but they consider the effect on coronary morbidity as a sufficient cause for intervention, and they are confident that longer periods of intervention may also lead to a reduction of mortality.

In the mentioned overview (Ravnskov 1992) the overall number of non-fatal coronary heart disease was decreased by a significant 0.32 per cent (10.4 per cent relative to the control group). As total mortality is the only measure which is absolutely free of bias this small difference as regards a soft end-point appears to be an insufficient argument for causality, much less for intervention.

The idea that morbidity is improved faster than mortality is also contradicted by the findings in the Framingham study. Between 1950 and 1970 cardiovascular mortality decreased from 86 to 49 per 1000, while the baseline prevalence increased from 117 to 165 per 1000. These authors thought that a shorter time would be necessary to reduce mortality than to reduce incidence (Sytkowski & al 1990).

Angiographic trials

Trials using morbidity and mortality as end-points are expensive because large numbers of test individuals are necessary to reach statistical significance. Therefore, trials using angiographic changes as end-point have been popular.

In conflict with the observational studies mentioned above (Bemis & al 1973, Shub & al 1981, Kramer & al 1983) it has been claimed that progress in atheroma growth can be inhibited by lowering of the serum cholesterol concentration.

The alleged vascular changes on the few angiographs which have been published (Brown & al 1990) may have been due to vasodilation as well, however. Furthermore, it has been shown that variations in plaque size may occur without corresponding differences in the diameter of the lumen, and early stages of atherosclerosis is compensated by an enlargement of the lumen area. In fact, at less than 40 percent stenosis of the area between the lumen and the internal elastic lamina the lumen area is overcompensated (Glagov & al 1987). This means that a secular dilatation of a coronary vessel may be due both to an increase and a decrease of atherosclerosis, which evidently makes it impossible to evaluate degree of, or changes of, atherosclerosis by a method which only depicts the lumen area.

Only in two of the angiographic studies have a sufficient number of deaths been reported to allow a statistical evaluation. In one of them the number of cardiac events was equal in the drug and the control group (Cashin-Hemphill & al 1990); in the other study ileal bypass was used as intervention in patients with familial hypercholesterolemia and the result bears therefore no relevance to the general population.

CONCLUSION

A great number of clinical and epidemiological studies, and experiments on human beings disprove that an excess of saturated fatty acids in the diet, or an imbalance between dietary saturated and polyunsaturated fatty acids, or a high cholesterol concentration, are causally related to coronary heart disease. Furthermore, a low blood cholesterol concentration is associated with increased

death due to various non-cardiovascular diseases, and overviews have shown that intervention in groups of individuals with high cholesterol concentrations has resulted in a significant increase in violent deaths and in non-cardiovascular deaths. Cholesterol campaigns should therefore be stopped immediately.

REFERENCES

Anderson KM, Castelli WP, Levy D. 1987. Cholesterol and mortality. 30 years of follow-up from the Framingham study. JAMA 257:2176-80.

Bassett DR, Abel M, Moellering RC, et al. 1969. Coronary heart disease in Hawaii: dietary intake, depot fat, "stress," smoking, and energy balance in Hawaiian and Japanese men. Am J Clin Nutr 22: 1483-1503.

Bemis CE, Gorlin R, Kemp HG, Herman MV 1973. Progression of coronary artery disease. A clinical arteriographic study. Circulation 47:455-64.

Brown G, Albers JJ, Fisher LD, et al. 1990. Regression of coronary artery disease as a result of intensive lipid-lowering therapy in men with high levels of apolipoprotein B. N Engl J Med 323:1289-98.

Burr ML, Fehily AM, Gilbert JF et al. 1989. Effects of changes in fat, fish, and fibre intakes on death and myocardial reinfarction: diet and reinfarction trial (DART). Lancet 2:757-61.

Cabin HS, Roberts WC. 1982. Relation of serum total cholesterol and triglyceride levels to the amount and extent of coronary arterial narrowing by atherosclerotic plaque in coronary heart disease. Am J Med 73:227-34.

Cashin-Hemphill L, Mack WJ, Pogoda JM et al. 1990. Beneficial effect of colestipol-niacin on coronary atherosclerosis. A 4-year follow-up. JAMA 264:3013-7.

Cornfield J, Mitchell S. 1969. Selected risk factors in coronary disease. Arch Environ Hlth 19:382-94.

Craig WY, Palomaki GE, Haddow JE. 1989. Cigarette smoking and serum lipoprotein concentrations: an analysis of published data. BMJ 298:784-8.

Dattilo AM, Kris-Etherton PM. 1992. Effects of weight reduction on blood lipids and lipoproteins: a meta-analysis. Am J Clin Nutr 56:320-8.

Day J, Carruthers M, Bailey A, Robinson D. 1976. Anthropometric, physiological and biochemical differences between urban and rural Maasai. Atherosclerosis 23:357-61.

Dayton S, Pearce ML, Hashimoto S, et al 1969. A controlled clinical trial of a diet high in unsaturated fat in preventing complications of atherosclerosis. Circulation 40,suppl II:1-63.

Dimsdale JE, Herd JA. 1982. Variability of plasma lipids in response to emotional arousal. Psychosom Med 44:413-30.

367

Dorr AE, Gundersen K, Schneider JC, et al 1978. Colestipol hydrochloride in hyper-cholesterolemic patients-effect on serum cholesterol and mortality. J Chron Dis 31:5-14.

Finegan A, Hickey N, Maurer B, Mulcahy R. 1968. Diet and coronary heart disease: dietary analysis on 100 male patients. Am J Clin Nutr 21:143-8.

Garcia-Palmieri MR, Sorlie P, Tillotson J, et al. 1980. Relationship of dietary intake to subsequent coronary heart disease incidence: the Puerto Rico heart health program. Am J Clin Nutr 33:1818-27.

Glagov S, Weisenberg E, Zarins CK, et al. 1987. Compensatory enlargement of human atherosclerotic coronary arteries. N Engl J Med 316:1371-5.

Gordon T, Kagan A, Garcia-Palmieri M, et al. 1981. Diet and its relation to coronary heart disease and death in three populations. Circulation 63;500-15.

Gordon DJ, Probstfield JL, Garrison RJ, et al. 1989. High-density lipoprotein cholesterol and cardiovascular disease. Four prospective American studies. Circulation 79:8-15.

Gore I, Hirst AE, Koseki Y. 1959. Comparison of aortic atherosclerosis in the United States, Japan, and Guatemala. Am J Clin Nutr 7:50-4.

Gotto AM, LaRosa JC, Hunninghake D, et al. 1990. The cholesterol facts. A summary of the evidence relating dietary fats, serum cholesterol, and coronary heart disease. A joint statement by the American Heart Association and the National Heart, Lung, and Blood Institute. Circulation 81: 1721-33.

Gurr MI. 1992. Dietary lipids and coronary heart disease: old evidence, new perspective. Prog Lipid Res 31:195-243.

Hjermann I, Byre KV, Holme I, Leren P. 1981. Effect of diet and smoking intervention on the incidence of coronary heart disease. Report from the Oslo study group of a randomized trial in healthy men. Lancet 2:1303-10.

Jacobs D, Blackburn H, Higgins M, et al. 1992. Report of the conference on low blood cholesterol: mortality associations. Circulation 86:1046-60.

Kannel WB, Gordon T. 1970. The Framingham diet study: diet and the regulation of serum cholesterol. The Framingham study. An epidemiologic investigation of cardiovascular disease. Section 24, Washington DC.

Keys A. 1970. Coronary heart disease in seven countries. Circulation 41, suppl 1:1-211.

Kramer JR, Kitazume H, Proudfit WL, et al. 1983. Progression and regression of coronary atherosclerosis: relation to risk factors. Am Heart J 105:134-44.

Kromhout D, Coulander CDL. 1984. Diet, prevalence and 10-year mortality from coronary heart disease in 871 middle-aged men. The Zutphen study. Am J Epidemiol 119:733-41.

Kushi LH, Lew RA, Stare FJ, et al. 1985. Diet and 20-year mortality from coronary heart disease. The Ireland-Boston diet-heart study. N Engl J Med 312:811-8.

Landé KE, Sperry WM. 1936. Human atherosclerosis in relation to the cholesterol content of the blood serum. Archiv Pathol 22:301-12.

Lapiccirella V, Lapiccirella R, Abboni F, Liotta S. 1962. Enquête clinique, biologique et cardiographique parmi les tribus nomades de la Somalie qui se nourissent seulement de lait. Bull Wld Hlth Org 27: 681-97.

Mann GV, Shaffer RD, Anderson RS, Sandstead HH. 1964. Cardiovascular disease in the Masai. J Atheroscl Res 4:289-312.

Marmot MG, Syme SL. 1976. Acculturation and coronary heart disease in Japanese-Americans. Am J Epidemiol 104:225-47.

Marmot MG, Booth M, Beral V. 1982. International trends in heart disease mortality. Atheroscl Rev 9:19-27.

Mathur KS, Patney NL, Kumar V, Sharma RD. 1961. Serum cholesterol and atherosclerosis in man. Circulation 23:847-52.

McGee DL, Reed DM, Yano K, et al. 1984. Ten-year incidence of coronary heart disease in the Honolulu heart program. Relationship to nutrient intake. Am J Epidemiol 119:667-76.

Moore MC, Guzmán MA, Shilling PE, Strong JP. 1976. Relation of selected dietary components to raised coronary lesions. Dietary-atherosclerosis study on deceased persons. J Am Diet Ass 68:216-23.

Muldoon MF, Manuck SB, Matthews KA. 1990. Lowering cholesterol concentrations and mortality: a quantitative review of primary prevention trials. BMJ 301:309-14.

Naito HK. 1976. Effects of physical activity on serum cholesterol metabolism. Cleveland Clin Quart 43:21-49.

National Research Council. 1989. Diet and health. Implications for reducing chronic disease risk. Washington D.C. National Academy Press.

Newman WP, Freedman DS, Voors AW, et al. 1986. Relation of serum lipoprotein levels and systolic blood pressure to early atherosclerosis. The Bogalusa study. N Engl J Med 314:138-44.

Nitter-Hauge S, Inge I. 1973. Relation between blood lipid levels and angiographically evaluated obstructions in coronary arteries. Br Heart J 35:791-5.

Paterson JC, Armstrong R, Armstrong EC. 1963. Serum lipid levels and the severity of coronary and cerebral atherosclerosis in adequately nourished men, 60 to 69 years of age. Circulation 27:229-36.

Paul O, Lepper MH, Phelan WH, et al. 1963. A longitudinal study of coronary heart disease. Circulation 28:20-31.

Ravnskov U. 1991. An elevated serum cholesterol level is secondary, not causal, in coronary heart disease. Med Hypoteses 36: 238-41.

Ravnskov U. Cholesterol lowering trials in

coronary heart disease: frequency of citation and outcome. 1992. BMJ 305:15-9.

Reed DM, MacLean CJ, Hayashi T. 1987. Predictors of atherosclerosis in the Honolulu heart program. 1. Biologic, dietary, and lifestyle characteristics. Am J Epidemiol 126:214-25.

Resch JA, Okabe N, Kimoto K. 1969. Cerebral atherosclerosis. Geriatrics Nov:111-23.

Scrimshaw NS, Guzmán MA. 1968. Diet and atherosclerosis. Lab Invest 18:623-8.

Shaper AG. 1962. Cardiovascular studies in the Samburu tribe of Northern Kenya. Am Heart J 63:437-42.

Shub C, Vlietstra RE, Smith HC, et al. 1981. The unpredictable progression of symptomatic coronary artery disease. A serial clinical-angiographic analysis. Mayo Clin Proc 56: 155-60.

Smith RI. 1991. The cholesterol conspiracy. St. Louis. Warren H. Green.

Smith JG. 1992. Cholesterol lowering treatment and mortality. BMJ 305:1226-7.

Stampfer MJ, Colditz GA, Willett WC & al. 1991 Postmenopausal estrogen therapy and cardiovascular disease. Ten-year follow-up from the nurses' health study. N Engl J Med 325: 756-62.

Stanhope JM, Sampson VM, Prior IAM. 1980. The Tokelau Island migrant study: serum lipid concentrations in two environments. J Chron Dis 34:45-55.

Stehbens WE. 1988. Flaws in the lipid hypothesis of atherogenesis. Pathology 20:395-8.

Sytkowski PA, Kannel WB, D'Agostino RB. 1990. Changes in risk factors and the decline in mortality from cardiovascular disease. N Engl J Med 322:1635-41.

The Coronary Drug Project Research Group. 1972. The coronary drug project. Findings leading to further modifications of its protocol with respect to dextrothyroxine. JAMA 220:996-1008.

WHO MONICA Project. 1989a. WHO MONICA Project: Assessing CHD mortality and morbidity. Int J Epidemiol 18:S38-S45.

WHO MONICA Project. 1989b. WHO MONICA Project: Risk factors. Int J Epidemiol 18: S46-S55.

Worth RM, Kato H, Rhoads GG, et al. 1975. Epidemiologic studies of coronary heart disease and stroke in Japanese men living in Japan, Hawaii and California: mortality. Am J Epidemiol 102:481-90.

Yano K, Rhoads GG, Kagan A, Tillotson J. 1978. Dietary intake and the risk of coronary heart disease in Japanese men living in Hawaii. Am J Clin Nutr 31:1270-9.

Yerushalmy J, Hilleboe HE. 1957. Fat in the diet and mortality from heart disease. A methodologic note. N Y State J Med 57:2343-54.

Zukel WJ, Lewis RH, Enterline PE, et al. 1959. A short-term community study of the epidemiology of coronary heart disease. A preliminary report of the North Dakota study. Am J Publ Health 49:1630-9.

Dairy Products in Human Health and Nutrition, Serrano Ríos et al. (eds) © 1994 Balkema, Rotterdam, ISBN 90 5410 359 0

Child nutrition and cardiovascular risk

I. Villa Elízaga
Pediatric Department, University Clinic of Navarra, Pamplona, Spain

J. I. Gost Garde
Trace Element Unit, Department of Pediatric, School of Medicine, University of Navarra, Pamplona, Spain

R. Elcarte López
Pediatric Service 'Virgen del Camino' Hospital, Pamplona, Spain

ABSTRACT: In this study, we analize the main risk factors (Hypertension, hypercholesterolaemia, and obesity) of cardiovascular disease (CVD) in the Childhood, and the current nutritional situation in Spain, considering, mainly, the studies realize in our research group.

1. CARDIOVASCULAR RISK

Cardiovascular disease (CVD) is the main cause of morbidity and mortality in the developed countries, and the most promising approach to checking its advance now lies in the prevention of certain pathological conditions, beginning in childhood (Elcarte et al. 1991).

Paediatrics should not restrict its scope merely to curing disease. Our ambition should be to enable the adolescent to embark upon adulthood in perfect health, that is, to ensure that today's children, the men and women of tomorrow, are sound in mind and body.

The growing interest in this pathology within the paediatric age group has drawn attention to the following factors (Elcarte et al. 1992):

1. The anatomical/pathological basis of CVD, the atherosclerotic plaque, is formed in the first stages of life (OMS 1982, Stong et al. 1969).

2. The relationship between risk factors in children and any pathological lesions (Newman et al. 1986, Burke et al. 1987).

3. The relationship between the latter in children and those of their relatives (Ayman et al. 1984, Annest et al. 1983, Muñoz et al. 1980, Laskarzewski et al. 1981, Blumenthal et al. 1975, Schrott et al. 1979).

4. Tracking, or the tendency of these factors to remain within the same percentile in the long term (Newman et al. 1986, Burke et al. 1987, Berenson et al. 1987, Voller et al. 1981, Ibsen 1981, Berenson 1980, Frerichs et al. 1979, Clarke 1978, Lloyd et al. 1982, Stark et al. 1981).

5. The high prevalence of these factors observed in studies of different child populations (Lauer et al. 1975, Rudas 1980, Frerichs et al. 1976, Plaza et al. 1986).

6. Epidemiological studies of recent years indicate that hypertension, smoking, hypercholesterolaemia and obesity, the main risk factors associated with a quantifiable increase in the likelihood of suffering from CVD (Stamler 1973), are due in part to behaviour traits which start in childhood (OMS 1982).

These factors have been singled out (Stamler 1973) because of their influence on the genesis of CVD, the consistency of the findings in this field over a wide range of studies, the cardiovascular risk factor entailed by each one of the above aspects, their frequency among the population, and the fact that they are all either preventable or curable.

Research into the aetiology and prevention of CVD finds its starting place in descriptive epidemiological studies of high-risk populations, and retrospective and prospective clinical studies of patients who have had CVD (Puska et al. 1981).

This research has brought to light the great variations in the incidence of these diseases and their mortality rates among the various populations studied. Similarly, the differences between professional, socio-economic, religious and ethnic groups have also been subjected to scrutiny. These studies have confirmed that the main risk factors involved in this pathology are interrelated (OMS 1984).

Environmental factors seem to go most of the way towards accounting for cardiovascular risk; none the less, it must be remembered that the agents in question act on individuals who have a given genetic predisposition (Puska et al. 1981).

The studies mentioned above (Stamler 1973) enabled us to identify the series of risk factors set out in table I.

At present controversy rages over whether the factors implicated in the pathogenesis of CVD in adults are equally significant in childhood. This is due to the need to bear in mind the definition of a risk factor, its potential developments and dynamic character (Spyckerelle et al. 1984).

With respect to the age at which these disorders

Table I
Classification of the risk factors for cardiovascular disease
1. Genetic predisposition.
2. Environmental factors.
   I. Major factors.
      a. High blood pressure.
      b. Hyperlipaemia.
      c. Smoking.
   II. Other risk factors
      a. Obesity.
      b. Physical inactivity.
      c. Character type Λ.
      d. Diabetes.
3. Biological factors independent of exogenous influences, *risk markers*.
   I. Age (direct relationship).
   II. Sex (male predominance).
4. Factors under investigation.
   I. Hyperuricaemia.
   II. Plasma insulin level.
   III. Plasma copper and zinc.
   IV. Socio-economic status.

appear, comparative studies of various populations (Strong et al. 1958, Galindo et al. 1961) have shown that fatty deposits in the aorta set in during the first decade of life in all populations.

In general, these lesions spread and the fatty deposits increase in size and number as the child grows (Kannel et al. 1972).

Underlying the nutritional practices of many infants and children is the concept that "obesity equals good health", in spite of the different nutritional needs of each child. This concept establishes artificial points of reference and produces nutritional models which are inappropriate to the requirements of the individual metabolism (Voller et al. 1981).

The eating habits and patterns of physical exercise which are partly responsible for hypercholesterolaemia, hypertension and obesity are thus established from childhood onwards.

The introduction of pre-cooked solid foods has raised the average salt intake among infants from 9 to 60 mg/day, a level of consumption which is in excess of the child's requirements. This early introduction does not only raise the intake of solids, ut is also formative in encouraging a taste for salt. Although foods of this kind already contain sodium, parents frequently add more salt in order to adjust them to their own tastes (Voller et al. 1981).

It can therefore be seen that dietary habits can be established from a very early age, leading to an excess of calories, salt, cholesterol, saturated fatty acids and so on, which within a few years may result in the emergence of some cardiovascular pathology in childhood.

1.1. High blood pressure in childhood

1.1.1. High blood pressure and cardiovascular disease.

Many epidemiological studies have shown high blood pressure to be a risk factor for premature atherosclerosis, independent of and additional to other factors (Stamler 1973, WHO 1975). Studies in different population groups have provided evidence that such disease is reduced when high blood pressure is controlled (Hypertension detection and follow-up program cooperative group 1979, 1982).

As has already been indicated, high blood pressure in childhood points towards a propensity to CVD in adult life. This is shown by the phenomenon of aggregation within family groups, and that of tracking. Furthermore, blood pressure can be regulated from the earliest years by adjusting the food intake or the amount of physical exercise taken.

1.1.2. Familial tendencies in blood pressure: genetic or environmental?

One of the most widely studied aspects of blood pressure in both children and adults is that of familial predispositions and their possible genetic or environmental origin (Cassimos et al. 1982, Clarke et al. 1986).

Blood pressure may in fact be the product of both types of influence, and while the genetic influence tends to predominate in the first stages of life, interaction with environmental factors increases as the child matures (Szlo et al. 1979).

1.1.3. Tendencies in blood pressure tracking

Among all the variables associated with blood pressure (height, weight, etc.) none has greater predictive value than the initial blood pressure readings, even when the tests are followed up over very long periods of time. Systolic pressure seems to be of greater predictive value than diastolic pressure (Rosner et al. 1987).

The results of blood pressure tracking in childhood have been confirmed by several studies (Voors et al. 1978, 1979, Shear et al. 1986). Other authors, however, have questioned this phenomenon (Clarke et al. 1978, Hofman et al. 1983). André et al. (1986) found results which were positive, but of such a slight nature as to justify preventive measures of a dietary nature only.

1.1.4. High blood pressure and salt in the paediatric diet

First, epidemiological studies have shown that populations with low salt intake (1-10 g/day) have a low incidence of high blood pressure, while those in which large quantities of this substance are ingested (5-55 g/day) show a greater incidence of high blood pressure (Dahl 1972).

Secondly, it is widely known that a reduction in the sodium intake lowers blood pressure levels in hypertense subjects (Dahl 1972, Freis 1973).

It should be remembered that as salt intake in childhood is much higher than which is necessary for growth and other physiological functions, a reduction in the sodium intake can safely be recommended, at least in the case of children who fall into the highest percentiles for blood pressure within their sex and age group.

1.1.5. Physical exercise and blood pressure in the paediatric age group

The relationship between blood pressure and physical exercise in childhood is discussed in several studies, including that of Fraser et al. (1983) who found that systolic and diastolic pressure was lower in children who performed more physical activity than average. This was true for both sexes and all age groups.

On the other hand, there is some indication that vigorous physical activity may reduce raised blood pressure levels in children (Dwyer 1983).

1.2. *Hyperlipaemia in childhood*

1.2.1. Lipids and cardiovascular disease

A close relationship exists between blood lipids and the development of atherosclerosis. The hypothesis that hypercholesterolaemia is an important risk factor in CVD rests on two types of study.

It has been proven, both experimentally (Wissler et al. 1983) and clinically (Stamler et al. 1972, Kannel et al. 1971), and by means of longitudinal and transverse studies (comparing different populations) that a direct relationship exists between the level of cholesterolaemia and the frequency of CVD, although no critical threshold dividing healthy from diseased subjects can be fixed (Stamler et al. 1986).

Secondly, monitoring programmes, which postdate the above surveys, demonstrate that when the cholesterol level is lowered, the incidence of CVD falls (Lipid Research Clinic Program I y II, 1984, Frick et al. 1987, Blankenhorn et al. 1987).

As far as lipoproteins are concerned, their importance in the pathogenesis of atherosclerosis has been suggested ever since Gofman et al. in 1950.

Several epidemiological studies carried out in the last few years have confirmed the atherogenic role of LDL and the antiatherogenic role of HDL (Stamler et al. 1986, Lipid Research Clinic Program 1984).

This relationship between LDL and atherosclerosis has been demonstrated in experimental models in primates (Rudell et al. 1985) and other animals (Goldberg et al. 1983).

Subjects with familial hypercholesterolaemia don't degrade LDL by the receptor physiological way, so, LDL plasmatic concentration increase (Goldstein et al. 1982).

The results of prospective studies (Goldbourt et al. 1979, Gordon et al. 1977), as well as the low morbidity/mortality associated with ischaemic cardiopathy observed in subjects with hyperalphalipoproteinaemia (Glueck et al. 1975), or in some situations in which an increase in HDL is inherent, such as in sportsmen (Lethone et al. 1978), women of childbearing age (Krauss 1982), cases of weight loss in obesity (Carmena et al. 1984) or intake of monounsaturated fats (Ascaso et al. 1987), have led specialists to hypothesize that HDL may have an anti-atherogenic or protective effect to check the development of atherosclerotic plaque.

Hyperlipaemia in childhood is a risk factor for CVD in adult life, as such conditions also display the phenomena of familial aggregation and tracking. Similarly, the lipid levels in the blood can be regulated from the earliest years by sanitary and dietary measures and by physical exercise.

1.2.2. Familial tendencies to hyperlipaemia: genetic or environmental?

In the case of hyperlipaemia, familial tendencies exist, as has been shown by different authors (Biadaioli et al. 1982, Ibsen et al. 1982).

Ibsen et al. (1982) show that familial predispositions towards hypercholesterolaemia are greater than those found for blood pressure, smoking and lack of physical activity.

The tendencies found (Schrott et al. 1979, Snidreman et al. 1985, Sveger et al. 1987, Lee et al. 1986, Bodurtha et al. 1987, Ruiz Moreno et al. 1986) could be due to genetic (Andersen et al. 1982, Masana 1988) and/or environmental factors (Marmot et al. 1975).

1.2.3. The phenomenon of the tracking of lipids in childhood

Evidence clearly suggests that the levels of cholesterol and other lipoproteins show the phenomenon of tracking to a significant extent (Kwiterovich et al. 1986).

Studies (Clarke et al. 1978, Orchard et al. 1983) have shown that tracking is present in childhood. LDL was found to have a higher tracking factor than HDL and VLDL (Berenson et al. 1983).

1.2.4. Lipids and child nutrition

When the effects of diet on lipid and plasmatic lipoprotein concentrations are analysed, some problems arise: first, the considerable individual variation in the effects of diet; and second, the difficulty of analysing the effects of each nutrient in isolation (Masana 1988).

The existing correlation between atherosclerosis and dietary intake provides evidence that high saturated fatty acid and cholesterol consumption is associated with high blood cholesterol levels; more recently, it has been shown that these are also associated with raised LDL levels (Glueck 1979, 1979, McGill 1979, 1979).

On analysis of all available data, we can maintain that every 100 mg/1000 calories of cholesterol in the diet produces a 10 mg/dl increase in blood cholesterol (Mattson et al. 1972).

Saturated fatty acids produce an increase in the LDL concentrations, whereas polyunsaturated fats reduce these concentrations (International Collaborative Study Group 1986); on the other hand, the saturated fats have greater potential to modify these concentrations.

It is likewise well known that saturated fatty acids, with the exception of stearic acid, reduce plasmatic HDL concentrations (Bonanome et al. 1988). Polyunsaturated fatty acids tend to reduce blood cholesterol levels.

Monounsaturated fatty acids, of significance in the Mediterranean region because of the consumption of olive oil, have a role parallel to that of the polyunsaturated fatty acids (Sola et al. 1987).

In childhood, a significant correlation has been found between the type of food ingested and the variations in plasma lipids (Morrison et al. 1980, Vartiainen et al. 1986, Puska et al. 1982).

In infants, the rapid postnatal rise in lipids poses important questions as to whether the composition of breast milk or its substitutes affects the postnatal increase in lipids, and whether dietary habits in infancy affect the responses found in later childhood and in adult life.

In 1976 the American Academy of Pediatrics recommended that the fat content in infant milk formulas should provide at least 30% of the total energy, and that linoleic acid should account for no less than 1.7% (5% of the fatty acids).

The dietary recommendations for infants were initially determined by the American Academy of Pediatrics (AAP) in 1983. Subsequently more restrictive recommendations were published by the American Heart Association (AHA) (Weidman et al. 1983) and by the National Institute of Health Conference (NIH) (1985).

The AHA recommends that the total intake of fats should account for 30% of the calories. This 30% should include 10% or less saturated fatty acids, 10% polyunsaturates, and less than 10% monounsaturates. The daily intake of cholesterol should be 100 g/1000 kcal, and should not exceed 300 mg/day. These recommendations are similar to those put forward at the NIH Conference in 1984.

At present, the American Academy of Pediatrics (AAP) (1986) recommends that infants should be breast fed, and should be given formula milk plus supplementary feeding from 4 to 6 months onwards. After the initial stage, a varied diet is recomended. The AAP indicate the need to assess children from families with a predisposition towards hyperlipaemia from age 2 onwards. For children from families in which such conditions are not present, slight changes in diet are recommended in order to reduce the consumption of saturated fats, cholesterol and salt. The AAP's most recent report reflects a further swing towards the viewpoint represented by the AHA.

1.3. *Obesity in childhood*

1.3.1. Obesity and cardiovascular disease

Some epidemiological studies in adults covering long periods of time define obesity as a primary risk factor for certain types of ischaemic cardiopathy in young men (Rabkin et al. 1977, Keys et al. 1972). Other surveys (Kannel et al. 1976) nevertheless suggest that the obese subject is at a lower risk of CVD than the hypertense or hypercholesterolaemic subject. It is thought that the risk potential which has long been associated with this pathology in fact results from the obese subject's propensity to hypercholesterolaemia, hypertension, carbohydrate intolerance and a sedentary lifestyle. It is these associations which raise the risk of CVD.

In recent years, this pathology in childhood has been on the increase in developed countries, including Spain (Bueno 1985, 1988). The relationship between obesity and high blood pressure in children has also become more prevalent (Gortmarker et al. 1987).

As is the case with hypertension and hyperlipaemia, obesity in childhood is a risk factor for CVD in adult life, and the phenomena of familial aggregation and tracking are found. This condition may likewise be modified by environmental means, changing the diet or exercise habits.

1.3.2. Aetiology of obesity

Obesity is a disorder of the energy metabolism caused by an intake in excess of the required amount. Many factors have a bearing on its origin. The latest theories implicate both genetic (Valls 1987, Dietz 1986, Stunkard et al. 1986, Zonta et al. 1987) and environmental factors.

The environmental factors which influence obesity are diet and physical exercise.

1. Diet
Excessive calorie intake is one of the main causes of obesity at any age. In general, the obese child has a hypercalorific diet which is poor in fruit and vegetables, and consumes food at all times of day. In this, he is influences by acquired eating habits, the family environment, and the mass media.

In a recent study, Kramer et al. (1985) reached the

conclusion that weight and adiposity at one year are determined by the following: birth weight, sex, duration of breast feeding, and age at which solids were introduced. Parental obesity has no effect. At 24 months, the weight depends on birth weight (principal factor in prediction), duration of breast feeding (which has a protective role against obesity), mother's weight, and sex (boys weigh more, but girls are more obese, their tricipital fold being lárger).

2. Physical activity

The overweight subject tends to cut down on physical exercise, and as obesity becomes more pronounced it leads to an increasingly sedentary lifestyle.

Physical exercise represents one third of the normal energy output, and it is the best means of increasing thermogenesis; moreover, the thermogenic response to exercise is greater (Segal et al. 1985).

1.3.3. Phenomenon of tracking in childhood obesity

The classic notion that childhood nutrition is responsible for later obesity is based on the hypothesis that there are two critical periods in the development of adipose tissue in man: the first begins before birth and lasts until the end of the first year of life, and the second occurs in adolescence. It is thought that a proliferation of adipose cells, established during this period of time as a result of over-eating, predisposes the individual to obesity at some later date. Acording to this hypothesis, the number of fat cells never decreases, and weight loss is explained as a reduction in the size of the adipose cells.

2. THE CURRENT SITUATION IN SPAIN

With the aim of devising a set of standard procedures and dietary recommendations relating to the risk factors for CVD (high blood pressure, hyperlipaemia and obesity), the role of these factors in the aetiology and pathogenesis of cardiovascular disease was studied (Elcarte et al. 1991, 1992).

The conclusions of our research are based on an epidemiological study carried out by our group over 5829 Navarrese children of both sexes, chosen at random, aged between 4 and 17 years. From the results of this study, we concluded that $23.68 \pm 0.63\%$ of the paediatric population of Navarra presented one of the three cardiovascular risk factors studied, the prevalence of high blood pressure, hypercholesterolaemia, hyperlipaemia and obesity, considered independently, being $7.17 \pm 0.34\%$, $21.07 \pm 0.54\%$, $15.70 \pm 0.49\%$ and $3.96 \pm 0.26\%$ respectively.

Two risk factors rarely coincided, the prevalence being 1.19%, 0.79% and 1.00% for hypertense and

hyperlipaemic children, hypertense and obese children, and hyperlipaemic and obese children respectively.

Oncly 0.25% of the paediatric population (age 4-17) studied presented all three pathological conditions.

The existence of a correlation between the three pathologies studied was confirmed.

A significant association was found between obesity and hypertension and obesity and hyperlipaemia measured by LDL/HDL>2.2. An obese subject has 5.19 more probability of having high blood pressure (5.03, if the effect of hyperlipaemia on this association is eliminated), and 2.60 (2.49 if the effect of hypertension on this association is eliminated) more probability of being hyperlipaemic (LDL/HDL>2.2) than a non-obese subject.

A hypertense subject is 1.36 times more likely to be hyperlipaemic (LDL/HDL>2.2) than a non-hypertense subject. This association disappears if the effect of obesity on it is eliminated.

Subjects who are hypertense and overweight are 1.81 times more likely to be hyperlipaemic than inviduals who do not have these conditions.

A hypertense, hyperlipaemic child is 8.47 times more likely to be obese than is one which displays neither pathology.

A hyperlipaemic, overweight child is 3.83 times more likely to be hypertense than is one which displays neither pathology.

The high prevalence of hyperlipaemia in the paediatric population of Navarra, pedominantly in male adolescents, and the raised blood pressure findings, again in adolescent males, indicate that if no preventive health care measures are undertaken, the children and teenagers of today may have high rates of CVD-related mordibity and mortality in adult life.

We can thus conclude that healthy dietary habits provide the most satisfactory basis for the prevention of all potential risk factors involved in the genesis of cardiovascular disease.

Research carried out in developed countries (Swan 1983, Dupin et al. 1984) show that the last 50 years have seen dramatic changes in nutritional habits. These changes are characterized by an increase in the consumption of animal proteins to the detriment of vegetable proteins, a reduction in the intake of complex carbohydrates and an increase in those which are rapidly absorbed, and a sharp rise in lipid intake, which is mainly accounted for by animal fats.

Although this period has seen an improvement in major health care indices such as life expectancy, child mortality and growth, which is thought to be partly related to nutritional changes, these same developments may well have led to a raised frequency of certain diseases such as tooth decay, hypertension, obesity, arteriosclerosis, and some types of neoplasm (Langley-Danysz 1984, McLaren et al. 1982).

Most researchers agree that dietary habits are formed in childhood and persist in good measure in adult life, and that the processes which lead to the diseases mentioned above probably also start during childhood or adolescence.

It is hard to control all the factors which influence dietary habits, and only if different research groups pool their resources can new perspectives on old problems be won (Gutierrez et al. 1985), which can gradually enable us to understand the behaviour of the population.

Habits exist which are deeply rooted in the population and prove difficult to eradicate; these may be part of something as difficult to quantify as the 'general popular culture', which it would be very difficult to influence.

As healthy dietary patterns are thought to be formed at an early age, more and more studies are being published on the forms of nutrition which are appropriate at any given stage in the child's development.

It would thus seem to be logical, in view of present scientific knowledge, to conduct research into children's dietary habits in order to introduce any suitable modifications at an early stage, should aberrations in their diet be found.

With the aim of combatting the pernicious effects of poor diet, many countries first attempt to assess the real state of dietary intake within the population, and then, on the basis of the data obtained, hold health education campaings on the subject of nutrition and, in some cases, enrich certain foodstuffs with special nutrients. In Spain we have patchy information at our disposal (Bueno 1983, Sarriá et al. 1984, Tojo et al. 1975, Martinez et al. 1987, Farré et al. 1990, Moreiras-Vasela et al. 1984) on the reality of the Spanish diet, and it would therefore be appropriate to carry out research in areas which might broaden our knowledge of present-day dietary habits and the role which these play in the development of certain hight-incidence diseases.

One particularly important study was that carried out by Salas et al. (I, 1985), consisting of a survey based on interviews which was designed to provide a profile of the intake of a particular population (that of Reus), the socio-economic structure of which makes it fairly representative of the urban nuclei of Catalonia. Broadly speaking, this study brought to light excessive sugar consumption, with high levels of meat, fish, eggs, pulses and fats, and low consumption of milk, other dairy products, fruit, cereals and root vegetables.

Meat, fish and eggs have in common the fact that they are rich in proteins of high biological value. Most such foodstuffs have a protein content of 10 to 20%, as well as containing the amino acids which are essential for adults. The main difference between them lies in their lipid content (1-25%), although the quality of the lipids is much the same in all of them: saturated fatty acids predominate (SFA) over the unsaturated fatty acids, and cholesterol and uric acid are present to a variable degree. The study mentioned above (Salas et al., II, 1985) shows that among middle-aged people, men ate an excess of meat (231.8 ± 38.3 g/day), whereas women consumed much less (157.1 ± 21.3 g/day); meat consumption was high in children (112.6 ± 13.0 g/day) and low in the elderly (110.7 ± 34.4 g/day). Consumption of eggs and fish was high for all age groups. The intake of pulses was higher than in other developed countries.

In developed countries, high consumption of milk and dairy products has been observed, which has increased over the last few decades, a rise which has particularly affected dairy products and which is more pronounced in certain age groups than in others. The importance of a large intake of milk and dairy products is obvious, as these foods are high in proteins of excellent biological values and rich in vitamins A, D and B$_2$ and in calcium. The main drawback is that they contain saturated fatty acids (SFA) which are associated with the aetiology of atherosclerosis.

The latter study (Salas et al., III, 1985) showed that a relatively low consumption of milk and dairy products during the years of growth, even though it was in these years that the milk intake was at its highest. In the second year of life, 30% of the population studied no longer drank milk. Milk consumption reached a peak in the 7-10 age group (246.8 ± 30.9 g/day), and after this, the second heaviest milk consumers were those aged over 65 (173.0 ± 79.1 g/day). The frequency of milk consumption stood between 52 and 81%.

The intake of dairy products tended to decrease with age after a reaching its peak at the age of 2 years (98.9 ± 37.8 g/day), dropping to its lowest point in the 51-65-year age group (25.5 ± 8.6 g/day), then increasing in persons aged over 65. Intake levels were raised between the ages of 2 and 6, and it was after the sixth year that a marked decline in the consumption of dairy products set in, which ranged from 56-90%.

In general, smaller amounts of this category of food was consumed in the population subjected to study than in data obtained from France (Dupin et al. 1984, Serville 1980) and Canada (Rapport de Nutrition Canada 1973, 1973). An intake level of around half that recommended was found in all the age groups questioned.

Fat intake (oils and margarines) was low in the second year of life, rising to a peak between the ages of 16 and 20 (62.1 ± 16.5 g/day), and again in the 51-65 age group.

The consumption of green vegetables also tended to rise to a maximum between the ages of 51 and 65, with intake levels of between 90-100%; there was a noticeable shortfall in this area in individuals aged under 30.

In developed countries, the total intake of carbohydrates, starches and natural sugars tends to diminish, whereas consumption of refined sugars generally increases.

In this survey (Salas et al., IV, 1985) it was noted that the quantity of cereals consumed was small, being greater for men than women. The highest cereal intake was found between the ages of 7 and 20. The population of under 15 consumed a large quantity of sugars, the peak age for this being between 7 and 10 years. Fruit intake tended to rise with age, reaching a maximum in those over 65.

A more recent study of the school-age population of Madrid over a three-year period (1989-92) (Lopez Mondedeu et al. 1993) reflected the progressive abandonment of the Mediterranean diet in favour of a diet containing a large amount of precooked and industrially-manufactured foods with a high saturated fat and cholesterol content.

This survey found that the consumption of eggs, fats, green vegetables, pulses and fruits coincided with the amounts recommended for the population in question by the Spanish Health Ministry. None the less, the consumption of fish, potatoes, cereals and dairy products was much lower than the recommended level, even though the amounts consumed tended to be somewhat greater than in the Reus study (Salas et al., I, II, III, IV, 1985).

The consumption of meat products exceeded the recommended amounts, and the intake of sweets, snacks and manufactured products was also high; this implies that the diet of the children studied contained too much protein and fat, at the expense of the products listed above.

In addition to studying the overall consumption of food in certain population centres, this survey includes partial studies of given foodstuffs, paying special attention to the amounts of milk and dairy products consumed.

A recent study, also concerning Navarra, on child nutrition in the first year of life, shows that the basic characteristics of breast feeding in our area are as follows: an initial rate which is acceptable, although somewhat lower than that described in category I of the OMS report; breast feeding is then generally abandoned at some time during the first three months of life; and natural lactation is practically non-existent after the age of six months.

According to this study (Sanchez Valverde 1990), 71% of children are fully breast-fed during the first month of life, while 20% are given milk formulas, 6% mixed feeding, and 3% cow's milk. After the age of two months, only 50% of infants are breast-fed. Full breast-feeding is only maintained by 50% of mothers after the first month of life.

In general, it was noted that the results of this survey were lower than those currently found in most developed countries such as the Scandinavian regions (Stählberg 1985, Persson et al. 1985, Barros et al. 1986), the United States (Feinstein et al. 1986, Kurinji et al. 1988), Britain (Fomon 1976), France (Antier et al. 1982), Italy (Minetti et al. 1980) and Australia (Gracey et al. 1985).

A close association exists between the duration of lactation and the age at which complementary feeding is introduced (OMS 1985, Ribó et al. 1983, Gray-Donald et al. 1985, Ekwo et al. 1983).

Before the age of 4 months, the introduction of complementary feeding would not seem to be justified

(ESPGAN 1982, Jones 1984, Vitoria 1986, Ballabria 1987, American Academy of Pediatrics 1983, Ros 1986, Turkewitz et al. 1986). Among the infants studied, 19% were introduced to other foodstuffs before this age, whereas 78.6% began complementary feeding towards the age of 6 months.

On a worldwide scale, the time at which complementary feeding is introduced is found to be related to the economic development of the nation in question (OMS 1985). In third-world countries, it is very late, taking place at the age of about twelve months (Ajenifuga 1987, Ramachandran 1987, Ahmad 1987). Developed countries have gone from the extremely early introduction of complementary feeding, coinciding with the lowest rates of breast-feeding (Ballabriga et al. 1987, Manzella et al. 1984, Persson et al. 1984), to the somewhat later introduction which is found in the most recent studies (Quandt 1984, Casares et al. 1987).

The average age at which complementary feeding was started was 4.5 ± 1.2 months. The first food given was most frequently fruit (45.6%), followed by gluten-free cereals (33.6%), which coincides with other publications concerning Southern Europe (Ballabuga et al. 1987). Ninety-three per cent of mothers gave their children fruit 3 or more times a week; the other 7% did so sporadicaly.

The earliest starting date for complementary feeding in this study was found among mothers who acted under the influence of their own experience, and those in a rural environment.

Complementary feeding was started earlier in infants who had been breast-fed for shorter periods of time (Quandt 1984, Perez-Choliz et al. 1986, Whitehead et al. 1986), as in our study group.

The commonest method of giving cereals, according to this study (Sanchez Valverde 1990), was by adding them to the milk formula which the child was taking: 60% gave gluten-free cereals, 52% mixed cereals. The average age at which these were introduced was 5.1 ± 1.49 months.

The mean age for the introduction of gluten was 7.29 ± 2.07 months; that for green vegetables was 5.91 ± 1.28 months. It was calculated that 96% of mothers gave vegetables on 3 days every week. Beans and pulses were first given at around 12 months.

It is recommended that proteins of high biological value should be added to the diet after the age of 5 months (Ballabriga et al. 1987), or between 6 and 8 months (Jones 1984). In Europe generally, however, it is usual to introduce such proteins earlier (Ballabriga et al. 1987), and this tendency has been noted in Spain (Muñoz 1986, Paidos '84, Garcia et al. 1981).

First of all, meat is given, followed by fish, with offal and eggs being added around the age of one year.

Prior to the age of 6 months meat was introduced in 20.5% of cases, and the overwhelming majority of infants incorporated meat into their diets at around the 6-month stage. The chief sources of protein were chicken, beef and lamb. Fish was found to follow an introduction curve parallel to that of meat, at a delay of only 1 to 2 months.

Finally, infants were first ofered eggs at an average age of 9.66 months.

Continuation milk formulas were consumed by 70.7% of the population, and were generally introduced between 4 and 6 months of age. They were generally given until around 12 months, to be followed by the period during which the intake of cow's milk is at its highest.

It is recommended that dairy products should be introduced between 6 and 8 months (Jones 1984), and consumption of these products is reported to be on the increase in industrialized countries at the present time (Toenz et al. 1980).

The milk derivate introduced most commonly was yoghurt (78.1%), followed by cheese (10.6%).

From the age of 6 months onwards, it is recommended that infants should drink a minimum of 500 cc/day of milk (ESPGAN 1982). When we consider each dairy product independently, none of them manages to reach the required level to cover the dietary needs adequately. However, if all are considered together, 86.9% of the population surveyed ingested over half a litre of milk and/or dairy products.

This survey (Sanchez Valverde 1990) found a high consumption of sacarose and others sugared products.

Milk and dairy products undoubtedly make an important contribution in terms o energy and nutrition, and should be considered essential in the diet of children, adolescents and adults alike.

Studies relating to dairy product consumption have been published, covering several different areas of Spain. Our own group carried out a survey of this kind in a region of Aragon, comprising over 400 people (45% children and 55% adults).

The data obtained from this study (Escribano Subías 1990) led us to conclude that it was a community with high levels of milk and dairy product consumption. Ninety-nine per cent of the children and 90% of the adults questioned drank at least one glass of milk a day. The average intake among the children was calculated as being 483.05 ± 27.88 cc/day, a very high figure which is close to the recommendations on child nutrition which suggest half a litre per day as being the required amount. These findings were very similar to those encountered in Canada and France (Serville 1980, Canada Department of National Health 1973), areas in which there is a tradition of consuming large quantities of dairy products. Among the adults, the figure was 354.63 ± 13.4 cc/day.

Analysis of milk consumption by age group reveals a peak between 7-9 years, with 490.21 ± 45.65 cc/day, in contrast to 340 ± 72.53 cc/day found in the group of adolescents. The latter group repeatedly presented lower indices of milk and dairy product consumption, although this did stay fairly close to the higher end of the scale, as up to 88% of the adolescent population consumed at least 250 cc of milk per day. This high level of consumption also

came to light in a study of the adolescent population of Zaragoza (Saragossa) by Ros et al. (1989) in which up to 84% of the subjects questioned drank at least one glass of milk a day. In the study by Salas et al. of the population of Reus (Salas et al., I, II, III, IV, 1985), only 70% of teenagers drank milk. These figures provide evidence of the high level of milk consumption among the Aragonese population, which approaches that found in other areas of the world where dairy products are traditionally popular (figures 1 and 2).

According to the study mentioned above, almost all children drank full-cream milk (95%), generally accompanied by some soluble product. The most popular additive was cocoa (60%). In 26%, sugar was added to the milk, and in 7% it was added to coffee. Milk was consumed without any type of additive in 4.7% of cases.

Regarding the origin of the milk, 64% of the children studied drank fresh milk which had not been processed or packaged, as was to be expected in a traditional, society with a high level of milk production and consumption. When this phenomenon was contrasted with the corresponding figures in adults, we found that only 40% of the latter drank non-processd milk, and that they were more likely to drink skimmed (22.88%) or semi-skimmed milk (4.34%).

The consumption of cheese increased progressively with age, whereas intake of yoghurt, butter and petit suisse decreased.

Cheese consumption was widespread among this population group, 73.8% of children and 90% of adults being regular consumers. The rate of consumers among children would exceed that among adults if petit suisse were included as cheese instead of as a separate entity.

The children in the group ate soft cheese and cream cheese from preference (80%), while the adult consumption figures were divided more or less evenly between soft and cream cheeses and matured cheeses.

The adults ate an average of 220.4 ± 44.5 g/week, as compared to 177.45 ± 17.38 g/week for children. Peak consumption occurred in adolescence, with 232.34 g/week and 94.12% of consumers. In the study by Ros et al. (1989), 54% of teenagers ate cheese every day. In this age group the lower milk intake was found to be supplemented y greater cheese consumption.

The packaging of petit suisse has made it, out of all yoghurts and soft cheeses, the favourite milk product of many young children. It is rich in proteins, lactose and fats, and has a high calorie content; up to the age of 9, consumption figures are high, but they then drop sharply to a consumption level of almost zero in the adult population. From age 4 to 6 years, 59% ate petit suisse regularly, with an average of 5.57 units per week, almost one a day.

Butter was the dairy product which had suffered the greatest decline. The launching of non-dairy margarines into the market had dealt a blow to butter consumption. Relatively high consumption indices

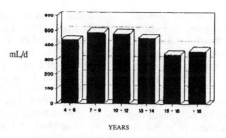

mL/d

YEARS

Diferences in consumption according to age

FIGURE 1. MILK CONSUMPTION IN THE POPULATION

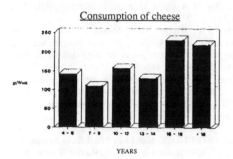

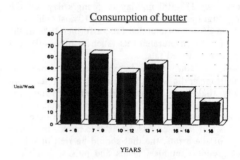

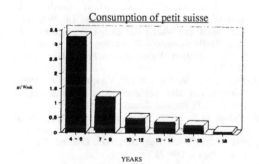

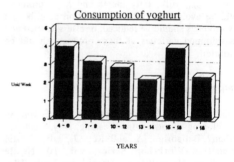

FIGURE 2. CONSUMPTION OF DAIRY PRODUCTS IN

THE POPULATION

were found for these margarines, standing at 45.45%, but with a low intake level (59.23 g/week). For adults, the index of consumers was low, only 15.78%, and consumption genuinely low (20.21 g/week).

Yoghurt, along with cheese, was the dairy product which maintained the highest consumption level in the different age groups, with the maximum intake being found among the youngest subjets (72.73%), falling in adolescents (64.7%) and adults (42.1%). The mean intake varied from 4 to 6 tubs per week, one per day being the norm.

The consumption of lactose followed a course parallel to that of milk consumption, as the latter is the main form in which dairy products are taken. Its highest peak was in the 7-9-year age group, with 25.85 g/day, and its minimum among adolescents, with 16.65 g/day.

3. SUMMARY

On the lines of the above findings, the

epidemiological studies show the need for various preventive measures to be applied to the whole community, preferably from childhood onwards. At this age it is possible to prevent the formation of fat deposits and/or halt their development into other more serious disorders, as this is a moment which could be described as critical in the aetiology of atherosclerosis. A suitable lifestyle should be encouraged in children and adolescents, encompassing a diet which is balanced in terms of energy and nutrition, exercise, giving up harmful habits, and so on.

General dietary recommendations establish that carbohydrates should provide 50-55% of the total energy component of the diet, fats 30-35%, and proteins 10-18%. The cholesterol intake should be no higher than 275-300 mg/day or 5 mg/k/day. Of the energy ingested in the form of fats, 10% should be in the form of polyunsaturated fats, a further 10% in the form of monounsaturated fats (such as olive oil), and the rest as saturated fats.

Owing to the gradual move away from the Mediterranean die towards one which resembles more closely that found in industrialized countries, the Spanish paediatric population is now consuming a diet which is high in energy and contains an excess of proteins and saturated fats. In order to reduce the raised intake of these fats, the diet should be rich in salads, fruit, green vegetables, beans and pulses, white and oily fish, vegetable oils and lean meat; foods which are high in cholesterol and saturated fatty acids, such as cakes, egg yolk, fatty meats and meat products should be avoided, and the consumption of milk and dairy products should be reduced, or else skimmed and semi-skimmed varieties of these products should be substituted.

REFERENCES

Ahmad, A. 1987. Supplementary infant feeding in developing countries. In: Weaning, why, what and when? Ballabriga, A. and Rey, J., eds., Nestlé Nutrition Workshop Series, vol. 10. Nestlé Nutrition. Vevey/Raven Press, New York, 197-204.

Ajenifuja, B. 1987. Weaning practices in developing countries. In: Weaning, why, what and when? Ballabriga, A. and Rey, J. eds. Nestlé Nutrition Workshop Series, vol. 10. Nestlé Nutrition. Vevey/Raven Press, New York, 205-10.

American Academy of Pediatrics. Committee on Nutrition. 1976. Commentary on breast-feeding and infant formulas, including standars for formulas. Pediatrics; 57: 278-91.

American Academy of Pediatrics. Committee on Nutrition. 1983. Hacia una dieta prudente para los niños. Pediatrics (Ed. Esp.); 15: 70-1.

American Academy of Pediatrics. Committee on Nutrition. 1983. Toward a prudent diet for children. Pediatrics; 71: 78-80.

American Academy of Pediatrics. Committee on Nutrition. 1986. Prudent life-style for children dietary fat and cholesterol. Pediatrics; 78: 521-5.

Andersen, G.E., Petersen, M.B. and Povey, M. 1982. Genetics of serum lipids and lipoproteins. A study of twins at birth and 3-5 years of age. Acta Paediatr. Scand. 72: 805-8.

André, J.L. Deschamps, J.P., Petit, J.C. and Guéguen R. 1986. Change of blood pressure over five years in childhood and adolescence. Clin. Exp. A8 (4&5): 539-45.

Annest, J.L., Sing, C.H.F., Biron, P. and Mongeau, J.G. 1983. Familial aggregation of blood pressure and weigh in adoptive families. Am. J. Epidemiol., 117: 492-506.

Antier, E. and Amiel-Tison, C. 1982. Breast feeding. Results of a study in a maternity hospital. Ann. Pediatr., 29: 482-7.

Ascaso, J.S., Serrano, S., Martínez Valls, J. et al. 1987. Efecto del aceite de oliva en la dieta sobre las lipoproteinas plasmáticas de alta densidad. Rev. Clin. Esp., 180: 486-8.

Ayman, D. 1984. Heredity in arteriolar essential hypertension: A clinical study of blood pressure in 1.524 members of 277 families. Arch. Intern. Med., 53: 792-802.

Ballabriga, A. and Rey, J. 1987. Weaning, why, what and when? Nestlé Nutrition Workshop Series, vol. 10. Nestlé Nutrition. Vevey/Raven Press, New York.

Ballabriga, A., and Schmidt, E. 1987. Actual trends of the diversification of infant feeding in industrialized countries in Europe. In: Weaning, why, what and when? Ballabriga, A., and Rey, J., eds. Nestlé Nutrition Workshop Series, vol. 10. Nestlé Nutrition. Vevey/Raven Press, New York, 129-51.

Barros, F.C., Victora, C.G. Vaughan, J.P. 1986. Breastffeding and socioeconomics status in souther Brazil. Acta Paeditr. Scand. 75: 558-62.

Berenson, G.S. 1980. Serum lipids and lipoproteins at birth, 6 months and one year. In: Cardiovascular risk factors in chilfren. Berenson, G.S. ed. Oxford: Univ. Press, 166-78.

Berenson, G.S., Epstein, F.H., Glueck, C.J., Lewis, B., Wissler, R.W. and McGill, H.C. Jr. 1983. Summary and recommendations of the conference on blood lipids in children: optimal levels for early prevention of coronary artery disease. Pre. Med. 12: 728-40.

Berenson, G.S., Srinivasan, S.R., Freedman, P.S., Radhakrishnamurthy, B. and Dalferes, E.R. Jr. 1987. Atherosclerosis and its evolution in childrood. Am. J. Med. Sci. 249: 429-40.

Biadaioli, R., Bertini, G., De Martino, M., Appendino, C., Praiesi, F. and Vierucci, A. 1982. Fattori rischio per la malattia aterosclerotica in età pediatrica. Min. Ped. 34: 683-689.

Blankenhorn, D.H., Nesim, S.A., Johnson, R.L., Sanmarco, M.E., Azen, S.P. and Cashin-Hemphil, L. 1987. Beneficial effects of combined colestipol-niacin therapy in coronary atherosclerosis and coronary venous bypass grafts. JAMA 257: 3233-40.

Blumenthal, S. and Jesse, M.J. 1975. Risk factors for coronary heart disease in children of affected families. J. Pediatr., 87: 1187-93.

Bodurtha, J.N., Schieken, R., Segrest, J. and Nance, W.E. 1987. High density lipoproteins - cholesterol subfractions in adolescent twins. Pediatrics 79: 181-9.

Bonanome, A. and Grundy, S.M. 1988. Effect of dietary stearic acid on plasma cholesterol and lipoprotein levels. N. Engl. J. Med. 318: 1244-8.

Bueno, M. 1983. Necesidades nutritivas durante el crecimiento y desarrollo. Bol. S. Aragonesa Ped., 77-80.

Bueno, M. 1988. Obesidad. En: Tratado de Pediatría, Cruz, M., ed. Barcelona, Expaxs.

Bueno, M., Fernández, J. and Sarria, A. 1985. Paidos'84, 1984. Estudio espidemiológico sobre nutrición y obesidad infantil. Danone, S.A. Móstoles (Madrid).

Burke, G.L., Arcilla, R.A., Culpepper, W.S., Webber, L.S., Chiang, R.A. and Berenson, G.S. 1987. Blood pressure and echocardiographic measures in children: The Bogalusa heart study. Circulation 75: 106-114.

Canada Department of National Health and Welgare, Otawa. 1973. Nutrition Canada National Survey: nutrition, a national priority. Otawa: Information Canada.

Carmena, R., Ascaso, J.F., Tebar, J. and Soriano, F. 1984. Changes in plasma high density lipoproteins after body high reduction in obese women. Int. J. Obesity 8: 135-40.

Casares, I., Valbuena, L., Rodríguez, P., Bombin, J.M., Gamarra, C. and Cadenas, A. 1987. Estudio de la evolución en la introducción de la alimentación complementaria a nivel urbano extrahospitalario. An. Esp. Pediatr. 27 (Suppl. 27): 46-52.

Cassimos, C.H.R., Aivazis, V., Karamperis, S., Varlamis, G. and Katsouyannopoulos, V. 1982. Arterial blood pressure serum lipids and cardiovascular complications in families of hypertensive children. Acta Paediatr. Scand., 71: 235-8.

Clarke, W.R., Schrott, H.G., Burns, T.L., Sing, C.F. and Laver, R.M. 1986. Aggregation of blood pressure in the families of children with labile high systolic blood pressure: The Muscatine study. Am. J. Epidemil., 123: 67-80.

Clarke, W.R., Schrott, H.G., Leaverton, P.E., Connor, W.E. and Laver, R.M. 1978. Tracking of blood lipids and blood pressures in school age children: The Muscatine study. Circulation 58: 626-33.

Dahl, L.K. 1972. Salt and hypertension. Am. J. Clin. Nutr., 25: 231-44.

Dietz, W.H. 1986. Prevention of chilhood obesity. Pediatr. Clin. North Am. 33: 823-35.

Dupin, H., Hercberg, S. and Lagrange, V. 1984. Evolution of the French diet: Nutritional aspects. World Rev. Nutr. Diet 44: 57-84.

Dwyer, T. 1083. An investigation of the effects of daily physical activity on the health of primary school students in South Australia. Int. J. Epidemiol. 12: 308-13.

Ekwo, E.E., Dusdieker, L.B. and Booth, B.M. 1983. Factors influencing initiation of breast-feeding. Am. J. Dis. Child. 137: 375-7.

Elcarte López, R., Villa Elízaga, I. and Sada Goñi, J. 1991. Manual práctico para la prevención de las enfermedades cardiovasculares desde la infancia. Sociedad Nestlé A.E.P.A. Esplugas de Llobregat (Barcelona).

Elcarte López, R., Villa Elízaga, I., Sada Goñi, J., Sola Mateos, A., Elcarte López, T. and Gascó Eguiluz, M. 1992. Factores de riesgo cardiovascular en la población infanto juvenil de Navarra. Premio Amagoia sobre Nutrición Infantil 1991. In: Premios Nutrición Infantil 1991. Sociedad Nestlé A.E.P.A. Esplugas de Llobregat (Barcelona), 267-368.

Escribano Subías, J. 1990. Hipolactasia primaria tipo adulto en la comarca del Cinca medio. Tesis doctoral. Universidad de Navarra.

European Society of Pediatric Gastroenterology and Nutrition. ESPGAN. 1982. Guideliness on infant nutrition III. Recommendations on infant nutrition. Acta Paediatr. Scand. 302: 1-27.

Farré, R., Pérez, A., Rodrigo, S., Frasquet, M. and Frasquet, I. 1990. Encuesta dietética en el parvulario de la Universidad Politécnica de Valencia. An. Esp. Pediatr. 32: 122-6.

Feinstein, J.M., Berkelhamer, J.E., Gruzska, M.E., Wong, L.A. and Carey, A.E. 1986. Factores relacionados con la interrupción precoz de la lactancia materna en una población urbana. Pediatrics (Ed. Esp.) 22: 138-42.

Fomon, S.J. 1976. Historia reciente y tendencias actuales. In: Nutrición Infantil. Fomon, S.J., ed. Editorial Interamericana. México 1-18.

Fraser, G.E., Phillips, R.L. and Harris, R. 1983. Physical fitness and blood pressure in school children. Circulation 67: 405-12.

Freis, E.D. 1973. Salt, volume and the prevention of hypertension. Circulation 53: 589-95.

Frerichs, R.R., Srinivasan, S.R., Webber, L.S. and Berenson, G.S. 1976. Serum cholesterol and triglyceride levels in 3.445 children from a biracial community: The Bogalusa heart study. Circulation 54: 301-9.

Frerichs, R.R., Weber, L.S., Voors, A.W., Srinivasan, S.R. and Berenson, G.S. 1979. Cardiovascular risk factor disease, risk factor variables in children at two successive years: The Bogalusa heart study. J. Chronic Dis. 32: 251-62.

Frick, M.H., Elo, O., Haapa, K., Heinonen, O.P., Heinsalmi, P., Helop, H., Muttenen, J.K., Kaitanieme, P., Koskinen, P., Manninen, V., Maenpaa, H., Malkonen, M., Manttara, M.,

Norolas, T., Pasternack, A., Pikkarainen, J., Romo, M., Sjoblom, T. and Nikkila, E.A. 1987. Helsinki heart study: Primary prevention trial with gemfibrocil in middle aged men with dyslipidemia. N. Engl. J. Med., 317: 1237-45.

Galindo, L., Arean, V., Strong, J.P. and Baldizon, C. 1961. Atherosclerosis in Puerto Rico. Arch. Pathol. 72: 367-74.

García, A., Paredes, C., Codoñes, C., Iranzo, A. and De Miguel, A. 1981. Reflexiones acerca de la alimentación infantil. Desde la lactancia hasta el beikost. In: Premios de Nutrición Infantil 1980. Ed. Sociedad Nestlé A.E.P.A. Barcelona, 47-75.

Glueck, C.J. 1979. Appraisal of dietary fat as a cousative factor in atherogenesis. Am. J. Clin. Nutr. 32: 2637-43.

Glueck, C.J. 1979. Dietary fat and atherosclerosis. Am. J. Clin. Nutr. 32: 2703-11.

Glueck, C.J., Fallat, R.W., Millet, F., Garaside, P., Elston, R.C. and Go, R.C.P. 1975. Familial hiperalfalipoproteinemia studies in 80 kindreds. Metabolism 24: 1243-65.

Gofman, J.W., Lindgren, F.T. and Elliot, H. 1950. The role of lipids and lipoproteins in atherosclerosis. Science 111: 155.

Goldberg, I.J., Le, N.A., Ginsberg, H.N. and Paterniti, Jr. 1983. Metabolism of apoprotein B in cynomolgus monkeys. Am. J. Physiol. 244: 196-201.

Goldbourt, U. and Medalie, J.H. 1979. High density lipoproteins cholesterol and incidence of coronary heart disease. Epidemiol. 109: 296-308.

Goldstein, J.L. and Brown. M.S. 1982. LDL receptor defect in familial hypercholesterolemia. Med. Clin. North Am. 66: 335-62.

Gordon, T., Catelli, W.P., Hjortland, M.C., Kannel, W.B. and Dawber, T.R. 1977. High density lipoprotein as a protective factor against coronary heart disease. The framinghan study. Am. J. Med. 62: 707-14.

Gortmaker, S.L., Dietz, W.H., Sobol, A.M. and Wehlwr, C.A. 1987. Increasing pediatric obesity in the United States. Am. J. Dis. Child 141: 535-40.

Gracey, M. and Hitchock, N.E. 1985. Studies of growth of australian infants. In: Nutritional needs and assesment of normal growth. Gracey, M., ed. Nestlé Nutrition Workshop series vol. 7. Nestlé Nutrition. New York: Raven Press, 139-64.

Gray-Donald, K., Kramer, M.S., Munday, S. and Leduc, D.G. 1985. Efectos de los suplementos de leche artificial intrahospitalarios sobre la duración de la lactancia materna. Un estudio clínico controlado. Pediatrics (Ed. Esp.) 19: 204-7.

Gutierrez, M. and Gallí, A. 1985. Lactancia materna. Promoción mediante capacitación del equipo de salud. Bol. Of. Sanit. Panam. 98: 1-7.

Hofman, A. and Valkenburg, H.A. 1983. Determinants of change in blood pressure during childhood. Am. J. Epidemiol. 117: 735-43.

Hypertension detection and follow-up program cooperative group. 1979. Five-year findings of the hypertension mortality of persons with high blood pressure, including mild hypertension. JAMA; 242: 2562-71.

Hypertension detection and follow-up program cooperative group. Five-year findings of the hypertension and follow up program. 1982. III. Reduction in stroke incidence among persons with high blood pressure. JAMA; 247: 633-8.

Ibsen, K.K. 1981. Blood pressure in danish children and adolescents. Acta Paedieatr. Scand. 70: 27-31.

Ibsen, K.K., Lous, P. and Andersen, G.E. 1982. Coronary heart risk factor in 177 children and young adults whose fathers died from ischemic heart disease before age 45. Acta Paediatr. Scand. 71: 609-13.

International collaborative study group. 1986. Metabolic epidemiology of plasma cholesterol. Lancet; 2: 991-6.

Jones, F. 1984. Normal infant feeding. In: Manual of Pediatric Nutrition. Kelts, D.G., Jones, E.G., eds. Little brown an Company. Boston/Toronto 125-38.

Kannel, W.B. and Dawer, T.R. 1972. Atherosclerosis as a pediatric problem. J. Pediatr. 80: 544-54.

Kannel, W.B., Castelli, W.P., Gordon, T. and McNamarra, P.M. 1971. Serum cholesterol, lipoproteins, and the risk of coronary heart disease. The Framinghan study. Ann. Intern. Med. 74: 1-12.

Kannel, W.B., McGee, T. and Gordon, R. 1976. A general cardiovascular risk profiles. The Framingham study. Am. J. Cardiol. 38: 46-51.

Keys, A., Aravanis, C., Blackburn, H., Van Buchem, Fsp., Buzina, r., Djodjevic, B.S., Fidanza, F., Karvonen, M.J., Menotti, A., Puddu, V. and Raylor, H.L. 1972. Coronary heart disease: Overweight and obesity as risk factors. Ann. Inter. Med. 77: 15-27.

Kramer, M.S., Barr, R.G., Leduc, D.G., Boisjoly, C. and Pless, I.B. 1985. Infant determinants of childhood weight and adiposity. J. Pediatr. 107: 104-7.

Krauss, R.M. 1982. Regulation of high density lipoproteins levels. Med. Clin. North Am. 66: 403-30.

Kurinji, N., Shiono, P.H. and Rhoads, G.G. 1988. Incidencia y duración de la lactancia materna en mujeres de raza negra y blanca. Pediatrics (Ed. Esp.) 25: 203-6.

Kwiterovich, P.O. Jr. 1986. Biochemical, clinical, epidemiologic, genetic, and pathologic data in the pediatric age group relevant to the cholesterol hypothesis. Pediatrics 78: 349-62.

Langley-Danysz, P. 1984. Cancer: Los riesgos de la alimentación. Mundo Científico 33: 170-82.

Laskarzewski, P.M., Morrison, J.A., Kelly, K., Khoury, P., Mellies, M. and Glueck, C.J. 1981. Parent-child coronary heart disease risk factor associations. Am. J. Epidemiol., 114: 827-35.

Lauer, R.M., Connor, W.E., Leaverton, P.E., Reiter, M.A. and Clarke, W.R. 1975. Coronary heart disease risk factors in school children: The Muscatine study. J. Pediatr., 86: 697-706.

Lee, J., Laver, R.M. and Clarke, W.R. 1986. Lipoproteins in the progeny of young men with coronary artery desease: children with increased risk. Pediatrics 78: 330-7.

Lethone, A. and Vilkari, J. 1978. Serum triglycerides and cholesterol and high density lipoprotein cholesterol in highly physically active men. Acta Med. Scand. 204: 111-4.

Lipid Research Clinic Program. 1984. The lipid research clinics coronary primary prevention trial results. I. Reduction in incidence of coronary heart disease. JAMA 251: 351-64.

Lipid Research Clinic Program. 1984. The lipid research clinics coronary primary prevention trial results. II. The relationships of reduction in incidence of coronary heart disease to cholesterol lowering. JAMA 251: 365-74.

Lloyd, J.K. and Wolff, O.H. 1982. Surnutrition et obesité. In: Prévention chez l'enfant des problémes de santé du futur adulte. Falkner, F. OMS.

López Mondedeu, C. 1993. Estudio C.A.E.N.P.E. (en prensa).

Manzella, M. and Scotto, E. 1984. Indagazione epidemiologica sul tipo d'allatamento in due communi della provincia de Palermo. Min. Pediatr. 36: 87-91.

Marmot, M.G., Syme, S.L., Kagan, A., Kato, H., Cohen, J.B., and Belsky, J. 1975. Epidemiologic studies of coronary heart disease and stroke in japanese men living in Japan, Hawai and California: prevalence of coronary and hypertensive heart disease and associated risk factors. Am. J. Epidemiol. 103: 514-25.

Martínez, C., Brines, J., Codoñer, P., García, A. and Nuñez, F. Cuantificación del consumo de nutrientes en 113 escolares de la comunidad Valenciana: resultados de 452 encuestas dietéticas. Bol. Soc. Cast. Ast. Leon. Pediatr. 28: 281-8.

Masana, L. 1988. Regulación de la concentración de colesterol LDL: Hipercolestorelemias. En: Lipoproteinas plasmáticas y aterosclerosis coronaria. Barcelona. Editorial M.C.R., S.A., 2: 145-80.

Mattson, F.H., Erickson, B.A. and Kligman, A.M. 1972. Effect of dietary cholesterol in man. Am. J. Clin. Nutr. 25: 589-94.

McGill, H.C. Jr. 1979. Apprisal of cholesterol as a causative factor in atherogenesis. Am. J. Clin. Nutr. 32: 2632-6.

McGill, H.C. Jr. 1979. The relationship of dietary cholesterol to serum cholesterol concentration and to atherosclerosis is man. Am. J. Clin. Nutr. 32: 2664-702.

McLaren, D.S. and Burman, D. 1982. Textbook of Paediatric Nutrition. Nueva York: Churchill Livingstone.

Minetti, C., Zoppi, G., Conforti, G. and Venzano, V. 1980. L'allatamento materno oggi. Un'indagazione statistica nella citá di Genova. Min. Pediatr. 132: 543-6.

Moreiras-Varela, O., Carbajal, A., Blázquez, M.J., Cabrera, L. and Martínez, A. 1984. La alimentación en la escuela y en el hogar de niños madrileños: estudio piloto. Rev. Esp. Pediatr. 40: 257-66.

Morrison, J.A., Larsen, R. and Glatfelter, L. 1980. Nutrient intake: Relationships with lipids and lipoproteins in 6-19 year old children the Princeton school district study. Metabolism 29: 133-40.

Muñoz, J., Salazar, N., Pérez, M., Dapeña, J. and Gómez, I. 1986. Estado actual de la alimentación del lactante en nuestro medio. An. Esp. Pediatr., 26: 64-70.

Muñoz, S., Muñoz, H. and Zambrano, F. 1980. Blood pressure in a school age population. Distribution, correlations, and prevalence of elevated values. Mayo Clinic Proc., 55: 623-32.

National Institute of Health. 1985. Lowering lood cholesterol to prevent heart disease. Jama; 253: 2080-6.

Newman, W.P., Freedman, D.S., Voors, A.W., Gard, P.D., Srinivasan, S.R., Cresanta, J.L., Williamson, G.d., Webber, L.S. and Berenson, G.S. 1986. Relation of serum lipoproteins and systolic blood presure to early atherosclerosis: The Bogalusa heart study. N. Engl. J. Med., 314: 138-44.

OMS. 1982. Prevención de la cardiopatía coronaria. Serie de Informes Técnicos 678. Ginebra.

OMS. 1984. Le programme europeén de L'OMS relatif aux maladies cardiovasculares. La Sante publique en Europe-15 (Bureau Regional de L'Europe), Copenhague.

OMS. 1985. Cantidad y calidad de la leche materna. Informe sobre el estudio en colaboración de la OMS acerca de la lactancia materna. Ed. Organización Mundial de la Salud. Ginebra.

Orchard, T.J., Donahue, R.P., Kuller, L.H., Hodge, P.N. and Drash, A.L. 1983. Cholesterol screening in childhood: does it predict adult hypercholesterolemia? The Beaver County experience. J. Pediatr. 103: 687-91.

Paidos'84. 1985. Estudio epidemiológico sobre nutrición y obesidad infantil. Ed. Danone S.A.

Pérez-Chóliz, V., García, M.A., Castro, A. and Pérez, J.M. 1986. Evolución de la alimentación con beikost en nuestro medio: estudio estadístico. Premios de Nutrición Infantil 1986. Ed. Nestlé A.E.P.A. Barcelona, 319-98.

Persson, C.A. and Samuelson, G. 1984. De la lactancia natural a la comida familiar habitual. Alimentación en tres comunidades suecas. Acta Paediatr. Scand. (Ed. Esp.), 1: 721-9.

Persson, L.A. 1985. Infant feeding and growth. A longitudinal study in three Swedish communities. Ann. Hum. Biol. 12: 41-52.

Plaza, I., Otero, J., Muñoz, M.T., Baeza, J., Ceñal, M.J., Ruiz-Jarabo, C., Parra, M.J., Orellana, M.A., Puga, M., Asensio, J., Madero, R., Sánchez, J., Mariscal, R.P. and Dominguez, J. 1986. Estudio de Fuenlabrada: Factores de riesgo cardiovascular en niños y adolescentes. Rev. Lat. Cardiol., 7: 387-93.

Puska, P., Tnomilehto, J., Salonen, J., Nissinen, A., Virtamo, J., Björkquist, S., Kostela, K., Neitiiaanmärki, L., Takalo, T., Kotte, T.E., Mäki, J., Sipila, P. and Varvikko, P. 1981. The north Karelia project: Evaluation of a comprensive community programme to control cardiovascular disease in 1972-1977 in north Karelia, Finland. WHO, Copenhagen.

Puska, P., Variainen, E., Pallonen, V., Salonen, J.T., Poyhid, P., Koskela, K. and McAlister, A. 1982. The north Karelia youth proyect: Evaluation of two years of intervention on health behavior and CVD risk factors among 13 to 15 year old children. Prev. Med., 11: 550-70.

Quandt, S.A. 1984. The effect of beikost on the diet of breast-fed infants. J. Am. Diet Assoc. 84: 47-51.

Rabkin, S.W., Mathewson, Fal. and Hsu, P.N. 1977. Relation of body weight to development of ischemic heart disease in a cohort of young north american men after a 26 year observation period: The Manitobva study. Am. J. Cardiol. 39: 452-8.

Ramachandran, P. 1987. The Indian experience. In: Weaning, why, what and when? Ballabriga, A. and Rey, J., eds. Nestlé Nutrition Workshop Series, vol. 10. Nestlé Nutrition. Vevey/Raven Press, New York, 187-96.

Rapport de Nutrition Canada au Ministere de la Sante Nationale et du Bien-etre Social. 1973. Nutrition Canada. Food consumption patterns report. Ottawa: Information Canada.

Rapport de Nutrition Canada au Ministere de la Sante Nationale et du Bien-etre Social. Nutrition Canada. 1973. Enquete Nationale. Ottawa: Information Canada.

Ribó, M.A., Golobart, M., Castella-Ribo, M.A. and Mazamontero, J.M. 1983. Prácticas de nutrición infantil en el primer año de vida y nivel de conocimientos de las madres. In: Premios de Nutrición Infantil 1983. ed. Nestlé A.E.P.A. Barcelona, 400-39.

Ros, L. 1986. Alimentación complementaria: Cuando debe indicarse. Como hacerlo. Ventajas e inconvenientes del tiempo y de la forma de iniciarla. Dietética en Pediatría extrahospitalaria. Mesa redonda. An. Esp. Pediatr., 25 (Supp. 26): 1-14.

Ros, L. Alimentación y hábitos alimentarios de los adolescentes. 1989. Distinción Wander. Accésit. Ed. S.A.E. Wander.

Rosner, B., Cook, N.R., Evans, D.A., Keough, M.E., Taylor, J.O., Polk, B.F. and Hennekens, C.H. 1987. Reproducibility and predictive values of routine blood pressure measurements in children comparison with adult values and implicatins for screening children for elevated blood pressure. Am. J. Epidemiol. 126: 1115-25.

Rudas, B. 1980. L'incidence des facteurs de risque des maladies cardiovasculaires chez des ecoliers "Etude Viennoise". Med. et Nutr., 16: 237-41.

Rudell, L.L., Bond, M.G. and Bullock, B.C. 1985. LDL heterogenicity and atherosclerosis in non human primates. Ann. Ny. Acad. Sci. 454: 248-53.

Ruiz Moreno, M., Gutierrez, M.T., Rincon, P., Alvarez-Sala, L. and Camps, M.T. 1986. Hipercolesterolemia moderada en niños. ¿Indice de patología familiar? An. Esp. Pediatr. 25: 322-8.

Salas, J., Font, I., Canals, J., Guinovart, L., Sospedra, C. and Martí Henneberg, C. 1985. Consumo, hábitos alimentarios y estado nutricional de la población de Reus: I. Consumo global por grupos de alimentos y su relación con el nivel socioeconómico y de instrucción. Med. Clin. (Barc.) 84: 339-43.

Salas, J., Font, I., Canals, J., Guinovart, L., Sospedra, C. and Martí Henneberg, C. 1985. Consumo, hábitos alimentarios y estado nutricional de la población de Reus: III. Distribución por edad y sexo del consumo de leche, derivados de la leche, grasas visibles, vegetales y verduras. Med. Clin. (Barc.), 84: 470-5.

Salas, J., Font, I., Canals, J., Guinovart, L., Sospedra, C. and Martí Henneberg, C. 1985. Consumo, hábitos alimentarios y estado nutricional de la población de Reus: IV. Distribución por edad y sexo del consumo de raices y tubérculos, cereales, azúcares y frutas. Med. Clin. (Barc.) 84: 557-62.

Salas, J., Font, I., Canals, J., Guinovart, L., Sospedra, C. and Martí Henneberg, C. 1985. Consumo, hábitos alimentrios y estado nutricional de la población de Reus: II. Distribución por edad y sexo del consumo de carne, huevos, pescado y legumbres. Med. Clin. (Barc.) 84: 423-7.

Sánchez-Valverde Visus, F. 1990. Alimentación durante el primer año de vida en Navarra. Colección: Investigación. Gobierno de Navarra. Departamento de Salud.

Sarriá, A., Fleta, J. and Bueno, M. 1984. El adolescente obeso. MDP Monografías de Pediatría 17: 65-77.

Schrott, H.G., Clarke, W.R., Wiebe, D.A., Connor, W.E. and Laver, R.M. 1979. Increased coronary mortality in relatives of hypercholesterolemic school children: The Muscatine study. Circulation 59: 320-6.

Segal, K.R., Gutin, A.M. and Pi-Sunyer, F.X. 1985. Thermic effect of food at rest, during exercise in lean and obese men of similar body weight. J. Clin. Invest., 76: 1107-12.

Serville, Y. 1980. Rations d'alimens. In: Manuel de l'alimentation humaine: Les bases de l'alimentation. Tremoliéres, J., Serville, Y., Jacquod, R. and Dupin, H. eds. Paris, ESF ed. 444-54.

384

Shear, C.L., Burke, G.L., Freeditan, D.S. and Berenson, G.S. 1986. Value of childhood blood pressure measurements and family history in predicting future blood pressure status: Results from 8 years of follow up in the Bogalusa Heart Study. Pediatrics 77: 862-9.

Snidreman, A., TEng, B., Genest, J., Cianflone, K., Wacholder, S. and Kwiterovich, P. Jr. 1985. Familial aggregation and early expression of hyperaprobetalipoproteinemia. Am. J. Cardiol. 55: 291-5.

Sola, R., Masana, L. and Sarda, P. 1987. Determinantes metabólicos de las concentraciones de colesterol en el hombre. Importancia de los factores dietéticos. Med. Clin. (Barc.) 89: 811-5.

Spyckerelle, Y. and Deschamps, J.P. 1984. Le riske cardiovasculaire chez l'enfant et l'adolescent. Centre de Medicine Preventive-Vandoeuvre-Les-Nancy. Maloine, S.A., ed. Coeur 15:715-28.

Stählberg, M.R. 1985. Lactancia natural y factores sociales. Acta Paediatr. Scand. (Ed. Esp.) 2: 37-40.

Stamler, J. 1973. Epidemiology of coronary heart disease. Med. Clin. North Am., 57: 5-46.

Stamler, J., Berkson, D.M. and Lindberg, H.A. 1972. Risk factors: Atherosclerotic diseases. In: Pathogenesis of atherosclerosis. Wissler, R.W., and Geer, J.C., eds. Baltimore, Maryland, Williams and Wilkins.

Stamler, J., Wenworth, D. and Neaton, J.A. 1986. Is relationship between serum cholesterol and risk of premature death from coronary heart disease continuos and graded? JAMA 256: 2823-8.

Stark, D., Atkins, E., Wolff, O.H. and Douglas, J.W.B. 1981. Longitudinal study of obesity in the National survey of health and development. Br. Med. J. 283: 13-7.

Strong, J.P. and McGill, H.C. Jr. 1969. The pediatric aspects of atherosclerosis. J. Atheroscler. Res., 9: 251-65.

Strong, J.P., McGill, H.C. Jr., Tejada, C. and Holman R.L. 1958. The natural history of atherosclerosis: Comparasion of early aortic lesions in New Orleans, Guatemala, and Costa Rica. Am. J. Pathol. 34 (14): 731-44.

Stunkard, A.J., Sorensen, T.I.A. and Hanis, C. 1986. An adoption study of human obesity. N. Engl. J. Med. 314: 193-8.

Sveger, T., Fex, G. and Borgefdrs, N. 1987. Hyperlipidemia in school children with family histories of premature coronary disease. Acta Pediatr. Scand. 76: 311-5.

Swan, P.B. 1983. Food consumption by individuals in the United States: Two major surveys. Ann. Rev. Nutr. 3: 413-32.

Szklo, M. 1979. Epidemiologic Paterns of blood pressure in children. Epidemiol. Rev., 1: 143-69.

Toenz, O. and Schwaninger, U. 1980. Infant feeding practices in Switzerland 1978. Part II. Artificial feeding. Schweitz Med. Wochenschr. 110: 1522-31.

Tojo, R., Iglesias, H., Alonso, M.C., Esquete, C. and Iglesias, J.L. 1975. Nutritional status of school children in Galicia (Northwertern Spain). A biochemical, anthropometric, psycometric and socio-economic survey nutrition, growth and development. Mod. Probl. Paediatr. 14: 247-63.

Turkewitz, D. and Baztan, C. 1986. Infant and child nutrition: controversies and recommendations. Postgrad. Med. 79: 151-4.

Valls, A. 1987. Obesidad primaria del niño. An. Esp. Pediatr. 27: 65-9.

Vartiainen, E., Puska, P., Petinen, P., Hissinen, A., Leino, U. and Vusitalo, V. 1986. Effects of dietary fat modifications on serum lipids and blood pressure in children. Acta Paediatr. Scand. 75: 396-401.

Vitoria, J.C. 1986. Alimentación infantil en el primer año de vida. An. Esp. Pediatr. 25: 481-8.

Voller, R.D. Jr. and Strong, W.B. 1981. Pediatric aspects of atherosclerosis. Am. Heart 101: 815-36.

Voors, A.W., Webber, L.S. and Berenson, G.S. 1978. Blood pressure of children, aged 2 1/2 years, in a total biracial community: The Bogalusa Heart Study. Am. J. Epidemiol. 107: 403-11.

Voors, A.W., Weber, L.S. and Berenson, G.S. 1979. Time course studies of blood pressure in children: The Bogalusa Heart Study. Am. J. Epidemiol. 109: 320-34.

Weidman, W., Kwiterovich, P., Jesse, M.J. and Nugent, E. 1983. AHA committee report: Diet in the healthy child. Circulation 67: 1411A-14A.

Whitehead, R.G., Paul, A.A. and Ahmed, E.A. 1986. Weaning practics in the United Kingdom and variations in anthropometric development. Acta Paedatr. Scand. 323: 14-23.

WHO. 1975. Fifht report on the world health situation 1969-1972. Official records of the WHO 225.

Wissler, W.R. and McGill, H.C. Jr. 1983. Conference on blood lipids in children: Optimal levels for early prevention of coronary artery disease. Prev. Med. 12: 868-902.

Zonta, L.A., Jayakar, S.D., Bosisio, M., Galante, A. and Pennetti, V. 1987. Genetic Analysis of human obesity in an italian sample. Hum. Hered. 37: 129-39.

7 Intestinal flora, lactose intolerance and hypoallergenic formulas

Dairy Products in Human Health and Nutrition, Serrano Ríos et al. (eds) © 1994 Balkema, Rotterdam, ISBN 90 5410 359 0

Dairy products and intestinal flora

J.C. Rambaud, Y. Bouhnik & Ph. Marteau
Service de Gastroentérologie et Unité INSERM U 290, Hôpital Saint-Lazare, Paris, France

ABSTRACT : Relationships between diary products and intestinal flora include lactose malabsorption and fermented milks. Lactose malabsorption results in an osmotic fluid flow in the small intestine. In the colon, malabsorbed lactose is more or less completely fermented, depending on the oral load. Resulting VFAs and lactic acid are readily absorbed and sodium transport is stimulated. This results in decreased osmotic load and diarrhea. Lactose/lactulose fermentation may be enhanced by adaptation to these sugars with lactic acid bacteria overgrowth, hence a reduced diarrhea in response to a lactulose load. Milks fermented with yogurt bacteria, *Bifidobacteria* and other genii are among the most frequently used probiotics. Lactose is better absorbed from yogurt than from milk in malabsorbers because of *in vivo* bacterial lactase activity and slower gastric emptying. Probiotics have some effects on colonic indigenous flora, and especially modify some enzymatic activities in a way probably beneficial for the host.

Relationships between dairy products and the intestinal flora encompass two main topics which have in common a single denominator : lactose. In one case, this sugar is more or less malabsorbed, and fermented by large intestinal microflora. This occurs in the vast majority of humans. In the other case, milk lactose is fermented *in vitro* by bacteria isolated from the intestinal flora and which are thought to beneficial for human health. These living bacteria ingested daily in fermented milks are by far the most frequently used probiotics.

1 LACTOSE MALABSORPTION.

Acquired lactase deficiency is a physiological state present in most of the world adult population (Flourié 1987). Secondary lactase deficiency due to small intestinal villus injury is, by comparison with acquired deficiency, a very rare pathological state (Flourié, 1987). In spite of lactose malabsorption, a large percentage of people with acquired lactase deficiency do consume milk with little or no adverse symptoms (Newcomer 1984). A brief recall of the pathophysiology of lactose intolerance is necessary before discussing the mechanisms of lactose tolerance in malabsorbers, and especially the role of colonic flora. Lactose is a small osmotically active molecule, whose malabsorption results in the accumulation of water and electrolytes in the duodenum and jejunum (Christopher 1971, Rambaud 1988), which are highly permeable to osmotic water flow. These movements of fluid increase the speed of transit in the small bowel (Lades 1982), reducing lactase hydrolysis by residual lactose activity (Rambaud 1988). Thus, a significantly increased flow rate of fluid is delivered to the large intestine (Christopher 1971, Bond 1976). In the absence of other solutes in the test solution, 30 % of the ileal fluid solutes are lactose on a molar basis (Bond 1976). Noteworthy, these alterations in the small bowel function midly affect the absorption of nutrients other than lactose itself (Debongnie 1979).

The role of the colon and its microflora in lactose intolerance has mainly been studied in volunteers receiving the non absorbable disaccharide lactulose. The reason for this is, as seen later, that the residual absorption of lactose varies among lactase deficient subjects, whereas lactulose malabsorption is always 100 %.

When lactose or lactulose reaches the colon, it is more or less completely fermented by the resident flora into volatile fatty acids (VFA), lactic acid, CO_2, H_2 and CH_4 in methane-producers (Grimble 1989). The consequences of this fermentation process are the following.

The catabolism of unabsorbable sugars in readily absorbable VFA (Ruppin 1980) and lactic acid (Hamer 1989) reduces the osmotic load, and thus suppresses or decreases diarrhea which would have resulted from unmodified ileal output. This effect is enhanced by the simulatory effect of VFA on sodium absorption (Ruppin 1980). The protective role on diarrhea of sugar fermentation has been clearly shown by comparing the diarrheas resulting from isoosmolar loads of the unfermentescible and unabsorbable polyethylene glycol 4000 and of lactulose (Hamer 1989). Also, in piglet's transmissible gastroenteritis, newborn animals with few established colonic bacteria have more diarrhea than older ones (Argenzio 1984). It has been shown that non absorbed organic fatty acids (SCFA) or residual sugars are responsible for diarrhea when the lactulose load is moderate or high, respectively (Hamer 1989). Beside its effects on colonic osmotic load, sugar fermentation could also play a role in modulation of colonic transit, as seen later.

Contrary to its beneficial action on diarrhea, colonic fermentation of sugars is thought to be responsible for adverse effects. There is no doubt that excess of gas results from the fermentation process. Most gases diffuse through the colonic mucosa and are expired in breath, but a variable proportion, depending on the quantities formed per unit of time in the colonic lumen, are expelled through the anus (Christle 1992). It is likely that gas and bloating are also responsible for borborygmi although the latter result in fact from the mixing of gas and intestinal fluid contents, and thus may be due at least in part to fluid excess (Rambaud 1988). Abdominal pains are also usually assigned to excess gas, due to colonic wall strain and mecanoreceptors stimulation. However, small bowel distension by the increased luminal fluid content could also play a role. Indeed, in 2 lactose malabsorbers, it has been shown that the colonic perfusion with a lactose solution did not induce pain, whereas oral ingestion of the lactose solution was painful (Christopher 1971). Moreover, disturbed small and large intestinal motility could also play a role in the pain process. Finally, excessive production of the poorly metabolized D-lactic acid may have deleterious effects (Flourié 1990).

How do so many lactase deficient subjects tolerate milk in spite of the above intestinal disturbances ? Several mechanisms have been emphasized : a) the degree of lactase deficiency varies from one subject to another and may be mild, allowing a normal or nearly normal milk consumption (Bond 1976) ; b) as, for a given lactase deficency level, events occuring in the small and large intestine are lactose - load dependent (Ravich 1983) an empirical adjustment of lactose consumption may occur to suppress or minimize adverse effects ; c) frequent ingestion of milk during the course of the day (Lisker 1976) and at meals (Solomons 1985) distribute the lactose load and dilute it with other foods, reducing the osmotics effect, hence slowing the transit and increasing lactose hydrolysis due to residual lactase activity.

Together with these mechanisms, we have shown that colonic flora can adapt to a non diarrheogenic chronic load of lactulose (Florent 1985) and that this adaptation has a beneficial effect on the diarrhea induced by a large load of the sugar (Flourié 1993). In the first experiment (Florent 1985), volunteers ingested 20 g of lactulose twice a day during 7 days. They had no diarrhea. Stool weight and composition remained the same at the beginning and at the end of lactulose administration, except for a sharp rise of ß-galactosidase. Caecal intubations showed at the 7th day, compared to the first one, a marked fall in fecal fluid pH, a faster disappearance of lactose and of its constitutive hexoses, an increased concentration of VFA and D and L lactic acids, with a dome-shaped curve for lactic acid indicating lactic acid catabolism. Among VFAs, there was a rise of the percentage of acetic acid, whereas H_2 pulmonary excretion fell. Thus, a 7 day load of a non diarrheagenic dose of lactose induced a faster bacterial catabolism of this sugar and a change in the metabolic pathways characteristic of lactic acid fermentation.

In the second experiment (Flourié 1993), we made the hypothesis that the same 7 day load of 40 g/d lactulose could reduce diarrhea induced by the morning ingestion of 60 g of lactulose. We did find a significant fall of stool number and weight, and of sugar "units" fecal excretion. VFA and lactic acid fecal outputs were unchanged, showing that the excess SCFA due to increased fermentation of lactulose had been absorbed. Once again there was a drop of H_2 pulmonary excretion. Colonic transit time was markedly longer, whereas ileal intubation showed that the chronic lactulose load had no effect on the small bowel handling of the 60 g lactulose. It cannot be settled whether the slower colonic transit merely reflected the decrease of the osmotic load or was also due to alterations in colonic motility per se, related to changes in the SCFA pattern. Whatever its mechanism, the slower transit increases the efficiency of bacterial fermentation and of SCFA absorption.

Thus, adaptation of the colonic flora to a lactulose load is able to reduce the effects of an acute load of this sugar. What about lactose itself ? In a preliminary double blind design (Arrigoni 1992) we studied the effect in lactose malabsorbers of the ingestion during 15 days of 17 d/d lactose compared to 17 g to the completely absorbed saccharose. Subjects received 50 g of lactose in water before and after the adaptation period. In the lactose group there was an improvement of nearly all symptoms of lactose intolerance, including the number of stools. However, stool weight remained unchanged. There was clear evidence of bacterial adaptation to lactose, i.e. decreased H_2 pulmonary excretion and increased fecal ß-galactosidase activity during the 50 g lactose load. However, the saccharose group, although showing no signs of adaptation, behaved in all other points in the same manner as the lactose group. Thus, although present, the effects of lactose adaptation were masked by the well known acclimatization to repeated challenge. Moreover, there was no apparent modification on the single parameter not influenced by this effect, i.e. stool weight. At present, the reason for this finding remains obscure. It is opposite to the study of an infant with congenital lactose malabsorption in whom a lactose containing diet during a 3 week period resulted, by comparison with the first days, in a decreased stool volume and disaccharide content, and in a sharp rise of lactic acid excretion, whereas no adaptation had occured in the small intestine (Launiala 1968). Bacteriological data on lactose intolerance or even maldigestion and on lactulose fermentation are very scanty).

It is well known that in breast-fed young infants, lactic-acid forming bacteria, especially faecal streptococci and Bifidobacterium bifidum, increase in stools (Weijers 1961). However, the rise is small and of no diagnostic value. In adults, as shown by our first experiment (Florent 1985), effects of malabsorbed lactose or lactulose are limited to (or depending of the load predominate in) the caecum and right

Table 1 Products of glucose metabolism by colonic flora

Microorganisms	Products
Non-sporing strickly anaerobes bacteria	
Bacteroides spp	acetate, succinate, propionate
Fusobacterium spp	acetate, butyrate
Bifidobacterium spp	lactate, acetate, ethanol
Propionibacterium spp	lactate, acetate, propionate
Spore-forming anaerobic bacteria	
Clostridium butyricum	butyrate, acetate, formate
Clostridium perfrigens	butyrate, acetate, formate
Lactic acid bacteria	
Lactobacillus spp	lactate, acetate, ethanol
Streptococcus spp	lactate, acetate, ethanol
Facultative organisms	
Escherichia coli	lactate, acetate, formate, ethanol

From M.J. Hill 1983. In J. Delmont (ed) Milk intolerances and rejection 22-26. Basel : Karger.

colon, hence the failure of many workers to detect the effect of lactulose on the faecal flora (Hill 1983).

When a single dose of lactose/lactulose is initially given, it will stimulate the growth of all lactose-fermenting organisms (table 1) at the expense of non-lactose fermenters. The low pH resulting from lactulose/lactulose fermentation strongly favours the growth of lactic acid bacteria (streptococci, lactobacilli). Good production of ß-galactosidase and antagonistic effects on other species also favour lactic acid bacteria growth (Hill 1983). Thus, while initially all organisms able to utilize lactose/lactulose will do so, resulting in the formation of a wide range of VFA and large amounts of gas, with time the increasing dominance of lactic acid bacteria will increase the amount of lactic and acetic acid formed, and gas production will decrease (Hill 1983).

These theoretical considerations are in complete agreement with our findings with the non diarrheogenic dose of lactulose. The dome-shaped form of lactic acid concentration in the caecum of our volunteers suggests also that lactic-acid utilizing bacteria are also operating at these low pH (Florent 1985).

2 PROBIOTICS IN FERMENTED MILKS

Probiotic is defined as a live microorganism feed supplement which beneficially affects the host by improving its microbial ecosystem (Fuller 1991). As a reminiscence of old times, most probiotics are still intestinal bacteria given as fermented milk. They mainly include yogurt bacteria, Lactobacillus spp and Bifidobacterium spp.

2.1 Transit and implantation of probiotics

To exert biological activities on the host's intestinal microflora and other characteristics, a candidate probiotic must be present at the aimed site at a sufficient concentration, i.e. at least 10^5 (small bowel) - 5.10^7 (large intestine) microorganisms per g. This can be achieved either through implantation, or through transit of continuously fed bacteria. In order to allow a sufficient number of bacteria to reach the small and large intestine, a transit action requires several conditions depending on the inoculum, the viability, the stability and the bacterial membrane resistance, especially for gastric acid and bile salt injuries (Conway 1987). Implantation, if possible in adults, would require additional conditions: host specificity, adhesion properties to the mucosa, non immunogenicity and resistance to the "barrier" action of the host flora (Conway 1987, Ducluzeau 1992). To date, all attempts to colonize the adult intestine with a non pathogenic exogenous bacteria have failed, although several authors erroneously claimed successful attempts. Implantation of a "good flora" seems to be an attainable goal in new borns, whose barrier to colonization is not established. A few apparently successful attempts have been reported, such as the oral administration of plasmid free E.coli avoiding further colonization by plasmid harboring E.coli strains (Duval-Iflah 1982). Recently, attemps to colonize the gut with a strain of Bifidobacterium bifidum was successful in a small percentage of neonates (Hudault 1993).

In adults, bacteria only transit in the gut without implantation and their survival mainly depends on their genius. Bididobacterium sp in fermented milk induces a large increase in bifidobacteria fecal excretion, corresponding to a 30 p.cent survival of the inoculum (Bouhnik 1992) (figure).

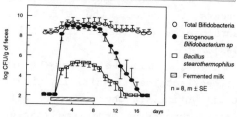

FECAL CONCENTRATIONS OF BIFIDOBACTERIA FOLLOWING FERMENTED MILK INGESTION

Bouhnik et al. Gastroenterology 1992 ; *102* : 875-8.

This ratio is also found in the distal ileum (Marteau 1992), indicating neither bacteriolysis, nor multiplication in the colon. This is due to the bacteriostatic effect of the resident flora. This bacterium or B. Longum could be used for its proper intrinsic biological and bacteriological properties or, in the future, as a vector of cloned useful genes. Fecal lactobacillus counts slightly increased after ingestion of fermented milk, but no attempts were made to distinguish the exogenous strain from the indigenous ones. However, ileal intubation showed that 1.5 p.cent of ingested *Lactobacillus acidophilus* reached the colon (Marteau 1992), and this ratio was much higher than that obtained with ingestion of yogurt *L. bulgaricus* in ileostomits (Lindwall 1984). Similar figures were found in the duodenum, indicating that yogurt bacteria lysis occurred in the upper gut (Pochart 1989).

L.casei strain GG, a human strain resistant to acid and bile salts, was recovered from stools of most volunteers when ingested inoculum was $1.5.10^9/d$, and persisted after various antibiotic treatments (Siitonen 1990).

2.2 Luminal effects of probiotics

It has been shown with the use of hydrogen breath test that lactase deficient subjects digested lactose more efficiently in fresh yogurt than in milk (Kolars 1984). This has been attributed to the high bacterial lactase activity in *L.bulgaricus* and *S.thermophilus* (Kolars 1984) and was confirmed by the persistence of a significant level of bacterial lactase activity in the small intestine following yogurt consumption (Marteau 1990). However, the slower gastric emptying of yogurt compared to milk also plays a role in yogurt properties.

The ability of some exogenous microorganisms to hydrolyze some substrates could also have potentially harmfull effects, such as deconjugation of bile salts in the small intestine by *Bifidobacterium sp*.

2.3 Parietal effects of probiotics

In a double blind study, ingestion of fresh yogurt for 8 d in lactase deficient subjects failed to modify the duodenal mucosal lactase activity (Lerebours 1989). However, there is no basal residual lactase activity in the duodenum of these subjects, and yogurt bacteria could stimulate lactase activity more distantly.

Among other possible actions of probiotics, effects on the immune system, owing to findings in animal models, should be considered. Current knowledge in human is scanty, although high doses of lyophilized *L.bulgaricus* and *S.thermophilus* were shown to increase serum gamma-interferon and circulating NK cells (De Simone 1989). These systemic effects imply translocation of the exogenous bacteria.

2.4 Effects of probiotics on pathogens and indigenous flora

Since some probiotic strains are well known to be antagonist *in vitro* to pathogens or indigenous bacteria, several authors attempted to assess this effect of these microorganisms *in vivo*. In several but not all studies *Lactobacillus spp* administration induced a decrease in fecal count of *E.coli*. Administration of a *B.longum* strain was accompanied by a decrease in *Bacteroides sp*, *clostridia* and *E.coli* (Rambaud 1993). Attemps to cure or prevent the symptoms of infectious diarrheas by probiotics

Table 2. Effects of lactic acid bacteria ingestion on fecal bacterial enzymatic activities in humans

Reference	Ingested bacteria	Quantity	Azoreductase	Nitroreductase	Glucuronidase
Ayebo 1980	L.acidophilus*	10^9	ND[+]	ND[+]	↓**
Goldin 1984	L.acidophilus*	10^9	↓**	↓**	↓**
Pedrosa 1990	L.acidophilus*	10^9	↓**	↓**	↓**
Pedrosa 1990	L.bulgaricus and S.thermophilus	5.10^8	-[s]	-[s]	-[s]
Marteau 1990	L.acidophilus + Bifidobacterium sp + Streptococcus sp	10^9-10^{10}	-[s]	↓**	-[s]
Bouhnik (unpublished)	Bifodobacterium sp	10^{10}	-[s]	↓**	↓**

* no effect with milk or killed bacteria
[+] not done
** : p < 0,05 ; [s] : no effect

have given variable results ; however the elimination of the pathogen was not obtained (Rambaud 1993). Lactobacillus GG seemed to be effective in preventing new attacks of relapsing pseudo-membranous colitis. Prevention of antibiotic-induced diarrhea by S.boulardii, a B.longum strain and Lactobacillus GG has also been clearly shown, but the mechanisms involved remain unknown (Rambaud 1993).

The effects of probiotics on indigenous flora are much more appearent when enzyme activities are studied in feces. A few studies using a Lactobacillus strain showed that ß-glucuronidase, azoreductase and nitroreductase fecal outputs decreased.Similar results have been obtained with Bifidobacterium sp and two mixtures containing L.acidophilus, S.thermophilus and L.bulgaricus in the one, and L.acidophilus and Bifidobacterium sp in the other (table 2).

The relevance of these data on prevention of colonic carcinoma remains to be proven.

3. CONCLUSION

Intestinal flora has a physiological role in the digestion of lactose in lactase-deficient subjects. This colonic digestion reduces the diarrhea due to lactulose ingestion, which mimicks lactose consumption by lactose intolerance patients. In turn, lactose/lactulose ingestion modify the colonic flora by promoting the growth of lactic acid bacteria. Intestinal bacteria fermenting lactose are widely used as probiotics in the form of fermented diary products. They are able to promote small intestinal lactose absorption in lactase deficient-sujets and modify the colonic flora echosystem in a way which could be beneficial to the host. Selecting with the help of genetic engeneering new microorganism which would transit at a high rate in the gut is currently an active field of research.

REFERENCES

Argenzio, R.A., Moon, H.W., Kemeny, L.J. & S.C. Whipp 1984. Colonic compensation in transmissible gastroenteritis of swine. Gastroenterology 86 : 1501-1509.

Argenzio, R.A. & C.E. Stevens 1984. The large bowel - a supplementary rumen ? Proceed. Nutr. Soc. 43 : 13-23.

Arrigoni, E., Pochart, P., Flourié, B., Marteau, P., Franchisseur, C. & J.C. Rambaud 1992. Does a prolonged lactose ingestion induce clinical and colonic metabolism adaptation in lactose intolerant subjects ? Gastroenterology 102 : 197 abstract.

Ayebo, A.D., Angelo, I.A. & K.M. Shahani 1980. Effect of ingesting *Lactobacillus acidophilus* milk upon fecal flora and enzyme activity in humans. Milchwissenschaft 35 : 730-733.

Bond, J.H. & M.D. Levitt 1976. Quantitative measurement of lactose absorption. Gastroenterology 70 : 1058-1062.

Bouhnik, Y., Pochart, P., Marteau, P., Arlet, G. Goderel, I. & J.C. Rambaud 1992b. Fecal recovery in humans of viable *Bifidobacterium* sp ingested in fermented milk. Gastroenterology 102 : 875-878.

Christl, S.U., Margatryod, P.R., Gibson, G.R. & J.H. Cummings 1992. Production, metabolism, and excretion of hydrogen in the large intestine. Gastroenterology 102 : 1269-1277.

Christopher, N.L. & T.M. Bayless 1971. Role of the small bowel and colon in lactose-induced diarrhea. Gastroenterology 60 : 845-852.

Conway, P.L., Gorbach, S.L. & B.R. Goldin 1987. Survival of lactic acid bacteria in the human stomach and adhesion to intestinal cells. J. Dairy Sc. 70 : 1-12.

Debongnie J.C., Newcomer A.D., McGill D.B., & S.F. Philips 1979. Absorption of nutrients in lactase deficiency. Dig. Dis. Sci. 24 : 225-231.

Ducluzeau, R. & P. Raybaud 1989. Les interactions bactériennes dans le tube digestif. Rev. Scient. Tech. Off. Int. Epiz 8 : 291-311.

Duval-Iflah, Y., Ouriet, M.F., Moreau, C., Daniel, N., Gabilan, J.C. & P. Raibaud 1982. Implantation précoce d'une souche d'*Escherichia coli* dans l'intestin de nouveaux-nés humains : effet de barrière vis-à-vis de souches de *E.coli* antibiorésistantes. Ann. Microb. (Institut Pasteur) 133A : 393-408.

Florent, C., Flourié, B., Leblond A., Rautureau, M., Bernier, J.J. & J.C. Rambaud 1985. Influence of chronic lactulose ingestion on the colonic metabolism of lactulose in man (an in vivo study). J. Clin. Invest. 75 : 608-613.

Flourié, B., Briet, F., Florent, C., Pellier, P., Maurel, F & J.C. Rambaud 1993. Can diarrhea induced by lactulose be reduced by prolonged ingestion of lactulose ? Am. J. Clin. Nutr (in press).

Flourié, B., Florent, C., Desjeux, J.F. & J.C. Rambaud 1987. Défaut en lactase et intolérance au lactose. Cah. Nutr. Diet. XXII : 367-371.

Flourié, B., Messing, B., Bismuth, E., Etanchaud, F., Thuillier, F. & J.C. Rambaud 1990. Acidose D lactique et encéphalopathie au cours d'un syndrome du grêle court à l'occasion d'un traitement antibiotique. Gastroenterol. Clin. Biol. 14 : 596-598.

Fuller, R. 1991. Probiotics in human medicine. Gut 32 : 439-442.

Goldin, B.R. & S.L. Gorbach 1984. The effect of milk and lactobacillus feeding on human intestinal bacterial enzyme activity. Am. J. Clin. Nutr. 39 : 756-761.

Grimble, G. 1989. Fibre, fermentation, flora and flatus. Gut 30 : 6-13.

Hamer, H.F., Santa Ana, C.A., Schiller, L.R. & J.S. Fortran 1989. Studies of osmotic diarrhea induced in normal subjects by ingestion of polyetheline glycol and lactulose. J. Clin. Invest. 84: 1056-1062.

Hill, M.J. 1983. Bacterial adaptation to lactase deficiency. In J. Delmont (ed). Milk intolerances and rejection : 22-26. Basel : Karger.

Hudault, S., Bridonneau, C., Raibaud, P., Chabarret, C. & M.F. Vial 1993. Establishment of *Bifidobacterium bifidium* in the intestine of human neonates : relationship with the bifidus factors found in the stools. Proceed. Nutr. Soc. (in press).

Kolars, J.C., Levitt, M.D., Aouji, M. & S.A. Savaiano 1984. Yogurt : an autodigesting source of lactose. N. Engl. J. Med. 310 : 1-3.

Ladas, S., Papanikos, J. & G. Arapakis 1982. Lactose malabsorption in breek adults : correlation of small bowel transit time with the severity of lactose intolerance. Gut 23 : 968- 973.

Launiala K 1968. The mechanism of diarroea in congenital disaccharide malasorption. Acta Paediat. Scand. 57 : 425-432.

Lerebours, E., N'Djitoyap Ndam, C., Lavoine, A., Hellot, M.F., Antoine, J.M. & R. Colin 1989. Yogurt and fermented-then pasteurized milk : effects of short-term and long-term ingestion on lactose absorption and mucosal lactase activity in lactase-deficient subjects. Am. J. Clin. Nutr. 49 : 823-827.

Lindwall, S. & R. Fonden 1984. Passage and survival of *L.acidophilus* in the human gastrointestinal tract. Int. Dairy Fed. Bul. 21 : 179.

Lisker R.L., Aguilar L. & S.C. Zavada 1978. Intestinal lactase deficiency and milk drinking capacity in the adult. Am. J. Clin. Nutr. 31 : 1499-1503.

Marteau, P., Flourié, B., Pochart, P., Chastang, C., Desjeux, J.F. & J.C. Rambaud 1990. Effect of the microbial lactase activity in yogurt on the intestinal absorption of lactose : an *in vivo* study in lactase-deficient humans. Br. J. Nutr. 64 : 71-9.

Marteau, P., Pochart, P., Bouhnik, Y., Zidi, S., Goderel, I. & J.C. Rambaud 1992. Survie dans l'intestin grêle de *Lactobacillus acidophilus* et *Bifidobacterium sp* ingérés dans un lait fermenté : une base rationnelle à l'utilisation de probiotiques chez l'homme. Gastroenterol. Clin. Biol. 16 : 25-28.

Newcomer, A.D. & D.B. McGill 1984. Clinical importance of lactase deficiency. N. Engl. J. Med. 310: 42-43.

Pedrosa, M.C., Golner, B., Goldin, B., Baraket, S., Dallal, G. & R.M. Russel 1990. Effect of Lactobacillus acidophilus or yogurt feeding on bacterial fecal enzymes in the elderly. Gastroenterology 98 : A439.

Pochart, P., Dewit, O., Desjeux, J.F. & P. Bourlioux 1989. Viable starter culture, ß-galactosidase actibity, and lactose in duodenum after yogurt ingestion in lactase-deficient humans. Am. J. Clin. Nutr. 49 : 828-831.

Pochart, P., Marteau, P., Bisetti, N., Goderel, I., Bourlioux, P & J.C. Rambaud 1990. Isolement des bifidobactéries dans les selles après ingestion prolongée de lait au bifidus. Médecine et Maladies Infectieuses 20 : 75-78.

Rambaud, J.C. 1988. Physio-pathologie de l'intolérance aux disaccharides. In J.C. Rambaud et R. Modigliani (eds) L'intestin grêle physiologie, physio-pathologie et pathologie : 70-80. Amsterdam : Excerpta Medica.

Rambaud, J.C., Bouhnik, Y., Marteau, P. & P. Pochart 1993. Manipulation of the human gut microflora. Proc. Brit. Nutr. Soc. (in press).

Ruppin, H., Bar-Meir, S., Soergel, K.H., Wood, C.M. & M.G. Schmitt Jr 1980. Absorption of short-chain fatty acids by the colon Gastroenterology 78 : 1507-1508.

Ravich, W.J. & T.M. Bayless 1983. Carbohydrate absorption and malabsorption. Cli. In Gastro-enterol 12 : 335-356.

Siitonen, S., Vapaatalo, H., Salminen, S., Gordin, A., Saxelin, M., Wikberg, R. & A.L. Kirkkola 1990. Effect of *Lactobacillus* GG yogurt in prevention of antibiotics associated diarrheoa. Ann. Med. 22 : 57-59.

Solomons, N.W., Guerrero, A.M. & B. Torun 1985. Dietary manipulation of post-prandial colonic lactose fermentation. I. Effect of solid food in a meal. Am. J. Clin. Nutr. 41 : 199-208.

Weijers, H.A., Van de Kamer, J.H., Dicke W.K. & J. Ijsseling 1961. Diarrhoea caused by deficiency of sugar splitting enzymes. I. Acta Paediatr. 50 : 55-71.

Dairy Products in Human Health and Nutrition, Serrano Ríos et al. (eds) © 1994 Balkema, Rotterdam, ISBN 90 5410 359 0

Lactose intolerance: Dietary management

D.A. Savaiano
College of Human Ecology, University of Minnesota, Minn., USA

ABSTRACT: Lactose is the primary sugar in virtually all mammalian milks. It is readily digested in the small intestine by a lactase enzyme in nearly all infants. However, up to 70% of the world's population experiences a genetically programmed loss of the majority of intestinal lactase activity following weaning, usually between the ages of three and five years. The preferred term to describe this loss of lactase activity is "lactase nonpersistence". Lactase nonpersistent individuals retain some residual lactase activity which allows for the digestion in the upper intestine of small amounts of lactose. Undigested lactose moves to the colon where it undergoes bacterial fermentation. Intolerance symptoms such as flatulence, bloating and acute diarrhea may result from excessive undigested lactose and its fermentation. Variability in bacterial fermentation and intestinal transit, and the use of exogenous sources of beta-galactosidase activity (yogurts and tablets) appear to influence tolerance to lactose. Hence, symptoms may be eliminated or reduced with dietary management that includes: 1) limiting milk consumption to one glass at a time 2) drinking milk with other foods rather than alone (thus slowing gastrointestinal transit) 3) eating yogurts (that contain microbial beta-galactosidase activity) instead of fluid milk 4) using beta-galactosidase enzyme drops or tablets to predigest the lactose in milk or to supplement the body's own lactase and 5) possibly eating small amounts of dairy foods each day to adapt the colonic bacteria, thus limiting excessive gas production.

INTRODUCTION:

Dairy foods are an important source of high quality protein, riboflavin and calcium in the diets of children and adults in the United States, Canada, Europe, and other countries with a dairy industry. However, up to 70% of the world's population may develop gastrointestinal symptoms including excessive flatulence, pain and acute diarrhea following the consumption of lactose-containing dairy foods. Young mammals, including humans, have a high level of lactase activity in the lining of their upper intestine, as they depend on lactose as the primary carbohydrate in their diet. As mammals mature and are weaned, lactase activity in the intestine is greatly reduced. Like other mammals, most humans (approximately 70%) lose the majority of their intestinal lactase activity after weaning. Individuals who lose their intestinal lactase have been described as lactase-deficient, lactase nonpersistent, lactose malabsorbers or lactose maldigesters. Interestingly, a small portion of the world's population (approximately 30%; including descendants of some African and Middle

Eastern tribes and most Northern Europeans) have apparently adapted to maintain the lactase enzyme. Research strongly suggests that this adaptation is genetically controlled, permanent, and is related to the development of dairying in these regions of the world several thousand years ago (1). For those individuals who maintain the lactase enzyme, eating dairy foods will not cause lactose intolerance symptoms. But, individuals who are lactase nonpersistent will maldigest a significant portion of a dietary load of lactose in the small intestine. Lactose which is not digested in the small intestine reaches the large intestine where it is fermented by the microflora, forming lactic acid, short chain fatty acids (SCFA), hydrogen gas and in some individuals, methane. The SCFAs are rapidly absorbed by the intestine and are a source of energy. Presumably, when the lactose concentration of the large intestine exceeds the ability of the bacteria to digest it, osmotic pressure results in increased motility, pain, loose stool and diarrhea. This presentation is designed to provide an overview of the recent research findings relating to the dietary management of lactose intolerance.

LACTOSE INTOLERANCE SYMPTOMS ARE RELATED TO THE AMOUNT OF LACTOSE CONSUMED

Scientists and clinicians have recognized for some time that the majority of lactose maldigesters will not develop symptoms of intolerance following the consumption of a single 225ml (8 ounce) serving of milk containing approximately 12g of lactose. Newcomer and McGill (2), Savaiano and Levitt (3) and recently Scrimshaw and Murray (4) have reviewed the research findings relating dose of lactose to the development of symptoms with the uniform conclusion that, at most, only one-fifth to one-third of maldigesters will develop symptoms following consumption of one glass of milk. Further, the level of symptom response to one glass of milk is not very different from that observed with lactose-free, flavored placebo beverages (5), although such controls may be criticized for their high osmotic loads. Increasing the dose of lactose to 24g (the amount or lactose found in two glasses of milk) increases the incidence of symptoms to a range close to 50%. Increasing the dose further, toward 50g of lactose (the amount of lactose in approximately one liter of milk) increases the incidence and severity of symptoms to a point where almost all lactose maldigesters experience symptoms. Historically, a 50g lactose load has been used to test for the presence of lactose maldigestion. Unfortunately, the extensive and relatively severe symptoms resulting from this unphysiologic lactose load have tended to develop and reinforce the misconception that any lactose load will cause symptoms in lactose maldigesters. A corollary to this misconception is the unfounded belief that all dairy foods will cause lactose-intolerance symptoms. Lactose is a water soluble disaccharide which remains primarily with the whey portion of dairy foods. As such, hard cheeses (with the whey removed from the curds) contain very little lactose (3). Cottage cheese, ice creams and yogurts contain reduced amounts of lactose relative to milk, and therefore cause fewer symptoms. A special attribute of yogurt, its microbial beta-galactosidase which assists the digestion of lactose in vivo, will be discussed later.

INGESTION OF LACTOSE WITH OTHER NUTRIENTS REDUCES INTOLERANCE

Food consumed (both quantity and type) along with lactose is a second important factor in determining the incidence of symptoms. In controlled experiments evaluating lactose intolerance, researchers have typically fed lactose in water or milk. Such experimental designs probably result in a higher incidence of symptoms than the typical consumer might experience, since consumers often drink milk with other foods. In 1973, Leichter demonstrated improved digestion and tolerance to lactose consumed in whole milk as compared to skim milk or water (6). Pirk and Scala (7) reported that in maldigesters, stomach emptying is delayed with lactose (versus sucrose) feeding whereas small intestinal transit is more rapid. Chocolate milk also appears to delay stomach emptying, presumably due to the greater osmotic load (8). The delay in gastrointestinal transit of lactose by other nutrients appears to be significant in slowing maldigestion and improving tolerance. Both Solomons et al. (9) and Martini and Savaiano (10) have published experiments showing delayed transit of lactose to the colon (as measured by breath hydrogen) when lactose is consumed with a meal. In the Martini and Savaiano study, both the severity and incidence of symptoms were reduced three-fold so that only 25% of subjects experienced symptoms of any kind following a 20g lactose load consumed with a breakfast meal (10).

LACTOSE DIGESTION FROM YOGURTS AND OTHER FERMENTED DAIRY FOODS

Since the work of Gallagher et al. (11) and Alm (12) in the 1970s, it has been suggested that fermented dairy foods may be tolerated better than similar unfermented products. Several reasons were typically invoked to explain the phenomenon including; the lower lactose levels found in these foods (12) and the contribution to digestion that lactic acid bacteria might make (13). Work by Kilara and Shahani (14) and Goodenough and Kleyn (15) indicated that the bacteria used in yogurt cultures (*Streptococcus thermophilus and Lactobacillus bulgaricus*) contain a beta-galactosidase activity and that this activity could possibly enhance lactose digestion in vivo in the rodent gastrointestinal tract. Such findings led Kolars et al. (16) and Gilliland and Kim (17) to evaluate lactose digestion from yogurt containing controlled amounts of lactose. In January of 1984, both groups reported a significant improvement in lactose digestion as measured by breath hydrogen production. In addition, Kolars et al. were able to demonstrate a significantly improved tolerance with yogurt feeding, and the presence of yogurt beta-galactosidase activity in the duodenum of yogurt-fed subjects (16). The enhanced digestion of and tolerance to lactose from yogurt has been replicated by several investigators (18-25).

The mechanism by which the yogurt-borne microbial beta-galactosidase can facilitate lactose digestion in vivo in the gastrointestinal tract is not completely understood. It appears that an intact microbial cell structure is critical for the survival of the enzyme during gastric digestion (19). Sonication or heating to disrupt the cell structure significantly increases maldigestion while reducing the survival of the enzyme in vitro (17,19). The pH of the stomach may be a second critical factor since the yogurt culture beta-galactosidase is rapidly destroyed in vitro at pHs $\leq$ 3.0 (19). Yogurt is an excellent buffer of acid, due to its casein, lactate and calcium phosphate content. This buffering capacity may keep portions of the stomach above pH 3.0 following ingestion of a yogurt meal (19). Once the intact yogurt bacteria enter the small intestine, bile acids are hypothetically able to disrupt the cell structure, releasing enzyme into the lumenal contents. In vitro, bile will disrupt yogurt bacteria, releasing beta-galactosidase activity (17). However, the in vivo action of physiological concentrations of bile acids on yogurt bacteria has not been demonstrated. Recently, Marteau et al. (26) reported that approximately one-fifth of the yogurt lactase activity reached the terminal ileum. This activity, plus the reported slow oral-caecal transit of yogurt, resulted in greater than 90% of the lactose in yogurt being digested in the small intestine.

The beta-galactosidase from yogurt culture is sensitive to freezing. After one week, beta-galactosidase activity fell to 34% of the original activity when yogurt was frozen at -14 C and to 73% of the original activity when frozen at -70 C (20). Most commercially manufactured frozen yogurts in the U. S. apparently contain little or no beta-galactosidase activity (20), but some products may contain activities similar to that observed with the freezing of fresh yogurt (27). The lack of U.S. standards for frozen yogurt production makes promoting the efficacy of these products for lactose maldigesters difficult.

LACTOSE DIGESTION FROM UNFERMENTED ACIDOPHILUS MILK

Several research groups have evaluated the ability of unfermented milk containing *Lactobacillus acidophilus* to modify lactose digestion and the development of intolerance symptoms (18,28-31). *L.acidophilus* strain NCFM has been most extensively studied in the United States. This strain is derived from human fecal samples, has been available commercially for several years, and synthesizes a beta-galactosidase (32,33). In 1981, Payne et al. (28) reported no improvement in lactose maldigestion after feeding commercially available acidophilus milk for one or eight days. Unfortunately, the number of viable lactobacilli and the beta-galactosidase activity of the product were not evaluated. Utilizing defined acidophilus products with 10^6, 10^7, or 10^8 viable NCFM strain lactobacilli per ml, Kim and Gilliland in

1983 showed a moderate but significant reduction in initial breath hydrogen production (approximately 15-20ppm) with the 10^6 (two experiments) and 10^8 doses but no improvement with the 10^7 dose (29). Unfortunately, Kim and Gilliland did not report intolerance symptoms nor did they measure the beta-galactosidase activity of the products. Newcomer et al., also in 1983, reported no improvement in intolerance symptoms with the substitution of acidophilus milk (10^6 cells/ml of the NCFM strain) for milk in mixed diets of lactose malabsorbers (30). Milk (or acidophilus milk) intakes varied from 1/4 to 4 1/2 glasses per day in a randomized, double-blind cross-over design. Each treatment lasted for one week. Symptoms were identical for the acidophilus milk and control milk periods. No estimate of lactose malabsorption was made in this study.

A potential variable which could alter the activity of beta-galactosidase in the intestinal tract is the bile sensitivity of the strain. Gilliland et al. (34) have shown that growth rates of *L. acidophilus* strains vary considerably in bile-containing media. Theoretically, a bile-sensitive strain would be more likely to release its beta-galactosidase in vivo, thereby aiding lactose digestion. In accord with this hypothesis, McDonough et al. reported the improved digestion of lactose from sonicated acidophilus milk (21). The product was formulated from frozen concentrates (NCFM strain, 10^8 cells/ml) and sonicated to disrupt the cell structure just prior to consumption. The release of beta-galactosidase reduced breath hydrogen production from 28ppm to 12ppm, suggesting that bile sensitive strains, where beta-galactosidase is release in vivo, could be effective in improving lactose digestion. Lin et al. (31) recently reported that strains differences exist in the ability of *L. acidophilus* to improve lactose digestion. While strain NCFM was ineffective, strain LA-1 caused a modest improvement in lactose digestion, when fed at 10^8 cfu/ml. Unpublished data from our laboratory confirm that both strains LA-1 and ADH can moderately improve lactose digestion when fed at concentrations of at least 10^8 cfu/ml.

ENZYME TABLETS:

An additional approach to prevent intolerance symptoms is the use of commercially available lactose-digesting enzyme tablets. Several brands are commonly available in the United States. If instructions are followed, these products are effective in reducing and/or eliminating symptoms. The tablets are either added to milk the night before drinking to predigest most of the lactose or they are taken with the dairy food (sprinkled over ice cream for example) and work in the stomach or intestine to supplement the body's lactase just like yogurt. Experiments confirm the effectiveness of these enzyme preparations either as a means of producing low-lactose milk (28,35-38) or as a dietary adjutant (39-42). We recently evaluated the effectiveness of three commercial brands currently available in the U.S. market (43). All products were evaluated for beta-galactosidase activity. Dose-response studies were conducted with one of the products. When 6000 IU of enzyme activity was fed to maldigesters along with milk containing 20g of lactose, digestion of lactose was uniformly enhanced three-fold, regardless of the brand or tablet form of the product. Feeding 3000 IU of enzyme activity with 20g of lactose resulted in a stoichiometric increase in maldigestion, as measured by breath hydrogen. Symptom-responses correlated well with hydrogen production. However, when 6000 IU of beta-galactosidase activity was fed with 50g of lactose in water, the added lactose load appeared to overwhelm the ability of the enzyme to aid digestion. Digestion and tolerance were not improved when the higher dose of lactose was fed.

COLONIC ADAPTATION TO LACTOSE:

Lactase-deficient persons who routinely eat lactose-containing foods adapt to exhibit fewer symptoms (44-48). Such observations result, in part, from research aimed at determining if the mammalian small intestinal lactase can adapt to the long-term ingestion of lactose. It appears that the mammalian lactase is a non-adaptable enzyme (44,49). However, incidental to these findings, researchers noted that both rodents and humans exhibit fewer symptoms of intolerance after "adapting" to a lactose-containing diet. Studies in rodents (50), chickens (51) and pigs (52,53) also show that the large intestine bacteria adapt to ongoing lactose-containing diets. Fecal microbial beta-galactosidase increases three to six-fold in such experiments. Concurrent with this increase in lactose-digesting capacity is a reduction in malabsorption symptoms. Whether this increased enzyme activity is due to induction in existing microbes or an alteration in the microbial population is not known.

In humans, Florent et al. (54) have completed elegant work showing similar adaptation to lactulose. Lactulose is a non-digestible disaccharide of fructose and galactose. Administration of 20g of lactulose twice per day for 8 days resulted in a six-fold increase in fecal beta-galactosidase activity, increased cecal ^{14}C-lactulose oxidation, lactic acid and SCFA production, and a reduction in breath hydrogen production. In a follow-up study (54), adaptation to lactulose resulted in slower transit times and reduced

incidence of diarrhea from a single lactulose load. Similar controlled studies with lactose-feeding have recently been reported by Arrigoni et al. (56), and Hertzler and Savaiano (57). In both reports, significant reductions in hydrogen production and increases in fecal beta-galactosidase activities were observed with adaptation to lactose, but improved symptom-response to a lactose load (as compared to sucrose or dextrose-feeding in the control periods) was not demonstrated following adaptation. Thus, the physiological relevance of colonic adaptation to lactose has not been clearly demonstrated.

Studies suggest that lactose digestion may improve during pregnancy (58) (when milk consumption might be increased) and worsen with aging (59) (when milk consumption might decline). The role of the large intestine bacteria in these reported adaptations is unknown. A recent comparison of adult and elderly Asian-American maldigesters (who consumed similar amounts of lactose in their daily diets) demonstrated little difference in the metabolism of lactose (60). Additional research is needed in order to determine if the intestinal bacteria hold the key to preventing the gastrointestinal intolerance symptoms that can occur in lactase-deficient persons.

REFERENCES

1. Simoons, F.J., Digestive Diseases 23(11):963-980, 1978.
2. Newcomer, A.D. and McGill, D.B., Clinical Nutrition 2(3):53-58, 1984.
3. Savaiano, D.A. and Levitt, M.D., J. Dairy Sci. 70:397-406, 1987.
4. Scrimshaw, N.S. and Murray, E.B., Amer. J. Clin. Nutr. 48(4):1083-1159, 1988.
5. Unger, M. and Scrimshaw, N.S., Nutr. Res. 1:227-233, 1981.
6. Leichter, J., Amer. J. Clin. Nutr. 26:393-396, 1973.
7. Pirk, F. and Scala, I., Digestion 5:89-99, 1972.
8. Welsh, J.D. and Hall, W.H., Dig. Dis. 22(12):1060-1063, 1977.
9. Solomons, N.W., et al., Amer. J. Clin. Nutr. 41:199-208, 1985.
10. Martini, M.C. and Savaiano, D.A., Amer. J. Clin. Nutr. 47:57-60, 1988.
11. Gallagher, C.R., et al., JADA 65:418-419, 1974.
12. Alm, L., J. Dairy Sci. 65:346-352, 1982.
13. Speck, M.L., J. Food Prot. 40(12):863-865, 1977.
14. Kilara, A. and Shahani, K.M., J. Dairy Sci. 59:2031-2035, 1976.
15. Goodenough, E.R. and Kleyn, D.H., J. Dairy Sci. 59(4):601-606, 1976.
16. Kolars, J.C., et al., NEJM 310(1):1-3, 1984.

17. Gilliland, S.E. and Kim, H.S., J. Dairy Sci. 67:1-6, 1984.

18. Savaiano, D.A. et al., Amer. J. Clin. Nutr. 40:1219-1223, 1984.

19. Martini, M.C. et al., Amer. J. Clin. Nutr. 45:432-436, 1987.

20. Martini, M.C. et al., Amer. J. Clin. Nutr. 46:636-640, 1987.

21. McDonough, F.E., et al., Amer. J. Clin. Nutr. 45:570-574, 1987.

22. Dewitt, O., et al., Nutrition 4(2):131-135, 1988

23. Rao, D.R., et al., Fed. Proc. 46:4035, 1987.

24. Dewitt, O., et al., J. Trop. Pediatr. 33:177-180, 1987.

25. Wytock, D.H. and DiPalma, J.A., Amer. J. Clin. Nutr. 47:454-457, 1988.

26. Marteau, P. et al., Brit. J. Nutr. 64:71-79, 1990.

27. Martini, M.C. and Savaiano, D.A., unpublished results.

28. Payne, D.L. et al., Amer. J. Clin. Nutr. 34:2711-2715, 1981.

29. Kim, H.S. and Gilliland, S.E., J. Dairy Sci. 66:959-966, 1983.

30. Newcomer, A.D., et al., Amer. J. Clin. Nutr. 38:257-263, 1983.

31. Lin, M-Y. et al., J. Dairy Sci. 74:87-95, 1991.

32. Premi, L., et al., Applied Microbiology 24(1):51-57, 1972.

33. Toba, T., et al., J. Dairy Sci. 64:185-192, 1981.

34. Gilliland, S.E., et al., J. Dairy Sci. 67:3045-3051, 1984.

35. Jones, D.V., et al., Amer. J. Clin. Nutr. 29:633-638, 1976.

36. Turner, S.J., et al., Amer. J. Clin. Nutr. 29:739-744, 1976.

37. Gudmand-Hoyer, E. and Simony, K., Amer. J. Dig. Dis. 22:623-625, 1977.

38. Iwasaki, T. and Kawanishi, G., In: milk intolerances and rejection, 1983.

39. Rosado, J.L., et al., Gastroenterology 87:1072-1082, 1984.

40. Solomons, N.W., et al., Amer. J. Clin. Nutr. 41:209-221, 1985.

41. Rosado, J.L., et al., J. Amer. Coll. Nutr. 5:281-290, 1986.

42. Barillas, C. and Solomons, N.W., Pediatrics 79:766-772, 1987.

43. Lin, M-Y., et al., Dig. Dis. Sci., in press.

44. Gilat, T., et al., Gastroenterology 62:1125-1127, 1972.

45. Reddy, V. and Pershad, J., Amer. J. Clin. Nutr. 25:114-119, 1972.

46. Habte, D., et al., Acta Paediatr. Scand. 62:649-654, 1973.

47. Latham, M.C., unpublished results, 1978, as reported by (4).

48. Sadre, M. and Karbasi, K., Amer. J. Clin. Nutr. 32:1948-1954, 1979.

49. Fisher, J.E., Amer. J. Physiol. 188:49-53, 1957.

50. Kim, K.I., et al., J. Nutr. 109:856-863, 1979.

51. Siddons, R.C. and Coates, M.E., Br. J. Nutr. 27:101-112, 1972.

52. Ekstrom, K.E., et al., J. Anim. Sci. 42(1):106-113, 1976.

53. Engstrom, M.A., et al., J. Anim. Sci. 48(6):1349-1356, 1979.

54. Florent, C., et al., J. Clin. Invest. 75:608-613, 1985.

55. Florent, C., et al., Gastroenterology 99(5):1417, 1986.

56. Arrigoni, E. et al. Gastroenterology 102:A197, 1992

57. Hertzler, S. and Savaiano D.A. FASEB J. 7:3 A583, 1993

58. Villar, J., et al., Obstet. Gynecol. 71:697-700, 1988.

59. Saltzberg, D.M., et al., Dig. Dis. Sci. 33(3):308-313, 1988.

60. Suarez, F. and Savaiano, D.A. FASEB J. 7:3 A583, 1993.

Dairy Products in Human Health and Nutrition, Serrano Ríos et al. (eds) © 1994 Balkema, Rotterdam, ISBN 90 5410 359 0

Milk based hypoallergenic infant formulas

J.C. Monti
Nestlé Research Centre, Lausanne, Switzerland

ABSTRACT: Cow milk infant formula with reduced allergenic potential can be obtained by a combination of enzymatic hydrolysis and heat treatments. Hypoallergenic formulas based on a whey protein hydrolysate have excellent nutritional quality and good organoleptic characteristics which allow their use during long periods for prevention of allergic disorders in newborns.

1 INTRODUCTION

Allergy to cow milk proteins was estimated to vary between 2-7% of the newborns according to Bock (1987). Sampson (1992) reported that the peak of food hypersensitivity occurs about 1 year of age rising to 3-4% of the population. The incidence of allergic manifestations is higher in the population "at risk" composed of babies having atopic relatives. Elemental diets and extensive protein hydrolysates have been used during the last 40 years for therapy of allergy to cow milk. These kinds of products are not convenient for use as prophylactic over a long period due to their particular biological properties and cost. In this paper we resume the technology applied in industry to obtain milk based hypoallergenic formulas destined to the prevention of allergy.

2 MILK PROTEINS AS A BASE FOR HYPOALLER-GENIC (HA) FORMULA

During the 70's the first adapted formulas were launched. In these products the ratio caseins/whey proteins, which is about 80/20 in cow's milk, was adapted to 30/70 or 40/60. These formulas have higher digestibility and nutritional value compared with dried cow's milk. In fact, the whey proteins have higher PER and NPU than caseins and vegetable proteins and no limiting amino acids (see Table 1).
Rigo (1989) compared the plasma amino acid composition of full-term newborn fed human milk, adapted formula or a whey hydrolysate based formula. The plasmatic amino acid profile of the infants fed with whey hydrolysate was close to that of the group fed

Table 1. Biological properties of protein from different origins. PER: Protein Efficiency Ratio; NPU: Net Protein Utilisation

PROTEIN	PER	NPU	LIMITING amino acid
CASEIN	100	77.3	methionine
WHEY	121	91.2	none
SOY	69	59	methionine
WHEAT	9,7	47.7	lysine, methionine

human milk, with the exception of the threonine concentration which was higher in this group. In addition to the nutritional value, other metabolic effects of the whey proteins have been demonstrated. In a recent study, Nagaoka (1991) determined in the rat the influence of the diet on the plasmatic concentration of cholesterol. The rats fed with whey proteins has a cholesterol level significantly lower than the animals fed caseins. Similar results were obtained with infants: four groups of newborns aged 4-8 weeks were nourished with human milk and artificial formulas in which the ratio caseins/whey proteins was 82/18, 66/34 and 50/50, the liquid composition being exactly the same. In this study Tseng (1990) showed that the group receiving the formula 82/18 had plasmatic cholesterol concentration significantly higher than the other groups. The triglycerides blood concentration was inversely proportional to the casein content. These results suggest that the concentrations

Table 2. Physicochemical characteristics of the main milk proteins. (*) Hydrolysis is efficient after heat denaturation of the protein. B-LG: B-Lactoglobulin, A-La: a-lactalbumin, BSA: bovine serum albumin, IgG: Immunoglobulins G.

CHARACTERISTIC	CASEINS	B-lg	A-LA	BSA	IgG
% on milk	0.3	0.3	0.15	0.04	0.05
% of total proteins	80	9	4	2	2
Suceptibility to heat denat.	low	high	medium	high	high
Suceptibility to hydrolysis	high	high	high	low(*)	low(*)

of cholesterol and triglycerides in the blood are influenced by the proteins independently of the lipid composition.

Taking into account the above mentioned reasons the protein composition of a baby formula, hypoallergenic or not, should be one in which whey proteins are predominant.

3 ANTIGENICITY/ALLERGENICITY REDUCTION BY INDUSTRIALLY APPLIED MEANS

Allergenicity of the individual cow milk proteins was extensively studied, the results being controversial. B-Lactoglobulin is the most abundant whey protein and it has not been found, so far, in human milk. Hambreus (1977) and Baldo (1984) reported this protein as the major cow's milk antigen. Many attempts were made in order to eliminate a "major" allergen of milk; for example Kuwata (1985) proposed a method to obtain a formula similar to human milk by elimination of the B-lactoglobulin. The procedure consisted of the precipitation of this protein by using iron chloride. This formula cannot be considered as hypoallergenic because the other milk proteins such as a-lactalbumin or immunoglobulin are also allergenics. In fact the allergenicity of a protein depends on multiple factors going from the individual susceptibility to "see" or not an antigenic site, the state (native, denatured, intact or not) of the protein, the presentation of the antigenic site, etc. The cumulation of the results of laboratory and challenge tests indicates that no individual protein can be considered as the major antigen as mentioned in a recent paper by Savilahti et all (1992) It was also demonstrated by Adams (1991) that there is a cross-reactivity between a-lactalbumin and B-lactoglobulin with human IgE.

There are roughly two kinds of antigenic sites in proteins: conformational epitopes related to the spatial structure and sequential epitopes related to the amino acid

sequence of the protein. Heat treatments lead to a relative decrease of allergenicity by "disruption" of the spatial structure of the proteins.

It is evident that this process is not efficient in decreasing the antigenicity of proteins such as caseins, which have a low degree of ordered structure (Table 2).

On the contrary, heat treatment could be an approach to decrease allergenicity of whey proteins like B-lactoglobulin or serumalbumin which have an ordered structure. Heppell (1984) suggested the obtention of an all whey hypoallergenic formula by heating the proteins at 100-115° C during at least 30 min. The heat treated whey failed to sensitize guinea-pigs when administered orally. Even if this kind of process is realistic on an industrial scale, it leads to a very important reduction of water solubility of the proteins and hence the in-vitro controls of the reduction in antigenicity of the product are very limited.

Enzymatic hydrolysis, which destroys conformational and sequential epitopes, is the one most realistic and industrial process to decrease protein antigenicity. The caseins that we stated above do not lose antigenicity by heat treatment but are easily hydrolysed by proteases. The susceptibility to hydrolysis of whey proteins is not equal for each one, B-lactoglobulin and a-lactalbumin are easily degraded by trypsin/chymotrypsin without preliminary heat denaturation (Jost et al, 1991). On the contrary, serumalbumin and immunoglobulin are not hydrolysed by the same enzymatic preparation without previous thermal denaturation.

The molecular weight of the peptides obtained by hydrolysis with trypsin/chymotrypsin is comprised between 500 and 1000 D. Poulsen et al (1978) demonstrated that peptides obtained by hydrolysis of whey proteins having a molecular weight below 1500 D exhibited very low allergenic potential as determined by the passive cutaneous anaphylaxis test in the rat.

Table 3. Flow sheet of the manufacture of HA formula according to patent: Jost et al. (1988). DWL: Demineralised whey liquid; DWP: Demineralised whey powder.

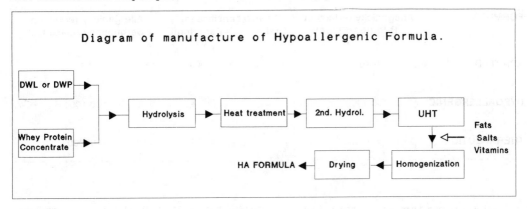

One can reduce the length of the peptides by using enzymes of broad specificity or enzyme mixtures. The specificity of the enzyme influences the organoleptic characteristics of the hydrolysate. Peptides having hydrophobic amino acids as C-terminal are generally bitter. Mercier et al (1972) proposed that the bitterness of a peptide can be predicted on the basis of the hydrophobicity of the amino acids. Related also with the length and amino acid composition of peptides is the stability of the fat emulsions. Jost and Monti (1982) showed that the peptides obtained by action of trypsin/chymotrypsin have significantly higher tensioactivity than the peptides obtained by the hydrolysis with non-specific proteases.

Resuming an industrially applicable process to obtain a hypoallergenic formula could be by the combination of hydrolysis of whey proteins and heat treatments.

A protein hydrolysate obtained by using a porcine trypsin preparation according to the process schematised above, was devoid of sensitisation capacity when administered orally to guinea pigs (Pahud et al 1985). To sensitise the animals it is necessary to administer this hydrolysate by the parental way.

The enzyme used during the process constitutes a new antigen. Heat inactivation destroys catalytic activity but only partially its allergenicity. The denatured enzyme must hence be eliminated by a separation process like ultrafiltration or, even better, by using temperature conditions which lead to the autodigestion of the protease.

4 QUALITY

Each batch of hydrolysate has to be controlled by physicochemical, immunochemical and immunological tests. Among the most currently used physicochemical methods we can mention electrophoresis and high pressure liquid chromatography.

Electrophoresis is used to detect the presence of intact proteins or large polypeptides in the range of ug/ml. The chromatographic methods are currently used to establish the peptide profiles of the hydrolysates.

With the immunochemical methods it is possible to quantify the residual antigenicity of a protein hydrolysate. These tests are the radioimmunoassay (RIA) or Enzyme linked immunosorbent assay (ELISA), which both have detection limits in the range of ng-pg of antigen. As shown in Table 4, the hypoallergenic formulas typically exhibit a reduction of antigenicity expressed, in this case, as equivalents of B-lactoglobulin comprised between 100 - 1000 times as compared with the unhydrolysed protein.

An in-vitro test which mimics an allergic reaction is the H3-serotonin release test using rat mast cells sensitised with antibodies directed towards the B-lactoglobulin as described by Fritsche (1990), who found that enzymatically hydrolysed milk formulas had 100 - 1000 times lower mast cell-triggering capacity than unhydrolysed protein (see Table 4).

5 ANIMAL TESTING

In view of their use in infant formulas the protein hydrolysates are tested on animal models to obtain an in vivo indication of the allergenicity reduction. Pahud et al (1985) tested a whey protein tryptic hydrolysate on a guinea pig model. The animals were fed with different cow's milk intact protein preparations which induced anaphylactic sen-

Table 4. Residual antigenicity and allergenicity of HA formula compared with an adapted and a therapeutic formula.

FORMULA	Antigenicity reduction B-Ig (RIA/ELISA)	In-vivo sensitisation Oral	Parenteral	Allergenicity reduction Serotonine release test
ADAPTED	5-10	+ +	+ +	1-10
HYPOALLERGENIC	100-1000	-	+	100-1000
THERAPEUTIC	> 10000	-	-	>100000

sitisation in more than 90% of the guinea pigs. The trypsin hydrolysed whey protein was devoid of sensitising capacity by oral way. The same hydrolysates have to be injected to induce sensitisation in animals (see Table 4).

6 CLINICAL TESTING

Concerning the biological value of whey hydrolysate based formulas, a clinical study showed that the weight gain curve of the new-borns fed with the hydrolysate was almost identical to the curve of the infants receiving mother's milk (Guesry et al 1991).
The same hydrolysate was tested by Chandra and Harmed (1991) on its ability to present atopic disorders in infants with a family history of atopic disease. The study showed a lower incidence of allergy in the groups fed hydrolysate or breast milk, compared with the groups receiving soy formula or cow milk.

7 CONCLUSION

Hypoallergenic formulas based on a partial hydrolysate of milk whey proteins prove to be efficient in the prevention of food allergy. The preventive effect is obtained by the use of the formula during 6 months or longer. This long period of use is almost unrealistic for the semi-elemental diets due to their poor organoleptic characteristics and their biological properties too far removed from the original proteins.

REFERENCES

Adams, S.L., Bardett, D., Walsh, R.J.H., Hill,D.J:, and Howden, M.E.H. 1991. Immunology and Cell Biology 691: 191-197

Baldo, B.A. 1984. Milk allergies. Australian Journal of Dairy Technology 27: 120-128
Bock, S.A. 1987. Prospective appraisal of complaints of adverse reactions to foods in children during the first 3 years of life. Pediatrics 79: 683-688
Chandra, R.K. and Hamed, A. 1991. Cumulative incidence of atopic disorders in high risk infants fed whey hydrolysate, soy, and conventional cow milk formulas. Annals of Allergy 67: 129-132
Fritsché, R. and Bonzon, M. 1990. Determination of cow milk formula allergenicity in the rat model by in vitro mast cell triggering and in vivo IgE induction. International Archives of Allergy and Applied Immunology 93: 289-293.
Guesry, P.R., Secretin, M.C., Jost, R., Pahud, J.J. and Monti, J.C. 1991. Milk formulae in the prevention of food allergy. Allergy Proceedings 12: 221-226
Hambraeus, L. 1977. Proprietary milk versus human breast milk. A critical approach from the nutritional point of view. Pediatrics Clinical North American 24: 17-25
Heppel, L.M.J., Cant, A.J. and Kilshaw, P.J. 1984. Reduction in the antigenicity of whey proteins by heat treatment. A possible strategy for producing and hypoallergenic infant formula. British Journal of Nutrition 51: 29-36
Høst, A. and Halken, S. 1990. A prospective study of cow milk allergy in Danish infants during the first 3 years of life. Allergy. 1990. 45: 587-596
Jost, R., Meister, N. and Monti, J.C. 1988. Procédé de préparation d'un hydrolysat de protéines et de lactosérum et d'un aliment hypoallergénique. European Patent 1988 No. 0 322 589 A1
Jost, R. 1988. Physicochemical treatment of food allergens: Application to cow's milk proteins. Food Allergy. Ed. by Reinhardt, D. and Schmidt, E. Nestlé Nutrition Workshop Series. Raven Press 17: 187-197

Jost, R. and Monti, J.C. 1982. Emulgateurs peptidiques obtenus par l'hydrolyse enzymatique partielle de la protéine sérique du lait. Le Lait. 617-618/619-620: 521-530

Jost, R., Monti, J.C. and Pahud, J.J. 1991. Reduction of whey protein allergenicity by processing. Nutritional and Toxicological Consequences of Food Processing. Edited by Friedman. Plenum Press, New York 23: 309-320

Kwata, T., Pham, A.M., Ma, C.Y. and Nakai, S. 1985. Elimination from whey to simulate human milk protein. Journal of Food Science 50: 605-609

Mercier, J.C., Grosdaude, F. and Ribadeau-Dumas, B. 1972. Primary structure of bovine caseins. A review. Milchwissenschaft 27: 402-408

Nagaoka, S., Kanamam, Y. and Kuzuya, Y. 1991. Effects of whey protein and casein on the plasma and liver lipids in rat. Agricultural and Biological Chemistry 55: 813-818

Pahud, J.J., Monti, J.C. and Jost, R. 1985. Allergenicity of whey proteins: its modification by tryptic in vitro hydrolysis of the protein. Journal of Pediatric Gastroenterology and Nutrition 4: 408-413

Poulsen, O.M. and Hau, J. 1987. Murine passive cutaneous analphylaxis for the all-or-none determination of allergenicity of bovine whey proteins and peptides. Clinical Allergy 17: 75-83

Rigo, J., Velroes, A. and Senterre, J. 1989. Plasma amino acid concentration in term infants fed human milk, a whey predominant formula, or a whey hydrolysate formula. Journal of Pediatrics 115: 752-755

Sampson, H.A. 1992. Food Allergy and the role of immunotherapy. Journal of Allergy and Clinical Immunology. 151-152

Savilahti, E. and Kuitunen, M. 1992. Allergenicity of cow milk proteins. The Journal of Pediatrics 121: 512-519

Tseng, E., Potter, S.M. and Picciano, M.F. 1990. Dietary proteins source and plasma lipid profiles of infants. Pediatrics 85: 548-552.

8 Calcium, osteoporosis and dairy products

Dairy Products in Human Health and Nutrition, Serrano Ríos et al. (eds) © 1994 Balkema, Rotterdam, ISBN 90 5410 359 0

Factors affecting bone metabolism and osteoporosis: Calcium requirements for optimal skeletal health in women

J.A. Kanis

Department of Human Metabolism and Clinical Biochemistry, University of Sheffield Medical School, UK

Summary. There is a great deal of uncertainty concerning the requirements of calcium for skeletal health. Some argue that all mixed diets contain sufficient calcium whereas others suggest that most of the world's population is calcium deficient. This paper reviews the sources of these conflicting views and the assumptions on which both are based.

Key words: Bone density – Bone resorption – Calcium, dietary – Osteoporosis.

The recommended daily allowances (RDA) of calcium for healthy women varies from country to country, ranging from 400 to 1500 mg daily [1]. The World Health Organization recommended an allowance of 400 to 500 mg daily [2], but this has been repeatedly challenged. Many consider a daily intake of 800 to 1000 mg is required to keep the young healthy population in skeletal balance for calcium [3–12]. The allowance recommended is higher in women after the menopause. It is a widely held view that the RDA should be 1000 mg in premenopausal and 1500 mg in postmenopausal women [6, 13–18]. This view is endorsed by many institutions concerned with osteoporosis, including prestigious bodies in both Europe and the USA [19–21].

A recent review and subsequent correspondence drew attention to the difficulties in interpreting the calcium requirements from epidemiological and balance studies [22, 23]. The authors of the review argue that most of the world's population consume less than 500 mg daily, and that there is little convincing evidence that countries with lower dietary intakes are disadvantaged in regard to osteoporosis. Indeed, they contend that calcium is sufficiently abundant in most mixed diets for arguments based on the RDA to be misleading and largely irrelevant to public health. This has been vigorously challenged by Nordin and Heaney [6] who defend an RDA of 1000 mg in young healthy adults, largely on the basis of the same evidence as reviewed by Kanis and Passmore [24].

These diametrically opposing views based on the same data must, to say the least, be confusing to uninformed readers. The purpose of this paper is to draw attention to the differences and examine their foundations. To understand them it is first necessary to review some aspects of bone remodelling in adult women and the ways in which these are disturbed in osteoporosis.

Bone Remodelling

In adults in whom longitudinal growth has ceased, more than 95% of the skeletal turnover is accounted for by remodelling of bone. Remodelling comprises a series of discrete events

well characterized morphologically but not well understood physiologically [25]. The process is important for self-repair of skeletal tissue. When remodelling is inhibited spontaneous fractures occur, presumably because of the inability of the skeleton to repair fatigue damage [26].

In the adult, bone is made up of cortical (or compact) tissue and trabecular (or spongy) bone. Approximately three-quarters of the skeleton is accounted for by cortical bone, the remainder by trabecular bone. Although trabecular bone accounts for a minority of skeletal mass, its surface to volume ratio is much higher than that of cortical bone. Since bone remodelling is surface-based, the metabolic activity of trabecular bone is ten times greater than that of cortical bone. The remodelling cascade (Fig. 1) is a highly ordered sequence of cellular events comprising a resorption phase whereby old bone is removed, followed by bone formation and mineralization. The phase involving osteoclast activation and osteoclastic bone resorption results in formation of a resorption (erosion) cavity. Mononuclear cells are found deep within resorption bays. This is presumed to represent a late event in the resorption sequence [27]. These cells may be responsible for the signals that ultimately attract osteoblasts to the sites of resorption (reversal phase). The attraction of osteoblasts to sites of resorption is termed coupling [28]. Coupling ensures that osteoblasts are attracted almost exclusively to sites of resorption, after which they synthesize an uncalcified osteoid matrix which undergoes mineralization several days later.

In the healthy adult who is neither gaining nor losing bone, the rate of bone resorption must equal the rate of new matrix formation and mineralization. Approximately 5 mmol of calcium is resorbed from bone daily. This is matched by deposition of an equal amount during bone formation. Thus, the net flow of calcium from bone to extracellular fluid attributable to bone remodelling is close to zero. At any one time approximately 10%–15% of bone surface is undergoing remodelling, the remaining surface being relatively quiescent.

It is important to recognize that accretion of calcium into bone occurs after matrix production, not before. Thus skeletal demands for calcium are governed by the rate of matrix synthesis rather than the other way round. If the skeletal demands for calcium are not met, then hypocalcaemia and defective mineralization of bone will follow. Thus low dietary intakes of calcium induce osteomalacia in mammals [29, 30], including man [31, 32]. The question arises whether low dietary intakes of calcium might decrease bone matrix synthesis in man. Most evidence suggests that this is not so, since calcium supplementation decreases rather than increases the turnover of bone [33]. This suggests that under normal conditions the skeletal requirements for calcium are governed by the rate of matrix synthesis, rather than by the availability of calcium.

It is nevertheless possible that severe calcium deficiency

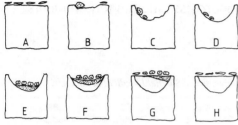

Fig. 1. Steps in the remodelling sequence of trabecular bone. Early in the remodelling sequence osteoclasts are attracted to a quiescent bone surface (a) and excavate a resorption cavity (b, c). Mononuclear cells smooth off the resorption cavity (d) which forms a site attracting osteoblasts, which synthesise an osteoid matrix (e). Continuous new bone matrix synthesis (f) is followed by calcification (g) of the newly formed bone. When complete, lining cells once more overlie the trabecular surface (h).

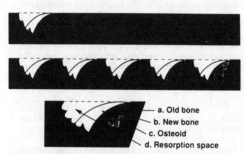

a. Old bone
b. New bone
c. Osteoid
d. Resorption space

Fig. 2. Effect of bone turnover on bone and calcium balance. Upper panel depicts normal bone remodelling activity occurring on 15% of the trabecular surface. Resorption space (d) occupies 2% of the bone volume, and a somewhat smaller amount is occupied by osteoid (1.5%) accounting for 3.5% of the bone volume. When bone turnover is increased fivefold (without affecting the balance between formation and resorption), the resorption space and osteoid space increase to 17.5% of bone volume. In addition, new bone formed at each site is not completely mineralized, increasing the mineral deficit so that trabecular density is decreased by 20%.

might decrease the rate of matrix synthesis in man. In longstanding hypoparathyroidism, hypocalcaemia can result in osteomalacia [34] but bone mass is characteristically not reduced. This is not, however, an adequate model of calcium deficiency since although serum concentrations and intestinal absorption of calcium are low, so too is the rate of bone remodelling. In growing animals severe privation of dietary calcium gives rise to osteoporosis [30], but the relevance of these observations to the more modest variations in dietary intakes in infancy, adolescence and young adulthood is not known.

Bone Remodelling and Skeletal Mass

Consideration of this remodelling process is important for understanding the relationships between the various aspects of skeletal balance and calcium requirements. In health and in a number of metabolic bone disorders there is a close quantitative relationship between the amount of bone formed and that lost by bone resorption. For example, in Paget's disease, where bone remodelling may be augmented as much as tenfold, skeletal balance is usually close to zero, indicating that the high rates of bone formation are accompanied by an equally high rate of bone resorption. In many metabolic bone disorders, including postmenopausal osteoporosis, accelerated rates of bone resorption are attributable to increased activation rates of osteoclastic bone resorption, so that at any one time more bone remodelling units are extant on bone surfaces, and a proportionately greater surface of bone is occupied by all the phases of bone remodelling.

An increase in the turnover of bone has several consequences. Since the process of bone remodelling implies a net deficit of bone (until resorption cavities are completely infilled), the skeletal volume missing at any one time will increase in proportion to the number of functional bone remodelling units (Fig. 2). This skeletal deficit, termed the resorption space, amounts to approximately 0.76% of total body calcium. On the basis of these considerations, Parfitt [25] has calculated that a fivefold increase in bone turnover would produce a negative balance of 30 g, or a decrease in total body bone volume of 3% under steady-state conditions.

A further consequence of increased skeletal remodelling relates to the turnover time of the skeleton. The amount of calcium normally removed by bone resorption is 250 mg daily, from a total body calcium of 1 kg. Thus, for the whole skeleton the average turnover time is 11 years, or 9% per annum. It is, however, much more rapid at trabecular sites than at cortical sites because of the higher surface activity of the former. If bone turnover is accelerated a proportionately greater amount of bone volume is occupied by young rather than old bone. In this regard, it is important to recognize that mineralization proceeds for many months after completion of the bone remodelling sequence. Thus the proportion of immature and incompletely mineralized bone will increase if turnover is increased, and result in a decrease in bone mineral content. A third consequence of increased remodelling is that the osteoid in the incompletely formed bone remodelling units at any one time is not mineralized. Thus the calcium space exceeds the resorption space by a small but fixed proportion.

For these three reasons the mineral content of bone may be profoundly influenced by changes in bone turnover. In the trabecular bone of the ilium, a fivefold increase in turnover would decrease the actual bone volume by 20% and the mineral content by a factor of almost two. This process is entirely reversible when bone turnover is decreased.

Transient and Steady States with Respect to Calcium Nutrition

In the healthy adult whose dietary calcium is decreased, the turnover of bone is increased because of an increase in activation frequency. Conversely, if high amounts of calcium are ingested bone remodelling is decreased. A great deal of circumstantial evidence suggests that the mechanism for this is related to hormonal changes in calcium metabolism. Thus during calcium depletion serum calcium tends to fall, which stimulates the secretion of parathyroid hormone and the synthesis of calcitriol. Parathyroid hormone may be the hormone responsible for the increased activation of bone remodelling. For the reasons outlined above it would be expected that a substantial decrease in calcium intake would be associated with a finite but reversible deficit in bone mineral content. Conversely, an increased intake of calcium would increase the net intestinal absorption of calcium. The small rise in plasma calcium would reduce parathyroid hormone secretion (and could increase that of calcitonin) [35] and thus the rate of bone turnover, giving rise to a small but finite increase in reversible bone mass. The reduction in parathyroid hormone secretion would be expected to reduce the synthesis of calcitriol and offset, to some extent, the effects of high dietary calcium levels.

For reasons explained elsewhere [33, 36] such changes in bone mineral content may take several years to be complete.

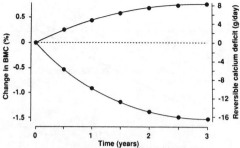

Fig. 3. Anticipated effects of doubling or halving bone remodelling in a young healthy adult on bone mineral content and on reversible calcium deficit. Reversible skeletal deficit of calcium resulting from changes in bone remodelling is based on a total body calcium of 1000g.

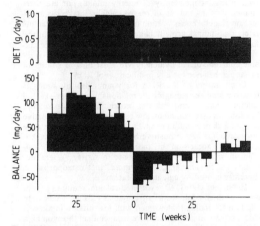

Fig. 4. Mean (± SEM) dietary calcium and calcium balance in healthy prisoners. Dietary calcium intake was decreased at time 0 when calcium balance became negative. Note the slow attenuation of negative calcium balance thereafter. (Data calculated from Malm [37].)

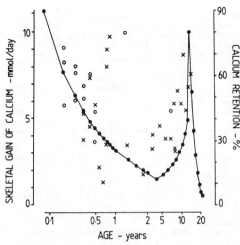

Fig. 5. Estimated daily skeletal gains of calcium females (solid circles) during growth (data from Mitchell (in 1939) [74]). Right ordinate shows the percentage of daily dietary intake of 500 mg that must be retained to ensure the maintenance of skeletal mass. Data points show observations from healthy children with high (x) or low (open circles; > 500 mg daily) intakes of calcium (data from the balance studies of Leitch (in 1937) [75]). Note the efficiency of calcium absorption of the age range shown, even on low calcium diets.

A view of the problem can be gained by examining the amount of calcium that must be retained for normal skeletal growth (Fig. 5). Peak requirements occur during the first month of life and during the adolescent growth spurt, when up to 400 mg of calcium may be retained daily. At other times, retention is much lower, less than 20 mg daily. Minimum skeletal requirements for calcium are dictated by these factors but actual requirements depend upon the amount in the diet, the efficiency of absorption and obligatory losses in the urine, faeces and sweat. The efficiency with which the body must retain calcium to cope with skeletal demands during growth may be computed for any dietary load and varies from 5%–80%. Children and young adults are usually capable of such adaptation [24] (Fig. 5).

These considerations suggest that changes in calcium nutrition during growth or in young adult women are associated with changes in bone remodelling and a small but reversible change in bone mineral content, of no clinical significance. Where then is the evidence that the requirement for calcium in healthy adults is 10–50 times greater than net skeletal gains of calcium? The evidence of a high requirement and its computation comes from epidemiological and from balance studies.

Requirements for Calcium in Healthy Young Women

A variety of epidemiological studies have shown an association between the life-time intake of calcium and either bone density or the risk of fracture in women [38–46]. However, many studies have shown no such association over a range of dietary intakes [47–58]. Which are we to believe? Is it right to ignore that half of the data which fails to satisfy a particular hypothesis [6]?

We must be suspicious of both conclusions and examine possible biases. A starting point is to ask what nutritional differences there were between populations. Answering this question is not straightforward since most studies omit such details. The most often cited and complete information avail-

It would be expected, therefore, that the calcium balance (intake minus total urinary, faecal and dermal excretion) would be negative for several years before the new equilibrium is attained (Fig. 3). Elegant studies by Malm [37] in healthy prisoners showed that calcium balance did indeed decrease. Over the ensuing year the balance for calcium became less negative. After a change in dietary calcium Malm's prisoners did not reach a new steady state of calcium balance even after 1 year or more of follow-up (Fig. 4; [24]). This indicates that it may take several years for a new steady state to be achieved. Adaptation may be associated with changes in major calcium regulating hormones. Not only are these responsible for the observed changes in bone remodelling rates, but they also regulate intestinal absorption of calcium to ensure that perturbations in extracellular concentrations of calcium are minimized.

The question arises whether in the healthy, and particularly in the developing skeleton, such adaptive mechanisms are adequate. Failure to adapt adequately to low dietary calcium would decrease the availability of calcium for the mineralization of bone.

Table 1. Nutritional and energy intakes (mean ± SD) in women from two Yugoslavian communities (100 in each group). Note the significant increase in energy intake in women taking the higher calcium diets despite the similarities in body weight. Data computed from Matkovic et al. 1979 [45]

	A High dietary calcium		B Low dietary calcium		A/B	P <
Calcium						
(mg/day)	876	± 280	395	± 276	2.22	0.001
Protein						
(g/day)	84.4 ±	19.5	56.9 ±	16.5	1.48	0.001
(kcal/day)	346 ±	80	233 ±	68	1.48	0.001
Fat						
(g/day)	92.6 ±	23.5	59.8 ±	21.2	1.55	0.001
(kcal/day)	861	± 219	556	± 197	1.55	0.001
Carbohydrate						
(g/day)	327	± 71	345	± 80	0.95	NS
(kcal/day)	1341	± 291	1415	± 328	0.95	NS
Body weight						
(kg)	68.8 ±	6.0	68.8 ±	6.0	1.00	NS
Total energy						
(kcal/day)	2548	± 539	2204	± 389	1.02	0.02
Waking energy						
expenditure						
(kcal/day)	2086	± 539	1742	± 389	1.20	0.02

Table 2. Calculated balance for calcium at ten levels of dietary intake

Calcium intake (mg/day)	Calcium balance (mg/day)				
	A	B	C	D	Mean ± SEM
100	− 30	− 100	0	− 90	− 33 ± 20
200	0	− 50	− 40	− 10	− 25 ± 12
300	− 40	− 10	− 60	+ 20	− 23 ± 18
400	− 20	− 40	− 60	− 20	− 35 ± 10
500	+ 20	− 40	0	− 30	− 13 ± 14
600	− 20	+ 50	+ 30	+ 40	25 ± 16
700	+ 60	+ 10	+ 50	+ 30	38 ± 11
800	+ 30	+ 30	+ 10	− 10	15 ± 10
900	0	− 10	+ 50	+ 40	20 ± 15
1000	0	+ 70	+ 20	+ 30	30 ± 15

able is that of Matkovic et al. [45] showing a relationship between calcium intake, bone mass and fracture from two communities in Yugoslavia. People of one community had a substantially higher calcium intake, greater bone mass and fewer femoral fractures. Evident in the paper but not commented on by the authors was the finding that where the calcium intake was higher, the energy intake was also higher (Table 1). The mean body weight in the two communities was identical. A lower energy intake in one population with a similar body weight to another indicates less physical activity in the former. Diminished activity is a well-recognized factor affecting skeletal mass. The data suggest that energy expenditure was 20% greater (assuming no difference in basal metabolic rate) between the communities in subjects with higher dietary intakes for calcium. This greater energy expenditure is equivalent to the activities of a blacksmith or a stone mason for 1 h daily, or to a daily 3-mile walk. A few studies have taken activity or energy expenditure into account, and they have shown a significant and independent relationship between calcium intake and bone density [40, 44, 59]. Although these studies are limited by their cross-sectional nature, it is important that the differences in the skeletal mass between subjects with high and low intakes of calcium are trivial, and readily accounted for by differences in the reversible calcium space.

There are no prospective controlled studies to show

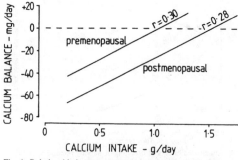

Fig. 6. Relationship between external balance and dietary intake of calcium in 207 untreated premenopausal and 41 untreated postmenopausal women. (Data from Heaney et al. [63].)

whether or not an increase in calcium intake increases peak bone mass independently of energy intake, nor are there studies showing that an increased calcium intake has an effect on skeletal consolidation or subsequent risk of fracture after longitudinal growth has ceased. These facts suggest that global recommendations concerning the RDA for calcium should not be made on the basis of the presently available epidemiological evidence. We must turn to studies of metabolic balance for any justification of RDA.

Computation of the RDA for young, healthy adults is based on studies examining the relationship between skeletal calcium balance and calcium intake. Many investigators have shown that women on low calcium diets are in negative calcium balance and, conversely, that women who consume large amounts are in positive balance [60–67]. The investigators have argued on this basis that the availability of calcium in many women is inadequate to satisfy skeletal demands for calcium and, furthermore, that osteoporosis is therefore caused by calcium deficiency.

Heaney et al. [61, 62] estimated calcium requirements in many healthy adult women from such balance studies. In addition to finding that women with low dietary intakes of calcium were in greater negative balance than those on high dietary calcium intakes, they noted a positive correlation between calcium intake and balance (Fig. 6). The intercept of the regression showed that requirements in women before the menopause were of the order of 1 g, and even greater in postmenopausal women.

The calculation of dietary requirements from balance studies in this way is a statistical artefact and this type of evidence that should no longer be forwarded to promote the view that large dietary intakes of calcium are required to maintain skeletal health. Some theoretical balance studies are presented in Table 2 in relation to forty cases where the dietary intake ranged from 100 to 1000 mg daily, in increments of 100 mg. Calcium balances were computed from differences between dietary intakes and total excretion of calcium. The total excretion of calcium was randomly selected under double-blind conditions by four investigators. Ten randomly chosen dietary assessments were randomly matched with 10 estimates of calcium output by each investigator. There was a highly significant positive correlation between calcium intake and balance in all 40 cases studied (Fig. 7; $r = 0.63$; $P < 0.001$). The mean requirement for calcium is normally computed from where the regression line describing this relationship intercepts with zero balance. The calcium intake in this example at zero balance was 550 mg daily. The RDA on the basis of the 95% confidence interval of this regression was 1300 mg daily.

The correlation between dietary intake and balance is an inevitable consequence of plotting the two dependent variables [68]. The artefact arises because calcium intake is used

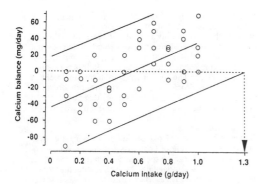

Fig. 7. Relationship between calcium balance and calcium intake for 40 randomly chosen dietary intakes matched to random excretion values. Diagonal lines describe the mean relationship of the regression with 95% confidence intervals.

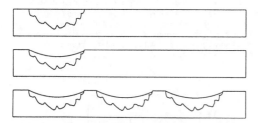

Fig. 8. Schematic representation of a trabecular bone surface to illustrate the effect of balance and remodelling on the rate of bone loss. Top panel shows infilling of a resorption bay with an equal volume of new bone. In osteoporosis less bone is deposited in resorption cavities (centre). If bone turnover is increased without altering this balance (lower panel), the rate of trabecular bone loss will increase in proportion to the increment in bone turnover.

in both sides of the equation (balance equals intake minus excretion). When dietary intake is high, a randomly chosen value for excretion is likely by chance to be low and the balance positive. Conversely, when intake is low, a randomly chosen value for excretion is likely to be higher, and the balance for calcium negative. Treating intake and balance as independent leads to spurious correlations. Such considerations suggest that the conclusions of all studies computing requirements from balance may be seriously flawed.

Skeletal disease in the context of osteoporosis implies fracture and, as mentioned previously, several epidemiological studies have shown an association between dietary intake of calcium and the risk of fracture. There is also an association between grey hair and hip fracture but this should not necessarily be taken as evidence that dyeing the hair will beneficially affect the natural history of fracture. The real problem lies in establishing the causality or otherwise of the relationships. The strength of attributing causality or otherwise depends in part on the plausibility of the association. This is weak in the case of advocating hair dye for the management of osteoporotic fracture but stronger in the case of calcium. The possible protective role of physical activity, however, emerges from all epidemiological data [48, 57, 58, 69, 70], and is certainly more plausible than that of calcium or hair dye. The RDA of young healthy women is therefore unknown, and recommendations should await the outcome of adequately controlled prospective studies outlined elsewhere [24].

Skeletal Metabolism after the Menopause

There is a great deal of evidence to indicate that osteoporosis is a disorder of bone remodelling. As previously discussed, the term coupling is used for the attraction of osteoblasts to sites of previous resorption. In osteoporosis, coupling appears to be intact. The progressive decrease in bone mass arises from an imbalance between the amount of mineral and matrix removed and that subsequently incorporated into each resorption cavity, so that skeletal mass decreases progressively. In postmenopausal and other types of osteoporosis there is evidence to suggest that the imbalance between

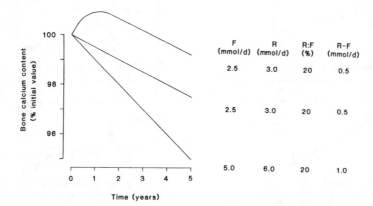

Fig. 9. Effects of altering bone turnover in osteoporosis. Relationship between bone mineral content with time is shown for a patient losing 1% of bone mass per year because of an imbalance of bone at remodelling sites. In terms of calcium flows, more calcium is resorbed (r; 6 mmol/day) than formed (f; 5 mmol/day), with a net deficit of 1 mmol/day, representing a skeletal loss of 1% per annum. If bone turnover is halved without altering the imbalance between the amounts formed and resorbed, the rate of bone loss is halved. Administration of calcium and inhibition of bone resorption permits continued formation at pre-existing resorption sites so that bone mineral content increases to fill in this resorption space. When bone formation decreases to match the prevailing rate of bone resorption, bone loss will occur once more, but at a slower rate than before treatment.

the amount of bone resorbed and that formed at each remodelling site arises from a decrease in the functional capacity of osteoblasts or in the recruitment of osteoblasts to previous resorption sites.

Irrespective of the mechanism, a finite deficit of bone is the end result of each remodelling sequence. If bone turnover is increased the number of bone remodelling units

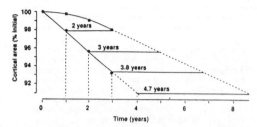

Fig. 10. Effect of pharmacological doses of calcium (1.5 g daily) in women after a surgical menopause. This 3-year placebo controlled study indicates that calcium significantly reduces the rate of bone loss. Dotted lines indicate the changes expected, assuming that a steady state has been reached. Solid horizontal lines denote the extent of the preservation of skeletal age with this pharmacological manipulation. (Data from Stepan et al. [71].)

present at any one time also increases. If the imbalance at each site remains constant, the result of increasing bone turnover will be to amplify the rate of bone loss (Fig. 8). There is now good evidence that oestrogen deficiency not only induces an imbalance at remodelling sites, but also increases the remodelling rate of bone [63]. In this way, bone loss is accelerated. The role of calcium in the treatment of established osteoporosis appears to arise from its ability to decrease bone turnover [5]. It seems likely that this is related to small increments in serum calcium and resulting decreases in the activation of bone turnover in much the same way as seen in younger women.

It would be expected that inhibition of bone turnover would decrease the rate of bone loss but not prevent it entirely. The reason for this expectation is related to the effect of calcium on bone remodelling. At each remodelling site a finite volume of bone is resorbed. In osteoporosis a somewhat lesser amount is formed. In terms of calcium transport, approximately 6 mmol of calcium are resorbed daily and 5 mmol put back by low formation in the several million remodelling sites This gives rise to a net deficit of 1 mmol of calcium per day (equivalent to bone loss of approximately 1% per annum). When bone turnover alone is decreased the number of remodelling sites also decreases, but the imbalance between formation and resorption at each remodelling site persists. Thus, if bone turnover were decreased by 50%, bone loss would be reduced from 1% to 0.5% per annum.

A number of observations have shown that calcium supplements may be associated with maintenance of or even an increase in skeletal mass but this is modest (2%–10% de-

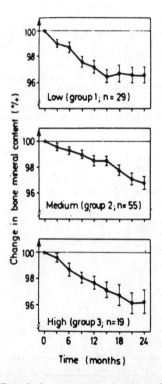

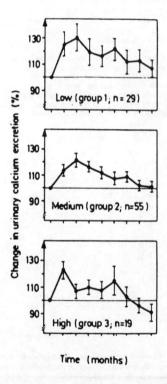

Fig. 11. Effects of a dietary supplement of calcium on forearm bone mineral and 24-h urinary excretion of calcium in postmenopausal women (mean ± SEM). The women were subdivided according to total daily calcium intake. Note the substantial increase in 24-h urinary excretion shortly after the start of treatment, an effect attenuated with continued treatment. Bone loss continued, indicating that osteoporotic women can adapt to changes in dietary intake but such adaptation, as in healthy males, takes several years to complete. (From Nilas et al. [52].)

pending on the site measured) and not sustained. The reason for the transient increase in bone mass is decreased activation of new remodelling sites. During the early stages of treatment bone formation continues at existing remodelling sites and bone mass increases transiently to fill in resorption space (Fig. 9). Since turnover is slow, the transient state can persist for up to 3 years. Recent studies of calcium supplements suggests that this is so [71] (Fig. 10).

Attainment of a new steady state after calcium treatment is very similar to the adaptation of young adults to changes in dietary intake. The process is slow and takes several years to be complete. If adaptation were complete, it would be expected that intestinal absorption of calcium would decrease, and that the increment in absorbed calcium would decrease with time. This is what is observed in prospective studies (Fig. 11), indicating that postmenopausal women are at least capable of adapting to increments in dietary intake.

The difference in adaptation between pre- and postmenopausal women is that in the latter bone loss persists but at a lower rate, since the balance of resorption and formation at remodelling sites remains unchanged. This imbalance which results from oestrogen deficiency is not reversed by calcium. In contrast, bone loss is completely halted by oestrogen by correcting of imbalance and thereby preserving bone mass, irrespective of when it is given after surgical castration or the menopause.

This and evidence reviewed elsewhere [22] suggests that calcium supplements can decrease the rate of bone loss in postmenopausal women. It should not be argued, however, that osteoporosis represents a calcium deficiency disease [5, 6, 64]. Although skeletal calcium losses are clearly attenuated by pharmacological manipulation of bone turnover, this argues that calcium deficiency causes osteoporosis only in the same sense that penicillin deficiency causes streptococcal infection. It is perhaps more appropriate to consider both as effective pharmacological interventions rather than causes of disease. The major cause of postmenopausal bone loss is oestrogen deficiency. A great deal of evidences suggests that the administration of oestrogens prevents this loss.

There are some analogies between calcium deficiency in osteoporosis and iron deficiency anaemia in chronic gastrointestinal bleeding. Chronic bleeding results in anaemia which is, in part, reversible by the administration of iron. In the same way, gonadal failure results in skeletal calcium loss. We should not, on this basis, argue that iron deficiency causes gastrointestinal bleeding, nor can iron stop bleeding, even though it is well recognized that supplementary iron reduces anaemia. In the same way, calcium deficiency does not cause osteoporosis, nor does it reverse the process, even though rates of bone loss can be attenuated.

For all these reasons, there is clearly a place for calcium supplementation for postmenopausal women at risk of osteoporosis. The rationale depends upon the assumption that a decrease in rate of bone loss decreases the risk of osteoporotic fracture. This is likely but is nevertheless a conclusion that is inferential. The interpretation of the only studies [72, 73] directly examining the effects of calcium on fracture rates is fatally flawed [36], and we must await the outcome of adequately designed prospective studies.

Acknowledgments. I am grateful to the Medical Research Council and to Rorer Central Research for their support. I thank Drs. S Adami, P Delmas, I Fogelman and M Kleerekoper for randomly and blindly selecting values for "dietary intake" and "total excretion of calcium" in the hypothetical balance studies.

References

1. Truswell AS, Irwin T, Beaton GH, et al. (1983) Recommended dietary intake around the world. Nutr Abstr Rev 53:939–1015
2. Food and Agricultural Organization and World Health Organization (1962) Calcium requirements. WHO Tech Rep Ser No 230
3. Heaney RP, Gallacher JC, Johnston CC, Neer R, Parfitt AM, Whedon GD (1982). Calcium nutrition and bone health in the elderly. Am J Clin Nutr 36:986–1013
4. Heaney RP (1982) Calcium intake, requirement and bone mass in the elderly. J Lab Clin Med 100:309–312
5. Nordin BEC, Morris HA (1989) The calcium deficiency model for osteoporosis. Nutr Rev 47:65–72
6. Nordin BEC, Heaney RP (1990) Calcium supplementation of the diet: justified by the present evidence. Br Med J 300:1056–1059
7. Anderson JJB (1990) Dietary calcium and bone mass through the life cycle. Nutr Today 25:9–14
8. Barrett-Connor E (1989) The RDA for calcium in the elderly: too little too late. Calcif Tissue Int 44:303–307
9. Dixon SJA (1980) Non-hormonal treatment of osteoporosis. Br Med J 286:999–1000
10. Epstein O (1987) The role of calcium in the prevention of osteoporosis. Int Med 12 (Suppl):30–32
11. Robinson CJ (1987) The importance of calcium intake in preventing osteoporosis. Int Med 12 (Suppl):28–29
12. Simonen O (1986) Osteoporosis: a big challenge to public health. Calcif Tissue Int 39:295–296
13. Heaney RP (1990) Calcium. In: Kanis JA (ed) Progress in basic and clinical pharmacology. Karger, Basel, pp 28–54
14. Avioli LV (1989) Calcium and the recommended allowance. Triangle 28 (Suppl 1):29–32
15. Nordin BEC, Need AG (1989) The rationale for calcium therapy in the prevention and treatment of osteoporosis. Triangle 28 (Suppl 1):49–56
16. Francis RM (1989) Calcium's role in preventing and treating osteoporosis. Geriatr Med 19:24–26
17. Johnson F, Francis RM (1989) Effective management of established osteoporosis. Geriatr Med 19:45–52
18. Riggs BL (1986) Involutional osteoporosis. N Engl J Med 314:1676–1686
19. Anonymous (1984) Osteoporosis Consensus Conference. National Institutes for Health. JAMA 252:799–802
20. National Osteoporosis Society (1990) Calcium. In: Recommended daily allowance. NOS Publication, Bath
21. Swedish National Board of Health and Welfare (1989) Prophylaxis and treatment of osteoporosis. In: Osteoporosis: pharmacological treatment and prophylaxis. Swedish National Board of Health and Welfare, Uppsala, pp 111–118
22. Kanis JA, Passmore R (1989) Calcium supplementation of the diet. Br Med J 298:137–140, 205–208, 673–674
23. Stevenson JC (1989) Calcium supplementation of the diet. Br Med J 298:1034
24. Kanis JA, Passmore R (1990) Calcium supplementation of the diet. Br Med J 300:1523
25. Parfitt AM (1983) the physiologic and clinical significance of bone histomorphometric data. In: Recker R (ed) Bone histomorphometry techniques. CRC Press, Boca Raton, Florida, pp 143–223
26. Frost HM (1960) Presence of microscopic cracks in vivo in bone. Henry Ford Hosp Bull 8:25–35
27. Baron R, Vignery A, Horowitz M (1983) Lymphocytes, macrophages and the regulation of bone remodelling. In: Peck WA (ed) Bone and mineral research annual. Elsevier, Amsterdam, pp 175–184
28. Kanis JA (1985) Osteoporosis. In: Butler WT (ed) The chemistry and biology of mineralised tissues. EBSCO Media, Birmingham, Alabama, pp 398–407
29. Pettifor JM, Marie PJ, Sly MR, du Bruyn DB, Ross F, Isdale JM, de Klerk WA, van der Walt WH (1984) The effect of differing dietary calcium and phosphorus contents on mineral metabolism and bone histomorphometry in young vitamin D-replete baboons. Calcif Tissue Int 36:668–676
30. Kalu DN, Masoro EJ (1990) Undernutrition as a modulator of general and bone aging in the rat. In: Simmons DJ (ed) Nutrition and bone development. Oxford University Press, Oxford New York, pp 93–113
31. Cundy TC, Kanis JA, Heynen G, Earnshaw M, Clemens TL, O'Riordan JL, Merrett AL, Compston JE (1982) Failure to heal vitamin D-deficient rickets and suppress secondary hyperparathyroidism with conventional doses of 1,25-dihydroxyvitamin D$_3$. Br Med J 284:883–885
32. Kooh SW, Fraser D, Reilly B, Hamilton JR, Gall DG, Bell L (1977) Rickets due to calcium deficiency. N Engl J Med 297:1264–1266
33. Parfitt AM (1980) Morphological basis of bone mineral measurements: transient and steady state effects of treatment in osteoporosis. Miner Electrolyte Metab 4:273–287

34. Nagant de Deuxchaisnes C, Krane SM (1978) Hypoparathyroidism. In: Avioli LV, Krane SM (eds) Metabolic bone disease. Academic Press, New York, pp 218–445
35. Nordin BEC, Marshall DH (1988) Dietary requirements for calcium. In: Nordin BEC (ed) Calcium in human biology. Springer, Berlin, pp 447–471
36. Kanis JA (1984) Treatment of osteoporotic fracture. Lancet i:27–33
37. Malm OJ (1958) Calcium requirement and adaptation in adult men. Scand J Clin Lab Invest 10 (Suppl 36)
38. Yano K, Heilbrun LK, Wasnich RD, Hankin JH, Vogel JM (1985) The relationship between diet and bone mineral content of multiple skeletal sites in elderly Japanese-American men and women living in Hawaii. Am J Clin Nutr 42:877–888
39. Hansen MA, Overgaard K, Riis BJ, Christiansen C (1991) Potential risk factors for development of postmenopausal osteoporosis examined over a 12 year period. Osteopor Int 1 (in press)
40. Anderson JJB, Tylavsky FA (1984) Diet and osteopenia in elderly caucasian women. In: Christiansen C, Arnaud CD, Nordin BEC, Parfitt AM, Peck WA, Riggs BL (eds) Osteoporosis. Glostrup Hospital, Copenhagen, pp 299–303
41. Nordin BEC (1966) International patterns of osteoporosis. Clin Orthop 45:17–30
42. Holbrook TL, Barrett-Connor E, Wingard DL (1988) Dietary calcium intake and risk of hip fracture: 14 year prospective population study. Lancett ii:1046–1049
43. Kamiyama S, Kobayashi S, Abe S, Takahashi E, Wakamatsu E, Kurashina S (1972) Osteoporosis prevalence and nutritional intake among the people in farm, fishing and urban districts. Tohoku J Exp Med 107:387–394
44. Kanders B, Dempster DW, Lindsay R (1988) Interaction of calcium nutrition and physical activity on bone mass in young women. J Bone Miner Res 3:145–149
45. Matkovic V, Kostial K, Simonovic I, Buzina R, Broderec A, Nordin BEC (1979) Bone status and fracture rates in two regions of Yugoslavia. Am J Clin Nutr 32:540–549
46. Sandler RB, Slemendra CW, LaPorte RE (1985) Postmenopausal bone density and milk consumption in childhood and adolescence. Am J Clin Nutr 42:270–274
47. Van Beresteijn ECH, van t'Hof MA, de Waard H, Raymakers JA, Duursma SA (1990) Relation of axial bone mass to habitual calcium intake and to cortical bone loss in healthy early postmenopausal women. Bone 11:7–13
48. Cooper C, Barker DJP, Wickham C (1988) Physical activity, muscle strength and calcium intake in fracture of the proximal femur in Britain. Br Med J 297:1443–1445
49. Donath A, Indermuhle P, Baud R (1975) Influence of the national calcium and fluoride supply and of a calcium supplementation on bone mineral content of health population in Switzerland. Proceedings of an international Conference on Bone Mineral Measurement. Department of Health, Education and Welfare, Washington, DE, p 67
50. Garn SM, Rohmann CG, Wagner B, Davila GH, Ascoli W (1969) Population similarities in the onset and rate of adult endosteal bone loss. Clin Orthop 65:51–60
51. Hegsted DM (1967) Mineral intake and bone loss. Fed Proc 26:1747–1754
52. Nilas L, Christiansen C, Rodbro P (1984) Calcium supplementation and postmenopausal bone loss. Br Med J 289:1103–1106
53. Riggs BL, Wahner HW, Melton LJ, Richelson LS, Judd HL, O'Fallon WM (1987) Dietary calcium intake and rates of bone loss in women. J Clin Invest 80:979–982
54. Smith RW, Frame B (1965) Concurrent axial and appendicular osteoporosis. Its relation to calcium consumption. N Engl J Med 273:73–78
55. Smith RW, Rizek J (1966) Epidemiological studies of osteoporosis in women of Puerto Rico and Southwest Michigan with special reference to age, race, nationality and other associated findings. Clin Orthop 45:31–48
56. Stevenson JC, Whitehead MI, Padwick M, Endocott JA, Sutton C, Banks LM, Freemantle C, Spinks TJ, Hesp R (1988) Dietary intake of calcium and postmenopausal bone loss. Br Med J 297:15–17
57. Stevenson JC, Lees B, Cust MP, Ganger KF (1989) Determinants of bone density in normal women: risk factors for future osteoporosis. Br Med J 298:924–928
58. Wickham CAC, Walsh K, Cooper C, Barker DJP, Margetts BM, Morris J, Bruce SA (1989) Dietary calcium, physical activity and risk of hip fracture: a prospective study. Br Med J 299:889–992
59. Kelly PJ, Pocock NA, Sambrook PN, Eisman JA (1990) Dietary calcium, sex hormones and bone mineral density in man. Br Med J 300:1361–1364
60. Harrison M, Fraser R, Mullan B (1961) Calcium metabolism in osteoporosis. Lancet i:1015–1019
61. Heaney RP, Recker RR, Saville PD (1977) Calcium balance and calcium requirement in middle aged women. Am J Clin Nutr 30:1603–1611
62. Heaney RP, Recker RR, Saville PD (1977) Menopausal changes in calcium balance performance. J Lab Clin Med 92:953–963
63. Heaney RP, Recker RR, Saville PD (1978) Menopausal changes in bone remodelling. J Lab Clin Med 92:964–970
64. Nordin BEC (1960) Osteoporosis and calcium deficiency. Proc Nutr Soc 19:129–137
65. Nordin BEC (1976) Nutritional considerations. In: Nordin BEC (ed) Calcium, phosphate and magnesium metabolism. Churchill Livingston, Edinburgh, pp 1–35
66. Nordin BEC, Polley KJ, Need AG, Morris HA, Marshall D (1987) The problem of calcium requirement. Am J Clin Nutr 45:1295–1304
67. Whedon GD (1959) Effects of high calcium intakes on bone, blood and soft tissue: relationship of calcium intake to balance in osteoporosis. Fed Proc 18:1112–1118
68. Cochran WG (1939) Long term agricultural experiments. J R Statist Soc 6 (Suppl):104
69. Cahalmers J, Ho KC (1970) Geographical variations in senile osteoporosis. J Bone Joint Surg 52B:667–675
70. Smith EL, Raab DM (1986) Osteoporosis and physical activity. Acta Med Scand 711 (Suppl):149–156
71. Stepan JJ, Pospichal J, Presl J, Pacovsky V (1989) Hydroxyapatite compound in surgically induced postmenopausal women. Bone 10:179–185
72. Nordin BEC, Horsman A, Crilly RG, Marshall DH, Simpson M (1980) Treatment of spinal osteoporosis in postmenopausal women. Br Med J 280:451–454
73. Riggs BL, Seeman E, Hodgson SF, Taves DR, O'Fallon WM (1982) Effect of the fluoride/calcium regimen on vertebral fracture occurrence in postmenopausal osteoporosis. Comparison with conventional therapy. N Engl J Med 306:446–450
74. Mitchell HH (1939) The dietary requirements of calcium and its significance. Actualités scientifiques et industrielles 18. Hermann and Company, Paris.
75. Leitch I (1937) The determination of the calcium requirements of man. Nutr Abstr Rev 6:553–578

Dairy Products in Human Health and Nutrition, Serrano Ríos et al. (eds) © 1994 Balkema, Rotterdam, ISBN 90 5410 359 0

The importance of Vitamin D for the prevention of osteoporosis

L.H.Allen

Department of Nutritional Sciences, University of Connecticut, Storrs, Conn., USA

ABSTRACT: The vitamin D status of older individuals is often poor, because of low intakes, inadequate exposure to ultraviolet radiation, and age-related changes in metabolism. Vitamin D deficiency induces PTH-stimulated bone resorption and adversely affects intestinal calcium absorption. In many studies, an increase in dietary or supplemental vitamin D has been effective in reducing bone loss of the elderly.

1 INTRODUCTION.

In this article we review current information concerning the role of vitamin D in the development of osteoporosis. Because of the focus of this symposium, most attention will be paid to the importance of adequate vitamin D status for the prevention of osteoporosis and for reducing bone loss in the elderly.

2 THE ROLE OF VITAMIN D IN CALCIUM ABSORPTION.

The process of calcium absorption is primarily regulated by the vitamin D endocrine system (Norman, 1990). In this system, vitamin D precursors are synthesized in the skin, or vitamin D is consumed in the diet. In the liver, cholecalciferol is hydroxylated to 25-hydroxycholecalciferol (25(OH)D), which can be regarded as the "storage" form of the vitamin in so far as serum levels are a reasonable reflection of vitamin D status. The kidney plays a central role in producing and regulating the synthesis of the two most important vitamin D metabolites. These are 1,25-dihydroxyvitamin D (1,25(OH)$_2$D) and 24,25 dihydroxyvitamin D (24,25(OH)$_2$D), produced from 25(OH)D by hydroxylase enzymes in the mitochondria and proximal tubules of the kidney. These enzymes are similar to other steroid hydroxylases and contain cytochrome P-450.

Many other vitamin D metabolites have been identified, but for the present discussion 1,25(OH)$_2$D$_3$ is the most important because it is the primary regulator of intestinal calcium absorption. Receptors for this hormone have been identified in the intestine, bone and kidney, as well as in many other organs where the hormone has functions ranging from regulation of the immune system to hormone synthesis.

At the intestinal level, vitamin D is necessary for the active transport of calcium. Cells in the duodenum and upper duodenum have vitamin D receptors in the cytoplasm and nucleus, which form a 1,25(OH)$_2$D$_3$-receptor complex. This complex interacts with genes in the nucleus so that new mRNA is produced that codes for a calcium-binding protein (CaBP, or calbindin). Calbindin probably helps to recognize calcium at the brush border of the intestinal cell, and in the absorptive process is internalized with the calcium by endocytosis.

In states of calcium deficiency, it is the vitamin D-dependent active transport system that responds by increasing the calcium absorptive efficiency of the intestine. Low serum calcium stimulates the synthesis of more parathyroid hormone (PTH), which in turn stimulates the renal 25(OH)D$_3$-1-hydroxylase to produce more 1,25(OH)$_2$D$_3$ from 25(OH)D$_3$. The higher levels of 1,25(OH)$_2$D$_3$ cause the production of more CaBP and hence promote the absorption of calcium. Conversely, in vitamin D deficiency, the synthesis of CaBP is markedly impaired so that the active transport of calcium is lower. Thus, adequate vitamin D status is crucial for the efficient absorption of dietary calcium by the active transport process. In addition, 1,25(OH)$_2$D$_3$ also stimulates calcium absorption by a non-genomic, "transcaltachia-mediated" process which appears to be involved with the minute-to-minute regulation of calcium uptake by the intestinal cells (Norman, 1990).

3 THE ROLE OF VITAMIN D IN BONE METABOLISM.

In addition to its indirect effects on bone through regulation of calcium absorption, 1,25(OH)$_2$D$_3$ acts directly on osteoblasts to stimulate osteocalcin synthesis. It also acts on osteoclasts to stimulate bone resorption (DeLuca, 1990). While severe vitamin D deficiency (i.e. serum 25(OH)D below 7 ng/mL) produces osteomalacia, milder vitamin D deficiency induces parathyroid-stimulated bone remodeling and osteoporosis, rather than osteomalacia (Parfitt 1983, Gallagher 1992). It is not known to what extent the benefits of improving vitamin D status act through a direct effect of the vitamin on bone, as well as on intestinal calcium absorption.

4 RISK FACTORS FOR VITAMIN D DEFICIENCY.

In general, serum 25(OH) concentrations provide the best estimate of vitamin D status. When these levels fall below approximately 25-30 ng/mL, but not above this, supplementation produces higher levels of $1,25(OH)_2D_3$ (Francis et al. 1983, Lawoyin et al. 1980, Zerwekh et al. 1983).

Low serum 25(OH)D levels occur quite frequently in the elderly, usually occurring more commonly than in younger individuals. In Missouri, levels were low in about 10% of healthy women, age 52-77 years (Villareal et al. 1991). In New Mexico, a southern state of the USA, values for a group of elderly (60 to 93 years) were 40% of those with a mean age of 32 years (Omdahl et al. 1982). In The Netherlands, 35% of residents in an aged people's home and a nursing home (men and women, mean age slightly over 80 years) had deficient levels, and an additional 44% had marginal levels (Lips et al. 1988). In Switzerland, where neither dairy products or margarine are fortified, between the ages of 25 and 74 years 6% of the population was vitamin D deficient and 34-95% had a relatively low concentration of 25(OH)D (Burnand et al. 1992). However, in this population aging did not affect serum levels of the metabolite.

As discussed below, Vitamin D deficiency usually results from a combination of low dietary intake of the vitamin and one or more environmental or biological factors that impairs vitamin D status. Table 1 provides a summary of the risk factors for vitamin D deficiency in the elderly. The most common causes of low 25(OH)D concentration in serum are low dietary intake in combination with low dietary intake.

Table 1. Risk factors for vitamin D deficiency in the elderly.

Residence at northern latitude
Limited exposure to sunlight
Reduced previtamin D synthesis in skin
Low dietary intake
Impaired $1,25(OH)_2D_3$ synthesis
Intestinal resistance to $1,25(OH)_2D_3$

4.1 Inadequate exposure to sunlight

Theoretically, adequate amounts of vitamin D can be produced by ultraviolet radiation (sunlight) on the skin. However, the amount of vitamin D obtained from this source is likely to be negligible during winter months at northern latitudes, due to the angle of the sun. This has been tested by exposing human skin cells to sunlight at different latitudes (Webb et al. 1988). At 52°N (Edmonton, Canada) no previtamin D_3 was produced between October and March; at 42°N (Boston) none was

formed between November and February; while further south (34°N, Los Angeles and 18°N, Puerto Rico), some previtamin was formed even in the middle of winter.

The relatively poor synthesis of vitamin D precursors in the skin during winter months explains the large seasonal fluctuations in serum 25(OH)D concentration. Depending on latitude and occupation, in free-living individuals the concentration of this metabolite will be lowest in December - January, while the highest concentrations are found in September to November (Devgun et al. 1981, Omdahl et al. 1982, Burnand et al. 1992).

Seasonal variations in $1,25(OH)_2D_3$ have also been reported in some studies (Bouillon et al. 1987) but not others (Krall et al. 1989). For the many elderly who have limited outdoor activities or who are institutionalized, this clearly causes their 25(OH)D levels to be even lower (Devgun et al. 1981) even when intakes meet recommendations (Egsmose et al. 1987). In the U.S.A., serum levels of 25(OH) fall by about 50% in winter months, suggesting that half of the circulating level is contributed by sunlight.

An important observation is that seasonal changes in 25(OH)D concentrations are inversely associated with changes in serum PTH, indicating that vitamin D status has compromised calcium absorption to the extent that PTH-regulated compensatory mechanisms have been stimulated (Krall et al. 1989, Villareal et al. 1991, Lukert et al. 1992). The higher PTH levels suggest that bone breakdown is occurring to maintain calcium homeostasis. This is supported by observed negative correlations between serum PTH levels and bone mineral changes both prior to, and 5 years after menopause in a population in which low vitamin D intake predicted elevated PTH (Lukert et al 1992). Serum alkaline phosphatase also varies seasonally and inversely with 25(OH)D (Omdahl et al 1982).

Krall et al. (1989) investigated these seasonal changes in relation to usual level of vitamin D intake, in a cross-sectional study of 333 elderly Boston residents. The subjects were healthy, free-living, and postmenopausal. As expected, serum PTH was higher after the winter months than after the summer. However, this was true only for those individuals who habitually consumed less than the recommended intake of 200 I.U. vitamin D per day. In the relatively small proportion of individuals who consumed more than this the seasonal PTH fluctuations did not seem to occur. As would be expected, and as observed in a number of studies, the correlation between dietary vitamin D intake and serum 25(OH)D was stronger during the winter, when the contribution of vitamin D synthesis in the skin was small. Lips et al. (1988) also observed that supplementation of the elderly with vitamin D only increased serum $1,25(OH)_2D_3$ levels in those with initially low 25(OH)D concentrations.

Aging also affects the capacity of the skin to produce vitamin D. Between the ages of about 20 to 80 years, there is a progressive, apparently linear reduction of previtamin D_3 in the epidermis (MacLaughlin and Holick, 1985), such that aging can halve the production of the previtamin in skin.

4.2 The importance of dietary vitamin D

Considering these seasonal fluctuations in vitamin D status, and the relatively high prevalence of deficiency that occurs in older individuals in winter months, it is apparent that dietary sources of the vitamin are inadequate to maintain optimal vitamin D status in many individuals. This is likely to be true for all age groups, but especially so in older individuals. Indeed, reported usual intakes of the vitamin among elderly populations show that they are about half of recommended levels in the U.S.A. and Canada where both milk and margarine are fortified with the vitamin (Omdahl et al. 1982, Delvin et al. 1988, Krall et al. 1989), and in Great Britain and The Netherlands where milk is not fortified (Lawson 1981, Lips et al. 1987). Even in the USA, a substantial proportion of older populations has an intake below 100 IU/day (Omdahl et al 1982).

In part, the explanation for these low intakes is that the only good natural dietary sources of the vitamin are egg yolks, fatty fish, and liver, foods not eaten in consistently large amounts by most populations. In many countries, fortification of milk provides the most important source of the vitamin, such that a moderate consumption of milk as a beverage can provide the recommended daily intake. However, it is important to recognize that many elderly do not obtain much of the vitamin from fortified milk, because of real or perceived gastrointestinal discomfort caused by drinking milk or consuming dairy products (Omdahl et al. 1982). Thus, even in countries such as the United States, where milk and other foods are fortified with the vitamin, the elderly often consume intakes that are so low as to compromise their vitamin D status. Fortification of margarine with the vitamin is relatively common, which may be helpful for those who consume this product.

The recommended dietary intake for this vitamin is 200 IU per day in the United States. However, there have been reports that this intake is inadequate to prevent vitamin D deficiency in a substantial proportion of older individuals (Krall et al 1989, Francis et al. 1983) especially if they are homebound (Gloth et al. 1991).

4.3 Other factors causing vitamin D deficiency

In many women, calcium absorption becomes less efficient with aging. While outside of the purpose of this review, it is important to note that this may be related not only to lower serum 25(OH)D levels in older individuals, but in some cases there may be impaired conversion of this metabolite to $1,25(OH)_2D_3$ (Slovak et al. 1981). Another relatively common situation in the more elderly may be higher serum levels of $1,25(OH)_2D_3$ resulting from both increased production and decreased metabolic clearance, despite which calcium absorption is impaired, indicating intestinal resistance to $1,25(OH)_2D_3$ (Eastell et al. 1991, Ebeling et al. 1992).

Elevated serum levels of $1,25(OH)_2D_3$ also increase the rate of catabolism of 25(OH)D, and may explain the development of vitamin D deficiency in a number of clinical disorders where there is calcium malabsorption (Clements et al. 1992). We have shown recently that the half-life of 25(OH)D is approximately halved by feeding low-calcium diets to young men for three weeks (Siu-Caldera et al. 1993).

Individuals with who have darker skins synthesize less previtamin D_3 than lightly-pigmented individuals during exposure to ultra-violet radiation. While this difference is more pronounced in Blacks (Clements et al. 1982), Indians and Pakistanis also need longer exposure to a dose of ultraviolet radiation to increase their serum 25(OH)D levels to the same extent as Caucasians (Lo et al. 1986).

The elderly also suffer more from health problems that might affect vitamin D metabolism. These include renal disease and intestinal malabsorption. Medications such as anticonvulsants may increase vitamin D requirements.

5. EPIDEMIOLOGICAL EVIDENCE LINKING VITAMIN D STATUS TO OSTEOPOROSIS.

The first type of epidemiological evidence linking vitamin D status to osteoporosis is the observed association between latitude of residence, season, and bone mineral content. In Northern latitudes the prevalence of hip fractures and osteoporosis is higher than in more southern regions. In addition, seasonal variation in bone mineral content has been demonstrated in women living in northern Europe (Krolner et al. 1983, Hyldstrup et al. 1986) and the United States (Bergstralh et al. 1990). Other studies have found no such seasonal variation (Overgaard et al. 1988). These observations raise the question of whether vitamin D status plays a role in seasonal bone loss.

Some estimates show that a major proportion of older individuals with hip fractures in Northern latitudes are vitamin D deficient. For example, in Great Britain (Aron et al. 1974, Jenkins et al. 1974) and Boston (Doppelt et al. 1983) this estimate is 30-40%. In a healthy group of 539 women, age 52-77 years, being screened for osteoporosis, closer to 10% had deficient 25(OH) levels (Villareal et al. 1991). In Israel, 30/95 patients with a proximal femoral fracture had deficient 25(OH)D values (Eventov et al. 1989).

In older female residents of the USA who were non-osteoporotic but had low serum 25(OH)D values, serum 25(OH)D levels were inversely correlated with PTH and low vertebral mass, compared to age-matched controls with normal 25(OH)D levels. Because women with low 25(OH)D had similar intakes of vitamin D to those with normal levels, this underlies the importance of sunlight in determining vitamin D status (Villareal et al. 1991).

Similar associations have been reported from England. In 138 non-osteoporotic women age 45-65 years there was a significant association between bone density at three sites (lumbar, neck, trochanter) and both 25(OH)D and PTH (negative) concentrations (Khaw et al 1992). In Copenhagen, serum 25(OH)D was related to spinal bone mass in early postmenopausal women but not in those with osteoporosis, but concentrations of both 25(OH)D and $1,25(OH)_2D_3$ were lower in women with fractures of the spine (Hartwell et al. 1990).

Nevertheless, there is some epidemiological evidence for an association between dietary vitamin D intake and bone mineral content. It should be borne in mind, however, that the interpretation of associations between observed intakes (and, to some extent, serum levels) of vitamin D and bone status may be confounded by the fact that where dairy products are the source of vitamin D, the intakes of calcium will covary with those of the vitamin. Sunlight exposure will also tend to obscure any relationship between intake and bone mineral.

Lukert et al who found a strong inverse relationship between serum 25(OH)D concentrations and PTH levels in perimenopausal women in Kansas, reported more loss of distal radius bone mineral content over 5 years in women with lower dietary D intakes (Lukert et al. 1992). Controlling for other confounding variables, vitamin D intake explained 26% of the change in bone mineral content over the five years in a group of 20 women. These subjects all had frequent exposure to the sun.

Finally, serum concentrations of $1,25(OH)_2D_3$ have also been reported as associated with decreased calcium absorption and negative calcium balance in osteoporotic patients (Gallagher et al. 1979). An additional perspective was added by an Israeli study in which Lidor et al. (1993) observed that serum levels of $1,25(OH)_2D_3$ in women over 45 did not reflect bone levels of this metabolite. In osteoporotic women with a mean age of 78 years, serum levels of $1,25(OH)_2D_3$ were within the normal range, while femoral bone levels were markedly reduced compared to non-osteoporotics.

6 VITAMIN D INTERVENTION STUDIES.

During the past few years information has accumulated on the effectiveness of providing vitamin D supplements to older individuals. Interestingly, to date far more work has been done to test the benefits of vitamin D metabolites than with vitamin D_2 or D_3. The supplementation approach provides the strongest evidence for a causal role of vitamin D in the bone loss of the elderly.

In The Netherlands, Lips et al. (1988) provided a supplement of 400 IU of vitamin D daily to elderly residents of a nursing home. This reduced serum levels of PTH and osteocalcin, suggesting that the supplement slowed down bone turnover.

Dawson-Hughes et al. (1991) investigated whether the relative vitamin D deficiency that they had observed in Boston residents during winter months, contributed to faster bone loss in this season. In a one-year trial with 249 older women, they also tested the effect of providing a placebo or 400 IU of vitamin D daily. An important aspect of this study was that the participants had to have a usual vitamin D intake < 100 IU/day. All participants were provided with 377 mg/day of calcium

primarily as calcium citrate malate, so that calcium intakes were currently adequate and would be less likely to confound the interpretation of the vitamin D effects. The mean age of the participants was 62 years and the average time since menopause was 13 years.

Measurements were made in June-July through December-January (when serum 25(OH)D levels are highest in this population) and in December-January through June-July (the period of relative vitamin D insufficiency). In the placebo group, bone mineral density of the spine increased during the high-D season, decreased during the low-D season, and did not change at all during the year (possibly because of the calcium supplementation). In the D-supplemented group, the increase in mineral content of the spine in the high-D period was similar to that in the placebo group, but loss in the low-D period was much lower (-0.54% compared with -1.22%) so that over the year the supplement increased mineral by 0.85% compared to 0.15% in the placebo group. The mineral content of the whole skeleton was not differentially affected by treatment. Subjects who were supplemented also had higher 25(OH)D and lower PTH levels in serum. This study shows that achieving the recommended level of vitamin D intake during winter months is important for conserving bone mineral in the spine. Although women with low levels of usual intake - below half of the recommended amount - were selected for the study, their intakes before supplementation were actually similar to those reported for many populations.

Using a more unusual approach, a Finnish group found that an annual intramuscular injection of 150,000-300,000 I.U. of vitamin D, reduced fracture rates in the upper limbs and ribs of women aged more than 85 years (Heikinheimo et al. 1992). Lower limb fracture rates were unaffected. It is encouraging that this intervention was effective even in these aged individuals. However, in both this study and one in the United States by Orwoll et al. (1990), vitamin D supplementation failed to slow down bone loss in older men, despite evidence for the existence of an association between decreases in serum 25(OH)D and increases in PTH in males.

7 INTERVENTIONS WITH VITAMIN D METABOLITES.

7.1 Treatment with 25(OH)D

Treatment with this metabolite has been successful in increasing calcium absorption in osteoporotic women who responded by increasing their serum levels of $1,25(OH)_2D_3$. However, some individuals showed neither of these responses, suggesting that this treatment is only successful in those who have adequate $25(OH)D_3$ hydroxylase activity (Zerwekh et al. 1983).

7.2 Treatment with $1,25(OH)_2D_3$

Serum levels of $1,25(OH)_2D_3$ have most often been reported as low in women with osteoporosis,

426

although in some cases they are high. Logically, and somewhat supported by evidence, calcitriol would be expected to have the greatest impact on individuals whose renal capacity to produce this metabolite is impaired (which is more likely to occur in the type II osteoporosis of the elderly), and whose serum levels of this metabolite, or calcium absorptive capacity, are initially low. There is some evidence to support this (Tilyard et al. 1992, Zerwekh et al. 1983). Trials of the effectiveness of $1,25(OH)_2D_3$ (calcitriol) for treating osteoporosis have produced mixed results. This is probably because of the different dose levels and population groups tested.

Examples of trials in which this metabolite was effective for osteoporotic women include: a three-year trial in Boston where there was a three-fold reduction in vertebral fractures compared to providing 1 g calcium/day (Tilyard et al. 1992); a two-year trial where treatment improved the calcium content of the radius and spine even though all subjects, including the placebo groups, were also supplemented with 400 IU vitamin D per day (Aloia et al. (1990); a two-year trial in osteoporotics where calcitriol increased spinal bone density and total body calcium compared to a placebo (Gallagher and Riggs 1990), and improved calcium absorption and fracture rates (Gallagher and Riggs, 1990); and a 1-8 year trial in Italy where calcium absorption was increased and fracture rates improved (Caniggia et al. 1990). However, Ott and Chestnut (1989) found $1,25(OH)_2D_3$ to be ineffective for increasing whole body calcium or reducing fracture rates.

Doses around 0.g ug/day produce little toxicity in osteoporotic patients, but treatment with 0.75-1.0 ug/day may produce hypercalcemia or hypercalciuria especially if calcium intakes are also high (Gallagher and Riggs 1990). However, some long-term trials with 1.0 ug/day have shown benefits but not ill-effects (Caniggia et al. 1990). In general, its use should probably be restricted to the treatment of serious osteoporosis, and those individuals believed to have problems with synthesizing or responding to this metabolite.

8. CONCLUSIONS.

The general conclusion from this review is that vitamin D status is important for the postmenopausal maintenance of bone mineral. Poor vitamin D status produces an increase in serum PTH and PTH-dependent changes in bone mineral content. Especially in northern latitudes, dietary sources alone provide inadequate amounts of the vitamin for many elderly women. The intake of these individuals needs to be increased by recommending higher consumption of the few foods naturally rich in the vitamin, including vitamin D-fortified milk or margarine when this is available. Fortified milk can be an important source of the vitamin, although it should be recognized that many elderly consume only small amounts.

Another strategy is to recommend vitamin D supplements to older individuals. While more long-term studies of their effectiveness are needed, relatively low intakes of supplemental vitamin D have been effective at reducing bone loss. Most intervention studies have shown that daily supplements of 400-800 IU will raise serum 25(OH)D concentrations to those of young adults (McKenna et al. 1985, Delvin et al. 1988), and bone mineral content of the spine has been maintained with a supplement of 400 IU/day if calcium intake is adequate. More information is needed concerning the appropriate level of intake and supplementation in the elderly, and recommended dietary intakes for those with minimal sunlight exposure may need to be higher than 200 I.U. per day.

REFERENCES

Aloia, J.F. 1990. Role of calcitriol in the treatment of postmenopausal osteoporosis. *Metabolism* 39(4 suppl 1): 35-38.

Aron, J.E., J.C. Gallagher, J. Anderson, L. Stasiak, E.B. Longton, B.E.C. Nordin & M. Nicholson 1974. Frequency of osteomalacia and osteoporosis in fractures of the proximal femur. *Lancet* 1: 229.

Bergstralh, E.J., M. Sinaki, K.P. Offord, H.W. Wahner & L.J. Melton 1990. Effect of season on physical activity score, back extensor muscle strength, and lumbar bone mineral density. *J. Bone Miner. Res.* 5: 371-377.

Bouillon, R.A., J.N. Auwerx, W.E. Lissens, & W.K. Pelemans 1987. Vitamin D status in the elderly: seasonal substrate deficiency causes 1,25-dihydroxycholecalciferol deficiency. *Am. J. Clin. Nutr.* 45: 755-763.

Burnand, B., D. Sloutskis, F. Gianoli, J. Cornuz, M. Rickenbach, F. Paccaud & P. Burckhardt 1992. Serum 25-hydroxyvitamin D: distribution and determinants in the Swiss population. *Am. J. Clin. Nutr.* 56: 537-542.

Caniggia, A., R. Nuti, F. Lore, G. Martini, V. Turchetti & G. Righi 1990. Long-term treatment with calcitriol in postmenopausal osteoporosis. *Metabolism* 39: 43-49.

Clemens, T.L., J.S. Adams, S.L. Henderson & M.F. Holick 1982. Increased skin pigment reduces the capacity of skin to synthesise vitamin D_3. *Lancet* 1: 74-77.

Clements, M.R., M. Davies, M.E. Hayes, C.D. Hickey, G.A. Lumb, E.B. Mawer & P.H. Adams 1992. The role of 1,25-dihydroxyvitamin D in the mechanism of acquired vitamin D deficiency. *Clin. Endocrinol.* 37: 17-27.

Dawson-Hughes, B., G.E. Dallal, E.A. Krall, S. Harris, L.J. Sokoll & G.Falconer 1991. Effect of vitamin D supplementation on wintertime and overall bone loss in healthy postmenopausal women. *Ann. Intern. Med.* 115: 505-512.

DeLuca, H.F. 1990. Osteoporosis and the metabolites of vitamin D. *Metabolism* 39(4 suppl 1): 3-9.

Delvin, E.E., A. Imbach & M. Copti 1988. Vitamin D nutritional status and related biochemical indices in an autonomous elderly population. *Am. J. Clin. Nutr.* 48: 373-378.

Devgun, M.S., C.R. Paterson, B.E. Johnson & C. Cohen 1981. Vitamin D nutrition in relation to season and occupation. *Am. J. Clin. Nutr.* 34: 1501-1504.

Doppelt, S.H., R.M. Neer, M. Daly, L. Bourvet, A. Schiller, M.F. Holick & H. Mankin 1983. Vitamin D deficiency and osteomalacia in patients with hip fractures. *Orthop. Trans.* 7: 512.

Eastell, R., A.L. Yergey, N.E. Vieiria, S.L. Cedel, R. Kumar & B.L. Riggs 1991. Interrelationships among vitamin D metabolism, true calcium absorption, parathyroid function, and age in women: evidence of an age-related intestinal resistance to 1,25 dihydroxyvitamin D action. *J. Bone Miner. Res.* 6: 125-132.

Ebeling, P.R., M.E. Sandgren, E.P. DiMagno, A.W. Lane et al. 1992. Evidence of an age-related decrease in intestinal responsiveness to vitamin D: relationship between serum 1,25-dihydroxyvitamin D_3 and intestinal vitamin D receptor concentrations in normal women. *J. Clin. Endocrinol. Metab.* 75(1): 176-182.

Egsmose, C., B. Lund, P. McNair, T. Storm & O.H. Sorenson 1987. Low serum levels of 25-hydroxyvitamin D and 1,25 dihydroxyvitamin D in institutionalized old people: influence of solar exposure and vitamin D supplementation. *Age Aging* 16: 35-40.

Eventov, I., B. Frisch, D. Alk, Z. Eisenberg & Y. Weisman 1989 *Acta Orthop. Scand.* 60: 411-413.

Francis, R.M., M. Peacock, J.H. Storer, A.E.J. Davies, W.B. Brown, B.E.C. Nordin 1983. Calcium malabsorption in the elderly: the effect of treatment with oral 25-hydroxyvitamin D_3. *Eur. J. Clin. Invest.* 13: 391-396.

Gallagher, J.C. 1992. Vitamin D metabolism and therapy in elderly subjects. *South Med. J.* 85(8): 2S43-47.

Gallagher, J.C., B.L. Riggs, J. Eisman, A. Hamstra, S.B. Arnaud & H.F. DeLuca 1979. Intestinal calcium absorption and serum vitamin D metabolites in normal subjects or osteoporotic patients. *J. Clin. Invest.* 64: 729-736.

Gallagher, J.C. & B.L. Riggs 1990. Action of 1,25-dihydroxyvitamin D_3 on calcium balance and bone turnover and its effect on vertebral fracture rate. *Metabolism* 39(4 suppl 1): 30-34.

Gloth, F.M., J.D. Tobin, S.S. Sherman & B.W. Hollis 1991. Is the recommended daily allowance for vitamin D too low for the homebound elderly? *J. Am. Geriatr. Soc.* 39: 137-141.

Hartwell D., B.J. Riis & C. Christiansen 1990. Comparison of vitamin D metabolism in early healthy and late osteoporotic postmenopausal women. *Calcif. Tissue Int.* 47(6): 332-337.

Heikinheimo, R.J., J.A. Inkovaara, E.J. Harju, M.V. Haavisto, R.H. Kaarela, J.M. Kataja, A.M-L. Kokko, L.A. Kolho & S.A. Rajala 1992. Annual injection of vitamin D and fractures of aged bones. *Calcif. Tissue Int.* 51: 105-110.

Hyldstrup, L., P. McNair, G.F. Jensen & I. Transbol 1986. Seasonal variations in indices of bone formation precede appropriate bone mineral changes in normal men. *Bone* 7: 167-170.

Jenkins, D.H., J.G. Roberts, D. Webster & E.O. Williams 1974. Osteomalacia in elderly patients with fractures of the femoral neck. *J. Bone Joint Surg.*(Br) 55B: 575.

Khaw, K.T., M.J. Sneyd & J. Compston 1992. Bone density parathyroid hormone and 25-hydroxyvitamin D concentrations in middle aged women. *BMJ* 305(6848): 273-277.

Krall, E.A., N. Sahyoun, S. Tannenbaum, G.E. Dallal & Dawson-Hughes 1989. Effect of vitamin D intake on seasonal variations in parathyroid hormone secretion in postmenopausal women. *N. Engl. J. Med.* 321: 1777-1783.

Krolner, B. 1983. Seasonal variation in bone mineral content after the menopause. *Calcif. Tissue Int.* 35: 145-147.

Lawoyin, S., J.H. Zerwekh, K. Glass & C.Y.C. Pak 1980. Ability of 25-hydroxyvitamin D_3 therapy to augment serum 1,25- and 24,25-dihydroxyvitamin D in postmenopausal osteoporosis. *J. Clin. Endocrinol. Metab.* 50: 593-596.

Lawson, D.E.M. 1981. Dietary vitamin D: Is it necessary? *J. Hum. Nutr.* 35: 61-63.

Lidor, C., P. Sagiv, B. Amdur, R. Gepstein, I. Otremski, T. Hallel 1993. Decrease in bone levels of 1,25-dihydroxyvitamin D in women with subcapital fracture of the femur. *Calcif. Tissue Int.* 52: 146-148.

Lips, P., F.C. van Ginkel, M.J. Jongen, F. Rubertus, W.J. van der Vigh & J.C. Netelenbos 1987. Determinants of vitamin D status in patients with hip fracture and in elderly control subjects. *Am. J. Clin. Nutr.* 46: 1005-1010.

Lips, P., A. Wiersinga, F.C. can Ginkel, M.J.M. Jongen, J.C. Netelenbos, W.H.L. Hackeng, P.D. Delmas, & W.G.F. van der Vijgh 1988. The effect of vitamin D supplementation on vitamin D status and parathyroid function in elderly subjects. *J. Clin. Endocrinol. Metab.* 67: 644-650.

Lo, C.W., P.W. Paris & M.F. Holick 1986. Indian and Pakistani immigrants have the same capacity as Caucasians to produce vitamin D in response to ultraviolet irradiation. *Am. J. Clin. Nutr.* 44: 683-685.

Lukert, B., J. Higgins & M. Stoskopf 1992. Menopausal bone loss is partially regulated by dietary intake of vitamin D. *Calcif. Tisse Int.* 51: 173-179.

MacLaughlin, J. & M.F. Holick 1985. Aging decreases the capacity of human skin to produce vitamin D_3. *J. Clin. Invest.* 76: 1536-1538.

McKenna, M.J., R. Freaney, A. Meade & F.P. Muldowney 1985. Prevention of hypovitaminosis D in the elderly. *Calcif. Tissue Int.* 37: 113-116.

Norman, A.W. 1990. Intestinal calcium absorption: a vitamin D-hormone-mediated adaptive response. *Am. J. Clin. Nutr.* 51: 290-300.

Omdahl, J.L., P.J. Garry, L.A. Hunsaker, W.C. Hunt & J.S. Goodwin 1982. Nutritional status in a healthy elderly population: vitamin D. *Am. J. Clin. Nutr.* 36: 1225.

Orwoll, E.S., S.K. Oviatt, M.R. McClung, L.J. Deftos & G. Sexton 1990. The rate of bone mineral loss in normal men and the effects of calcium and cholecalciferol supplementation. *Ann. Intern. Med.* 112(1): 29-34.

Ott, S.M. & C.H. Chestnut III 1989. Calcitriol treatment is not effective in postmenopausal osteoporosis. *Ann. Intern. Med.* 110: 267-274.

Overgaard, K., L. Nilas, J.S. Johansen & C. Christiansen 1988. Lack of seasonal variation in bone mass and biochemical estimates of bone turnover. *Bone* 9: 285-288.

Parfitt, A.M. 1983. Dietary risk factors for age-related bone loss and fractures. *Lancet* 2: 1181-1185.

Siu-Caldera, M.L., L.H. Allen, K.O. O'Brien, A. Yergey, R. Ray & M. Holick 1993. Low calcium intake reduces the half-life of 25(OH) vitamin D. *FASEB J.* 7: A284.

Slovak, D.M., J.S. Adams, R.M. Neer, M.F. Holick & J.T. Potts 1981. Deficient production of 1,25 dihydroxyvitamin D in elderly osteoporotic patients. *N. Engl. J. Med.* 3: 372-374.

Tilyard, M.W., G.F.S. Spears, J. Thomson & S. Dovey 1992. Treatment of postmenopausal osteoporosis with calcitriol or calcium. *New Engl. J. Med.* 326(6): 357-362.

Villareal, D.T., R. Civiyrlli, A. Chines & L.V. Avioli 1991. Subclinical vitamin D deficiency in postmenopausal women with low vertebral bone mass. *J. Clin. Endocrinol. Metab.* 72: 628-634.

Webb, A.R., L. Kline & M.F. Holick 1988. Influence of season and latitude on the cutaneous synthesis of vitamin D_3: Exposure to winter sunlight in Boston and Edmonton will not promote vitamin D_3 synthesis in human skin. *J. Clin. Endocrinol. Metab.* 67: 373.

Zerwekh, J.H., K. Sahkaes, K. Glass & C.Y.C. Pak 1983. Long-term 25-hydroxyvitamin D_3 therapy in postmenopausal osteoporosis: demonstration of responsive and nonresponsive subgroups. *J. Clin. Endocrinol. Metab.* 56: 410-413.

Dairy Products in Human Health and Nutrition, Serrano Ríos et al. (eds) © 1994 Balkema, Rotterdam, ISBN 90 5410 359 0

Nutrition and bone

P. Burckhardt

University Hospital, Lausanne, Switzerland

ABSTRACT: Although genetics, hormones, and age are the principal determinant of bone mass, nutrition and physical activity as well show significant correlation with bone mass. Nutrition influences bone growth and maturation and becomes again increasingly important during senescence. Most knowledge is derived from research on Calcium and Vitamin D supplementation, while strictly nutritional aspects have been studied less. Calcium is provided by diary products for 40-50% in Western food, much less in Asia, and is equally well absorbed from some calcium-rich vegetables, wheat and mineral waters. Diary intake correlates with bone density in children and premenopausal women and with hip fracture incidence in elderly persons. Protein malnutrition inhibits bone growth and maintenance and is as frequent in the elderly as Calcium and Vitamin D insufficiency. High protein and salt intake stimulate Calcium excretion, while the potentially negative role of the P/Ca ration in food is debated. Trace elements show some correlation with bone density, but their exact role is still unknown. More long-term studies on the effects of controlled nutritional manipulation on bone density and fracture incidence are needed.

1 INTRODUCTION

Bone mass and density are conditioned by several factors, such as genetic factors, hormones, physical activity, general health, and nutrition. The respective role of these factors varies throughout life. Peak bone mass, i.e., the maximal bone mass obtained in early adult life, is a main predictor of bone health later in life. Although genetic factors account for about 80% of the peak bone mass (Johnston 1991), and are predominant during growth, nutrition is also important in this stage, as it allows full development of the genetically programmed possibilities (Heaney 1986). Although a secondary factor only, nutrition has the advantage over genetic factors, sex and age to be changeable. By that it offers the possibility of therapeutic and preventive interventions.

2 INFLUENCE OF NUTRITION ON BONE HEALTH

In childhood and adolescence, nutritional factors are of significant importance, although genetic factors are the main predictors of adult peak bone mass. Low Calcium intake delays the development of bone mass in adolescence (Grimston 1991), and Calcium supplementation promotes it slightly. Low Vitamin D intake leads to rachitism, a risk factor for low peak bone mass and for later osteoporosis. In general, low body weight (Slemenda 1990 b) and malnutrition result in low bone mass. Encountered in anorexia nervosa, it leads to osteoporosis (Treasure 1986, Rigotti 1984, Szmukler 1985), which is not necessarily reversible after normalization of body weight (Rigotti 1991). Although in anorexia nervosa malnutrition can hardly be dissociated from other significant risk factors for osteoporosis, such as low estrogen status, high cortisol secretion, low physical activity, it appeared that the duration of the disease and of that of inadequate Calcium intake were the best predictors of bone loss (Hay 1992).

After puberty, when growth is already completed, bone density can still increase (Tylavsky 1989). It is therefore conceivable that nutrition is important for bone development beyond the strict period of growth. This explains why low Calcium intake in puberty and adolescence correlates with a relatively low bone density (Grimston 1991). Later catch up seems to be possible, as shown in rats (Thomas 1991).

In early adult life, i.e., during the third decade of life, bone mass is still slightly increasing, and this increase is stimulated by a relatively high Calcium intake and by physical activity (Recker 1992). Within physiologic limits, the maintenance of bone health during adult life does not depend on nutrition; Calcium intake is not directly related to bone mass, and not more important than physical activity. In fact, both factors influence the maintenance of the bone mass in combination (Mazess 1986, Halioua 1989, Kanders 1988). During the early postmenopausal years, during which bone loss is accelerated, Calcium has even no significant influence on bone loss.

But later in life, especially during senescence, nutritional factors become increasingly important. Nutritional deficiencies are more frequent, absorptive efficiency deteriorates, adaptive mechanisms decline. For these reasons, Vitamin D deficiency (discussed in a previous chapter) is frequent in elderly, institutionalized persons, with a tendency to secondary hyperparathyroidism, which in turn accelerates bone loss. In this situation, supplementation with vitamin D and Calcium inhibits hyperparathyroidism, and increases bone quality, while supplementation with proteins reinforces general health and accelerates mobilization of patients who suffered from hip fracture (Delmi 1990). In general, it should be kept in mind that with increasing age the influence of life conditions and habits on bone health also increases. For this reason, differences linked to nutrition are small during young adulthood and increase thereafter (Matkovic 1979). Life long nutritional habits are more important for bone health than those of a given period of life (Halouia 1989)

3 SPECIFIC ROLE OF NUTRIENTS ON BONE METABOLISM

Bone formation is performed by osteoblasts, and bone resorption by osteoclasts, which are controlled by hormones, cytokines and growth factors. Nutritional factors influence these cells as long as they act on these hormones and cytokines, except Vitamin D. Nutritional constituents can vary the blood levels of phosphorus and of Calcium, which again influences secretion of parathyroid hormone and of the activation (hydroxylation) of vitamin D, and they can influence intestinal absorption or renal handling of minerals which are essential for bone. For these reasons, various nutritional constituents influence Calcium balance in different ways, as summarized in Table 1, and may by that modify bone metabolism. Vitamin D and lactose act mainly as promoters of Calcium absorption; phosphate, fibers, fat, and oxalate inhibit Calcium absorption; proteins, sodium and eventually caffeine are reported to enhance urinary Calcium excretion and by that to decrease Calcium balance.

Table 1. Nutritional influences on Calcium balance

Calcium	Absorption	Excretion	Balance
a) Vitamin D	↑	↔,↑	(+)
b) Lactose	↑	↔	(+)
c) Phosphate	↓	↓	?
d) Fibers	↓	↔	-
e) Fat	↓	↔	-
f) Oxalate	↓	↔	-
g) Protein	↔,↓	↑	-
h) Natrium	↔	↑	-

The manipulation of each of the above-mentioned nutrients is supposed to influence bone health and for many of them data are conclusive enough for practical deductions and dietary recommendations.

a) Vitamin D:
Vitamin D promotes intestinal Calcium absorption and mineralization of bone matrix. Its role is described in a previous chapter. It can be produced by the healthy organism under ultraviolet irradiation, but it often becomes deficient in the institutionalized or home-bound elderly, and by that contributes to secondary hyperparathyroidism and accelerated bone loss. Nutritional or pharmacological substitution decreases bone loss and fracture incidence.

b) Lactose:

Lactose enhances intestinal Calcium absorption (Cochet 1983), but this effect is not specific and is also exerted by glucose and galactose in subjects with normal lactase (Griessen 1989). Lactose deficiency was associated with osteoporosis (Birge 1967, Finkenstedt 1986), but is also frequently found in non-osteoporotic subjects. It causes osteoporosis rather through milk intolerance and by that through low Calcium intake, than through real Calcium malabsorption.

c) Phosphate:

High phosphate intake theoretically lowers calcium balance - at least in some animal models (Breslau 1988) - and stimulates the secretion of parathyroid hormone and, by that, bone resorption. The ratio of phosphorus over Calcium in nutrients has been thought to be of significance for bone health . It is high, i.e., of negative influence, in soft drinks, meat, and many fast-foods. Despite these theoretic considerations experimental data is again scarce. On the other hand, a low phosphorus intake seems to enhance the negative effect of high protein intake on Calcium balance, and a relatively high phosphorus + protein + Calcium intake may protect bone mass and decrease fracture risk (Matkovic 1979). Therefore, the Calcium over phosphorus ratio in food may be important, as shown in perimenopausal women (Lukert 1987); later in life Vitamin D intake becomes predominant.

d) Fibers:

Fibers decrease intestinal Calcium absorption, but not to an extent that diminishes the nutritional value of Calcium-rich vegetables.

e) Fat:

Dietary fat specifically decreases Calcium absorption only in case of fat malabsorption, where a high intestinal content of fat enhances formation of Calcium soaps which are eliminated with the feces. High fat intake, in itself, is not known to lower the Calcium balance, but it is usually associated with low Calcium intake, except in the case of regular consumption of fatty cheeses.

f) Oxalate:

Oxalate prevents Calcium from being absorbed which explains, together with the phytin content, why Calcium absorption from spinach is low (see below). There are no other foods in Western nutrition with an oxalate content sufficiently high to prevent the absorption of an otherwise high Calcium content.

g) Proteins:

See below

h) Sodium:

High salt intake increases urinary Calcium excretion (Breslau 1982, Castelmiller 1985), with a close correlation between Na and Calcium excretion and , by that, may enhance negative Calcium balance and osteoporosis (Nordin 1991). Salt restriction might therefore decrease bone loss. This is a still appealing hypothesis, because in continental countries salt intake has increased 10-fold over about 150 years and this might have influenced Calcium balance and the secular trend towards increased frequency of osteoporosis.

i) Alcohol

Alcoholism is a nutritional cause of osteoporosis. Alcoholics have decreased bone density and an increased fracture incidence (Spencer 1986, Bikle 1985, Diamond 1989). Alcohol inhibits osteoblasts and is associated with poor nutrition and with liver disease, all interfering with bone health.

k) Trace elements

The importance of trace elements for bone health is still unknown. Some data point to Iron, Zinc and Magnesium as significant factors (Angus 1988, for review see Rico). The contribution of milk and milk products is significant for Zinc and Iodine, while the concentrations of trace elements in formulas are generally higher, except for Selenium (Flynn 1992).

4 DAIRY PRODUCTS

In Western countries, dairy products represent the main source of nutritional calcium, 55% and 46% of the total Calcium intake in adolescents and young adults, respectively and still 42% in 60-65 year-old women (Pennington in Anderson 1991). This explains why Ca intake is generally high in, for example, Holland; in a Swiss mountain region (Oberwallis) it reaches even 1.7 g/day in men (personal communication). Higher Ca intake in the form of dairy products is related to higher bone density in American school children (Anderson 1991a), and bone mass before menopause was also found to be related to milk intake during childhood and adolescence

(Sandler 1985). During adolescence Calcium intake decreases in the US., because adult food is relatively Calcium poor (US Dept. of Health 1979, Abraham 1991). As most of the alimentary Calcium is provided by dairy products, the average Calcium intake is significantly higher in countries with a high intake of dairy products. Indeed, young adults in Canada take ca. 1500 mg per day (Grimston 1991), in Denmark normal subjects take 1240 mg (Hasling 1991), still more than young Swiss, who take ca. 1000 mg. On the other side, in Asian countries, where only ca. 20-30% of the alimentary Calcium is provided by dairy products, the average intake is much lower, e.g., 540 mg in China (Chen 1989), and 300-500 mg in Hong Kong Chinese (Pun). Although dairy products can supply the whole need for Calcium, man and animals do not depend upon this source. In the Paleolithicum the Calcium intake of man was estimated 1579 mg per day, and this without milk products (Eaton 1985).

In children there is a positive correlation between Calcium intake an Calcium retention, which is necessary for growth (Matkovic 1991). This applies to adolescents with an intake of up to 1500 mg Calcium and to young adults for up to 1000 mg. In twin studies, increased Calcium intake during growth promoted bone development (Slemenda 1990 a) and a relatively high consumption of diary products during school age was associated with a significantly higher bone density of the radius (Anderson 1991). This effect seems to remain as premenopausal women who had regular milk intake during childhood and adolescence showed higher bone density than women who did not (Sandler 1985). Supplementation with ca. 650 mg Calcium as dairy products, decreased bone loss in premenopausal women (Baran 1990) without any increase in blood lipids and modified positively Calcium balance in adult women (Recker 1985). When a cohort of elderly people was followed for over 10 years, it appeared that a high intake of dairy products was even associated with a lower incidence of hip fractures (Holbrook 1988).

Calcium from milk is as well absorbed as Calcium from commercialized Calcium salts (Sheikh 1987, Fritsch 1987), in some cases even better, but there are important individual differences (Recker 1988). at a dose of 200 mg of Calcium, absorption is about 30% (Heaney

1988). Lactose enhances Calcium absorption (Schuette 1989), which explains why the addition of milk increases the absorption of Calcium from fruits and vegetables (Fairweather-Tait 1989, Allen 1982). But lactose is not necessary. Calcium absorption from yogurt is not lower than that from milk, or even higher (Dupuis 1964) and that from cheese is at least comparable (Recker 1988). The absence of lactose in these two dairy products is even an advantage in lactose deficiency with milk intolerance. There is some doubt whether the ingestion of fatty cheeses facilitates the formation of unabsorbed Calcium soaps, but this has not been demonstrated. Altogether dairy products remain the main source of nutritional Calcium of Western adults, despite the sharp decrease of milk consumption after childhood. However, in Asian countries, it is difficult to include dairy products in sufficient quantities in daily food (Fujita 1991, Pun).

5 CALCIUM FROM WHEAT AND VEGETABLES

Although dairy products are the main nutritional sources of Calcium, some vegetables are also rich in Calcium, such as spinach, kale and broccoli, but they are generally not consumed in great enough quantities to cover the needs for Calcium. The absorbability of this Calcium depends mainly on the content of fibers, oxalate and phytate. This has been extensively examined (Weaver 1991a). First, Calcium absorption from spinach, which contains 126 mg Calcium/100 g, is low (about 5%, compared to about 30% from milk) (Heaney 1988a). This has been explained by the high oxalate content. Indeed, absorption of Calcium oxalate was 10-14%, that of milk 36-39%, and that of a mixture of both was 26.5% (Heaney 1989), while that from kale, a oxalate-poor and Calcium-rich (212 mg/100 g) vegetable, from the same family as broccoli, was 40.9% (Heaney 1990). Not only these vegetables, but also grain (Weaver 1991b) provide slightly better absorbable Calcium than milk, despite their fiber and phytic acid content. Only when phytic acid is highly concentrated, such as in extruded wheat bran cereal or soybeans (Heaney 1991), is Calcium absorption lower than from milk.

For the Asian kitchen "bean curd sheet" (136 mg Calcium/100g), broccoli (105 mg/100 g), shrimp paste and sardines are recommended (Pun 1991). But, except for "bean curd" and eventually broccoli, these nutrients are not regularly consumed and, if ever, only in small quantities. For this reason they cannot cover the needs for Calcium.

In general, most foods provide Calcium that is comparable in absorption to milk, but either their Calcium content is relatively low, or they cannot replace dairy products in sufficient quantities because of their relatively low palatability.

6 MINERAL WATERS

Mineral waters, in Europe especially from alpine regions, may be valuable sources of Calcium and other minerals with Calcium contents up to 500 mg per liter. They can be substitutes for milk in lactose intolerant adults (Halpern 1991). The Calcium content of water shows important regional variations. In Europe it lies between 3 mg/1 (Charrier, France) and 597 mg/1 (Aproz Cristal, Switzerland). For this reason, Calcium intake can vary by 50% only because of the water and this might condition the average Calcium intake of a whole region (Matkovic 1979). Furthermore, the Calcium content of the water is related to that of the ground which, in turn, influences that of the vegetables and, partially, also of the milk.

7 PROTEINS

Protein supply certainly is essential for bone growth. During childhood, severe protein malnutrition has negative effects on the skeleton: it reduces endochondral bone growth, increases endosteal bone loss and leads to osteopenia and to increased fractures (for review: Orwoll 1992). Although protein deficiency is rarely isolated, but associated with other nutritional deficiencies, low concentrations of certain growth factors, and eventually high cortisol levels, etc., animal data and clinical observations (Garn 1964) refer to protein deprivation as to a specific factor. In American children radial bone mineral density was found to correlate with protein as well as Calcium intake (Chan 1987). But adaptation

mechanisms, such as a decrease in calciuria, partially prevent bone loss or growth delay until protein deprivation becomes severe. In adults, under nutrition goes along with low bone mass, but protein malnutrition is only part of such situations.

In the elderly, protein intake often falls below the daily allowances of 0.8 g/kg and the average serum albumin levels decrease with age. In some studies, bone mineral density correlated with protein intake (Tylavsky 1988), but this is not a constant finding. Protein intake can hardly be identified separately. The positive effect of a protein supplement on the recovery of patients with hip fracture (Delmi 1990) might again be due to additional nutrients, but supports the hypothesis that protein malnutrition is frequent in elderly patients and that it not only affects general health, but also bone density and strength.

On the other hand, high protein intake increases urinary Calcium excretion and there is large evidence that this Na-independent hypercalciuric effect of proteins is not compensated by increased intestinal Calcium absorption (for review: Orwoll 1992). Therefore, the hypothesis is discussed that high protein intake might decrease Calcium balance (Heaney 1982) and lead to lower bone density and to higher fracture risk. Although this is questioned by others (Spencer 1983), an analysis of 34 studies from 16 countries showed a strong positive correlation between estimates of dietary animal protein intake and fracture incidence (Abelow 1992). Racial differences might have contributed to this observation, and the potential influence of high protein intake in the incidence of osteoporosis remains controversial even though its effect on Calcium metabolism is well documented. For protein rich nutrients, a relatively high protein over Calcium ratio is recommended, such as that found in dairy products.

REFERENCES

Abelow, B.J., T.R. Holford, K.L. Insogna. 1992. Cross-cultural association between dietary animal protein and hip fracture. Calcif. Tissue Int. 50:14-18.

Abraham, S., et al. Dietary intake findings. United States, 1976-1980, Hyattsville, MD:

National Center for Health Statistics, US Department of Human Services.

Allen, L.H. 1982. Calcium bioavailability and absorption: a review. Am. J. Clin. Nutr. 35:783-808.

Anderson, J.J.B., R.C. Henderson. 1991a. Dietary factors in the development of peak bone mass. In Nutritional Aspects of Osteoporosis. P. Burckhardt and R.P. Heaney (eds). Serono Symposia. Raven Press, vol. 85, 3-19.

Anderson, J.J.B., F.A. Tylavsky, L. Halioua, J. Lacey, J.A. Reed. 1991b. The assessment of calcium intake. In Nutritional Aspects of Osteoporosis. P. Burckhardt and R.P. Heaney (eds). Serono symposia. Raven Press, vol. 85, 105-114.

Angus, R.M., P.N. Sanbrook, N.A. Pocock, J.A. Eisman. 1988. Dietary intake and bone mineral density. Bone and Min. 4:265-277.

Baran, D.T., A. Sorensen, J. Grimes, R. Lew, A. Karellas, B. Johnson, J. Roche. 1990. Dietary modification with dairy products for preventing vertebral bone loss in premenopausal women. A three-year prospective study. J. Clin. Endocrinol. Metab. 70:264-270.

Bikle, D.D., H.K. Genant, C. Cann. 1985. Bone disease in alcohol abuse. Ann. Int. Med. 103:42-48.

Birge, S.J., H.T. Keutmann, P. Quatrecasas et al. 1967. Osteoporosis, intestinal lactose deficiency and low dietary calcium intake. NEJM 276:445-448.

Breslau, N.A., J.L. McGuire, J.E. Zerweh, C. Pak. 1982. The role of dietary sodium on renal excretion and intestinal absorption of calcium and on vitamin D metabolism. 55:369-373.

Breslau, N.A., L. Brinkley, K.D. Hill, C.Y.C. Pak. 1988. Relationship of animal protein-rich diet to kidney stone formation and calcium metabolism. J. Clin. Endocrinol. Metab. 66:140-146.

Castelmiller, J.M., R.P. Mensink, L. van der Heyden L. et al. 1985. The effect of dietary sodium on urinary calcium and potassium excretion in normotensive men with different calcium intakes. Am. J. Clin. Nutr. 41:52-60

Chan, G.M., R. McInnes, G. Gill 1987. Nutritional factors affecting bone mineral status in children. Clin. Res. 35:277A.

Chen, J.D. 1989. Some nutrition policies in China. Am. J. Clin. Nutr. 1989; 49:1060-1062. The Korean RDA 1980. 3rd Rev. Ed., Seoul, Korea; FAO/WHO Korean Assn.

Cochet, B., A. Jung, M. Griessen et al. 1983. Effect of lactose on intestinal calcium absorption in normal and lactose deficient subjects. Gastroenterology. 84:935-940.

Colombi, A., D. Steiger. 1989. Mineralwasser als Lebensmittel. Schweiz. Aerztezeitung. 47:2006-2007.

Delmi, M., C.H. Rapin, J.M. Bengoa et al. 1990. Dietary supplementation in elderly patients with fractured neck of the femur. Lancet. 335:1013-1016.

Diamond, T., D. Stiel, M. Lunzer et al. 1989. Ethanil reduces bone formation and may cause osteoporosis. Am. J. Med. 86:282-288.

Dupuis, Y. 1964. Ann. Bull. Féd. Int. Lait. III:36-43.

Eaton, S.B., M. Konner. 1985. Paleolithic nutrition: a consideration of its nature and current implications. NEJM. 312:283-289.

Fairweather-Tait, S.J., A. Johnson, J. Eagles, S. Ganatra, H. Kennedy, M.I. Gurr. 1989. Studies on calcium absorption from milk using a double-label stable isotope technique. Br. J. Nutr. 62:379-388.

Finkestedt, G., F. Skrabal, R.W. Gasser. 1986. Lactose absorption, milk consumption, and fasting blood glucose concentrations in women with idiopathic osteoporosis. Br. Med. J. 292:161-162.

Flynn, A. 1992. Minerals and trace elements in milk. Adv. Food Nutr. Res. 36:209-252.

Fritsch, C., J.D. Aubert, A.F. Jacquet, P. Burckhardt. 1987. Evaluation of intestinal calcium absorption by balance studies in normal volunteers: milk versus calcium gluconolactate. In Osteoporosis. C. Christiansen, J.S. Johannsen, B.J. Riis (eds). P. 271-273.

Fujita, T. 1991. Osteoporosis - East and West. Calcif. Tissue Int. 48:151-152.

Garn, S.M., M.A. Guzman, B. Wagner. 1964. subperiostal gain and endosteal loss in protein-caloric malnutrition. Am. J. Phys. Anthrop. 30:153-156.

Griessen, M., P.V. Speich, F. Infante et al. 1989. Effect of absorbable and nonabsorbable sugars on intestinal calcium absorption in humans. Gastroenterology. 96:769-775.

Grimston, S.K., K. Morrison, J.A. Harder, D.A. Hanley. 1991. Bone mineral density and calcium intake in children during puberty. In

Nutritional Aspects of Osteoporosis. P. Burckhardt and R.P. Heaney (eds). Serono Symposia. Raven Press, vol 85, 77-89.

Halioua, L. & J.J.B. Anderson. 1989. Lifetime calcium intake and physical activity habits: independent and combined effects on the radial bone of healthy premenopausal Caucasian women. Am. J. Clin. Nutr. 49:534-541.

Halioua, L., J.J.B. Anderson. Lifetime calcium intake and physical activity habits: independent and combined effects on the radial bone of healthy premenopausal Caucasian women. Am. J. Clin. Nutr. 1989; 49:534-54

Halpern, G.M., J. Van de Water, A.M. Delabroise et al. 1991. Comparative uptake of calcium from unit and a calcium-rich mineral water in lactose intolerant adults: implications from a treatment of osteoporosis. Am. J. Prev. Med. 7:379-383.

Hasling, C., P. Charles, F. Haagehooj Jensen, L. Mosekilde. 1990. Calcium metabolism in postmenopausal Osteoporosis: the influence of dietary calcium and net absorbed calcium. J. Bone. Min. Res. 5:939-946.

Hay, P.J., J.W. Delakunt, A. Hall et al. 1992. Predictors of osteopenia in premenopausal women with anorexia nervosa. Calcif. Tissue Int. 50:498-501.

Heaney, R.P. & R.R. Recker. 1982. Effects of nitrogen, phosphorus, and caffeine on calcium balance in women. J. Lab. Clin. Med. 99:46-55.

Heaney, R.P. 1986. Calcium, bone health, and osteoporosis. In Bone and Mineral Research 4. Peck, W.A. (ed). Elsevier Science Publ. B.V. 255-301.

Heaney, R.P., C.M. Weaver, R.R. Recker. 1988a) Calcium absorbability from spinach. Am. J. Clin. Nutr. 47:707-709.

Heaney, R.P., R.R. Recker & S.M. Hinders. 1988b. Variability of calcium absorption. Am. J. Clin. Nutr. 47:262-264.

Heaney, R.P. & C.M. Weaver. 1989. Oxalate: effect on calcium absorbability. Am. J. Clin, Nutr. 50:830-832.

Heaney, R.P. & C.M. Weaver. 1990. Calcium absorption from kale. Am. J. Clin. Nutr. 51:656-657.

Heaney, R.P., C.M. Weaver, M.L. Fitzsimmons. 1991. Soybean phytate content: effect on calcium absorption. Am. J. Clin. Nutr. 53:745-747.

Holbrook. T.L., E. Barrett-Connor & D.L. Wingard. 1988. Dietary calcium and risk of hip fracture: a 14-year prospective population study. The Lancet. 1046-1049.

Johnston, C.C. & C.W. Slemenda. 1991. The relative importance of nutrition compared to the genetic factors in the development of bone mass. In: Nutritional Aspects of Osteoporosis. P. Burckhardt and R.P. Heaney (eds), Serono Symposia. Raven Pes. Vol 85, 21-26.

Kanders, B., D.W. Dempster, R. Lindsay: Interaction of calcium nutrition and physical activity on bone mass in young women. J. Bone and Min. Res. 1988; 3, 2:145-149.

Lukert, B.P., M. Carey, B. McCarty et al. 1987. Influence of nutritional factors on calcium regulating hormones and bone loss. Calcif. Tissue Int. 40:119-125.

Matkovic, V., K. Kostial, I. Simonovic, R. Buzina, A. Brodarec & B.E.C. Nordin. 1979. Bone status and fracture rates in two regions of Yugoslavia. Am. J. Clin. Nutr. 32:540-549.

Matkovic, V. 1991. Calcium metabolism and calcium requirements during skeletal modeling and consolidation. Am. J. Clin. Nutr. 54:245-260.

Mazess, R.B., H. Barden, M. Towsley, V. Engle: Bone mineral density of the spine and radius in normal young women. J. Bone and Min. Res. 1986; 1: abstr. 234, 118.

Nordin, B.E.C., A.G. Need, H.A. Morris, M. Horowitz. 1991. Sodium, Calcium, and Osteoporosis. In Nutritional Aspects of Osteoporosis. P. Burckhardt and R.P. Heaney (eds). Serono Symposia. Raven Press, vol. 85, 279-295.

Orwoll, E.S. 1992. The effects of dietary protein insufficiency and excess on skeletal health. Bone. 13:343-350.

Pun, K.K., L.W.L. Chan, V. Chung & F.H.W. Wong. 1991. Calcium content of common food items in Chinese diet. Calcif. Tissue Int. 48:153-156.

Pun, K.K., L.W.L. Chan, V. Chung, F.H.W. Wong: Calcium and other dietary constituents in Hong Kong Chinese in relation to age and osteoporosis. J. Appl. Nutr.

Recker, R.R. & R.P. Heaney. 1985. The effect of milk supplements on calcium metabolism, bone metabolism and calcium balance. Am. J. Clin. Nutr. 41:254-263.

Recker, R.R., A. Bammi, J. Barger-Lux & R.P. Heaney. 1988. Calcium absorbability from milk products, an imitation milk and calcium carbonate. Am. J. Clin. Nutr. 47:93-95

Recker, R.R., K.M. Davies, S.M. Hjuders et al. 1992. Bone gains in adult young women. JAMA 268:2403-2408.

Rico, H. 1991. Minerals and Osteoporosis. Osteoporosis Int. 2:20-25.

Rigotti, N.Y., S.R. Nussbaum, D.B. Herzog & R.M. Neer. 1984. Osteoporosis in women with anorexia nervosa. N.E.J.M. 311:1601-1606.

Rigotti, N.A., R.M. Neer, S.J. Skates, D.B. Herzog & S.R. Nussbaum. 1991. The clinical cause of osteoporosis in anorexia nervosa. A longitudinal study of cortical bone mass. JAMA 265:1133-1138.

Sandler, R.B., C.W. Slemenda, R.E. LaPorte, J.A. Cauley, M.M. Schramm, M.L. Baresi, A.M. Kriska. 1985. Postmenopausal bone density and milk consumption in childhood and adolescence. Am. Clin. J. Nutr. 42:270-274.

Schuette, S.A., J.B. Knowles, H.E. Ford. 1989. Effect of lactose or its component sugars on jejunal calcium absorption in adult man. Am. J. Clin. Nutr. 50:1084-1087.

Sheikh, M.S., C.A. Santa Ana, B.S.M.J., Nicar, L.R. Schiller, J.S. Fordtran. 1987. Gastrointestinal absorption of calcium from milk and calcium salts. NEJM 317:532-536.

Slemenda, C., C.C. Johnston, S.L. Hui. 1990a. Patterns of bone loss and physiologic growing. Third Int. Symp. on Osteoporosis, Copenhagen. Abstr. 363.

Slemenda, C.W., S.L. Hui, C. Longcope, H.W. Ellman, C.C. Johnston. 1990b. Predictors of bone mass in perimenopausal women. Ann. Int. Med. 112:96-101.

Spencer, H., L. Kramer, M. de Bartolo et al. 1983. Further studies on the effect of a high protein diet as meat on calcium metabolism. Am. J. Clin. Nutr. 37:924-929

Spencer, H., H. Rubio, E. Rubio et al. 1986. Chronic alcoolism. Frequently overlooked cause of osteoporosis in men. Am. J. Med. 80:393-397.

Szmukler, G.I., S.W. Brown, V. Parson & A. Darby. 1985. Premature loss of bone in chronic anorexia nervosa. Br. Med. J. 290:26-27.

Thomas, M.L., D.J. Simmons, L. Kidder, M.J. Ibarra : Calcium metabolism and bone mineralization in female rats fed diets marginally sufficient in calcium: effects of increased dietary calcium intake. Bone Miner 1991; 12:1-14.

Treasure, J., I. Fogelman & G.F. Russell. 1986. Osteopenia of the lumbar spine and femoral neck in anorexia nervosa. Scott. Med. J. 31:206-207.

Tylavsky, F.A., J.J.B. Anderson. 1988. Dietary factors in bone health of elderly lactovovegetarian and omnivorous women. Am. J. Clin. Nutr. 48:842-849.

Tylavsky, F.A., A.D. Bortyz, R.L. Hancock, J.J.B. Anderson. 1989. Familial resemblance of radial bone mass between premenopausal mothers and their college-age daughters. Calcif. Tissue Int 45:265-272.

US Department of Health, Education and Welfare Publ. (PHS) 79-1657, 1979.

Weaver, C.M., B.R. Martin & R.P. Heaney. 1991a. Calcium absorption from foods. In Nutritional Aspects of osteoporosis. P. Burckhardt & R.P. Heaney (eds). New York, Raven Press. Vol 85, 133-139.

Weaver, C.M., R.P. Heaney, B.R. Martin et al. 1991b. Human calcium absorption from whole wheat products. J. Nutr. 121:1769-1775.

Dairy Products in Human Health and Nutrition, Serrano Ríos et al. (eds) © 1994 Balkema, Rotterdam, ISBN 90 5410 359 0

Dietary calcium as a possible anti-promoter of colorectal carcinogenesis

R. Van der Meer, M.J.A.P. Govers & J.A. Lapré
Department of Nutrition, Netherlands Institute for Dairy Research (NIZO), Ede, Netherlands

J.H. Kleibeuker
Department of Gastroenterology, University Hospital Groningen, Netherlands

ABSTRACT: Epidemiologic studies indicate that the high incidence of colorectal cancer in Western countries is associated with a high dietary intake of fat. Several studies also indicate that dietary calcium may inhibit this promotive effect of a high fat diet. We investigated in biochemical, animal, and human studies the possible protective mechanisms of dietary calcium. Our in vitro studies show that calcium phosphate precipitates bile acids and fatty acids and thus inhibits their cytolytic activity. The animal studies show that dietary calcium phosphate precipitates colonic bile acids and fatty acids and inhibits luminal cytolytic activity. In addition, calcium inhibits the release of an epithelial cell marker (alkaline phosphatase) as well as colonic epithelial proliferation. Also in healthy human volunteers, supplemental dietary calcium inhibits colonic cytolytic activity and the release of the epithelial cell marker. These mechanisms may explain the anti-proliferative effect of dietary calcium observed in most, but not all, clinical studies of patients at risk for colorectal cancer.

1 INTRODUCTION AND HYPOTHESIS

Colorectal cancer is the second most common cause of cancer deaths in Western societies. Only mortality from lung cancer in males and from breast cancer in females is more common (Waterhouse et al. 1982). The incidence of colorectal cancer is strongly related to age, both in high and low risk countries (Figure 1). This long latency period of colorectal cancer, probably reflects a sequence of slowly reacting cellular transformations in the protective surface layer (epithelium) of colon mucosa.

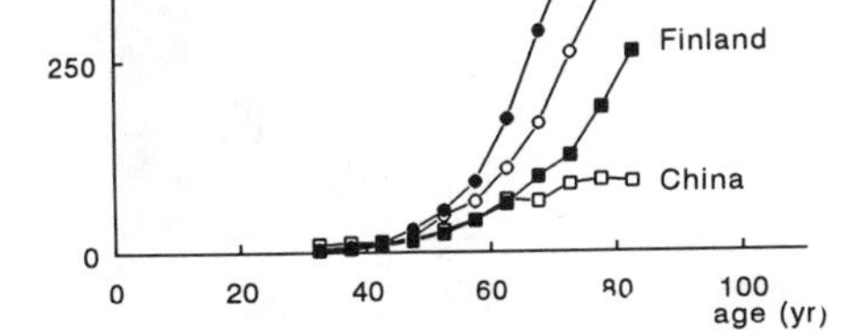

annual incidence per 100,000

Figure 1. Age dependence of the incidence of colorectal cancer in high-risk and low-risk countries (Waterhouse et al. 1982).

For this multistage development of colorectal cancer Lipkin (1974) described the following sequence of events. First, in normal colon mucosa, replication of epithelial cells becomes stimulated. Subsequently, these so called hyperproliferative cells may accumulate and transform to adenomatous polyps. Eventually these adenomas may transform to invasive and malignant carcinomas. Thus adenomas can be considered as the precursors of carcinomas. Studies of the molecular genetics of colorectal cancer (Fearon and Jones 1992) indicate that these phenotypical transformations most likely result from the accumulation of multiple mutations in tumor suppressor genes and oncogenes in the affected epithelial cell.

Migration from low to high risk countries drastically increases the incidence of colorectal cancer (Haenszel and Kurihara 1968). This implies that differences in incidence are not due to differences in genetic background and indicates that the frequency of cellular mutations is modulated by environmental factors. Epidemiological studies (Weisburger and Wynder 1987, Willett 1989) suggest that diet is an important modulator of colorectal carcinogenesis. Especially the high intake of fat in Western societies is associated with an increased risk of colorectal cancer (Carroll 1984, Willett et al. 1990), which may be due to a dietary fat-induced increase in fecal excretion of bile acids and fatty acids. Epidemiologic studies also indicate that dietary calcium (Garland et al. 1985, Sorenson et al. 1988), as well as milk consumption (Rosen et al. 1988), is negatively associated with the incidence of colorectal cancer between and within populations with a similar high intake of dietary fat.

Current hypotheses of the etiology of colorectal

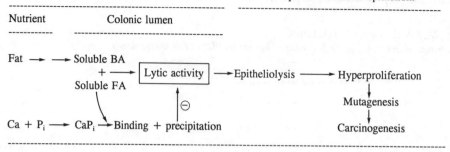

Figure 2. Proposed mechanism of the protective effect of dietary calcium on colon cancer risk.

cancer focus on the molecular interactions between bile acids, fatty acids, and calcium in the colonic lumen, because of the epidemiologic observations mentioned above. Bile acids and fatty acids are hydrophobic surface-active compounds which may damage colonic epithelial cells and thus induce a compensatory increase in proliferation of crypt cells. This epithelial hyperproliferation may increase the frequency of mutations in tumor suppressor genes and oncogenes and thus promote colorectal tumorigenesis. Newmark et al. (1984) proposed that these effects of bile acids and fatty acids on colonic epithelium could be inhibited by soluble calcium in the intestinal lumen. They hypothesized that Ca^{2+} precipitates these surfactants in the colonic lumen and thus prevents their detrimental, cytolytic, effects. They also suggested that dietary phosphate should inhibit this favorable effect of Ca^{2+}, due to the formation of insoluble calcium phosphate. However, they did not present direct experimental evidence supporting these proposed interactions between bile acids, fatty acids, calcium and phosphate. With regard to these intestinal interactions we proposed a modified hypothesis (Figure 2). Our working hypothesis implies that, in the intestinal lumen, dietary calcium and phosphate form an insoluble calcium phosphate (CaP_i), which precipitates and thus inactivates bile acids and fatty acids. As schematically illustrated in Figure 2, this precipitation may decrease the surfactant-dependent cytolytic activity. Consequently, epithelial proliferation as well as the expression of cellular carcinogenic mutations may be inhibited.

Because phosphate is far in excess of calcium in human diets, quantification of the proposed intestinal interactions between calcium, phosphate, bile acids, and fatty acids is relevant to a proper understanding of the antiproliferative effect of calcium. Moreover, in a typical Western diet about 70 % of dietary calcium is derived from milk and dairy products. These products contain equimolar amounts of calcium and phosphate. According to the hypothesis of Newmark et al. (1984) this implies that optimal prevention can only be realized with pharmaceutical preparations of calcium (like calcium carbonate). In contrast, our modified hypothesis implies that prevention can be accomplished using dietary calcium, supplied by milk and dairy products.

The present paper summarizes our research with regard to the molecular mechanisms of this modified hypothesis. First, we studied the molecular interactions between bile acids, fatty acids, calcium and phosphate in vitro because these interactions are difficult, if not impossible, to study in vivo. Subsequently the physiological relevance of these biochemical studies is ascertained in nutritional studies in animals and humans.

2 BIOCHEMICAL STUDIES

The cytolytic activity of bile acids and fatty acids and its interaction with calcium and phosphate was studied using erythrocytes as a cellular model system. By measuring hemolysis this model can adequately be used for the study of the molecular mechanisms of surfactant-induced cytolytic activity. First, we studied the effects of bile acid structure on lytic activity (Van der Meer et al. 1991). Figure 3 shows the lytic effects of different physiological mixtures of bile acids using the reciprocal of the concentration required for 50% lysis ($1/LC_{50}$) as measure for their cytolytic activity.

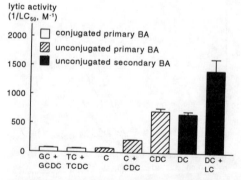

Figure 3. Lytic activity of the physiologically relevant primary and secondary bile acids. Lytic activity is defined as the reciprocal of the concentration required for 50% lysis. Mean$\pm$SD; n=6.

Cytolytic activity was increased by deconjugation and dehydroxylation which is probably due to an increased hydrophobicity of the unconjugated, secondary bile acids compared to their conjugated, primary counterparts. These effects of bile acid structure on cytolytic activity may be of relevance for the integrity of human intestinal mucosa. For instance, bile acids in bile and in the upper part of the small intestine are for about 75% composed of relatively non-lytic glycine- and taurine-conjugated primary bile acids cholate (GC and TC) and chenodeoxycholate (GCDC and TCDC) (Rossi et al. 1987). These bile acids are deconjugated and dehydroxylated by colonic bacteria. Consequently, more than 90% of the colonic bile acids consists of the hydrophobic, secondary bile acids deoxycholate and lithocholate which have a high lytic activity (Figure 3). In similar experiments we observed that also hydrophobicity of fatty acids is an important determinant of their cytolytic activity (Lapré et al. 1992). Moreover, low concentrations of bile acids synergistically stimulate fatty acid induced lytic activity with the same hydrophobic dependence as observed for bile acids alone. In particular, it appeared that the mixtures of lauric acid and the colonic bile acids DC and LC have a very high lytic activity (Figure 4).

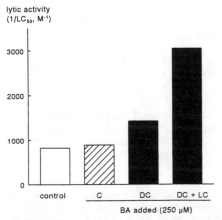

Figure 4. Effect of addition of 250 μM cholate (C), deoxycholate (DC) and deoxycholate/lithocholate (DC/LC; molar ratio 3:1) on lytic activity of laurate (control).

We also studied the effects of calcium and phosphate on the solubility and cytolytic activity of bile acids (Van der Meer and De Vries 1985, Van der Meer et al. 1991). Insoluble CaP_i binds and thus precipitates carboxylic bile acids. This binding inhibits the cytolytic activity, as is illustrated for deoxycholate (DC) in Figure 5. It should be noted that soluble calcium does not precipitate this bile acid but stimulates its cytolytic activity (Van der Meer et al. 1991). Insoluble CaP_i also lowers the solubility and cytolytic activity of fatty acids (Figure 5). Thus,

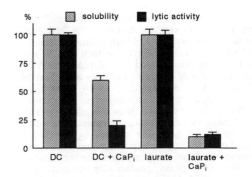

Figure 5. Effect of CaP_i on solubility and cytolytic activity of deoxycholate and laurate (2 mM).

Table 1. Estimation of CaP_i supersaturation of ileal and colonic contents of rat and man.

	μmol/g H_2O		Supersaturation*
	Ca	P_i	
Rat (low CaP_i)			
Ileum	16	15	0.8×10^2
Colon	30	25	2.5×10^2
Rat (high CaP_i)			
Ileum	310	140	1.4×10^4
Colon	900	420	1.3×10^5
Man (habitual)			
Ileum	30	17	1.7×10^2
Colon	190	115	7.3×10^3

* : Calculated as the concentration product of total Ca and P_i divided by the apparent solubility product of CaP_i at pH 7 (3×10^{-6} M^2).

insoluble CaP_i precipitates bile acids and fatty acids and decreases their cytolytic activity, consistent with the first step in our working hypothesis.
We feel that the qualitative effects of these model studies are relevant to the situation in vivo, because the precipitation of bile acids and fatty acids by CaP_i is solely dependent on their physicochemical characteristics. In addition, surfactant-induced lysis of erythrocytes is analogous to that of colonic epithelial cells in vitro (Lapré et al. 1992), which indicates that lysis of erythrocytes is a simple and physiologically relevant bioassay for the quantitation of the cytolytic activity of complex mixtures of surfactants.
Finally, to ascertain the physiological relevance of the effects of CaP_i, we investigated whether insoluble

calcium phosphate can be formed in the small and large intestine of rats and humans. Ileal and fecal samples of rats, fed low and high calcium phosphate purified diets, were analyzed for their Ca, P_i and water content (Govers and Van der Meer 1993). Ileostomy fluids of 4 persons and feces of 12 healthy volunteers (Van der Meer et al. 1990), all on their habitual diet, were used as samples of the luminal contents of ileum and distal colon, respectively. Total concentrations are calculated as the measured amounts of calcium and phosphate divided by the water content of these samples. Supersaturation with regard to insoluble calcium phosphate formation is calculated as the concentration product for calcium and phosphate, divided by its solubility product at pH 7.0 (Van der Meer and De Vries 1985). This pH value is a reasonable estimate of the pH value of the intestinal lumen (Fordtran and Locklear 1966). As shown in Table 1, ileal and colonic contents of rats fed a low CaP_i diet are 80 and 250 fold supersaturated with calcium phosphate. This supersaturation is at least 100-fold increased in rats fed the high CaP_i diet. In man, the intestinal CaP_i supersaturation is about 200 (ileum) and 7000 (colon). These results indicate that in rat and man the activity of Ca^{2+} may be low in ileum and will be extremely low in colon, because of the formation of insoluble CaP_i. It should be noted that the supersaturation data for man are in between those of rats fed low or high CaP_i diets, respectively. This shows that the human conditions can be mimicked in rats by increasing the CaP_i content of the diets.

3 ANIMAL STUDIES

The inhibitory effects of dietary calcium on (pre)malignant changes in colonic epithelium have been studied predominantly in rodents. Most tumor-induction studies showed that the promoter effect of a high-fat diet can be abolished by calcium supplementation (see e.g. Wargovich et al. 1990). Other studies used intrarectal instillation of, or perfusion with, bile acids or fatty acids to induce cellular damage and epithelial hyperproliferation (Rafter et al. 1986, Wargovich et al. 1984). Despite the protective effects of calcium found in these studies, their design precludes the normal intestinal interaction between calcium, phosphate, bile acids and fatty acids, and thus limits the physiological relevance of these studies. When dietary calcium was supplemented as calcium phosphate, colonic proliferation was drastically decreased by supplemental calcium (see e.g. Bird 1986). However, in none of these studies fecal parameters have been studied, thus providing no additional information on the molecular mechanism by which dietary calcium inhibits colonic proliferation and tumor formation.

Our experiments have been focused on the effects of dietary calcium on luminal parameters in relation to colonic epithelial proliferation. Table 2 summarizes the main results of our rat studies. In these experiments we used the concept of fecal water developed by Rafter et al. (1987). Fecal water represents that fraction of the feces which contains

the cytolytic surfactants, because only soluble surfactants are lytic (see above). In the first experiment increasing amounts of deoxycholate (DC) were added to the diet. This drastically increased the concentration bile acids in fecal water and stimulated cytolytic activity, measured with our hemolysis bioassay, and colonic proliferation. Cytolytic activity of fecal water and colonic proliferation were highly correlated (r=0.85, n=24) (Lapré and Van der Meer 1992).

Table 2. Summary of the results of our rat studies.

Treatment	Effect			
	BA/ FA	Lytic act.	ALP	Proli- feration
DC↑	↑	↑	n.d.	↑
$CaHPO_4$↑	↓	↓	n.d.	n.d.
$CaCO_3$↑	↓	↓	n.d.	n.d.
Na_2HPO_4↑	0	0	n.d.	n.d.
Type of fat $CaHPO_4$↑				
Butter	↓	↓	↓	↓
Sat.	↓	↓	↓	↓
PUFA	↓	↓	↓	0
Type of Ca Ca↑				
$CaCO_3$	↓	↓	↓	↓
$CaHPO_4$	↓	↓	↓	↓
Milk	↓	↓	↓	↓

↓: significant decrease; ↑: significant increase; 0: no significant effect; n.d.: not determined; DC: deoxycholate; BA/FA: concentration of bile acids and fatty acids in fecal water.

In the second experiment, we increased the amount of calcium phosphate in the diet from 20 μmol/g (which corresponds to about 400 mg Ca/day for humans) to 50 and 200 μmol/g diet. The concentration of soluble surfactants was decreased in a dose-dependent manner, and this resulted in a lower cytolytic activity of fecal water (Lapré et al. 1992). In the third experiment we addressed the question whether dietary phosphate inhibits the protective effects of dietary calcium. Increasing amounts of dietary calcium increased the fecal excretion of phosphate, indicating the intestinal formation of insoluble CaP_i. Calcium decreased the concentration of soluble bile acids and fatty acids and also the cytolytic activity of fecal water. Additional dietary phosphate had no effect, which indicates that phosphate does not inhibit the protective effects of calcium on luminal solubility and lytic activity of bile acids and fatty acids (Govers and Van der Meer 1993). In this study we also observed that calcium and phosphate were almost completely precipitated in colon and feces, which is consistent with the supersaturation data of Table 1. Subsequently, we investigated whether the type of dietary fat interferes with the protective effects of dietary calcium. Three different types of fat were used: butter, a saturated margarine and a polyunsaturated margarine. Supplemental calcium decreased the concentrations of soluble surfactants as well as the cytolytic activity of fecal water. These luminal effects resulted in a lower release of the epithelial cell marker alkaline phosphatase (ALP) and a lower colonic epithelial proliferation for the butter and saturated margarine, but not for the polyunsaturated margarine group (Lapré et al. 1993a). Whether this implies that polyunsaturated fatty acids induce hyperproliferation via an additional mechanism e.g. by stimulating protein kinase C is at present not known. Furthermore, this experiment showed that cytolytic activity as well as release of ALP are highly correlated with colonic epithelial proliferation (r=0.97 and 0.88, respectively). Finally, we studied whether the effect of calcium in milk is similar to that of inorganic calcium salts by supplementing the diets with equimolar amounts of calcium by means of $CaCO_3$, $CaHPO_4$ or milk. We found that supplemental calcium inhibited all luminal and epithelial parameters, irrespective of the type of calcium (Govers et al. 1993b).

Taken together, our animal experiments confirm earlier studies that have shown that dietary calcium inhibits colonic proliferation. They extend these studies by showing that this effect is not inhibited by phosphate and that milk calcium has a similar protective effect. In addition, they indicate that the protective effect of calcium is mediated by a decrease in solubility of colonic surfactants and an inhibition of epithelial cell damage, as illustrated for the butter containing diet in Figure 6. Because of the high correlations mentioned above, and the analogous results of our biochemical studies, we consider it most likely that this sequence of effects reflects causal relationships, consistent with our working hypothesis (Figure 2).

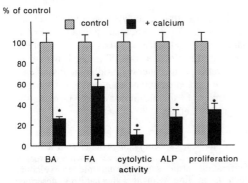

Figure 6. Effects of dietary calcium phosphate on luminal parameters and response of the colonic epithelium in rats (mean±SE;n=6).

4 HUMAN INTERVENTION STUDIES

To ascertain the relevance of the results of our biochemical and animal studies for human physiology, we first studied the intestinal association of calcium, phosphate and bile acids (Van der Meer et al. 1990). Because in human diets phosphate is far in excess of calcium, supplemental dietary calcium (without phosphate) may stimulate complexation with phosphate and/or bile acids. This increased complexation can only be measured as an increase in fecal excretion of phosphate and bile acids, provided that the intake of phosphate is maintained constant. Twelve healthy male volunteers were instructed to maintain their, calcium and phosphate constant, habitual diet during a period of two weeks. Before and after one week of supplementation with dietary calcium (35 mmol $CaCO_3$ = 1.4 g Ca/day) duodenal bile was sampled and feces and urine were quantitatively collected. Total fecal plus urinary excretion of phosphate and magnesium remained constant and more than 95% of the supplemental calcium was recovered showing an excellent compliance. This implies that the effects observed are solely caused by supplemental calcium and not by uncontrolled variations in dietary background.

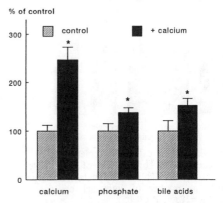

Figure 7. Effects of supplemental calcium on fecal output of calcium, inorganic phosphate and bile acids in healthy volunteers (mean±SE;n=12; *: P<0.05).

Figure 7 shows that calcium increased the fecal excretion of both phosphate (38%) and bile acids (53%) which indicates the intestinal formation of an insoluble complex of calcium, phosphate and bile acids. Using EDTA as a calcium chelator, it was shown that resolubilization of calcium resulted in an increase of soluble phosphate and of soluble bile acids. This shows that calcium, phosphate and bile acids are present in feces as an insoluble complex. Also in the control period significant amounts of phosphate and bile acids were complexed with calcium.

Supplemental calcium significantly changed the duodenal bile acid composition by decreasing the dihydroxy/trihydroxy ratio of bile acids. Because dihydroxy bile acids are more lytic than trihydroxy bile acids (Figure 3), this result suggests that calcium may lower the cytolytic activity of intestinal bile acids. Therefore, we isolated fecal water and determined its composition and cytolytic activity (Lapré et al. 1993b). Supplemental calcium did not alter the total bile acid concentration in fecal water but it decreased the ratio of hydrophobic to hydrophilic bile acids as shown in Figure 8. The concentration of soluble fatty acids was significantly decreased by calcium. In line with this decrease in fatty acid concentration and the shift from hydrophobic to hydrophilic bile acids, a decrease in neutral sterol (cholesterol + coprostanol) concentration was observed. These changes in fecal water surfactants show that, also in man, calcium causes a decrease in hydrophobic components of fecal water. In line with these results, a significant decrease in cytolytic activity of fecal water was observed. Also the ALP activity in fecal water as marker for intestinal cell-damage was significantly decreased by supplemental calcium which is consistent with our animal experiments (Lapré et al., 1993a).

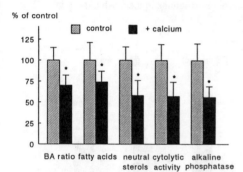

% of control

Figure 8. Effects of calcium supplementation in healthy volunteers on composition of fecal water, cytolytic activity and alkaline phosphatase activity in fecal water as marker of intestinal cell-damage (Mean±SE;n=12; *: P<0.05).

Recently, we studied whether these effects can be extended to calcium in milk products (Govers et al. 1993a). In a double-blind cross-over study, the habitual diet of healthy volunteers was supplemented with regular milk/yoghurt (30 mmol Ca/d) or placebo milk/yoghurt (3 mmol Ca/d). Supplemental milk Ca was completely (99%) recovered in feces + urine, whereas the total output of other minerals remained constant. Milk Ca significantly increased the total fecal excretion of phosphate, bile acids, and fatty acids, indicating intestinal CaP_i formation and precipitation of bile acids and fatty acids. Milk Ca also significantly inhibited the cytolytic activity of fecal water. These preliminary results suggest that the protective effects of milk Ca in colonic lumen are similar to those described above, but this is currently under investigation.

The design of these intervention studies is similar to that of the clinical trials studying the effect of calcium on colonic epithelial proliferation. This suggests that the mechanisms, described above, can be extrapolated to these trials. However, in humans, in contrast to rats, epithelial proliferation can only be measured in vitro, using mucosal biopsies from sigmoid (Kleibeuker et al. 1993) or rectum (other studies). For that reason, only patients at an increased risk of colon cancer, and not healthy volunteers, have been studied. The results in the different groups of patients are summarized in Table 3.

Table 3. Summary of clinical studies concerning the effect of calcium on epithelial proliferation in human subjects.

Characteristic subjects Author+year	n	Test per. (mo)	Ca dose (g/d)	Prol. M	E
FAP					
Lipkin 1989	7	3	1.4	T	↓
FCC					
Lipkin 1985	10	2	1.2	T	↓
Lipkin 1989	21	3	1.4	T	↓
FCC or adenomas					
Buset 1986	9	1.5	1.5	T	↓
Rozen 1989	35	1-3	1.4	T	↓
Adenomas					
Barsoum 1992	14*	2	1.3	C	↓
Wargovich 1992	20*	1	2.0	T	↓
Bostick 1993	21*	2	1.2	T	0
Kleibeuker 1993	17	3	1.5	B	↑
O'Sullivan 1993	20	1	1-2	B	↓
Resection					
Gregoire 1989	30*	1	1.2	T	0
Stern 1990	31*	9	1.2	T	0

* : Placebo-controlled study; other studies had an open design; FAP: Familial polyposis; FCC: Familial colorectal cancer kindreds; M: method used to measure proliferation rate; T:tritiated thymidine incorporation; B: bromodesoxyuridine incorporation; C: crypt cell production rate; E: effect of Ca treatment; ↓/↑: significant decrease or increase; 0: no significant effect.

Several studies, especially in patients with a family history of colorectal cancer, have shown a decreased proliferation after supplemental dietary calcium, which is in line with the mechanisms described above. The effects in patients with sporadic adenomas are, however, less clear. We consider it unlikely that these different results are due to differences in design and methodology of these studies. Apparently, in these patients, the protective effect of calcium on luminal cytolytic activity (Welberg et al. 1993) does not simply result in an inhibition of epithelial proliferation (Kleibeuker et al. 1993). Whether the ambiguous results in these patients are therefore due to different numbers of 'nonresponders', refractory to dietary intervention (Buset et al. 1986; Lipkin et al. 1989), in these populations cannot be determined because a specific characterization of the nonresponder phenomenon is not available. The absence of an inhibitory effect of calcium in patients after colonic surgery is probably less enigmatic. These operations may significantly alter bile acid metabolism (Cats et al. 1992; Cats et al. 1993) and thus probably interfere with the luminal effects of supplemental calcium.

Taken together, the results of the human studies show that dietary calcium has protective effects on the cytolytic surfactants in colonic lumen. However, an inhibition of epithelial proliferation is not yet unambiguously proven. We feel that research should be focused on the development of in vivo markers of hyperproliferation. In addition, more placebo-controlled studies of the effects of calcium on the epithelium of the whole colon and of the mechanisms of these effects are needed.

5 CONCLUSION

The biochemical and nutritional studies discussed here are consistent with the model presented in Figure 2. As shown in vitro, bile acids and fatty acids are precipitated by insoluble calcium phosphate. This precipitation drastically inhibits their cytolytic activity. In rats, a diet-induced increase in luminal surfactant concentration stimulates lytic activity of fecal water and intestinal cell-damage resulting in an increased proliferation. The increase in luminal surfactant concentration and lytic activity of fecal water can be counteracted by supplemental dietary calcium. Supplemental calcium in humans increases the formation of insoluble CaP_i in colonic lumen, decreases the concentration of soluble hydrophobic bile acids and fatty acids and decreases the lytic activity of fecal water. This sequence of effects offers a molecular explanation of the inhibitory effects of supplemental calcium on epithelial proliferation, observed in animals and several studies in humans. Final proof, however, is not yet available, because these inhibitory effects have not been observed in all clinical trials. More well-designed studies in patients and healthy volunteers are needed using a combined biochemical, nutritional and clinical approach to elucidate the complex mechanisms of the effects of calcium on colorectal carcinogenesis.

Acknowledgements. We gratefully acknowledge our colleagues at NIZO and the University Hospital for their contribution to the studies summarized here. Our work has been supported by the European Community, the Netherlands Organization for Scientific Research (NWO), Medical Sciences and the Dutch Cancer Society.

REFERENCES

Barsoum, G.H., C. Hendrickse, M.C. Winslet, D. Youngs, I.A. Donovan, J.P. Neoptolemos & M.R.B. Keighly 1992. Reduction of mucosal crypt cell proliferation in patients with colorectal adenomatous polyps by dietary calcium supplementation. Br. J. Surg. 79: 581-583.

Bird, R.P. 1986. Effect of dietary components on the pathobiology of colon epithelium: possible relationship with colon tumorigenesis. Lipids 21: 289-291.

Bostick, R.M., J.D. Potter, L. Fosdick, P. Grambsch, J.W. Lampe, J.R. Wood, T.A. Louis, R. Ganz & G. Grandits 1993. Calcium and colorectal cell proliferation: a preliminary randomized, double-blind, placebo-controlled clinical trial. J. Natl. Cancer Inst. 85: 132-141.

Buset, M., M. Lipkin, S. Winawer & E. Friedman 1986. Inhibition of human colonic epithelial cell proliferation in vivo and in vitro by calcium. Cancer Res. 46: 5426-5430.

Carroll, K.K. 1984. Role of lipids in tumorigenesis. J. Am. Oil Chem. Soc. 61: 1888-1891.

Cats, A., J.H. Kleibeuker, F. Kuipers, M.J. Hardonk, R.C.J. Verschueren, W. Boersma, R.J. Vonk, W.J. Sluiter, N.H. Mulder, B.G. Wolthers & E.G.E. De Vries 1992. Changes in rectal epithelial cell proliferation and intestinal bile acids after subtotal colectomy in familial adenomatous polyposis. Cancer Res. 52: 3552-3557.

Cats, A., F. Kuipers, E.G.E. De Vries, W. Boersma, N.H. Mulder, R.C.J. Verschueren & J.H. Kleibeuker 1993. Effects of partial colonic resections on intestinal bile acid metabolism. Gastroenterology 104: in press.

Fearon, E.R. & P.A. Jones 1992. Progressing toward a molecular description of colorectal cancer development. Faseb J. 6: 2783- 2790.

Fordtran, J.S. & T.W. Locklear 1966. Ionic constituents and osmolality of gastric and small-intestinal fluids after eating. Am. J. Dig. Dis. 11: 503-521.

Garland, C., R.B. Shekelle, E. Barrett-Conner, M.H. Criqui, A.H. Rossof & O. Paul 1985. Dietary vitamin D and calcium and risk of colorectal cancer: a 19 year prospective study in men. Lancet I: 307-309.

Govers, M.J.A.P. & R. Van der Meer 1993. Effects of dietary calcium and phosphate on the intestinal interactions between calcium, phosphate, fatty acids, and bile acids. Gut 34: 365- 370.

Govers, M.J.A.P., D.S.M.L. Termont, J.H. Kleibeuker & R. Van der Meer 1993a. Dietary calcium in milk products inhibits cytolytic activity of fecal water in healthy volunteers. Gastroenterology 104: in press.

Govers, M.J.A.P., D.S.M.L. Termont & R. Van der Meer 1993b. The mechanism of the anti-proliferative effect of milk mineral on rat colonic epithelium. Gastroenterology 104: in press.

Gregoire, R.C., H.S. Stern, K.S. Yeung, J. Stadler, S. Langley, R. Furrer & W.R. Bruce 1989. Effect of calcium supplementation on mucosal proliferation in high risk patients for colon cancer. Gut 30: 376-382.

Haenszel, W. & M. Kurihara 1968. Mortality from cancer and other diseases among Japanese in the United States. J. Natl. Cancer Inst. 40: 43-68.

Kleibeuker, J.H., J.W.M. Welberg, N.H. Mulder, R. Van der Meer, A. Cats, A.J. Limburg, W.M.T. Kreumer, M.J. Hardonk & E.G.E. De Vries 1993. Epithelial cell proliferation in the sigmoid colon of patients with adenomatous polyps increases during oral calcium supplementation. Br. J. Cancer 67: 500-503.

Lapré, J.A. & R. Van der Meer 1992. Diet-induced increase of colonic bile acids stimulates lytic activity of fecal water and proliferation of colonic cells. Carcinogenesis 13: 41-44.

Lapré, J.A., H.T. De Vries & R. Van der Meer 1991. Dietary calcium phosphate inhibits intestinal cytotoxicity. Am. J. Physiol. 261: G907-G912.

Lapré, J.A., D.S.M.L. Termont, A.K. Groen & R. Van der Meer 1992. Lytic effects of mixed micelles of fatty acids and bile acids. Am. J. Physiol. 263: G333-G337.

Lapré, J.A., H.T. De Vries, J.H. Koeman & R. Van der Meer 1993a. The anti-proliferative effect of dietary calcium on colonic epithelium is mediated by luminal surfactants and dependent on the type of dietary fat. Cancer Res. 53: 784-789.

Lapré, J.A., H.T. De Vries, D.S.M.L. Termont, J.H. Kleibeuker, E. G.E. De Vries & R. Van der Meer 1993b. Mechanism of the protective effects of supplemental dietary calcium on cytolytic activity of fecal water. Cancer Res. 53: 248-253.

Lipkin, M. 1974. Phase 1 and phase 2 proliferative lesions of colonic epithelial cells in diseases leading to colon cancer. Cancer Res. 34: 878-888.

Lipkin, M. & H. Newmark 1985. Effect of added dietary calcium on colonic epithelial-cell proliferation in subjects at high risk for familial colonic cancer. N. Engl. J. Med. 313: 1381-1384.

Lipkin, M., E. Friedman, S.J. Winawer & H. Newmark 1989. Colonic epithelial cell proliferation in responders and nonresponders to supplemental dietary calcium. Cancer Res. 49: 248-254.

Newmark, H.L., M.J. Wargovich & W.R. Bruce 1984. Colon cancer and dietary fat, phosphate, and calcium: a hypothesis. J. Natl. Cancer Inst. 72: 1323-1325.

O'Sullivan, K.R., P.M. Mathias, S. Beattie & C. O'Morain 1993. Effect of oral calcium supplementation on colonic crypt cell proliferation in patients with adenomatous polyps of the large bowel. Eur. J. Gastroenterol. Hepatol. 5: 85-89.

Rafter, J.J., V.W.S. Eng, R. Furrer, A. Medline & W.R. Bruce 1986. Effects of calcium and pH on the mucosal damage produced by deoxycholic acid in the rat colon. Gut 27: 1320-1329.

Rafter, J.J., P. Child, A.M. Anderson, R. Alder, V. Eng & W.R. Bruce 1987. Cellular toxicity of fecal water depends on diet. Am. J. Clin. Nutr. 45: 559-563.

Rosen, M., L. Nystrom & S. Wall 1988. Diet and cancer mortality in the counties of sweden. Am. J. Epidemiol. 127: 42-49.

Rossi, S.S., J.L. Converse & A.F. Hofmann 1987. High pressure liquid chromatographic analysis of conjugated bile acids in human bile: simultaneous resolution of sulfated and unsulfated lithocholyl amidates and the common conjugated bile acids. J. Lipid Res. 28: 589-595.

Rozen, P., Z. Fireman, N. Fine, Y. Wax & E. Ron 1989. Oral calcium suppresses increased rectal proliferation of persons at risk of colorectal cancer. Gut 30: 650-655.

Sorenson, A.W., M.L. Slattery & M.H. Ford 1988. Calcium and colon cancer: a review. Nutr. Cancer 11: 135-145.

Stern , H.S., R.C. Gregoire, H. Kashtan, J. Stadler & W.R. Bruce 1990. Long-term effects of dietary calcium on risk markers for colon cancer in patients with familial polyposis. Surgery 108: 528-533.

Van der Meer, R. & H.T. De Vries 1985. Differential binding of glycine- and taurine-conjugated bile acids to insoluble calcium phosphate. Biochem. J. 229: 265-268.

Van der Meer, R., J.W.M. Welberg, F. Kuipers, J.H. Kleibeuker, N. H. Mulder, D.S.M.L. Termont, R.J. Vonk, H.T. De Vries & E.G.E. De Vries 1990. Effects of supplemental dietary calcium on the intestinal association of calcium, phosphate, and bile acids. Gastroenterology 99: 1653-1659.

Van der Meer, R., D.S.M.L. Termont & H.T. De Vries 1991. Differential effects of calcium ions and calcium phosphate on cytotoxicity of bile acids. Am. J. Physiol. 260: G142-G147.

Wargovich, M.J., V.W.S. Eng & H.L. Newmark 1984. Calcium inhibits the damaging and compensatory proliferative effects of fatty acids on mouse colon epithelium. Cancer Lett. 23: 253-258.

Wargovich, M.J., D. Allnutt, C. Palmer, P. Anaya & L.C. Stephens 1990. Inhibition of the promotional phase of azoxymethane- induced colon carcinogenesis in the F344 rat by calcium lactate: effect of simulating two human nutrient density levels. Cancer Lett. 53: 17-25.

Wargovich, M.J., G. Isbell, M. Shabot, R. Winn, F. Lanza, L. Hochman, E. Larson, P. Lynch, L. Roubein & B. Levin 1992. Calcium supplementation decreases rectal epithelial cell proliferation in subjects with sporadic adenoma. Gastroenterology 103: 92-97.

Waterhouse, J., C. Muir, K. Shanmuguratman & J. Powell 1982. Cancer incidence in five continents, Vol 4. Lyon: IARC Sci Publ No 42.

Weisburger, J.H. & E.L. Wynder 1987. Etiology of colorectal cancer with emphasis on mechanism of action and prevention. In: Important advances in oncology (V.T. De vita S. Hellman & S.A. Rosenberg eds.): 197-220. Philadelphia: Lippincott.

Welberg, J.W.M., J.H. Kleibeuker, R. Van der Meer, F. Kuipers, A. Cats, H. Van Rijsbergen, D.S.M.L. Termont, W. Boersma-van Ek, R.J. Vonk, N.H. Mulder & E.G.E. De Vries 1993. Effects of oral calcium supplementation on intestinal bile acids and cytolytic activity of fecal water in patients with adenomatous polyps of the colon. Eur. J. Clin. Invest. 23: 63-68.

Willett, W. 1989. The search for the causes of breast and colon cancer. Nature 338: 389-394.

Willett, W.C., M.J. Stampfer, G.A. Colditz, B.A. Rosner & F.E. Speizer 1990. Relation of meat, fat, and fiber intake to the risk of colon cancer in a prospective study among women. N. Engl. J. Med. 323: 1664-1672.

Author index